The

Complete

Guide

to Protecting

and Improving

Your Health

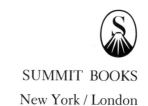

SUMMIT BOOKS

New York / London
Toronto / Sydney / Tokyo

The
Well
Adult

Mike Samuels, M.D.
and Nancy Samuels

Illustrated by Wendy Frost

*We dedicate this book to
all those who consciously work to change attitudes and habits
in order to promote health and healing.*

Summit Books
Simon & Schuster Building
Rockefeller Center
1230 Avenue of the Americas
New York, New York 10020

SUMMIT BOOKS and colophon are trademarks
of Simon & Schuster Inc.
Designed by Levavi & Levavi
Manufactured in the United States of America
1   3   5   7   9   10   8   6   4   2
1   3   5   7   9   10   8   6   4   2   pbk.
Library of Congress Cataloging-in-Publication Data
Samuels, Mike.
The well adult: the complete guide to protecting and improving
your health/Mike Samuels, Nancy Samuels.
p.   cm.
Bibliography: p.
Includes index.
ISBN 0-671-62540-3
ISBN 0-671-66952-4 pbk.
1. Health.   2. Self-care, Health.   I. Samuels, Nancy.   II. Title.
RA776.S2814   1988
613'.0434—dc19   88-24814
CIP

ACKNOWLEDGMENTS

We would like to thank all the people who contributed to the shaping of this book and the material it contains. We would like to thank our publisher, Jim Silberman, for being enthusiastic about an adult health book and continuing to support our work; Ileene Smith, Kate Edgar, and Dominick Anfuso for their editorial care and expertise in bringing this large and complex project to completion. Thanks to Wendy Frost for years of friendship and her images of health, and Meryl Levavi for careful laying out of the elements. As always, we are indebted to our agent, Elaine Markson, and to Geri Toma, for their wise counsel and just being there.

For this project, we especially want to thank those professionals who have discussed the work with us, and read sections of the manuscript and have given us invaluable comments, criticisms and suggestions: Dr. Fred Miller; Dr. Alan Datner; Charlotte Janis, NPA; Dr. Gail Altschuler; Dr. Charles Dailey; Dr. Joel Reiter; Dr. Howard Ort; Dr. David Sperling; Dr. Ray Bonneau; Dr. Ken Fye; Dr. Marion Rosenthal; Dr. Richard Bernstein; Dr. Jon Schwartz; and Skip Schwartz, EMT. Special thanks to Mickey Carpenter and Anita Duquette both for helping us select the art and for making the process easy. We'd also like to express our gratitude to Marshall and Phyllis Klaus, Joel and Charlotte Reiter, Hal Bennett, Charles Fox, and Jimmy Katz for support and wide-ranging book talk. As always, we want to thank our boys, Rudy and Lewis, who have grown up as this project has gone along; Linda and Hope for being supportive family members; and our parents, for whom we have come to have increasing love and respect as we've reached midadulthood ourselves.

CONTENTS

CHEST

MUSCULOSKELETAL

GASTROINTESTINAL

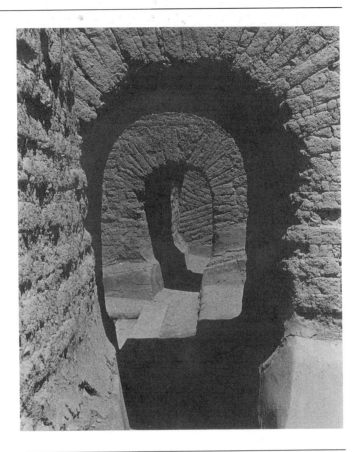

PART ONE

Delving Inward/Opening Up.
Photo by Michael Samuels.

Staying Well

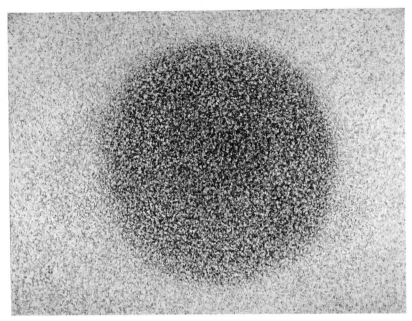

CHAPTER ONE

Taking Control of Your Health

W e believe that consciousness is the key to health. Our attitudes, more than events, determine the decisions and actions that affect our well-being. When we think positively, decide to be well, and make healthy practices part of our daily routine, we can actually alter the course of our lives, improving our health and creating a general sense of well-being. A sense of personal fulfillment is also a factor that we think is crucial to health during adulthood. When we pursue interests that we enjoy, that broaden our personality and allow for continued growth and development, we get in touch with our innermost feelings, which brings body and mind into balance and helps us heal. This process reduces stress and increases our sense of subjective well-being—the single factor that has been shown to be most important to health.

Health radiates from the center of consciousness. Richard Pousette-Dart. Radiance. 1962–63. Oil and metallic paint on canvas, 6'⅛" × 8'¼". Collection, The Museum of Modern Art, New York. Gift of Susan Morse Hilles.

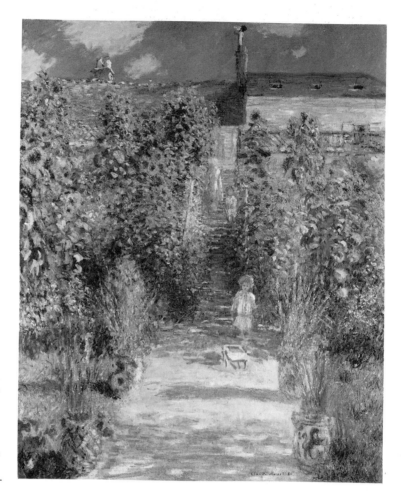

Interests that we enjoy bring our mind and body into balance and help us heal. Claude Monet. The Artist's Garden at Vetheuil. *1880. National Gallery of Art, Washington. Ailsa Mellon Bruce Collection.*

At a practical level, there is much that we can do ourselves to improve our own health, both by preventing disease and by dealing with illness effectively. This assertion is not just theoretical; there are so many studies that attest to this idea that the Department of Health, Education, and Welfare has set forth as a realistic goal a 25% reduction of deaths in the age group between 35 and 65, with a corresponding increase in longevity. We believe that the means to such a vast improvement in health and longevity is education. Through education we can transform our attitudes and philosophy towards healthy living.

A number of studies have demonstrated that when people understand how to prevent or deal with specific illnesses, and when they believe in their ability to take control of their health, both the frequency and the severity of many diseases decrease. One type of research has dealt specifically with disease prevention. Major studies of this type, including the Stanford Three Community Study, the Minneapolis Study, and the Karelia Project in Finland, have attempted to analyze the effect of health education on disease incidence and longevity. Typically, these studies deal with two groups of people, a control group that receives no intervention, and a matched experimental group that receives a well-designed health education program. To date, the largest projects have dealt with the prevention of heart disease. In these studies, the experimental group was informed about the major risk factors for heart disease—high cholesterol, smoking, untreated high blood pressure, stress, and sedentary life-style—and was encouraged to make related life-style changes. The initial results of the studies indicate that when educated, people are indeed more likely to make changes and take action to improve their risk status, and thereby increase their longevity.

A second type of research is designed to assess the effect of education on people who already have a specific illness. One example of this type of study is the Stanford Arthritis Study by psychologist Ann O'Leary. In this research project, the experimental group was given an arthritis self-management course, including information about the pathophysiology of arthritis and the relationship of stress, nutrition, and exercise to the disease. As compared to the control group, participants in the education group had a 25% reduction in pain, a 20% decrease in swollen joints, a 14% decrease in disability, an 18% decrease in depression, and a 20% increase in perceived sense of personal competence. Overall improvement correlated strongly with a positive outlook and a sense of control. Interestingly, the best predictor of improvement in the experimental group was a person's initial belief that he or she would improve.

In recent years, there has been a great deal of research on the relationship between attitude and health. Feelings of competence or self-efficacy, as well as skills in coping and decision-making, are increasingly recognized as playing a significant role in achieving optimal health. This whole area of research has stemmed from profound questions about the nature of health and illness.

The Nature of Health and Illness

With all the progress modern medicine has made, we still don't truly understand why people become ill. Many health theorists no longer feel that there is a distinct separation between health and illness, and they actually find themselves unable to define the terms precisely. For example, a person can feel well, yet have a blocked coronary artery that will soon cause chest pain; or have malignant cells that produce no symptoms yet and are therefore undetected. Illness does not spring full-blown from a condition of "total health"; rather, there is a latency period before symptoms occur in which risk factors are operating and physical changes are quietly taking place within the body. At the other extreme, there are times when people *feel* very ill, but actually have relatively little underlying pathology. For example, a person may be bedridden with low back pain, but have no evidence of disc degeneration or muscle damage. Ironically, in some cases a "well" person may be sicker than an "ill" person.

The most common definition of illness takes the view that health is the absence of symptoms of physical disease. One can see from the examples above that this definition is too superficial to be usable in medical terms. Carl Thoresen, a health psychologist from Stanford, says that this explanation is like defining wisdom as an absence of stupidity, or wealth as an absence of poverty. In the 1970s, the World Health Organization formulated a definition of health that has had great influence on subsequent medical thought. It defined health as a state of complete physical, mental, and social well-being. This definition, which almost enters the spiritual dimension, has been attacked as being too broad to be practical, because it includes experiences beyond the realm of medicine and beyond the control of the individual. Currently, many sociologists define health in a way that emphasizes people's ability to function within their own milieu—in particular, in terms of their family and job. This model views health as the ability to perform effectively.

Aaron Antonovsky, an Israeli medical sociologist, takes an intermediate position between the World Health Organization's definition of complete well-being and the old definition of absence of disease. He views health as a dynamic, continuous phe-

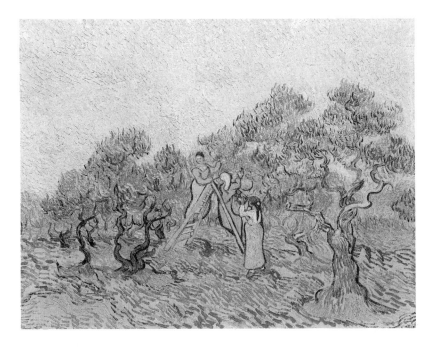

Health is the ability to work and function effectively. Vincent van Gogh. The Olive Orchard. 1889. National Gallery of Art, Washington. Chester Dale Collection.

nomenon, an ongoing process in which people move between imaginary poles of total wellness and total illness. The vast majority of people fit somewhere along this continuum, rather than at either of the poles. Like others before him, Antonovsky calls the pole of total wellness "ease," and the opposite pole "dis-ease." We likewise believe there is not a fixed, clear line between illness and health. We first dealt with an "ease–dis-ease" continuum in an earlier book, *Be Well* (1973). The concept that people's attitudes and actions will tend to move them to one end of the health spectrum or the other is key to the use of the present book.

Antonovsky calls his model a *salutogenic* one because it emphasizes the factors that make people healthy. By comparison, the *pathogenic* model, which is the prevailing view in Western medicine, concentrates on the factors that make people ill. It states that people are either one or the other—healthy or sick—but the normal state is health or order. According to this model, illness results when a particular cause—be it social, behavioral, biochemical, or bacterial—disrupts an organism's homeostasis or balance. Traditionally the pathogenic model has emphasized

Ease/Dis-ease Scale

Imagine a scale with ease at one end and dis-ease at the other, looking something like this:

EASE ☆ DIS-EASE
1 2 3 4 5 6 7 8 9 10 11 12

The feelings experienced along the scale range from joy and exhilaration at 1, to pain and suffering at 12. Most of us spend a good part of our lives in the center of the scale, with occasional movements back and forth between right and left ends.

Source: M. Samuels and H. Bennett, Be Well.

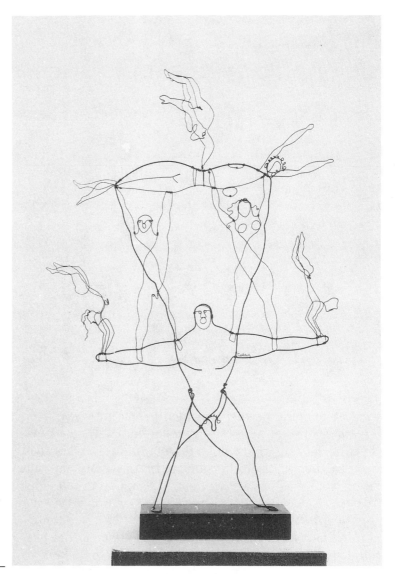

Health is a delicate balance involving social, psychological, and physical factors. Alexander Calder. The Brass Family. 1927. Brass wire. 64" × 41" × 8½". Collection, The Whitney Museum of American Art. Gift of the artist. 69.255.

only what people can do to prevent illness, whereas a main tenet of the salutogenic model holds that people can attempt to promote movement toward the healthy side of the continuum. Antonovsky notes that the things people can do are often rather general and not necessarily related to only one illness. The difference in theory is subtle, but the difference in practice is great. Thus, for example, instead of fearing stress because of its negative effects on health, the salutogenic model would emphasize those coping mechanisms and factors that can help to turn a stressful situation into a positive one.

Healthy Attitudes

At the center of the salutogenic model is a focus on successful coping—the answer to the question, "What makes a person healthier?" Antonovsky believes that the most important factor in health is what he calls a *sense of coherence*; that is, an ideology or way of looking at the world that gives people a sense of enduring confidence that their external and internal environments are predictable and that things will probably work out reasonably.

Antonovsky believes that when people have a sense of understanding about a situation, feel that they can deal with it, and are emotionally involved in it, they are more likely to engage in activities that are health-promoting, and less likely to engage in actions that are deleterious to health. In addition, people who have a sense of coherence to their lives are more likely to perceive stress as an opportunity, rather than a threat. Coherence is a concept that takes on new and increased meaning in the middle years of adulthood when disease often becomes more common, the meaning of life becomes a greater subject of concern, and wisdom becomes a natural goal (p. 75).

Studies by psychologists Albert Bandura and Suzanne Kobasa underscore the importance of a sense of control and positive expectations with regard to health. Bandura found that people's ability to deal with a stressful event correlated with their *perception* of how well they could cope with that event. The researchers termed this quality *self-efficacy*. They found that people's self-perception not only correlated with their emotional ability to cope, it even affected them physiologically. A strong sense of self-efficacy was associated with lower levels of stress hormones. Kobasa also defined a concept called *hardiness*, which dealt with commitment, control, and response to challenge. She studied two groups of middle-management executives under stress: one which reported few illnesses, and another which reported a high number of illnesses. Those executives who were not often ill had a clearer sense of values and a greater sense of control than did the executives who were frequently sick (see p. 55).

The more involved people become in setting up their own health program, the more successful their efforts are likely to be. A very interesting study by social psychologist Ellen Langer

Attitudes That Promote Health

COHERENCE: confidence that the world is predictable and life will work out reasonably.

SELF-EFFICACY: a perception that one is able to cope.

HARDINESS: a clear sense of values, and a sense of control.

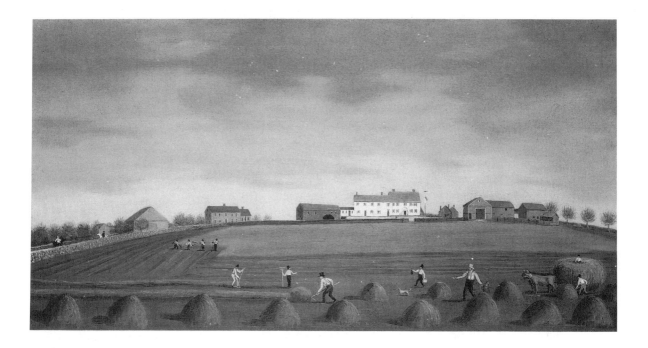

A sense that the external environment is predictable contributes to our health and well-being. Francis Alexander. Ralph Wheelock's Farm. c. 1822. National Gallery of Art, Washington. Gift of Edgar William and Bernice Chrysler Garbisch.

divided nursing home residents into two groups: one group who was encouraged to take personal responsibility for their own time and were encouraged to make suggestions regarding their own care; and another group who was told the staff would take care of them. Not only did the first group feel more interested, vigorous, and healthy a year and a half later, they had half the deaths of the second group. The more people take responsibility for their own lives and their health, the more healthy and vigorous they are likely to be.

Using This Book

This book provides a broad-based body of information on health and illness. The first part focuses on prevention. It gives information on the risk factors for the major diseases that cause death and disability in mid-adulthood. Then it addresses preventive medicine principles; health attitudes, stress, and personal fulfillment; nutrition and exercise; smoking, alcohol, and chemicals. Part I deals with the theories and studies that support suggested life-style changes, and includes charts that summarize the current research and recommendations in a form that is easy to scan.

In the second part of the book, we deal with more than 100 of the most common illnesses of the 35-to-65 age group. These illnesses are drawn from Health, Education, and Welfare Department statistics that list the reason for doctor visits in order of frequency. Each discussion contains information on the physiology and history of the illness, self-help advice, medical treatments, and prevention. Our emphasis in this section is on what people can do to actively cope with and improve their condition, as well as prevent or lessen recurrences. This emphasis is deliberate, because studies have shown—over and above any specific effects of medical treatment—that decision-making, goal-setting, and self-efficacy correlate with a reduction of immediate symptoms and with long-range improvement.

This book is designed to be equally useful for people who are well and for those who have a diagnosed condition. There are two ways to use the book—one for people who basically feel well but are interested in improving their health and living longer, and one for people who have an illness and want to deal with it more effectively. If you are basically healthy, begin by reading Chapters 2 and 3, "Preventive Medicine" and "Stress and Health." These chapters show the importance of risk factors and attitudes in relation to illness, as well as the importance of personal fulfillment in adulthood. Our hope is that by citing the studies which back up these assertions, we will help to encourage positive change.

The first step in any program involves learning basic facts about what affects health and how much you can do to change your health. From this must come an initial decision to be well. The second step involves choosing a health area on which to concentrate, and/or setting up specific health goals. Whether you are focusing on one or several goals, it is always important to set achievable goals and to work in steps. Beginning with small changes in one area prevents feeling overwhelmed and helps insure immediate success and reinforcement.

The choice of an area to work on or a disease to prevent is up to you, the individual. The decision may be made on the basis of interest, concern, family history, or intuition. If you are wor-

---

Using This Book

If you are basically healthy:
1. Learn about risk factors from Part I and make a decision to change your lifestyle accordingly.
2. Choose an area and set goals within it.
3. Implement changes, work to improve health attitudes, get support.

If you have an illness:
1. Read about your illness in Part II.
2. Commit yourself to whatever life changes are indicated and set appropriate goals.
3. Implement treatments recommended in the *Self-Care* and *Doctor* sections; work to make health attitudes positive, and get support.

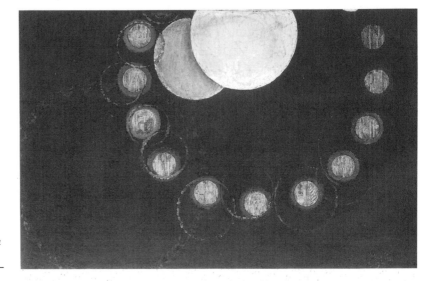

Improving health begins with a decision to be well. Frantisek Kupka. The First Step. *1909. Oil on canvas, 32¾" × 51". Collection,* The Museum of Modern Art, *New York. Hillman Periodicals Fund.*

ried that you may be at higher-than-average risk for a particular disease, read about that disease in Part II, in addition to reading the general prevention information in Part I. The Risk Assessment Questionnaire at the end of Chapter 2 can help you to accurately assess the general area or areas that are most important for you to concentrate on.

The final step is to implement those changes that will be of most benefit to you. A major factor in this regard involves dealing with your own health attitudes and getting support from others. Support can come from family, friends, physicians, therapists, counselors, or self-help groups. Although the framework of an individual program may start with this book, it should incorporate your own research, planning, and interests.

If you have an illness, the three overall steps remain the same: decide to be well, choose interventions and set goals, and implement the program. But you should begin with information in Part Two; read the discussion of the particular illness. Specific ideas for an individual program are included in the *Self-Care* and *Prevention* sections under each disease. Again, this is simply a beginning, and readers are encouraged to explore further in the bibliography and to take responsibility for and control over their own program. Often a part of the program may involve working actively with doctors and therapists. Although some illnesses

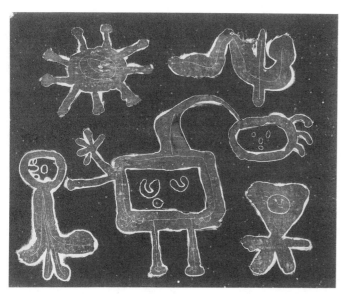

Joan Miro. The Family. 1953. Etching and aquatint, printed in color. Plate: 14¹⁵⁄₁₆″ × 17⁷⁄₈″. Sheet: 19¾″ × 25⁷⁄₈″. Collection, The Museum of Modern Art, New York. Gift of Abby Aldrich Rockefeller.

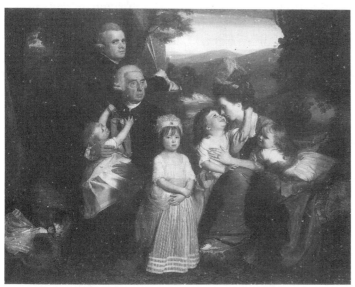

Families can be a great source of support—both when we are sick and when we are well. John Singleton Copley. The Copley Family. Circa 1776. National Gallery of Art, Washington. Andrew W. Mellon Fund.

may be more difficult to treat than others, we believe that in general you can help yourself feel better, control your symptoms more effectively, and, in many cases, heal yourself.

It is our belief that people who are actively involved in health education programs will, over time, have fewer illnesses and greater longevity. We also believe that a book is an excellent tool for involving people in health improvement. Thus, we think that readers of this book will actually enjoy better health than would a matched group who has the same risk factors and background, but is not reading material dealing with health education. We are interested in verifying this hypothesis by compiling the statistics from readers who complete the Health Risk Assessment Questionnaire (see p. 35) and send it in to be scored.

Previous studies have indicated that use of self-help medical books has resulted in fewer doctor visits. We believe that use of such books can lead to a great deal more than simply lowering the number of doctor visits, and, in fact, may result in less illness and greater longevity. Other studies have shown that people who are told they are being put in a special group generally work harder or do more than people in a matched control group. Thus readers who decide to become an active part of this experimental group are likely to be more motivated to make life-style changes that will result in improved health. We believe that this book can actually alter your health for years to come. It will do so if the material causes a change in your consciousness which will in turn motivate you to maintain a healthier life-style.

CHAPTER TWO

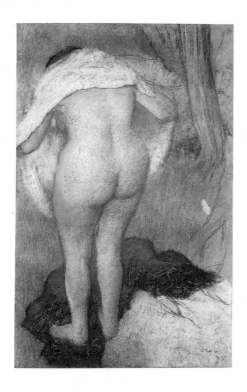

Preventive Medicine

W e believe that by midadulthood, most people are not only interested in feeling good in the present, they care about preventing diseases that might affect them in the future. By this age many of us are not in our best physical condition, and we may occasionally experience the type of aches and pains that did not trouble us in our 20s. One of the messages of this book is that this gradual decline is not wholly inevitable. By changing our attitudes and habits, we can take control of our health and increase our sense of well-being. Fortunately, those very changes that will make us feel better now will also help to prevent the illnesses that may be of concern to us in the future. By making positive changes that move us toward the "ease" end of the ease–dis-ease continuum, we can stop many disease pro-

For adults, health involves feeling good in the future as well as in the present. Edgar Degas. Girl Drying Herself. *Dated (18)85. National Gallery of Art, Washington. Gift of the W. Averell Harriman Foundation in memory of Marie N. Harriman.*

cesses before they even begin. Not feeling terrific in the present is a signal from the body that change is needed. Low energy, for instance, is not a necessary consequence of growing older, it's more likely the result of being under stress, being overweight, or not getting enough exercise.

Stopping illness before it begins is known as preventive medicine. It is the medicine of the future. In the last 20 years, many doctors and people in the medical community have undergone a tremendous change in consciousness and have come to realize that their focus must shift from *treating illness* to *preventing illness*. Studies have shown that most of the disease that occurs in midadulthood is unnecessary. Most disability and death that occurs during the years from 35 to 65 is preventable, and therefore it is *premature*. The great majority of deaths among men in middle age are attributable to only 10 causes: atherosclerotic heart disease, lung cancer, cirrhosis, automobile accidents, suicide, stroke, homicide, colon cancer, pneumonia, and alcoholism (see chart). These 10 killers are largely preventable. Thus, the message is that, in most cases, people in this age group should not be developing chronic diseases or dying.

What scientists are beginning to recognize is that much of the illness in these years is due to *life-style*, a factor that can be changed through individual initiative. In fact, researchers now believe that 80% of deaths in midadulthood are related to a relatively small number of life-style habits. Heart disease, includ-

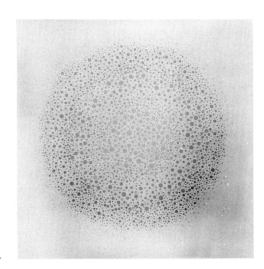

Changes in attitudes and habits affect our health and well-being. Paul Brach. New Day. 1967. Oil on canvas. 65" × 65". Collection, The Whitney Museum of American Art. Gift of Margery and Harry Kahn. 73.66.

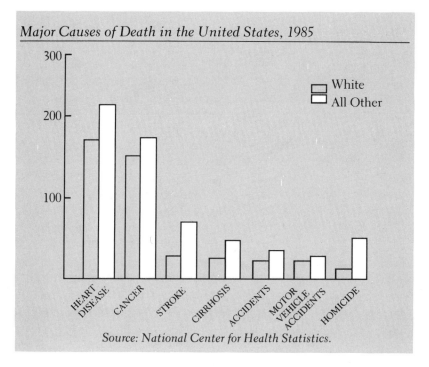

Major Causes of Death in the United States, 1985

White
All Other

HEART DISEASE · CANCER · STROKE · CIRRHOSIS · ACCIDENTS · MOTOR VEHICLE ACCIDENTS · HOMICIDE

Source: National Center for Health Statistics.

ing heart attacks and strokes—which together are by far the leading cause of death and disability for men 40–45—can largely be prevented by dealing with stress, changing nutritional habits, stopping smoking, getting reasonable exercise, and treating hypertension. Cancer, the second leading cause of death, can often be prevented in the long run by stopping smoking, making dietary changes, and avoiding exposure to occupational or environmental chemicals. Finally, cirrhosis, alcoholism, and a majority of accidents can be avoided by controlling the use of alcohol.

Why People Die: Primary Factors Affecting Cause of Death

CAUSE OF DEATH	LIFESTYLE	ENVIRONMENT	GENETICS	MEDICAL TREATMENT
Heart disease	54%	9%	28%	12%
Stroke	50%	22%	21%	7%
Cancer	37%	24%	29%	10%
Car accidents	69%	18%	1%	12%

Source: Adapted from G. Dever, "An Epidemiological Model for Health Policy Analysis."

Major Controllable Risk Factors for the 10 Leading Causes of Death

CAUSE OF DEATH	CONTROLLABLE RISK FACTORS
Heart disease	smoking, high blood pressure, high blood cholesterol, sedentary lifestyle, coronary-prone behavior (see p. 255)
Cancer	smoking; heavy alcohol consumption; environmental carcinogens; high-fat, low-fiber diet; exposure to sunlight
Stroke	high blood pressure, high blood cholesterol, smoking
Accident	heavy alcohol consumption, fires caused by smoking, hazards in the home, access to handguns
Pneumonia (due to influenza)	lack of flu shots (in high-risk people), smoking, heavy alcohol consumption, poor nutrition
Auto accident	heavy alcohol consumption, failure to use seat belts, poor automotive or roadway design
Diabetes (Type II)	obesity; a high-sugar, high-fat diet
Cirrhosis	longterm heavy alcohol consumption
Suicide	alcohol or drug abuse, stress, access to handguns
Homicide	alcohol or drug abuse, stress, access to handguns

From the standpoint of both individual health and national health, it is amazing to consider that in perhaps three out of four cases, death and disability in middle age can be avoided through a limited number of behavior changes that admittedly take effort and willpower, but are not impossible to achieve. None of these changes is dependent on new advances in medical technology, the development of new drugs or surgical techniques, or the building of prohibitively expensive medical facilities. Improvement is basically a matter of life-style changes and/or environmental changes. To make these changes we have to change our attitude and the way we look at the world. Belief in our own power to effect change is essential. We, not doctors, are largely responsible for creating our own state of health and well-being.

The Two Public Health Revolutions

Ironically, over the last 100 years, people have come to believe that science and technology have been, and continue to be, responsible for preventing most illness. Well into this century, the major killer worldwide has been communicable disease. In 1900, the leading causes of death in the U.S. were influenza, pneumonia, diphtheria, tuberculosis, and gastrointestinal infections. Eliminating communicable disease as the major killer represented the first revolution in public health. Most people, including health professionals, believe that these diseases were brought under control by medical means such as vaccination and antibiotics. Actually, new studies have shown that these diseases started to decline even before the introduction of the new drugs and vaccines (see charts). Medical epidemiologists now speculate that the most important cause of the decrease in these illnesses was social reform that led to improved nutrition and sanitation, including better storage and treatment of food and water, and more effective disposal of sewage. Medicine itself is estimated to have been responsible for as little as 10% of the work of eliminating infections. It is currently estimated that, at

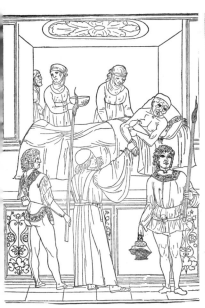

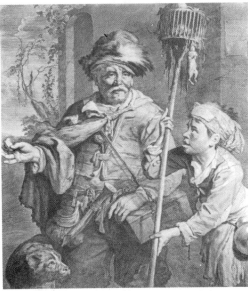

Social change, not medical technology, has resulted in eliminating most of the deadly communicable diseases of the past. Gentile Bellini. Visit to a Plague Patient. *Ca. 1495.*

Cornelius Visscher. The Rat Catcher. 1655. *Reproduced from* Medicine and the Artist *by permission of the Philadelphia Museum of Art.*

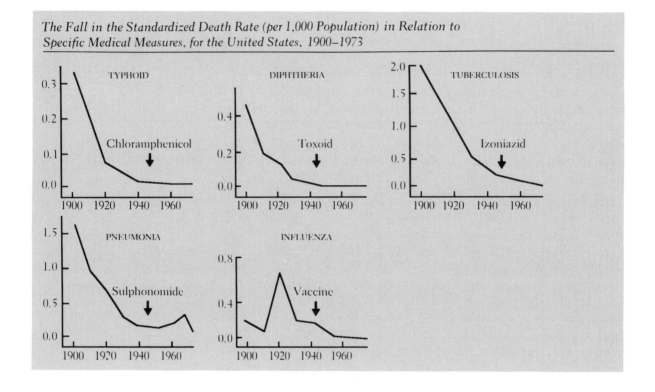

The Fall in the Standardized Death Rate (per 1,000 Population) in Relation to Specific Medical Measures, for the United States, 1900–1973

most, only 3.5% of the decline in deaths from communicable diseases since 1900 can be ascribed to medical measures.

At the turn of the century in this country, the average *life expectancy* was 49 years. By 1966, this figure had increased to 70 years. At first glance, it might appear from these statistics that middle-aged people were living longer, but in fact, virtually all of the increase in life expectancy is due to reductions in infant and child mortality. As of 1900, the *remaining life expectancy* for someone at age 65 was 11.9 more years. By comparison, in 1966, the remaining life expectancy for someone of 65 was 14 more years, an increase of only two years. Clearly, though we have made strides in reducing child mortality, we have not yet made equal progress against the diseases of midadulthood.

Unfortunately, the medical profession, including public health experts, attributed the gains of the first public health revolution to medical technology; specifically, to the application of the germ theory of disease. The basis of that theory, a classic tenet of Western medicine, is simple: one kind of germ causes one disease, and essentially, is cured by one type of drug therapy. The theory is not wrong, it just does not go far enough. In effect, the one-germ theory tends to stop researchers from seriously investigating personal behavior or environmental conditions as *underlying* factors in a multicausal explanation of disease. However, as most doctors would privately acknowledge, illness and healing depend greatly on the condition of the host—on how susceptible to disease a person is and how well his or her immune system is working. Although the germ theory recognizes the effect of external factors such as improved sanitation in reducing exposure to germs, it does not deal with internal influences such as the fact that better nutrition will improve person's resistance to disease, or that stress or other illness will increase a person's susceptibility.

Heart disease, cancer, alcoholism, and accidents have replaced communicable diseases as the leading causes of premature death and disability in adulthood. The challenge now is to find controls for these diseases, just as controls were developed for the communicable diseases that plagued people in the 19th century. Finding ways to deal with and ultimately prevent the present killers will constitute the *second public health revolution*. This revolution has the potential to be just as significant as the first in terms of reducing death and disability, but whereas the first revolution had the greatest effect on infants and children, the second will have its greatest effect on adults. Statistics show that the second revolution is already in progress. From 1960–1977, the remaining life expectancy for people 65 years of age rose from 14 to 16 years—as big a gain as had been achieved in the previous 60 years. This increase is largely the result of a significant decline in heart attacks. While the decline may in part be due to treatment, it is more likely that it is primarily due to people voluntarily lowering their fat and cholesterol intake.

The first public health revolution was chiefly based on social measures; the second revolution will probably be based on psycho-social changes; that is, on changes in consciousness and attitude that lead to changes in behavior. Whereas the first revolution involved life-style changes relating to hygiene, sanitation, and food storage, the second revolution will necessitate life-style modification with regard to stress and attitude, nutrition, exercise, smoking, alcohol consumption, and exposure to other harmful substances. This revolution will be more personal. Though its effects may be less immediate, its significance will be just as great.

Two Philosophies of Public Health

At present, the focus on life-style changes is divided into two schools or philosophies in the public health community. One group of experts believes that the primary factor relating to health is individual life-style and behavior. They believe that when people become educated about a particular health issue, they become motivated to change their habits and improve their health. The term for this view is *health promotion.*

The other group of experts believes that the social and economic environment is the main determinant of people's health

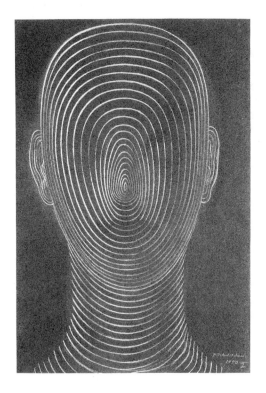

By focusing on a healthy lifestyle, we become motivated to improve our habits. Pavel Tchelitchew. Head. 1950. Colored pencil on black paper, 18⅞″ × 12½″. Collection, The Museum of Modern Art, New York. Purchase.

and habits, and that individuals are primarily influenced by the social structure at large. According to this philosophy, public health is achieved only by changing sociopolitical and economic structures through far-reaching social reform. Thus, people's life-styles change in response to broader cultural changes. This philosophy is called *health protection.* Implementing this philosophy might mean, for example, outlawing or heavily taxing cigarettes to get people to smoke less, or decreasing unemployment so as to lower levels of stress. By comparison, health promotion proponents might advocate teaching people to take responsibility for their own health by becoming educated about the risks of smoking, learning alternate ways of dealing with stress, and finally quitting smoking. No one disagrees with the validity of the two points of view, rather the argument centers around which one should receive the primary emphasis in public policy and funding.

Currently, the U.S. and Britain are committed to an emphasis on individual health promotion, unlike France and the Canadian province of Quebec, which are committed to emphasizing group health protection. The U.S. philosophy of health promotion was established during the Carter administration with the 1980 publication of the revolutionary document, *Healthy People.* This forward-looking report targeted cancer, heart disease, and accidents as the focus of the next public health revolution: "You, the individual, can do more for your own health and well-being than any doctor, any hospital, any drug, any exotic medical device . . . a wealth of scientific research reveals that the key to whether a person will be healthy or sick, live a long life or die prematurely, can be found in several simple personal habits. . ."[1]

The U.S. Department of Health, Education, and Welfare has set major health goals to be achieved by the year 2000. For people aged 25–65, the goal is to reduce overall deaths by 25%, a staggering challenge in the light of earlier improvements in mortality figures. The report proposed to do this, not by increasing medical expenditures or developing new technology, but by encouraging large numbers of individuals to make modest but significant life-style changes. The changes recommended by *Healthy People* include "elimination of cigarette smoking; reduction of alcohol misuse; moderate dietary changes to reduce in-

Two Philosophies of Public Health

HEALTH PROMOTION: lifestyle and behavioral changes are made voluntarily by individuals to create health.

HEALTH PROTECTION: social and economic reforms are implemented by government agencies to create health.

take of excess calories, fat, salt, and sugar; moderate exercise; periodic screening (at intervals determined by age and sex) for major disorders such as high blood pressure and certain cancers; and adherence to speed laws and use of seat belts . . . Additionally, it is important to emphasize that physical health and mental health are often linked. Both are enhanced through the maintenance of strong family ties, the assistance of supportive friends, and the use of community support systems."[2]

Health Promotion

The scientific evidence for health promotion is not only interesting, it is crucial to an understanding of the life-style changes that are discussed throughout this book. Health promotion is based on a series of studies that have established the relationship between people's life-styles and their health, with particular regard to heart disease and cancer. In the late 1940s, when epidemiologists realized that communicable disease had been replaced by chronic disease as the major threat to health, they undertook large population studies to determine what behavioral factors were linked with specific conditions. One of the first significant prevention studies was a 1952 smoking survey by the American Cancer Society which studied almost 200,000 men. During a four-year period, it was found that in comparison to nonsmokers, smokers died at an excessive rate due to lung cancer and heart disease.

Subsequent studies were bolder and more far-reaching. They followed very large populations in an effort to identify the causes of heart disease. Researchers interviewed large numbers of individuals who were healthy in order to establish their existing behavior patterns, then followed these people for a number of years in order to determine which of their behaviors was associated with later heart disease. The most famous of these studies, The Framingham Study, which dealt with 200,000 people in the town of Framingham, Mass., was first reported in 1957 and is still continuing today. By the early 1960s, evaluation of its data showed that high cholesterol levels, high blood pressure, smoking, obesity, sedentary life-style, diabetes, a high-fat diet, and family history were all associated with heart disease, and it labelled them *risk factors*. During the same time period, definitive studies found smoking to be a hazard to human health, posing a serious risk with regard to lung cancer and heart disease. The Surgeon General's Report on the dangers of smoking, published in 1964, was the first public health announcement to take a strong stand on health promotion.

In 1965, epidemiologists Lester Breslow and Lisa Berkman of UCLA issued The Alameda County Study, a groundbreaking report on 7,000 individuals who lived in one California county. For the study, they collated responses to a questionnaire on health practices. The questions were general; that is, they were not designed to find the causes of any particular disease, but what Breslow and Berkman found was staggering: a 45-year-old man who practiced six to seven health-promoting habits lived an *average of 78 years* whereas a man of the same age who practiced zero to three of the habits lived an *average of 67 years*. The health habits studied by Breslow and Berkman were so simple that today they seem almost obvious: three meals a day, at regular times, without snacks; a daily breakfast; moderate exercise two or three times a week; seven to eight hours of sleep a night; no smoking; maintaining a moderate weight; and no alcohol or moderate alcohol consumption. In follow-up studies, Breslow and Berkman found that the five most important factors were: smoking, physical activity, alcohol consumption, obesity, and sleeping patterns. Of these, the first three were tremendously significant. In the second study, it was found that people who had practiced only zero to two of the top five habits, as opposed to four to five, were almost three times as likely to have died during the nine-year period between the studies.

Breslow and Berkman's follow-up study also assessed the importance of "social networks" or "social support." The new questionnaire elicited information on marriage, contacts with close friends and relatives, church membership, and associations with nonchurch groups. People with intimate social relationships had much lower odds—almost one-third lower—of dying during the nine-year period studied. This striking relationship between health and intimacy is a generalized phenomenon that has also been demonstrated in relation to specific diseases (see p. 52). The Alameda Follow-up Study was one of the first to define a relationship between social factors and physical health. Subsequent work by Kobasa, Bandura, and Antonovsky has empha-

Simple Habits Found to Promote Health in the Alameda Study

- three meals a day, without snacks
- daily breakfast
- moderate exercise two to three times a week
- seven to eight hours of sleep per night
- no alcohol
- no smoking
- moderate weight

Source: Adapted from Breslow and Berkman, "Persistence of Health Habits and Their Relationship to Mortality."

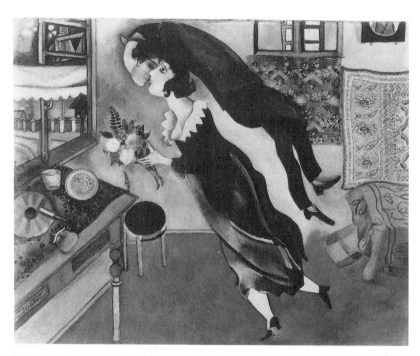

Intimacy is associated with greater longevity. Marc Chagall. Birthday. 1915. Oil on cardboard, 31¾" × 39¼". Collection, The Museum of Modern Art, New York. Acquired through the Lillie P. Bliss Bequest.

sized the importance of attitude as well as social support on states of health and well-being (see p. 53).

Armed with the knowledge that social and physical risk factors can negatively affect health, other researchers attempted to determine whether people can actually *improve* their health by undertaking positive life-style changes. The Stanford Three Community Study, begun in 1972 by Dr. J. Farquhar, was an attempt to assess the value of changes in health habits brought about by the intervention of educational television spots. The study recorded a significant decrease in smoking among people who received intensive education about the physical effects of smoking, and estimated that this decline would result in a 10% drop in deaths due to heart disease.

Another study, called The Multiple Risk Factor Intervention Trial, dealt with 12,000 people for a period of more than 10 years. It demonstrated that people who were educated about risk factors for heart disease showed a significant decrease in smoking and serum cholesterol levels as opposed to a group who received no education. No significant drop in death rate was shown, but this may have been due to the fact that the study did not cover a long enough period.

Finally, a study done in Karelia, Finland, illustrated that an entire community could radically change its health habits in response to health education. Karelia is in the area of Finland that has the highest heart disease rate in the world. In the 1970s, the townspeople had a high smoking rate, extremely high cholesterol levels due to a diet rich in dairy products and meat, and a significant amount of untreated high blood pressure. An intensive health promotion campaign was undertaken, and after five years, there was a significant drop in cigarette smoking, fat consumption, and untreated high blood pressure, as well as a much lower heart attack rate.

The tenets of the health promotion philosophy have been most dynamically summed up by John H. Knowles, former president of the Rockefeller Foundation, in a 1977 paper entitled, "The Responsibility of the Individual," an extremely influential work that is much quoted in public health textbooks. In his paper, Knowles states, "99% of us are born healthy and made sick as a result of personal misbehavior and environmental conditions. The solution to the problems of ill health in modern American society involves individual responsibility, in the first instance, and social responsibility through public, legislative, and private voluntary efforts, in the second instance. . . . Prevention of disease means forsaking the bad habits which many people enjoy—overeating, too much drinking, taking pills, staying up at night, engaging in promiscuous sex, driving too fast, and smoking cigarettes—or, put another way, it means doing things which require special effort—exercising regularly, going to the dentist, practicing contraception, ensuring harmonious family life, submitting to screening examinations."[3]

Health Protection

The second basic philosophy of preventive medicine is *health protection*, which as we've said, aims to alter political and economic structures. Health protection advocates do not deny that health habits such as smoking, drinking, and eating fatty foods affect illness patterns, but they feel that such health habits are often determined by forces beyond people's control, which can only be effectively addressed through widespread social changes. Leon Eisenberg, of Harvard Medical School, cogently voices the argument of the health protectionists: "The new converts to prevention, having discovered that behavior affects health, focus on the responsibility of the individual for illness prevention, by eating and drinking in moderation, exercising properly, not smoking, and the like. Surely, in the final analysis, it is the individual who carries out these actions. But what does it mean to hold the individual responsible for smoking when the government subsidizes tobacco farming, permits tax deductions for cigarette advertising and fails to use its taxing power as a disincentive to smoking? What does it mean 'to castigate the individual for poor eating habits when the public is inundated by advertisements for 'empty calorie' fast foods and is reinforced in present patterns of consumption by federal farm policy?"[4]

Advertising and public policy exert a powerful influence on our consciousness and health habits. Tom Wesselmann. Still Life Number Thirty-Six. *Oil, synthetic, polymer and collage of paper. 120″ × 192½″. Collection, The Whitney Museum of American Art. Gift of the artist. 69.151.*

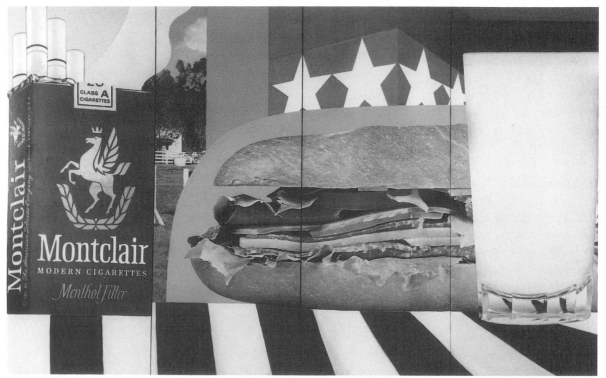

Health protectionists believe that telling individuals they are to blame for their health habits is simply blaming the victim. Health policy researcher Jean de Kervasdoue notes, "Exhorting the worker to exercise personal safety in the midst of hazardous working conditions, asking adolescents to exercise mature judgment in the face of sophisticated advertising and social pressures . . . , imploring poverty-stricken mothers to feed their malnourished children a more varied and nutritious diet, and encouraging those who live near toxic waste dumps or nuclear plants to jog, quit smoking, and reduce cholesterol intake, have not been demonstrated to be associated with positive health outcomes."[5]

There is considerable epidemiological evidence that supports the health protectionist view that the social environment interacts with personal risk factors or health habits to cause illness. The most dramatic example comes from studies which have found a direct relationship between socioeconomic status and health. There are two major studies that have graphically demonstrated a link between social class and life expectancy. The Matched Record Study of 1960, which compared 340,000 death certificates with census records, found that people of lower socioeconomic status generally died at a much younger age than people of higher status. The protective factor held true for profession alone (professional vs. blue-collar worker) and for wealth alone (high income vs. low income). The second major study, done by epidemiologists E. Kitagawa and P. Hauser, found that as formal education increased in years, people's mortality at a given age decreased, especially for the years between 25 and 65, during which span the decrease applied to most causes of death.

Research has also shown that during economic downturns, mortality from heart disease increases, alcohol consumption increases, and mental hospital admissions increase. Furthermore, the unemployment rate is directly reflected in the overall mortality, suicide, and homicide rates. Every 1% increase in the national unemployment rate is followed by 36,000 excess deaths over the next six years. All of these socioeconomic studies indicate to health protectionists that most of the factors affecting disease incidence are not solely under the control of the individual, but are strongly influenced, if not determined, by factors relating to the culture. Poverty makes it difficult for people to make healthy, responsible choices with regard to nutrition, exercise, chemicals, stress, and health attitudes.

A graphic comparison that health protectionists cite to illustrate their reasoning concerns governmental policy toward cigarettes, alcohol, and heroin. The government has made heroin illegal, and makes efforts to stop its import and prevent its sale. Heroin users are seen as victims and are not the primary focus of law enforcement activities. However, in terms of smoking and alcohol abuse, the government tells addicted individuals to stop what they're doing, while actively supporting alcohol and cigarette manufacturers with government subsidies or tax relief at the same time. As Kervasdoue observes, "This approach to the major public health problems of alcohol and cigarettes is equivalent to trying to change the behavior of the individual heroin addict, while subsidizing the activities of the heroin pusher."[6]

John B. McKinlay, a sociologist from Boston University, is a lucid spokesperson for health protection through legal and social reform. In his paper, "A Case for Refocusing Upstream: The Political Economy of Illness," he tells a story that graphically symbolizes the philosophy of the health protectionists and emphasizes the idea of preventing illness before it starts. In the story, a doctor is trying to explain the quandary of modern medicine: "You know," he says, "sometimes it feels like this. There I am standing by the shore of a swiftly flowing river and I hear the cry of a drowning man. So I jump into the river, put my arms around him, pull him to shore and apply artificial respiration. Just when he begins to breathe, there is another cry for help. So back in the river again, reaching, pulling, applying, breathing, and then another yell. Again and again, without end, goes the sequence. You know, I am so busy jumping in, pulling them to shore, applying artificial respiration, that I have *no* time to see who the hell is upstream pushing them all in."[7]

McKinlay says that this story has two meanings for him. First, that most of what a doctor does is treat illness that is already present. This process is referred to as *tertiary prevention*. The goal of tertiary prevention is to stop the disease from progressing and to reduce subsequent complications or impairment. McKinlay compares it to the job of pulling people out of the water. He feels that this kind of downstream effort is ultimately futile.

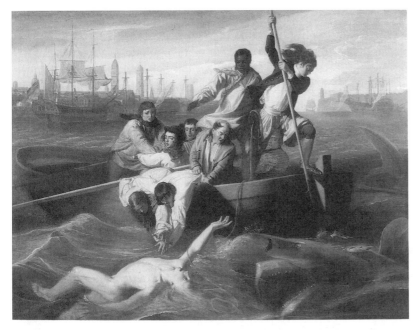

Some public health experts feel that doctors often spend so much time saving "drowning" people that they don't see who or what is pushing people in. John Singleton Copley. Watson and the Shark. 1778. *National Gallery of Art, Washington. Ferdinand Lammot Belin Fund.*

Treatment of illness is often difficult and is not always successful. The second point of the story is that we must refocus on who or what is pushing people into the river—in this case, McKinlay believes, "various individuals, interest groups, and large-scale, profit-oriented corporations."[8]

Secondary prevention consists of early intervention that reduces the likelihood of a disease progressing. The goal of secondary prevention is to identify and treat illness very early, while it will still respond to treatment, and is perhaps even asymptomatic. Examples of this are diagnosing and treating high blood pressure before it has caused a stroke or doing a lumpectomy before a small localized breast cancer found on a mammogram has spread.

Primary prevention includes both *health promotion* and *health protection*. It involves dealing with the root causes of illness. McKinlay considers primary prevention to be an "upstream effort." He makes the analogy that health protection is like stopping the manufacturers of illness from pushing people in, while health promotion is blaming people for not being able to swim after they have been pushed in the river. McKinlay does not disagree with educating people who are at risk for illness so that they'll lower their chances of getting ill, but he firmly states that part of this health education process should be to tell people the whole story, explaining the role played by those agents— whoever and whatever they are—that "push people into the stream."

We believe that health protection material is valuable because it helps to relieve people of guilt, and enables them to better understand that it is often difficult to give up negative life-style factors which are strongly supported by the government and/or the culture. Although the whole story is sometimes depressing, it can also be empowering because it helps us recognize and deal with our own resistances and motivations.

Health Risk Appraisals

Advocates of both the health prevention and the health protection philosophies believe that if the main risks for a disease are eliminated, the disease itself can be prevented. It is one thing to think about this theoretically, but another to put this into practice in our own lives. The Society of Prospective Medicine, a group devoted to health protection, has developed a program for the reduction or elimination of health risks. Its goals are to reduce health risks by fostering a healthy life-style before disease occurs. The major tool for achieving this change is a *health risk appraisal* or a *health hazard appraisal*, a questionnaire designed to quantify an individual's personal risks for major diseases, and to offer a personal prescription for reducing those risks. The first appraisal form, designed by Drs. Jack Hall and Lewis Robbins of Methodist Hospital in Indianapolis, grew out of The Framingham Study and the National Cancer Institute's earliest studies on the risks of smoking. From this data, researchers were able to develop probability tables linking causes of death by age, sex, and race to risk behaviors such as smoking, lack of exercise, etc. The tables produced, called the Geller Probability Tables, graphically show the average mortality risks for 20 major diseases and the specific risk factors or prognostic factors to which those diseases are linked.

Since its introduction in the early 1970s, the health risk appraisal has been increasingly fine-tuned into several standardized forms which have been widely adopted by public health groups, state government, and industry. The present forms include questions on life-style factors such as smoking, exercise, diet, alcohol consumption, driving, and stress. They also have questions pertaining to family health history, physical exam results, screening tests, and laboratory findings such as blood pressure, weight, rectal exam and occult blood test, Pap smear, and cholesterol.

An individual's responses are fed into a computer which compares them with the average risks from the Geller Tables for a person of similar age and sex. From this information, the computer generates a personal life expectancy based on individual risk factors and present life-style habits. In addition, the results show what a person's life expectancy would be if he or she made certain suggested changes designed to improve overall health. The hope is that seeing this comparison will motivate people to change deleterious habits before they produce serious or disabling disease.

Evidence from The Alameda County Study by Lester Breslow and Lisa Berkman indicates that the risk appraisal process actually predicted the chance of disease or death more accurately than insurance tables. Prospective medicine experts believe that most people are "intrigued" by their odds and curious to know how they compare with their peers. Health appraisal forms vary in how much educational information they include, and some are more graphic and easier to understand than others. Most physicians feel that the appraisal not only educates patients, it provides a basis for a doctor-patient dialogue on wellness. Currently many doctors believe that only a physician or trained health worker can fully and accurately interpret the questionnaires. Not only do the results then reflect physical and laboratory findings, but such evaluation allows for counseling and reinforcement that will lead to a set of specific goals for reducing risk factors. Many doctors feel that a skilled evaluation also deals with individual attitudes and differences more effectively than a self-scoring appraisal can.

We believe that health risk appraisals can help to change a person's consciousness and attitude toward their own health. By comparing people's individual risks with the average, they help people put their health needs in perspective. Setting healthcare priorities helps to motivate people and presents them with concrete, attainable goals that will have measurable results.

This book contains the Health Risk Appraisal developed by the Carter Center of Emory University and updated in collaboration with the Centers for Disease Control. The form is used by state health departments throughout the country. The reader is encouraged to fill it out and mail it in to be scored (see chart). In addition to life-style questions, the form calls for cholesterol, blood pressure, rectal, and Pap smear results, information that can only be obtained by a doctor's examination. Individuals should discuss the results of the appraisal with their doctor, who can help to put the data in the proper perspective, along with the results of the person's physical exam and history.

We believe that the Department of Health, Education, and Welfare's goal of a 25% reduction in deaths in the age range 35–65 is both possible and of the highest priority. The next four chapters of this book present in detail information on what you can do to feel better and be healthier. These chapters discuss studies that show the effect of life-style changes and spell out simple programs for healthy habits that will help to prevent major illness. Our goal is for every reader to have a greater sense of well-being and greater longevity.

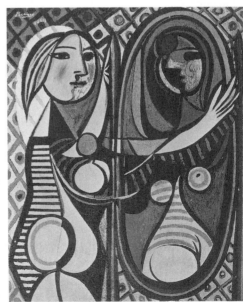

Assessing our own health risks can help to motivate us to change our lifestyle. Pablo Picasso. Girl Before a Mirror. *1932. Oil on canvas, 64″ × 51¼″. Collection, The Museum of Modern Art, New York. Gift of Mrs. Simon Guggenheim.*

Healthier People—Health Risk Appraisal

Send form and $5.00 to:
Michael Samuels, M.D.
P.O. Box 3728
San Rafael, CA 94912-3728

Health Risk Appraisal is an educational tool. It shows you choices you can make to keep good health and avoid the most common causes of death for a person your age and sex. This Health Risk Appraisal is not a substitute for a check-up or physical exam that you get from a doctor or nurse. It only gives you some ideas for lowering your risk of getting sick or injured in the future. It is NOT designed for people who already have HEART DISEASE, CANCER, KIDNEY DISEASE, OR OTHER SERIOUS CONDITIONS. If you have any of these problems and you want a Health Risk Appraisal anyway, ask your doctor or nurse to read the report with you.

DIRECTIONS: To have this form scored, have it photocopied and fill it out, then send it with a check for $5.00 to the address above. Include a stamped, self-addressed envelope. To get the most accurate results answer as many questions as you can and as best you can. If you do not know the answer leave it blank. Questions with a ★ (star symbol) are important to your health, but are not used by the computer to calculate your risks. However, your answers may be helpful in planning your health and fitness program. **Note:** This Health Risk Appraisal form is still being tested and improved. It may have mistakes or errors in it. If anything in your questionnaire or report doesn't seem right to you, ask a health person to help.

Please put your answers in the empty boxes. (Examples: ☒ or ☐125☐)

1. SEX	1 ☐ Male 2 ☐ Female
2. AGE	☐☐☐ Years
3. HEIGHT (Without shoes) (No fractions)	☐☐☐ Feet ☐☐☐ Inches
4. WEIGHT (Without shoes) (No fractions)	☐☐☐ Pounds
5. Body frame size	1 ☐ Small 2 ☐ Medium 3 ☐ Large
6. Have you ever been told that you have diabetes (or sugar diabetes)?	1 ☐ Yes 2 ☐ No
7. Are you now taking medicine for high blood pressure?	1 ☐ Yes 2 ☐ No
8. What is your blood pressure now?	☐☐☐ / ☐☐☐ Systolic (high number)/Diastolic (low number)
9. If you *do not* know the numbers, check the box that describes your blood pressure.	1 ☐ High 2 ☐ Normal or low 3 ☐ Don't know
10. What is your TOTAL cholesterol level (based on a blood test)?	☐☐☐ mg/dl
11. What is your HDL cholesterol level (based on a blood test)?	☐☐☐ mg/dl
12. How many cigars do you usually smoke per day?	☐☐☐ Cigars per day
13. How many pipes of tobacco do you usually smoke per day?	☐☐☐ Pipes per day

continued

14. How many times per day do you usually use smokeless tobacco? (Chewing tobacco, snuff, pouches, etc.) [   ] Times per day

15. CIGARETTE SMOKING
How would you describe your cigarette smoking habits?

1 ☐ Never smoked ☛ Go to 18
2 ☐ Used to smoke ☛ Go to 17
3 ☐ Still smoke ☛ Go to 16

16. STILL SMOKE
How many cigarettes a day do you smoke? [   ] Cigarettes per day ☛ Go to 18

17. USED TO SMOKE
a. How many years has it been since you smoked cigarettes fairly regularly? [   ] Years
b. What was the average number of cigarettes per day that you smoked in the 2 years before you quit? [   ] Cigarettes per day

18. In the next 12 months how many thousands of miles will you probably travel by each of the following?
(Note: U.S. average = 10,000 miles)
a. Car, truck or van: [   ] ,000 miles
b. Motorcycle: [   ] ,000 miles

19. On a typical day how do you *usually* travel?

(Check one only)

1 ☐ Walk
2 ☐ Bicycle
3 ☐ Motorcycle
4 ☐ Sub-compact or compact car
5 ☐ Mid-size or full-size car
6 ☐ Truck or van
7 ☐ Bus, subway, or train
8 ☐ Mostly stay home

20. What percent of the time do you usually buckle your safety belt when driving or riding? [   ] %

21. On the average, how close to the speed limit do you usually drive?

1 ☐ Within 5 mph of limit
2 ☐ 6–10 mph over limit
3 ☐ 11–15 mph over limit
4 ☐ More than 15 mph over limit

22. How many times in the last month did you drive or ride when the driver had perhaps too much alcohol to drink? [   ] Times last month

23. How many drinks of alcoholic beverages do you have in a typical week?

☛ (MEN GO TO QUESTION 33)

(Write the number of each type of drink)

[   ] Bottles or cans of beer
[   ] Glasses of wine
[   ] Wine coolers
[   ] Mixed drinks or shots of liquor

WOMEN
24. At what age did you have your first menstrual period? [   ] Years old

25. How old were you when your first child was born? [   ] Years old
(If no children write 0)

continued

26. How long has it been since your last breast x-ray (mammogram)?	1 ☐ Less than 1 year 2 ☐ 1 year ago 3 ☐ 2 years ago 4 ☐ 3 or more years ago 5 ☐ Never
27. How many women in your natural family (mother and sisters only) have had breast cancer?	☐ women
28. Have you had a hysterectomy operation?	1 ☐ Yes 2 ☐ No 3 ☐ Not sure
29. How long has it been since you had a Pap smear for cancer?	1 ☐ Less than 1 year ago 2 ☐ 1 year ago 3 ☐ 2 years ago 4 ☐ 3 or more years ago 5 ☐ Never
★30. How often do you examine your breasts for lumps.	1 ☐ Monthly 2 ☐ Once every few months 3 ☐ Rarely or never
★31. About how long has it been since you had your breasts examined by a physician or nurse?	1 ☐ Less than 1 year ago 2 ☐ 1 year ago 3 ☐ 2 years ago 4 ☐ 3 or more years ago 5 ☐ Never
★32. About how long has it been since you had a rectal exam? ☛ (WOMEN GO TO QUESTION 34)	1 ☐ Less than 1 year ago 2 ☐ 1 year ago 3 ☐ 2 years ago 4 ☐ 3 or more years ago 5 ☐ Never
MEN ★33. About how long has it been since you had a rectal or prostate exam?	1 ☐ Less than 1 year ago 2 ☐ 1 year ago 3 ☐ 2 years ago 4 ☐ 3 or more years ago 5 ☐ Never
★34. How many times in the last year did you witness or become involved in a violent fight or attack where there was a good chance of a serious injury to someone?	1 ☐ 4 or more times 2 ☐ 2 or 3 times 3 ☐ 1 time or never 4 ☐ Not sure
★35. Considering your age, how would you describe your overall physical health?	1 ☐ Excellent 2 ☐ Good 3 ☐ Fair 4 ☐ Poor
★36. In an average week, how many times do you engage in physical activity (exercise or work which lasts at least 20 minutes without stopping and which is hard enough to make you breathe heavier and your heart beat faster)?	1 ☐ Less than 1 time per week 2 ☐ 1 or 2 times per week 3 ☐ At least 3 times per week
★37. If you ride a motorcycle or all-terrain vehicle (ATV) what percent of the time do you wear a helmet?	1 ☐ 75% to 100% 2 ☐ 25% to 74% 3 ☐ Less than 25% 4 ☐ Does not apply to me

continued

★38. Do you eat some food every day that is high in fiber, such as whole grain bread, cereal, fresh fruits or vegetables?	1 ☐ Yes 2 ☐ No
★39. Do you eat foods every day that are high in cholesterol or fat, such as fatty meat, cheese, fried foods, or eggs?	1 ☐ Yes 2 ☐ No
★40. In general, how satisfied are you with your life?	1 ☐ Mostly satisfied 2 ☐ Partly satisfied 3 ☐ Not satisfied
★41. Have you suffered a personal loss or misfortune in the past year that had a serious impact on your life? (For example, a job loss, disability, separation, jail term, or the death of someone close to you.)	1 ☐ Yes, 1 serious loss or misfortune 2 ☐ Yes, 2 or more 3 ☐ No
★42a. Race	1 ☐ Aleutian, Alaska native, Eskimo or American Indian 2 ☐ Asian 3 ☐ Black 4 ☐ Pacific Islander 5 ☐ White 6 ☐ Other 7 ☐ Don't know
★42b. Are you of Hispanic origin such as Mexican-American, Puerto Rican, or Cuban?	1 ☐ Yes 2 ☐ No
★43. What is the highest grade you completed in school?	1 ☐ Grade school or less 2 ☐ Some high school 3 ☐ High school graduate 4 ☐ Some college 5 ☐ College graduate 6 ☐ Post graduate or professional degree
★44. What is your job occupation? (Check only one)	1 ☐ Health professional 2 ☐ Manager, educator, professional 3 ☐ Technical, sales or administrative support 4 ☐ Operator, fabricator, laborer 5 ☐ Student 6 ☐ Retired 7 ☐ Homemaker 8 ☐ Service 9 ☐ Skilled crafts 10 ☐ Unemployed 11 ☐ Other
★45. In what industry do you work (or did you) last work? (Check only one)	1 ☐ Electric, gas, sanitation 2 ☐ Transportation, communication 3 ☐ Agriculture, forestry, fishing 4 ☐ Wholesale or retail trade 5 ☐ Financial and service industries 6 ☐ Mining 7 ☐ Government 8 ☐ Manufacturing 9 ☐ Construction 10 ☐ Other

CHAPTER THREE

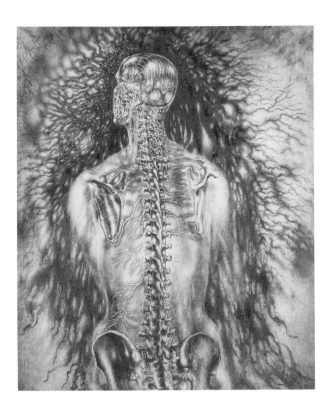

Stress
and Health

A n understanding of the connection between mind and
body is crucial to an understanding of health. Research
is increasingly finding that our thoughts, attitudes, feelings, and
philosophies play a major role in keeping us well, or producing
illness. Scientists are just beginning to unravel the links between
mind and body. They are delving deeper and deeper into how
thoughts in the mind affect the body through the autonomic
nervous system, the adrenal glands, and the immune system.
For years there have been a few researchers who thought that
happiness and depression affected health, but now that the roles
of specific physiological mechanisms are being brought to light,

*Scientists are learning more and more about the mysteries of the mind-
body connection. Pavel Tchelitchew. Anatomical Painting. c. 1945. Oil on
canvas, 56" × 46". Collection, The Whitney Museum of American Art.
Gift of Lincoln Kirstein.*

physicians are coming to realize that this research is an important new area in medicine.

The field of mind-body medicine has grown out of studies in psychosomatic medicine which found that people with certain personalities were more likely to get certain illnesses. For example, studies showed that businessmen under pressure were more likely to get ulcers than the average person. Early on, in the 1930s, the field of mind-body medicine focused on stress, specifically on how stress causes illness. Over the years, it was found that prolonged emotional stress was a risk factor for a wide variety of diseases—in particular, high blood pressure and heart disease. As a result of all this research, stress is presently regarded as one of the five main risk factors targeted for health education by the Department of Health, Education, and Welfare. Recently, there has been an exciting shift in research emphasis toward studying the factors that relieve stress and protect against stress-induced illness. Extensive work has been done on relaxation and meditation. Currently much study is being done on attitudes and outlooks that affect health. From this research will come programs to teach people how to cope with stress, and prevent or cure illness using mind-body tools.

Defining Stress

The term *stress* is widely used by psychologists, doctors, and lay people. Loosely defined, a stress situation can be any occurrence or event that causes a person to become anxious or upset, consciously or unconsciously, or any event that requires sufficient change in a person's routines so that they have to make adjustments. A number of more precise definitions have been used in specific contexts for research purposes, but a broad medical definition is useful for health promotion considerations.

In terms of health research, one of the most common definitions of a stress situation is one "in which the demands on individuals tax or exceed their adaptive capabilities."[1] From a psychological standpoint, a situation or event is considered stressful if a person perceives it as creating harm, loss, threat, or challenge. Stress researcher Milton Kaplan has a fascinating psychosocial definition of stress. He suggests that a characteristic common to most stressful situations is "the inability of the individual to obtain meaningful information that his actions are leading to desired consequences";[2] that is, the sense that one's actions will achieve one's desires or goals. This definition applies to situations of conflicting or ambiguous roles, blocked hopes or desires, or cultural dissonance.

In the broadest sense, harmful stress is anything in people's social-emotional world that causes them to feel distress or unease. People describe such situations as "difficulties," "hardships," or "problems," and they describe themselves, as a result, as being "anxious," "upset," "threatened," or "unsatisfied." Thus, stress not only relates to outside events, but more importantly to the way in which a person *perceives* those events. While most people would view the death of a loved person as a stressful event, only some people would view writing a report as very stressful. What is important is a person's perception of the events and of his or her ability to deal with them. According to this definition, even "positive" events can be anxiety-producing. For example, holidays and vacations are sometimes unsatisfying or upsetting. There are two reasons why such events can be stressful. First, the situation may require adaptation or change from normal routines. Secondly, for some reason people may have a feeling or expectation that they will have difficulty handling a particular situation.

Crucial to the new concept of stress is the idea that stress in itself is not harmful. What is harmful is the individual's feeling or perception that he or she cannot handle the situation. Psychologist David Ornstein and physician David Sobel have elucidated this point of view succinctly in their book, *The Healing Brain*: "The way we perceive and appraise the event, the availability and use of resources to cope with the challenge, have more to do with the outcome than the raw event itself. Stress, and its negative impact on health, derive from a mismatch between perceived environmental demands and perceived resources to adapt."[3] In other words, what one person might perceive as a fulfilling challenge, another might view as an overwhelming demand. Thus a given situation might be health-producing for one person, but unhealthy for another person.

Not stress itself, but the *perception* of stress, is what is unhealthy. The value of this distinction lies in the fact that we cannot eliminate all stress from our lives, but we can change the

Signs of Stress

tension, anxiety
agitation, restlessness, inability to relax
constant worrying
sense of time pressure
inability to concentrate
apathy, sadness
feelings of insecurity or worthlessness
feelings of powerlessness or inability to cope
frequent irritability, argumentativeness, and/or anger
defensiveness
arrogance, grandiosity
procrastination, chronic lateness
chronic fatigue
lack of sexual interest
sexual promiscuity
poor appearance
legal problems
crying spells
nervous indigestion
compulsive eating
compulsive smoking
headaches
neck and shoulder pain
use of tranquilizers or recreational drugs to relax
frequent illnesses or accidents

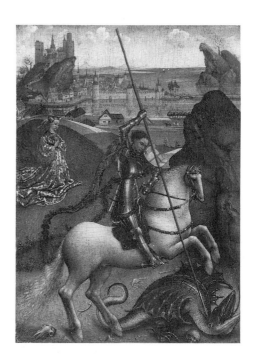

The fight or flight reaction prepares the body for emergencies, but wears the body down if sustained too long. Rogier van der Weyden. St. George and the Dragon. *1432. National Gallery of Art, Washington. Ailsa Mellon Bruce Fund.*

way we perceive the world. Response to stress is a normal human reaction that has an important survival aspect in evolutionary terms because it primes people for action when necessary. Early use of this concept stemmed from Walter Cannon's studies on the physiology of the *fight-or-flight-reaction* in the 1930s. Cannon's research dealt primarily with bodily reactions to emergency situations. When individuals encounter a situation that they *perceive* as dangerous, a series of predictable changes takes place within the body. Anxious thoughts excite nerve cells in the brain, which in turn send impulses out through the *autonomic nervous system.* Autonomic nerves go to virtually every part of the body—the digestive system, the heart and blood vessels, the uterus, and most importantly, to the adrenal glands.

How Stress Causes Illness

To understand the mechanism by which stress can cause illness, it is necessary to understand how stress affects the physiology of the body through the autonomic nervous system. This basic information makes it easier to grasp how complex social and psychological situations can have physical, as well as mental, effects. The autonomic nervous system has two parts: one part, called the *sympathetic*, is stimulated during stress or fight-or-flight; the other part, called the *parasympathetic*, is stimulated during relaxed, calm periods.

All of us have experienced sympathetic arousal, both acute and chronic. For example, in an acute situation, a fight-or-flight sensation is triggered when we feel like we're about to fall off a ladder or get into a car accident. Such rapid sympathetic arousal enables people to face or escape a danger, to mobilize themselves physically and mentally in a situation which requires them to act quickly. Throwing a spear at a lion during a hunt or running from a charging elephant are archetypal images of fight-or-flight. Modern life has replaced charging elephants and lions

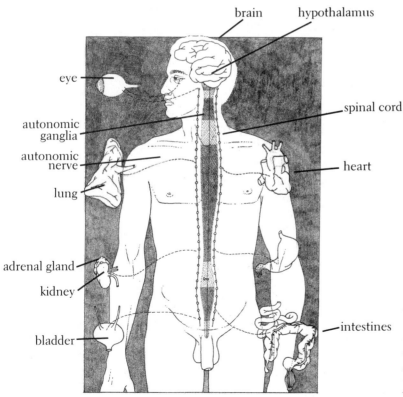

Sympathetic and parasympathetic nerves from the autonomic nervous system innervate all the organs of the body and affect blood flow, hormonal balance, heartbeat, breathing, and digestion. They are the basic hardware of the mind-body connection.

with job and family crises. Often such problems produce gnawing worries and "dis-ease" that are the symptoms of chronic sympathetic arousal. Long-standing sympathetic arousal not only keeps the body constantly "at the ready," it causes physiological changes that can lead to disease. Parasympathetic arousal, on the other hand, results from quiet, pleasurable activities like lying in the sun or listening to soft music. It results in warm, tranquil, relaxed feelings that cause physiological changes that promote health and prevent illness.

The arousal of either the sympathetic or the parasympathetic part of the autonomic nervous system affects the body's adrenal glands, which in turn produce hormones that sustain the initial reaction. During the fight-or-flight response, the core of the adrenals produce *adrenalin (epinephrine)*, which keeps a person galvanized for action. During relaxation, the outer portion of the adrenals produces *steroids*, which aid in keeping the body balanced in a healthy, smoothly functioning state.

In the last 30 years, doctors have learned a lot about how stress wears the body down. This concept comes directly from physiologist Hans Selye's research of the 1930s which showed that coping or dealing with stress can "cost" the body a great amount of energy and result in generalized physiological wear. If a person can cope successfully, the threatening situation is ended, and a long-term stress reaction does not take place, but when a person can't cope, long-term fatigue effects occur. The changes are greatest and most dangerous in health terms when stress is intense and long-lasting, and/or an individual's coping responses don't work or are perceived as not working.

A specific severe type of stress-illness relationship results in situations of "learned helplessness." People, and even animals, who believe that their actions have no effect on the outcome of a situation, that they have no control over their world, are more prone to illness. Animal studies have demonstrated the harm caused by learned helplessness. In these studies, two groups of mice were subjected to mild random electric shocks. Of the two groups, one was able to stop the shock by pressing on a lever, while mice in the second group received the same shocks, but had no means of controlling them. Researchers found that tumors introduced into the mice grew much more rapidly and were less likely to be rejected by the mice who were not able to control the shocks. Researchers have found that a sense of control, a feeling of being able to change a situation, reduces the negative effects of stress. Thus the effects of stress are more deleterious when stress is believed to be unpredictable or uncontrollable.

Studies also show that the most harmful types of stress are those that are prolonged, as well as uncontrollable. In such situations, people are particularly likely to eventually adopt patterns of learned helplessness; that is, they become passive and no longer make attempts to handle or relieve the stress they are under. At its most extreme, learned helplessness produces fear, depression, and disease. The concept of learned helplessness has even been used as a theoretical model to explain "taboo death" in which people die after hearing a powerful curse has been put on them. Such deaths have been documented in Australia and elsewhere. It has also been speculated that learned helplessness may be a factor in explaining why the death rate among matched groups is higher for people of low income.

Based on their studies of human and animal responses to stress, researchers have worked out a complex model of the physiological changes that ultimately cause illness. Stress plays an important role in infectious disease. Doctors have come to realize that in addition to exposure to a given germ, the spread

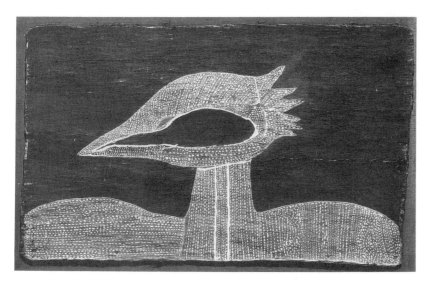

A powerful example of the mind-body connection involves taboo deaths *in which people die when a hex or spell is put on them. Primitive. n.d. Northern Australian Bark Painting. The Metropolitan Museum of Art, Michael C. Rockefeller Collection of Primitive Art. Bequest of Nelson A. Rockefeller, 1979.*

of infectious illness also depends on the *susceptibility* of the *host*. Stress, along with other factors such as diet, exercise, and genetics, determines how well a person's immune system will function in fighting a particular infection.

Researchers are beginning to investigate the specific pathways by which stress affects immunity. A variety of hormones and neurotransmitters that are influenced by a person's emotions and are under the brain's control have an impact on the immune system. The hypothalamus in the brain appears to participate directly in the regulation of antibody production. *Lymphocytes,* the special white blood cells that make antibodies, have receptor sites for many hormones, including estrogen, cortisol, and epinephrine. Other substances found in the blood, such as endorphins and prostaglandins, which are also affected by the emotions, can enhance or depress the immune system in complex ways. The stress hormones, triggered by sympathetic arousal, lower the white blood cells' ability to recognize germs and produce antibodies against them.

Theories on stress and the immune system have been borne out by studies of both humans and animals. These studies have shown that the immune changes produced by stress have medical significance. In the learned helplessness study in which mice were exposed to controllable or uncontrollable random shocks, the animals who could control the shock not only were better able to reject surgically implanted tumors, they had better immune function than the other group. Even more remarkably, the animals who could control the shock had higher immune function and were better able to reject tumors than rats who were subjected to no shock at all. In human studies, stress, bereavement, surgery, and sleep deprivation have all been shown to be associated with a decrease in immune response and an increase in the incidence of infectious disease. A viral study done on West Point cadets showed that those who were under stress were more likely to exhibit symptoms of a viral infection to which they had all been exposed. Immunologist Stephen Locke of Harvard found that students who were good at coping had higher immune functions than students who had difficulty coping. Two other studies showed that students who watched films about humor or altruism had better short-range immune functions than control groups. Studies such as these are the scientific basis for using relaxation and visualization to help cancer patients improve their immune functions.

The stress model is especially well documented for heart disease. When people perceive themselves as under stress, their sympathetic nervous system causes their heart rate and blood pressure to rise, which in turn causes the heart muscle itself to need more oxygen, because it is working harder. Since sympathetic nervous system arousal is designed to mobilize great amounts of energy, it profoundly affects the body's metabolism. Metabolic changes include the release of large amounts of glucose from the liver for energy, a decrease in water excretion from the kidney which raises blood pressure, and the release of free fatty acids into the bloodstream from adipose or fatty tissue. The result is that the blood, laden with fat molecules, is pushed through the arteries under high pressure, eventually producing tears and abrasions in the artery walls. Fatty acids become lodged in these tears. If stress is frequent or long-lasting, arteries can become sufficiently blocked to cause heart attacks and strokes. These effects are added to or minimized depending upon life-style factors such as smoking, exercise, dietary cholesterol, and inherited inability to handle cholesterol.

Animal studies show direct and unmistakable links between heart disease and stress in social situations. In one experiment, monkeys who were put into a variety of stressful situations became ill with high blood pressure, heart disease, and kidney failure. The stresses included electroshock, being confronted with a more aggressive animal, and being separated from a mate. In the Philadelphia Zoo, it was observed that animals who were put into assigned family groups rather than groups that were self-selected developed heart disease 10 times as often. Mice who were put into living situations that constantly required interaction with strangers developed high blood pressure, atherosclerosis, and kidney failure at higher rates. Other studies found that monkeys under stress had a higher incidence of atherosclerosis, while dogs under stress developed dangerous heart rhythms more often than a control group that was not stressed.

Human studies have also demonstrated a link between social stress and heart disease. The greatest amount of evidence has come from the studies of cardiologists Ray Rosenman and Meyer Friedman. Their Western Collaborative Group Study

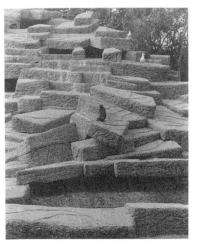

When a random collection of monkeys were grouped without respect to sex or social organization, a quarter of them died of stress-related diseases. Monkey Island. *Photo by Michael Samuels.*

Type A Characteristics

aggressive and hostile
competitive
compulsion to win at all costs
inclined to dominate in
    situations
irritable and easily aroused
often angry or hostile
angrily defends fixed opinions
often challenges others
makes angry generalizations
    about others
belligerent look
clenched jaw
angry frown
clenched fists
frequent use of obscenities

*Activities Recommended to
Counteract Type A Behavior*

walk and eat more slowly
listen to music for 15 minutes
    or more at a time
watch the sunset
look at trees
don't wear a watch
drive in the slow lane
listen to other people without
    interrupting them
make a point to smile at people
look for beauty

(1975) showed that a certain type of behavior, which they termed "Type A," was associated with an increased risk of coronary artery disease. Type A people are usually hostile, hard-driving, and have a tremendous sense of time urgency. Whereas initially, great importance was attached to time urgency, more recent research has identified hostility and anger as the most important aspects of Type A risk. Studies have shown that extreme Type A's have high blood levels of lipids and circulating stress hormones. Although several major studies have verified Rosenman and Friedman's results, other major studies have not. The relationship between the Type A personality and heart disease continues to be an important concept but needs further investigation.

Cardiologist Robert Elliot, author of the book *Is It Worth Dying For?*, has a similar but different theory about stress and heart disease. He believes that some people are "hot reactors"; that is, they perceive their environment as stressful and react to it with a rise in blood pressure (see chart). Elliot believes that stress is the major factor in heart disease and he has developed a special training program to help hot reactors to alter their perspective.

Psychologist James Lynch believes that stress causes heart disease through social factors such as loneliness, lack of human

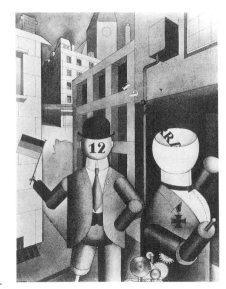

Loneliness and lack of human contact is a contributing factor in heart disease. George Grosz. Republican Automatons. 1920. Watercolor, 23⅝″ × 18⅝″. Collection, The Museum of Modern Art, New York. Advisory Committee Fund.

contact, and lack of love. The old expression "died of a broken heart" is proving to be more than folklore. Numerous studies done by Lynch show heart disease—including heart attacks, high blood pressure, and stroke—to be more common among single and divorced people than among those who are married. Lynch talks of the healing power of human contact and urges people to avoid loneliness and isolation. This concept is significant enough to have warranted an entire issue in *Circulation*, the journal of the American Heart Association.

The Value of Support

One of the greatest contributions to stress research was made by the Seattle psychiatrists Thomas Holmes and Richard Rahe. They set up a scale that ranked a variety of life events in terms of the degree of stress they produced, and the amount of coping they required. Holmes and Rahe asked a broad cross-section of people, including psychologists, teachers, and doctors, to rate many common events such as getting married, getting divorced, having a baby, changing jobs, moving, etc., in terms of stress. Holmes and Rahe used marriage as a reference point and assigned it an arbitrary value of 50 on a scale of 1 (low stress) to 100 (very stressful). They discovered a remarkable uniformity among the responses. In a subsequent survey in which people were asked about life events they found that people who had a high number of points due to recent life experiences had five times as great a chance of developing health problems. The study showed that the onset of illness is often correlated with a number of stressful life changes.

In the last few years, a shift has taken place in the study of stressful events and illness. Researchers realized that the complex nature of the subject warranted more than a simple response to the problem of "stress." This is not surprising, as common sense tells us that getting married or changing jobs does not affect everyone in the same way. Researchers have become aware of the fact that certain variables moderate a person's ability to deal with stress. These variables or moderators are referred to as *resistance resources* because they protect people against stress. The list of resistance resources that have been identified and studied is growing, but the main factors are support and hardiness.

Following the work of Holmes and Rahe, a number of landmark studies in stress research dealt with the effect that support has on people under stress. *Support* is a relatively new term in the health-care field and can be broadly defined as anything that makes a person feel good, function more effectively, and/or feel more optimistic. Support leads people to have a sense of being loved, nourished, and satisfied; it raises their self-esteem and makes them feel part of something larger than themselves. Support can come from close relationships with family and friends,

Stress Scale

LIFE EVENT	POINTS	LIFE EVENT	POINTS
___ Death of spouse	100	___ Son or daughter leaving home	29
___ Divorce	73	___ Trouble with in-laws	29
___ Marital separation	65	___ Outstanding personal achievement	28
___ Jail term	63	___ Spouse begins or stops work	26
___ Death of close family member	63	___ Starting or finishing school	26
___ Personal injury or illness	53	___ Change in living conditions	25
___ Marriage	50	___ Revision of personal habits	24
___ Fired at work	47	___ Trouble with boss	23
___ Marital reconciliation	45	___ Change in work hours, conditions	20
___ Retirement	45	___ Change in residence	20
___ Change in family member's health	44	___ Change in schools	20
___ Pregnancy	40	___ Change in recreational habits	19
___ Sex difficulties	39	___ Change in church activities	19
___ Addition to family	39	___ Change in social activities	18
___ Business readjustment	39	___ Mortgage or loan for lesser purchase	
___ Change in financial state	38	(car, TV, etc.)	17
___ Death of close friend	37	___ Change in sleeping habits	16
___ Change to different line of work	36	___ Change in number of family gatherings	15
___ Change in number of marital arguments	35	___ Change in eating habits	15
___ Mortgage or loan for major purchase		___ Vacation	13
(home, etc.)	31	___ Christmas season	12
___ Foreclosure of mortgage or loan	30	___ Minor violations of the law	11
___ Change in work responsibilities	29	Total score ___	

Reprinted from Thomas H. Holmes and Richard R. Rahe, "The Social Readjustment Rating Scale," Journal of Psychosomatic Research, *vol. 11.*

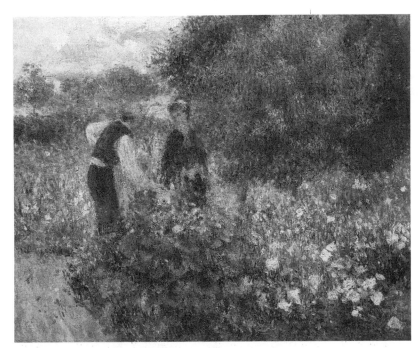

Social support gives people a sense of being loved, nurtured, and satisfied. Auguste Renoir. Picking Flowers. 1875. National Gallery of Art, Washington. Ailsa Mellon Bruce Collection.

from jobs or hobbies that give people positive feedback, and from systems of belief that give meaning to life.

One theoretical model of stress, designed by psychologist Irwin Sarason, holds that stressful situations result in, or involve, a "call to action." This call to action causes people to "appraise the situation" at hand in terms of their ability to successfully deal with it, based on their past life events and present social support. Depending on how people evaluate themselves and a given situation, they will have either self-preoccupying thoughts or task-oriented thoughts; that is, they will become anxious and worry, or they will make constructive plans for the future. Studies have shown that people are not as likely to become sick in response to many life changes or major life events if they have strong support systems. Support tends to counteract stress and protect people from the negative effects of stress. Support, in other words, is the functional opposite of stress. The classic study on the effect of support in counteracting stress was

Evaluating Support

- Do you confide in someone each day, once a week, less than once a week, never?
- Do you feel secure in your environment each day, once a week, less than once a week, never?
- Do you feel that you have some control over your environment each day, once a week, less than once a week, never?
- Do you feel that people approve of you each day, once a week, less than once a week, never?
- Does your support come from family, friends, groups, and/or community?
- Do you feel that you have enough money, usually, sometimes, never?
- Do you have a strong set of personal beliefs, a strong religious affiliation?

Why Social Support Increases Health

- gratifies emotional needs for security, affection, trust, intimacy, nurturing, a sense of belonging
- helps in appraising and defining reality
- makes people aware of shared norms of feeling and behavior
- increases group solidarity
- increases self-esteem through social approval

done by psychologist Katherine Nuckolls who queried several hundred pregnant women about intimacy, happiness, religion, economic support, and friendship patterns. Nuckolls found that women who had high life-change scores on the Holmes-Rahe Scale combined with strong support had one-third fewer complications with pregnancy and delivery than did a group who had high life-change scores but lacked strong support.

Since the Nuckolls study there have been many others confirming the fact that support helps to counteract disease patterns caused by stress. The Alameda County Study by Berkman and Breslow, which was very broad in scope, showed that people with social relationships involving marriage, contacts with close friends and relatives, or associations with church or nonchurch groups, had lower mortality rates than people who lacked these social connections. Marriage and friendship were stronger predictors than group associations, and the degree of intimacy was more important than the type of relationship involved. In the study, the most isolated people had twice the mortality of the people with the most intimate social relationships.

Other studies have shown that for all illnesses, divorced men and women have a higher death rate than those who are married, and single or widowed men have a higher death rate than those who are married. Becoming a widower is a particularly profound risk factor: men over 55 have a death rate 40% above the average during the first six months after their spouse's death. Among women the death rate is higher for single women than married women but not higher for widows. Finally, there have been several studies exploring the relationship between community cohesiveness and illness. In the closely knit Italian-American community of Roseto, Pennsylvania, the heart attack rate was found to be much lower than it was among a matched group of Italian Americans who moved to less cohesive communities, despite the fact that all the people in the study had a high-fat diet.

Several theories have been proposed to explain why support is so valuable in terms of health. A number of these focus on the ability of an individual to control or cope with a situation. Interactions within close relationships help people to define their roles and make situations less ambiguous. Strong social networks impart a sense of coherence and belongingness, increasing peo-

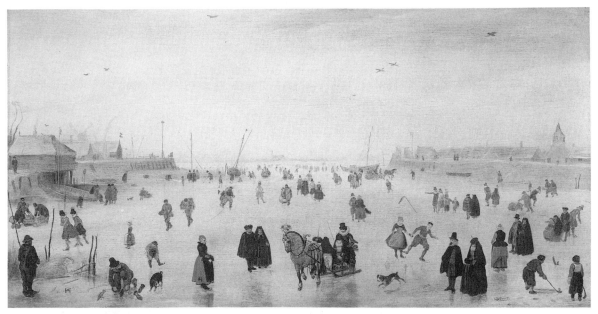

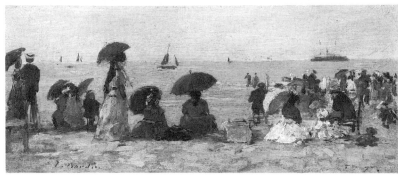

Studies show that community cohesiveness leads to lower rates of illness. Hendrick Avercamp. A Scene on the Ice. c. 1625. National Gallery of Art, Washington. Ailsa Mellon Bruce Fund.

Eugene Boudin. The Beach. Dated (18)77. National Gallery of Art, Washington. Ailsa Mellon Bruce Collection.

ple's confidence in the fact that their environment is predictable and there is a probability that things will work out (see chart).

Self-Efficacy

More recently, medical researchers have begun to study how different personality types deal with stress. We've all known people who seem to deal with certain stressful situations more easily than other people do. Scientists now think that the ability to cope may be the most important factor in dealing with stress.

Initially, this new line of research came from behavioral psychologists, not physicians. Psychologist Richard Lazarus put together a model dealing with the interactions between coping, stress, and illness. Lazarus theorizes that when people experience a life event, they appraise the situation in order to see if they need to act on it, and if they need to, they then assess whether or not they have the resources to deal with it. Lazarus believes that people naturally evaluate the balance between the demand and their own resources, and based on this, perceive the event either as a challenge that may lead to mastery and gain, or as a threat that may lead to harm or loss. If people see a situation as threatening, they feel stress. This stress involves both an emotional state and the release of stress hormones. If people are able to act in a constructive, coping manner, Lazarus believes they can slow and even reverse the effects of stress.

Stanford psychologist Albert Bandura did a study that lent the first objective support to Lazarus' theory. Bandura's study dealt with a group of women who were afraid of spiders. He assigned them a set of tasks involving increasing contact with spiders, and then questioned them as to how they assessed their ability to do the tasks. Like Lazarus, Bandura believes that people's perceptions that they cannot cope with a situation makes the event stressful. He called the women's perceived ability to cope with a situation *self-efficacy*. Bandura found that the greater the women's perceived self-efficacy, the less stress they felt with tasks, and the lower their levels of stress hormones. Conversely, the less women thought they would be able to deal with the tasks, the more stress they felt, and the higher their levels of stress hormones. These results were made even more significant by the next phase of the experiment. Bandura trained the women to increase their knowledge and control of the situation by teaching them about spiders and their handling. After the training, the women felt greater self-efficacy and, indeed, were able to undertake the same tasks without feeling stress or showing a rise in stress hormones. The implications of this study are far-reaching. The results show that by increasing a person's sense of self-efficacy and ability to cope, stress is reduced, stress physiology is changed, and, by extrapolation, one can speculate that stress-related diseases could also be reduced.

Hardiness

The next step in the research was to actually see if perceived coping skills would lead to a lower incidence of illness in the face of the same stressful situation. Social psychologist Suzanne Kobasa assessed this by studying the personality characteristics of people who seem to be resistant to the harmful effects of stress. Kobasa studied a large group of executives at a single company, during a time of great change and upheaval. She found that among the executives who showed the highest stress on the Holmes-Rahe scale, about half became ill and half remained healthy. These people differed in terms of personality, but were matched in every other way—income, background, age, job status, etc. Kobasa named the personality type of the healthy group *hardiness*. She divided hardiness into three components: *control*, *commitment*, and *challenge*. The healthy group, who exhibited high control, "believe and act as if they can influence the events taking place around them through what they imagine, say, and do."[4] In contrast, the unhealthy group tended to feel powerless, nihilistic, and poorly motivated. The healthy group were also

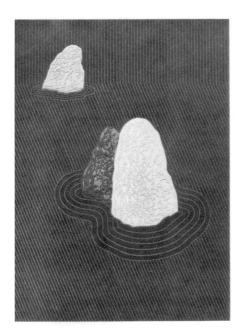

People who have a sense of control over their own lives and surroundings tend to be healthier. Arthur Okamura. Rock Garden. *Silkscreen print, 19″ × 26″. Collection, Michael and Nancy Samuels.*

committed; that is, they were actively involved in their life, and were curious and interested in people and things around them. Their commitment gave them a sense of purpose and an involvement with other people. Most of all, they were committed to themselves, in that they recognized their own values and goals, and their capacity to achieve them. The less healthy group, by comparison, generally felt alienated and found their environment boring and meaningless. Finally, the hardy executives viewed change as a challenge rather than a threat. They believed that they had the ability to cope with whatever alterations were necessitated. They were flexible and responded to the unexpected with interest. The hardy group approached stressful tasks with a sense of purpose, a belief in their own capacities and importance, and a vigorous posture. By contrast, the other group tended to see themselves as passive victims of threatening situations, with little ability to change the situation.

In other studies, Kobasa compared the effects of hardiness, exercise, and social support on people in stressful situations. She found that illness rates dropped with each additional resistance resource a person had, but her studies showed hardiness was a more important resource than exercise or social support. People who had all three factors working for them experienced only 10% of the illness reported by a group who had none of the resources. Kobasa's work confirms the conclusions of other studies on learned helplessness vs. control, loneliness vs. human contact, and the ability to cope vs. being overwhelmed. Without a question, Kobasa's findings are one of the keys to the new mind-body medicine.

Coherence

Another major theorist of mind-body medicine is Israeli medical sociologist Aaron Antonovsky. Like Kobasa, Antonovsky has done studies on personality aspects that help to keep people healthy. Working independently, Antonovsky came up with a set of coping variables very similar to those of Kobasa, but unlike her, he sees the coping qualities not as a personality type, but rather as a matter of philosophy or world outlook. Antonovsky calls the global orientation or world outlook that produces health a *sense of coherence*. He divides coherence into three parts: *comprehensibility*, *manageability*, and *meaningfulness*. Comprehensibility refers to the extent to which people see the world as making sense, as being structured, orderly, and having a predictable future. This does not mean that situations and events are either good or bad, merely that they are understandable and appear somewhat orderly. The opposite of high comprehensibility is a view of the world as being chaotic, random, and unpredictable. The second component, manageability, refers to the extent to which people feel they can meet the demands life puts upon them, or the extent to which they feel that they can cope with situations, either through their own resources or with the help of friends, loved ones, social agencies, or religious organizations. Again, this component in no way negates the idea that "bad" things happen to people. A sense of manageability protects people from feeling helpless, victimized, or treated unfairly. Meaningfulness is an emotional component that measures how much people care about and are involved with situations that confront them. A situation may range from a challenge that is very important to a person, to a burden that he or she would rather avoid.

Antonovsky believes that when people have a strong sense of coherence, they see life events as opportunities rather than threats, thereby minimizing stress and improving health. In addition, Antonovsky believes that people with a high degree of coherence are more likely to follow health-promoting activities such as exercising regularly and eating a nutritious diet, rather than harmful ones, because the meaningful nature of their lives gives them a reason to be healthy, and their coping skills give them the positive feeling that their efforts will be successful. Looked at from this perspective, health becomes a by-product of a meaningful, manageable life, rather than a goal in itself.

Feeling fulfilled is another factor that helps to counteract stress because it gives meaning to people's lives. In research over the last few years, fulfillment and life stages have become pertinent to health research. Insight, flexibility of character, and personal growth have been shown to be important factors in reducing stress, and therefore in preventing disease. Changes in self-concept influence people's perception of reality and their perception of what is stressful in their lives (see p. 71).

Coherence Factors

COMPREHENSIBILITY: the world appears orderly, the future seems predictable.

MANAGEABILITY: a feeling that one can cope.

MEANINGFULNESS: a sense of emotional involvement in one's experiences.

Coping with Stress

Ways to Reduce Life Stress

1. Identify major stressors: e.g., financial problems, marital problems, death in family, too many deadlines, overbooked schedule, lack of support.
2. Begin by changing the stresses that are easiest to deal with.
3. Set short- and long-term goals.
4. Do something to lower stress and/or feel good each day.
5. Get outside help with problems that are difficult to deal with by yourself.

As everyone knows, stress seems to be an inevitable part of modern life. There is stress in work, family life, even in hobbies and leisure activities. For people in midadulthood, there is stress in taking care of basic needs, raising children, paying for education, achieving job satisfaction, dealing with their mates, coping with bodily changes, helping elderly parents, and in evaluating their own pasts and futures.

There are two basic ways of dealing with stress: first, preventing or reducing stress itself, and second, improving one's ability to cope with stress. The first approach, stress prevention, basically involves changing the stressful setting and using specific problem-solving strategies. The second category includes increasing support and improving coping skills through activities such as psychotherapy, self-help groups, meditation, relaxation, imagery, and religion. All of these activities can help to affect philosophy, change personality, and increase fulfillment.

In the last 20 years researchers in the field of behavioral medicine have studied the physiology of various techniques for coping with stress. These techniques all serve to reverse the fight-or-flight response and stimulate the parasympathetic system, which opposes sympathetic arousal. The initial research was done by Dr. Herbert Benson of Harvard, who termed the opposite of the fight-or-flight response the *relaxation response*. Although relaxation seems like a deceptively simple process, the physiology of the relaxation response has subtle healing effects that are ultimately as powerful as the mobilization effects of the fight-or-flight response. These healing effects are both *physiological* and *psychological*. Although many of Benson's studies did not involve control groups, his basic findings revealed that the immediate physiological effects of the relaxation response involve a slower heart rate, a drop in the amount of blood pumped through the heart, lower blood pressure, slower breathing, a drop in oxygen consumption, a change in brain waves, and altered adrenal hormone levels. Psychologically, relaxation reduces fear and anxiety and replaces them with a sense of calmness and well-being. Relaxation also lessens a person's response to stressful stimuli. Because of the demonstrated changes

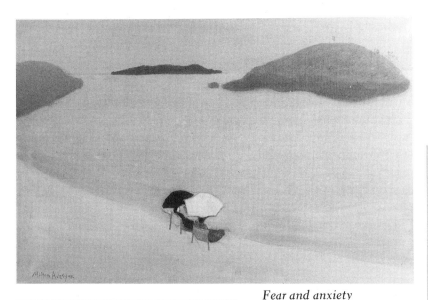

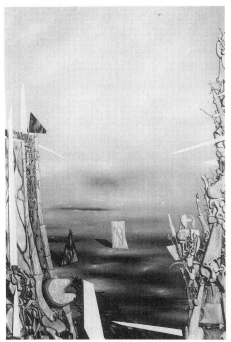

Fear and anxiety create one set of physiological responses; relaxation and a sense of security create the opposite effect. Above: Milton Avery. Sea Gazers. 1956. Oil on canvas. 30″ × 44″. Collection, The Whitney Museum of American Art. Lawrence H. Bloedel bequest. 77.1.3. Left: Yves Tanguy. Fear. 1949. Oil on canvas. 60″ × 40″. Collection, The Whitney Museum of American Art. Purchase. 49.21.

Activities That Help to Lower Stress

1. Discuss your concerns with friends.
2. Do something nice for yourself each day.
3. Exercise at least 15–30 minutes three to five times a week.
4. Get enough rest—go to bed early, or catnap during the afternoon or commute time.
5. Meditate 15–20 minutes a day.
6. Practice relaxation or imagery exercises 15–20 minutes a day.
7. Engage in hobbies or relaxing activities such as walking, gardening, or listening to music.
8. Change your pace and/or your routines.
9. Get outside help when the stress level is too great.

associated with the relaxation response, relaxation has become the most widely used technique for stress reduction.

Relaxation

Relaxation is characterized by turning inward—by concentrating on one's own body and mind, rather than on external events. Inherent in the relaxed state is a certain feeling of detachment; that is, a lack of concern for how things are going or how one is doing. Dr. Wolfgang Luthe, one of the originators of *autogenic training*, a German psychotherapeutic technique, has described the relaxed state as, "a casual, relaxed attitude involving minimal or no goal-directed voluntaristic efforts in the sense of energetic striving, and apprehensive tension-producing control of functions leading to the desired result."[5] Thus people do not so much actively "do" relaxation, as they permit it to happen. They merely "let go" and let relaxation take place. The lack of striving or goal-oriented activity in relaxation has a profound relationship to stress. First, by looking inward without a goal, a person forgets or puts out of mind any stressful thoughts. By engaging in a "goal-less" activity, people paradoxically gain control, in that they free themselves from having to accomplish a goal through their activities. As we've said, a sense that one's activities aren't achieving desired results is one of the causes of stress.

Interestingly, people are often uncertain as to how to identify feelings of relaxation. Although a certain minimum amount of muscle tension is necessary for functioning, it is common for people to hold their muscles in a slightly tense state without being aware of it even when resting or sleeping. The more nervous and tense people tend to be, the more likely they are to be unaware of constant, low-level tension because they have come to accept it as normal. Most people find they are least aware of low levels of tension in the muscles around the eye, jaw, neck and shoulders, or around the pelvis and lower back.

One of the best ways to differentiate between the feelings of relaxation and muscle tension was taught by physiologist Edmund Jacobson in his method called *progressive relaxation*. Jacobson instructed people to contract a single muscle or group of muscles by making a specific movement and holding it for a short period of time. When they let go after several moments, they would experience the feeling of relaxation in that muscle

Becoming Aware of Muscle Tension

To feel muscle tension, lie in a comfortable position with your hands resting at your sides. Raise one hand slightly by bending it at the wrist; you will feel the muscles in the top of your forearm contract and tense. If you let your hand go limp, these muscles will relax and your hand will drop. With practice, you will become aware of the subtle difference in feeling between a contracted muscle and a relaxed one. If you're not sure of the feeling of tension, rest the fingers of your other hand lightly on the top of your forearm and feel the muscle contract as you raise your hand.

group. The subtle contrast between the two feelings heightened people's awareness of the relaxed sensation. By methodically going through each of the muscle groups, people learn to distinguish deep relaxation from very small amounts of tension in every part of their body.

The maximum effects of relaxation can usually be achieved with only four to eight hours of instruction, and 20 minutes of practice a day. There are almost as many methods for learning to relax as there are instructors. Other methods for learning to relax have people follow a simple set of verbal or written instructions. No one method has proved superior. In fact, all the methods have great similarities. The common aspects that seem the most important are (1) a set of clear instructions that you trust, (2) a comfortable position in which your muscles can relax, (3) a passive attitude of allowing relaxation to take place, (4) a quiet place in which you won't be disturbed, and (5) a deep, regular rate of breathing.

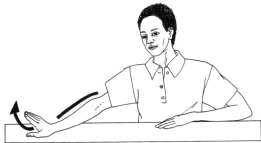

Tension in the muscles on top of the forearm can be felt when the hand is raised; relaxation is felt when the hand is dropped.

To do a relaxation exercise, find a quiet place where you can sit and not be disturbed.

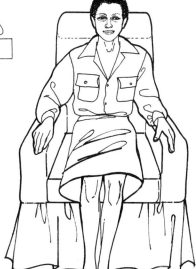

A Meditation Exercise

Find a tranquil place where you won't be disturbed. Sit in a comfortable position with your back relaxed and straight. Close your eyes. Inhale slowly and deeply, then exhale slowly and completely. As you breathe in and out, allow your body to relax. Breathe naturally and become aware of your breath as it enters your nostrils. As you breathe, keep your attention on this area of your nose and feel the sensations as each breath flows in and out. Maintain your attention on your breathing. If an outside thought, sensation, or sound enters your mind, note it for what it is without judgment ("thinking," "sound," or "sensation"), and return your attention to the breath in your nostrils. Continue to breathe naturally and keep your body relaxed. Imagine that you are like a watchman at a gate, who simply notes what passes in and out but does not follow it.

Whenever your mind wanders off and you lose track, simply return your awareness to your breathing.

Do this exercise for 15–20 minutes, once or twice a day. Initially you may want to set a timer in another room or just check your watch when you think 15–20 minutes have passed. Don't be concerned about how well you meditate. The point of the exercise is simply to keep your mind focused on breathing for the allotted time. Everyone's mind wanders. The goal is not to hold onto your thoughts but to be aware of your breathing. Some people find that it helps to say a word or a mantra such as "Om," "Lord," or "Peace" as they inhale and exhale. Alternatively, some people mentally say "one" or "in" as they inhale, and "two" or "out" as they exhale. The point is to focus; it is not so important what you focus on.

An Exercise for Relaxation

Find a tranquil place where you won't be disturbed. Sit with your legs uncrossed and your arms at your sides. Close your eyes; inhale slowly and deeply. Pause a moment. Then exhale slowly and completely. Allow your abdomen to rise and fall as you breathe. Do this several times. You now feel calm, comfortable, and more relaxed. As you relax, your breathing will become slow and even. Mentally repeat to yourself, "My feet are relaxing. They are becoming more and more relaxed. My feet feel heavy." Rest for a moment. Repeat the same suggestions for your ankles. Rest again. In the same way, relax your lower legs, then your thighs, pausing to feel the sensations of relaxation in your muscles. Relax your pelvis. Rest. Relax your abdomen. Rest. Relax the muscles of your back. Rest. Relax your chest. Rest. Relax your fingers and your hands. Rest. Relax your forearms, your upper arms, your shoulders. Rest. Relax your neck. Rest. Relax your jaw, allowing it to drop. Relax your tongue and cheeks. Relax your eyes. Rest. Relax your forehead and the top of your head. Now just rest and allow your whole body to relax.

You are in a calm, relaxed state of being. You can *deepen* this state by counting backward. Breathe in; as you exhale slowly, say to yourself, "Ten. I am feeling very relaxed. . . ." Inhale again and as you exhale, repeat mentally, "Nine. I am feeling more relaxed. . . ." Breathe. "Eight. I am feeling even more relaxed. . . ." Seven. "Deeper and more relaxed. . . ." Six. "Even more. . . ." Five (pause). Four (pause). Three (pause). Two (pause). One (pause). Zero (pause).

You are now at a deeper and more relaxed level of awareness, a level at which your body feels healthy, your mind feels peaceful and open. (It is a level at which you can experience images in your mind more clearly and vividly than ever before.) You can stay in this relaxed state as long as you like. To return to your ordinary consciousness, mentally say, "I am now going to move. When I count to three, I will raise my left hand and stretch my fingers. I will then feel relaxed, happy, and strong, ready to continue my everyday activities."

Autosuggestion, which can be taught in a short time, is one of the most popular methods for teaching relaxation today. In autosuggestion, the teacher initially recites the directions slowly. Then, after people have become familiar with the exercise, they can repeat the instructions to themselves mentally. In using any of the relaxation exercises we will give, people can have someone slowly read the directions out loud, tape record the exercise and play it back, or simply read the exercise over several times until they are familiar with the instructions. It is the concept and sequence of the exercise that is important, not memorizing it word for word.

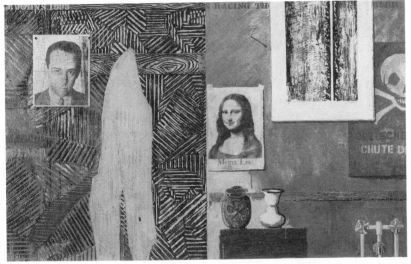

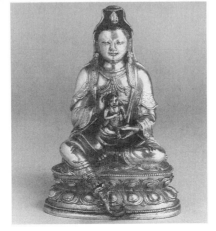

Meditation quiets the mind and produces a healing physiology within the body. Above: Jasper Johns. Racing Thoughts. 1983. *Encaustic and collage on canvas. 48″ × 75⅛″. Collection, The Whitney Museum of American Art. Purchase. 84.6. Right: Kuan Yin Bodhisattva. 17th–18th century. Asian Art Museum of San Francisco. The Avery Brundage Collection.*

People who are unfamiliar with methods like autosuggestion may feel a little awkward at first or even wonder if anything is happening. But doctors have found a measurable drop in muscle tension even the first time people practice relaxation. With more and more practice, people become aware of changes in sensation that they describe variously as feelings of heaviness, lightness, numbness, tingling, floating, or even the absence of feeling. Others describe warmth, coolness, or a radiating or pulsing sensation. The more people practice conscious relaxation, the better they become at it and the deeper the levels of relaxation they will achieve. Like learning to ski or ride a bike, relaxation becomes a habit ingrained in neuromuscular pathways.

Imagery and Healing

We believe that imagery is one of the most valuable healing techniques. Imagery involves picturing scenes or events in the mind's eye. People visualize all the time without being aware of it. They picture events from the past in their mind's eye, envi-

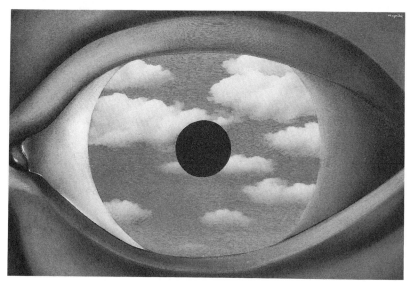

Imagery involves picturing scenes or events in the mind's eye. Rene Magritte. The False Mirror. 1928. Oil on canvas. 21¼″ × 37⅞″. Collection, The Museum of Modern Art, New York. Purchase.

sion plans and goals for the future, and conjure up solutions to problems that they are working on. Despite the fact that most people image constantly, they rarely make conscious use of this skill.

Seeing with the mind's eye is an inner process that has similarities with, and differences from, experience in the outer world. Like experiences in the outer world, seeing with the mind's eye can involve all our senses—vision, hearing, smell, touch, even body movement. Unlike experiences in the outer world, imagery feels like concentrating on a thought. Imagery's value in healing probably stems from several basic effects. First, the body responds physiologically to imagery in a manner similar to the way it responds to outer events. For example, if you imagine you are in a cozy, safe place, your heart beats slower, just as it would if you were really in such a place. Thus imagery gives us a tool that can be used to alter our physiology in a positive, healing way. Secondly, images often appear as symbols from our inner center, and can help us grow and achieve a sense of peace and fulfillment.

Imagery is widely used in counseling and psychotherapy in order to change attitudes and promote self-esteem, self-efficacy, and personal growth. The powerful effects of images have been used to good advantage in several other areas of modern medicine. The most dramatic uses involve cancer therapy. Imagery is currently being used to relieve the side effects of radiation and chemotherapy, to improve attitude and quality of life, and to strengthen the immune system and help shrink tumors. Imagery is also being used to treat high blood pressure, heart disease, asthma, and chronic pain. Imagery and relaxation are used extensively in natural childbirth techniques. Nurses are using imagery both in patient education and in therapeutic touch, a laying-on-of-hands technique.

Researchers have found that imagery works best when people are relaxed. Relaxation not only helps us clear our minds, it lowers the level of anxiety we feel about fearful and negative images. Since the same nerve and muscle pathways that are involved in a "real" action are also involved when we picture that activity in our mind, the more vividly we can picture a scene, the more our body reacts as if the events were actually taking place. Researchers have recorded changes in almost every

When to Use Relaxation

Relax your body and mind completely:

when you are worried
when you are upset, angry, or
 unhappy
when you feel stressed
when you are very tired
when you feel you are getting
 sick
when some part of your body
 hurts
just to make yourself feel good

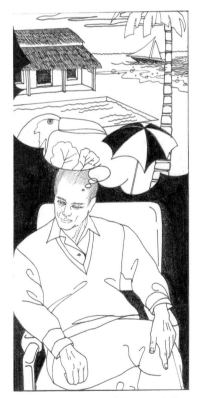

Imagining a peaceful scene helps to lower blood pressure, ease breathing, and reduce pain.

physiological system in response to imagery. When people picture running to catch a bus, their heartbeat and respiration actually rise and small electrical impulses are detectable in their running muscles. Conversely, when people picture themselves in a relaxing activity, such as lying on the beach, their breathing, heart rate, and muscle tension decrease.

Scientists are just beginning to study the effect of imagery on the body's physiology directly. Several very sophisticated experiments have documented how imagery affects the immune system. Psychologist Howard Hall had a group of people relax and imagine their white blood cells increasing in numbers and swimming like powerful sharks, attacking weak germs. The exercise lasted five minutes and the people were told to practice twice a day for a week. Blood tests before and after the imagery exercises showed that many people had a significant increase in immune system response. Researchers Wayne Smith and John Schneider of Michigan State did an even more remarkable study which demonstrated that imagery can specifically affect one type of cell. Subjects were shown slides of neutrophils, a special white blood cell, and then were directed to imagine their own neutrophils "picking up trash"; that is, eating foreign bodies in the tissues outside their bloodstream. Subjects concentrated on this image 20 minutes a day for six days, at which time a lower neutrophil count signaled that many of these cells had gone to work in tissues outside the bloodstream. Because of studies like these, doctors have become increasingly interested in ways that imagery can be applied to medical treatment.

In terms of use, we separate imagery techniques into two basic categories: receptive and programmed. *Receptive imagery*, which involves clearing the mind and letting images arise spontaneously, is one of the fundamental tools of psychiatry, providing access to inner feelings and ideas. Through receptive imagery, people can identify both the positive and the negative emotions they have about their jobs, families, or outside interests. This can help them to deal with their fears and anxieties, as well as make them more aware of their positive feelings. Currently, receptive imagery is used to help patients get in touch with their own symbols. For example, cancer therapists may ask their patients to imagine what their cancer looks like. These images are highly individualistic, and are therefore more meaningful to the patient than a generalized image. For example, one person might envision the cancer as a burning house, another as an insect eating away at the body. Psychologist Jean Achterberg has found that the pictures people draw of their tumors can help a physician predict how well a patient will do—knowledge that can be useful in choosing the type and amount of therapy that will be most effective.

Another form of receptive imagery involves meeting and talking with an inner advisor or spirit guide. Such inner figures have been used by American Indians for centuries. Psychologist Carl Jung evolved the use of inner guides in a therapy setting (see p. 78). Currently, inner guides are being used in medicine as well as psychiatry. The inner guide helps to open a person up to deep

How to Use Receptive Imagery to Get in Touch with Inner Feelings

- visualize how you'd like to spend your time at work, at home
- visualize how you'd like family relationships to be—how you'd like your children and partner to treat you, how you'd like to treat them
- visualize things that you could do to improve problem areas in your personal life, your family life, your work
- visualize situations that make you or family members sick or healthy
- visualize the most pleasurable family vacation or weekend that you can imagine

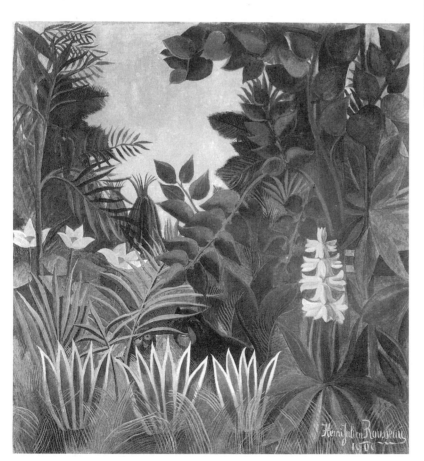

Receptive imagery involves clearing the mind and letting positive or negative images arise. It is used to help people get in touch with their own symbols. Henri Rousseau. The Equatorial Jungle. 1877. National Gallery of Art, Washington. Chester Dale Collection.

feelings about their illness. The guide offers advice and acts as a source of support. Many therapists who work with guides believe that they are a connection to the inner self which thinks in symbols. In *Healing Yourself,* Dr. Martin Rossman gives detailed instructions on using inner guides for healing.

Programmed imagery involves choosing and holding particular images, rather than letting images arise spontaneously. Like receptive imagery, programmed imagery has specific effects on people's mental and physical states and on their lives. Programmed imagery is useful in helping to achieve goals and make changes. Concentrating on positive images helps to strengthen confidence, increase peace of mind, and enhance joyful anticipation.

Programmed imagery is probably the most common type used for healing. Such imagery is often most powerful if it uses images that come from a person's inner self. Examples of programmed images include a wolf eating tumor cells, pain leaving the body like dark smoke coming out of a hole, eliminating bacteria by erasing them like dots on a blackboard, and picturing an infection filled with pulsing healing energy. Programmed imagery may involve either symbolic representations or actual physical anatomy drawings taken from books. Another type of programmed imagery involves picturing a person's entire body surrounded by white light or healing energy. In truth, most imagery work is a mixture of receptive and programmed; that is, people allow images to surface, then choose to concentrate on ones that are positive.

In terms of research, imagery is still a relatively new field of medicine, but one that holds great promise. Readers who are interested in using imagery for stress reduction and healing can use the exercises in this chapter, combining them with anatomical and physiological facts from Part II, which deals with specific illnesses. For example, if a person has low back pain, he or she might picture a cool green light soothing the area, or might picture the muscles around the vertebrae relaxing and tension on the nerves being relieved.

In this chapter we have tried to give a broad and inclusive view of what stress is, and how it can cause illness. It's important to realize that stress is not something outside ourselves, to be slavishly avoided because it causes illness. Rather, it is a combination of outside events and inner attitudes, perceptions, and

Find a place where you will be undisturbed, a place where you feel at ease. Make yourself comfortable. Let your eyes close. Breathe in and out deeply, allowing your abdomen to rise and fall. As your breathing becomes slow and even, you will feel relaxed. Imagine the relaxation in your whole body deepening by stages. You are now in a state in which your mind is clear and tranquil. You can visualize vividly and easily. Imagine that your mind is like a screen and you can see any image you choose. The image may be something you have seen, something you have imagined, something you would like to happen. Scan the image with your mind's eye and notice small details. The more closely you look at the image, the clearer and more vivid the details will become. When you visualize a scene, imagine you are really there. *Look* at your surroundings, *listen* to the noises, *smell* the air, *feel* the breeze. Be there. Enjoy all the sensations of the positive visualization you are holding. Experience your visualization as long as you wish. To return to your ordinary state, count slowly from one to three, and gently move some part of your body. Allow yourself to return slowly and open your eyes when you feel ready to do so. You will now feel rested and calm. You will be able to return to the positive image you held more and more readily each time you visualize it.

- do the *relaxation exercise* (see p. 62) to get yourself in a deeply relaxed state.

For any illness
- when relaxed, first picture your illness, then let the image of your illness turn into an image of healing.
- images that come from inside you are often the most vivid and powerful. Let go of images that make you frightened or uncomfortable.
- your images may be anatomical, symbolic, poetic, cartoonlike, etc., and may involve any or all of your senses. If you wish, you can make use of the anatomical and physiological information in the discussions on illnesses in Part II.
- picture the area bathed in white light; picture healing energy going to the injured area; picture the area as completely healed.
- imagine tension and pain leaving your body as you breathe out.
- imagine healthy immune cells engulfing bacteria or virus.
- imagine blood flow increasing to an injured area; imagine drugs getting in to heal an area or relieve the pain.
- imagine your body replacing damaged cells with new healthy cells.
- imagine the swelling in an area decreasing.
- imagine rough areas as smooth, hot areas as cool, and dry areas as moist.
- picture yourself active, healthy, relaxed, and involved in activities you enjoy.

For specific illnesses
- for allergies, picture your immune cells acting healthy and calm; imagine your mucous membranes as healthy and pink.
- for arthritis, imagine joint swelling and inflammation decreasing, imagine new cartilage growing wherever cartilage has broken down, imagine the joint moving smoothly and comfortably.
- for asthma, imagine your bronchial tubes widening so that air moves easily in and out of your lungs.
- for heart disease, picture your coronary arteries as smooth and open, easily bringing blood to all parts of the heart.
- for high blood pressure, picture all your blood vessels relaxing and imagine the blood flowing smoothly and easily throughout your body.
- for headache, picture the pain as smoke, and imagine it going out through the top of your head.
- for backache, imagine the muscles of your back feeling warm and becoming long and relaxed.
- for colds, imagine your mucous membranes shrinking down to stop a runny nose and make your breathing less stuffy.
- for cancer, picture white blood cells engulfing the cancer cells, picture radiation or chemotherapy destroying the cancer cells.

philosophies. In this regard, stressful events can be positive as well as negative; they can provide a framework for growth as well as illness. For example, moving can be a challenge which leads to new friends, interests, and work—a challenge that actually improves our life and heals our body. Or it can be a threat that brings upheaval, removes old supports, and causes illness. Fittingly, the tools that are best adapted to dealing with stress are the tools of personal growth and insight. If we can learn to deal with stress, whatever form it takes, we become that much stronger, feel better, and improve our health.

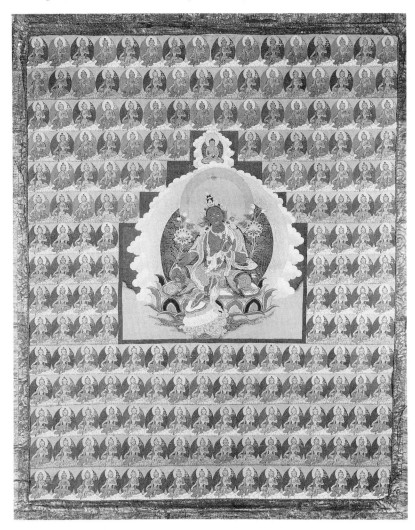

Holding a positive image, which helps focus our attention and create peace of mind, has long been a part of Buddhist tradition. Green Tara. 18th century. Asian Art Museum of San Francisco. The Avery Brundage Collection.

CHAPTER FOUR

Fulfillment and Health

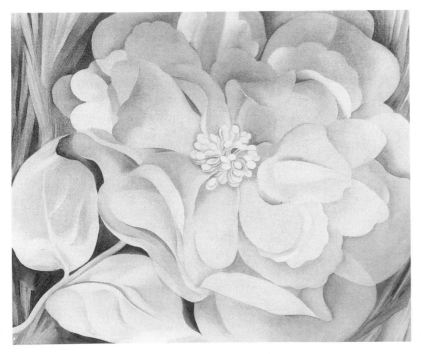

One of the central concepts of this book is that creative fulfillment in midadulthood is essential to maintaining health. A sense of fulfillment causes people to view the world in such a way that stressful events are transmuted into challenges. In essence, fulfillment changes people's perceptions, and it is our perceptions that color the way we see life. In the chapter on stress, we described in detail the physiological mechanisms by which stress causes illness. We believe that stress is one of the crucial factors in creating illness, and that a broad, inclusive theory on relieving stress in midadulthood is of great significance in terms of preventive medicine and optimum health. Creative fulfillment manifests itself as love of life, outside interests, and a sense of life as being meaningful.

The idea that a sense of fulfillment in midadulthood is neces-

Opening ourselves up helps to bring health and fulfillment to midadulthood. Georgia O'Keeffe. The White Calico Flower. 1931. Oil on canvas. 30″ × 36″. Collection, The Whitney Museum of American Art. Purchase. 32.26.

sary for health is not entirely new, but it has received little direct study or attention. Creative fulfillment has always been linked philosophically to mental health, but less study has been done on the relationship between creative fulfillment and physical health. In terms of physical health and fulfillment, midadulthood brings on a reassessment of life goals. Most psychiatrists and psychologists have concluded that spiritual growth is an essential element in the realignment of goals that must necessarily take place during this stage of life. When such a shift is not made, people find themselves in an antagonistic relationship to

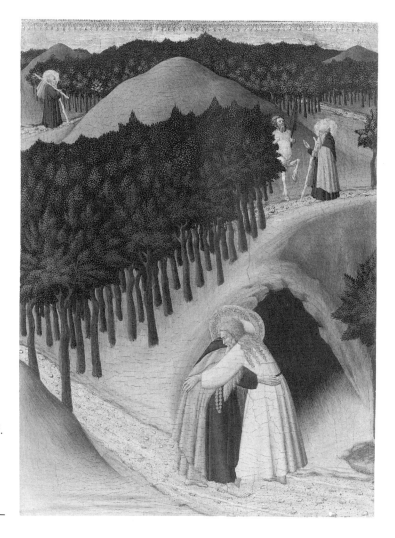

A quest that produces spiritual growth helps people to enjoy life and perceive events as challenging rather than stressful. Sassetta and assistant. Meeting of Saint Anthony and Saint Paul. 1440. *National Gallery of Art, Washington. Samuel H. Kress Collection.*

the world around them. Discord—a lack of harmony and balance—is likely to produce illness unless the internal strife is eventually resolved in some positive manner. When people feel fulfilled, they enjoy their life and they view external events as challenging, rather than stressful. Such a perception directly alters the physiology of stress and helps to prevent illness. This concept of fulfillment ties in with new theories about health and attitude. As we've discussed in the stress chapter, self-efficacy, hardiness, coherence, and spirituality all greatly affect our attitude and thus our reaction to stressful events.

To understand the concept of health and fulfillment in mid-adulthood, it is useful to look at the literature dealing with both life cycle and life crisis or transition. Life-cycle research has as its central theme the idea that the human life span is a cycle that naturally divides into stages, and that these stages, which are universally experienced, are determined both biologically through bioprograms stored in our genes, and sociologically through cultural patterns. Psychologists and psychiatrists don't agree on all points about the life cycle, but they acknowledge that the concept of dividing it into stages is useful in making generalizations about human behavior and health. They also agree that social/emotional growth does not proceed at an even pace, nor is it complete at the end of adolescence. Rather, human development proceeds with periods of rapid growth or jumps, followed by plateaus during which new skills and achievements are consolidated.

Up to the 1970s, most of the work on growth and development concerned childhood, because the prevailing view in the literature was that social and emotional growth took place *before* adulthood. But in the 1970s there was a sudden proliferation of studies focusing on growth stages that occurred universally in the *adult* years. Basically, the life cycle has been divided into four stages, which are sometimes likened to the seasons. The stages are: childhood and adolescence (spring), early adulthood (summer), middle adulthood (fall), and old age (winter). Each stage is thought to last about 20 years, and toward the end of one stage and the beginning of the next, major transitions are postulated. Some theorists believe that the transitions can be smooth and gradual; others believe the changes are abrupt and are likely to precipitate a personal life crisis.

Ancient Observations on the Stages of Life

at 30
THE TALMUD: attaining full strength
CONFUCIUS: planting one's feet firmly upon the ground
SOLON: having children

at 40
THE TALMUD: understanding
CONFUCIUS: no perplexities
SOLON: the mind broadens

at 50
THE TALMUD: giving counsel
CONFUCIUS: knowing the biddings of heaven
SOLON: tongue and mind are at their best

at 60
THE TALMUD: wisdom
CONFUCIUS: listening to heaven with a docile ear
SOLON: able but not nimble

Source: Adapted from D. Levinson, Seasons of a Man's Life.

The Stages of Life

The concept of adult development originated with the eminent Swiss psychologist, Carl Jung. As opposed to his colleague Sigmund Freud, who concentrated on childhood development, Jung's theory of the life cycle concentrated on the second half of life, or adulthood, and its relation to social institutions; in particular, to religion and mythology. Jung's theory of the stages of life is comprised of only three parts: childhood, youth, and adulthood. Jung believes that prior to puberty, a child's consciousness is tied to that of the parents—in a sense, the child has not even been psychically born at this point. The stage of youth is concerned with the demands of life, and extends from the end of puberty until middle life, which begins between the 35th and 40th year. Jung believes that the problems found in youth are often the result of one's clinging to childhood consciousness and a resistance to being involved in the world. In a way that parallels the world of physical matter, people tend toward inertia in their psychic development.

Between the ages of 35 and 40, Jung believes that there is an important change in the human psyche. This transformation can either be manifest as a gradual change in a person's character or as a marked transformation in traits, inclinations, and concerns. It is interesting to note that Jung observed a rise in the frequency of mental depression among men around the age of 40, and in women a little earlier. At midadulthood, there is a natural change in goals. The new goal is for people to achieve wisdom and harmony with their inner symbols. This is done through a process which Jung called *individuation*, which starts at about age 40 and continues for the rest of a person's life. According to Jung, neurotic disturbances in midadulthood—like earlier ones—are the result of inertia, that is, difficulty in initiating change, and represent a desire to carry into adulthood the psychology and goals of youth, the previous stage.

Jung's metaphor for the life cycle is the daily course of the sun across the heavens. The sun rises in the morning from unconsciousness into a world that widens as the sun climbs higher. The sun's goal is extension of its field of action, attainment of the greatest possible height. At noon, the sun begins its descent, into a reversal of the ideals and values of the first half of its journey. After middle life, people are not mounting and expanding, rather they are, or should be, contracting and devoting more time to their inner selves. One example of life cycle reversal that Jung gives is the natural tendency of a man to become more feminine in interests in the second half of life, and a woman to become more masculine.

Jung paralleled his three stages of life with stages of consciousness. In childhood, the first stage, Jung suggests that consciousness is in a chaotic state in which the ego is not separated from the unconscious. In youth, the second stage, the personality or ego develops, but is "monarchic" or "monistic"; that is, it is concerned only with itself. In the third stage, adulthood, the ego becomes divided or dualistic, and expands into the world.

Spiritual Growth as Healing

Jung believed that it is essential for people to undergo change during the third stage of life. "We cannot live the afternoon of life according to the programme of life's morning."[1] The significance of the morning lies in the development of personality, making one's way in the world, and having children, but the significance of the afternoon is quite different. During hunter-gatherer times, old people were the guardians of mystery and tribal lore. They were the keepers of the cultural heritage of the tribe and had the secrets of vision and wisdom. Jung believed that through visions, dreams, and intuition, people can get in touch with what he termed *archetypes*, primordial images that are inborn and are as old as history. According to Jung, wisdom consists of a return to knowledge of these archetypes and a life in harmony with them.

One of the major archetypes involves the concept of life after death. Jung felt that this archetype is of great significance in the third stage of life, but realized that his contemporaries often found it very hard to accept because it does not easily mesh with scientific theory. Jung believed that before the advent of modern science, religions were "schools for forty-year-olds" to help them ponder the meaning of life and develop a concept of life after death. "I have observed that a life directed to an aim is in general

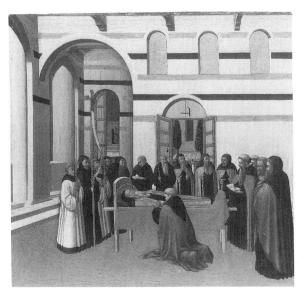 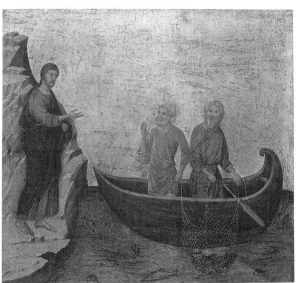

Carl Jung considered religions to be "schools for 40-year-olds" to help them ponder the meaning of life and death. Left: *Sassetta and assistant.* The Death of Saint Anthony. *1440. National Gallery of Art, Washington. Samuel H. Kress Collection.* Right: *Duccio di Buonisegna.* The Calling of the Apostles Peter and Andrew. *1308/1311. National Gallery of Art, Washington. Samuel H. Kress Collection.*

better, richer, and healthier than an aimless one, and that it is better to go forwards with the stream of time than backwards against it. . . As a doctor I am convinced that it is hygienic—if I may use the word—to discover in death a goal towards which one can strive, and that shrinking away from it is something unhealthy and abnormal which robs the second half of life of its purpose."[2] Jung also stated that he never observed a cure in the second half of life that did not involve some religious or spiritual change. Such a process inevitably entails changing attitudes, achieving feelings of fulfillment and self-control, and developing a personal myth or reason for being. A personal myth involves our own view of ourselves as important, as helping to make life better for people we love and for the world around us. Whether such myths are actually true or not, they are empowering. They provide a reason for living and help us to deal with change by transforming problems into challenges. Such myths are an integral part of all religious or spiritual philosophies.

Jung links fulfillment in midlife to understanding of one's own identity, including its inevitable end. Without this deep understanding, adulthood becomes fraught with problems and illness. The key to preventing these problems is the developmental process of individuation, through which people become better able to utilize their inner resources. Individuation reduces the stress of society's demands by having people concentrate on their inner world, and it defuses the unfulfilled demands of the unconscious by recognizing those demands. Central to this process is the idea that the unconscious archetypes or figures have their own inner-regulating or -directing tendencies. The inner Self that people discover is self-balancing, health-giving, and the source of creative images for personal growth. One technique Jung used to help people get in touch with these inner images was called *active imagination*, a form of imaginative meditation similar to what we call *receptive imagery*. When people listen to their innermost feelings, their personality matures and extends, and their psyche becomes more balanced and whole.

The themes of self-renewal and creative involvement are ones that are found again and again in the literature on growth, spirituality, midlife crisis, and most recently, health. We believe that getting deeply in touch with the inner Self is the first step toward healing and a major step toward preventing illness. Carl Jung has defined the Self as an organizing center or nuclear atom in our psychic system; an inventor, organizer, and source of images. Throughout the ages, shamans, religious thinkers, and philosophers have talked about an inner center or Self. The Egyptians referred to it as Ba-soul, the Greeks as daimon, the Romans as genius, and some American Indian tribes refer to it as inner companion or friend. Jung believes that the Self is an inner guiding factor, distinct from the conscious part of our personality, the Ego, which represents only a small part of a person's total psyche. When the Ego listens to the Self, we grow and heal, and in a sense, fulfill our own destiny.

The better we feel about ourselves, our bodies, and our lives, the better our bodies function and the healthier we feel. An important auxiliary concept that is developing in the mind-body field holds that when people are not fulfilling their own destiny, their inner Self becomes uncomfortable and uses illness to signal the external personality or Ego that something is wrong. Physicians who agree with this theory believe that illness can be a positive message for life change. Many times, the pain and suffering of illness is a catalyst that causes people to make fundamental, necessary changes in their lives. From this point of view, if we pay attention to our inner feelings and to slight feelings of

Changes Commonly Undergone by People Who Survive Life-Threatening Illnesses

- internal change as a result of meditation or prayer
- improved relationships with others
- significant change in dietary habits
- a sense of the spiritual
- a feeling that their recovery was the result of a struggle

Source: Dr. Kenneth Pelletier.

Growth Characteristics of People Who Have Survived Life-Threatening Illnesses

- playfulness that is nonpurposeful
- ability to lose track of time when absorbed
- innocent curiosity
- ability to observe without judging
- ability to accept criticism
- active imagination
- willingness to look foolish
- empathy for other people
- ability to see patterns
- trust and intuition
- good sense of timing
- cooperative nonconformity and independence
- self-ease in complex situations
- positive outlook
- confidence in adversity
- ability to find a positive outcome in unplanned or bad situations

Source: Adapted from Al Siebert, P.O. Box 535, Portland, Oregon 97207.

discomfort, we can often make changes that will prevent illness before it arises.

As the mind-body literature grows, more and more physicians are using spiritual growth techniques as a primary health tool to bring people into closer contact with their inner Self. The technique most commonly used to listen to the inner Self is meditation (see p. 62). The medical use of meditation is currently being pioneered by Dr. Joan Borysenko at the Harvard Mind-Body Clinic. Another powerful technique, based on Jung's concept of active imagination is the use of an inner guide or spirit guide. This ancient technique, which has historical roots in shaman-

---

An Exercise for Getting a Spirit Guide

Find a quiet space where you will be undisturbed, a place where you will feel at ease. Make yourself comfortable. Close your eyes. Inhale slowly and deeply; exhale slowly and completely. As you breathe in and out, allow your body to relax very deeply. Allow your abdomen to rise and fall as you breathe. Breathe in, and as you exhale, slowly say to yourself, "Three," three, three." See the numeral or the word "three" as you repeat it. Inhale again, and as you exhale, repeat and visualize the number "two." Inhale again, and as you exhale, repeat and visualize the number "one."

You are now in a calm and relaxed state of being; you can deepen this state by counting backward. Breathe in. As you exhale, say to yourself, "Ten, I am feeling very relaxed." Inhale again and as you exhale repeat mentally, "Nine, I am feeling more relaxed." Breathe. "Eight, I am feeling even more relaxed. Seven, deeper and more relaxed. Six, more relaxed. Five, deeper and more relaxed. Four, deeper and more relaxed. Three, deeper and more relaxed. Two, deeper and more relaxed. One, deeper and more relaxed."

You are now at a deeper and more relaxed level of awareness, a level where you feel healthy, peaceful, and open. Allow yourself to picture a place or a room where you can work in your inner world. The room can be as real as a studio, shop, or meadow, but it exists in your mind. Begin to look around. Notice whether you are outdoors or in a room. If you are in a room, notice how the walls, doors, and windows look. If you are out of doors, look closely at the trees, plants, and rocks. Because you are visualizing this space, there are no limits to what you may see in it. In this imaginary, protected space, you can meet an inner guide.

If you are inside, imagine a special door that slides open from the bottom to the top. Allow the door to slide open slowly. First you will see the guide's feet, then the legs, then the entire body. The guide may be a man or a woman, an animal or a plant, a strange being, or even a light or sound. Now ask the guide to communicate with you. You can even ask the guide's name and talk to the guide. If the guide begins to speak, let the information flow into your mind. It will sound like an inner conversation, but the guide's voice will be spontaneous. Ask the guide if you can talk further, and ask any questions about your life and health. Stay with your guide in your inner space as long as you wish. When you are ready to return to your ordinary state, count slowly from one to three and gently move some part of your body. Allow yourself to return to your everyday consciousness slowly, and open your eyes when you are ready to do so. You will feel rested and calm and will be able to return to your inner world and guide whenever you wish.

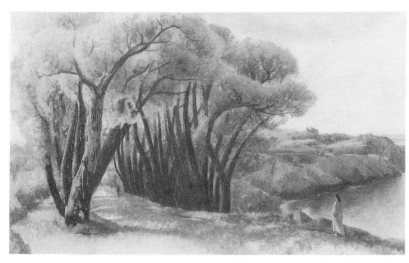

Voices from the unconscious are homeostatic; that is, they help to keep people true to their personal path. Leon Kroll. A Road Through Willows. *1933. Oil on canvas. 26″ × 42″. Collection, The Whitney Museum of American Art. Purchase. 34.17.*

Characteristics of People Who Get Ill and People Who Don't

LIKELY TO BECOME ILL	LESS LIKELY TO BECOME ILL
crisis-ridden	optimistic
under stress	has a purpose
dissatisfied	in life, a
unhappy	reason for
resentful	being
threatened	trusting
out of control	high self-
loaded with	esteem
responsi-	gets along
bility	well with
worried	peers
depressed	successful
frustrated	excited
helpless	interested
lonely	satisfied
grief-stricken	stimulated
confused	happy
feels	involved
abandoned	part of stable
lacks positive	social
feedback	structure
	has a sense of
	cohesion
	has social
	support,
	positive
	feedback

ism, involves creating an inner dialogue while one is in a relaxed physical and mental state. People can learn to talk to spirit guides about questions concerning life changes. The answers that arise will have special meaning because they come from a level that is deeper than our everyday, conscious concerns. Such voices are homeostatic and help to put people back on their path.

The Ages of Man

All life cycle theories deal with the concept of people changing and growing. One of the first comprehensive models of the life cycle, and the basis for many subsequent theories, is psychoanalyst Erik Erikson's "Eight Ages of Man," which was first published in 1950 in his classic work, *Childhood and Society*. Erikson's theory, which was based on cross-cultural studies, divides the life cycle into eight challenges, each of which is described in terms of two extremes of outcome. According to

Erikson's model, childhood and adolescence comprise the first five of the eight stages: (1) *basic trust* vs. *basic mistrust* (first year), (2) *autonomy* vs. *shame and doubt* (second and third year), (3) *initiative* vs. *guilt* (ages three to six), (4) *industry* vs. *inferiority* (age six to puberty), and (5) *identity* vs. *role diffusion* (puberty to adolescence). The sixth stage, *intimacy* vs. *isolation*, occurs in the first part of adulthood, and is succeeded by the seventh stage, *generativity* vs. *stagnation*. This seventh stage is the one that involves midadulthood. The eighth and final stage, *ego integrity* vs. *despair*, takes place in maturity.

Generativity vs. stagnation is Erikson's central concept of adulthood. The major concern of generativity is guiding the next generation. Generativity, which includes productivity and creativity, fulfills the adult's need to be needed. The concept generally involves children, but it can also involve the welfare of future generations or working with younger adults. Erikson believes that if people fail to develop this aspect of their personality during middle age, they often feel a pervading sense of stagnation and personal impoverishment. "Individuals, then, often begin to indulge themselves as if they were their own—or one another's—one and only child; and where conditions favor it, early invalidism, physical or psychological, becomes the vehicle of self-concern."[3] Thus, in 1950, Erikson glimpsed a crucial link between middle-aged fulfillment and physical, as well as mental, health. One can make the assumption, based on Erikson's line of thought, that if the middle-aged stage is not successfully resolved, feelings of stagnation and impoverishment would make people unhappy enough that the mind-body connection would produce illness. Such feelings result in alienation, boredom, depression, and loss of control, all of which have been shown to make people more susceptible to illness and less likely to heal. Erikson does not make much of the idea of crises between the various stages; in particular, he does not discuss the idea of a midlife crisis. However, he does state that only after an individual meets the challenges of the seventh stage, generativity, does the final stage, ego integrity vs. despair, begin.

In Erikson's model, the last stage deals with world order and spiritual sense, an acceptance of the dignity of one's own life. If people are not able to accept the accidental coincidences of their own life, their ego does not become integrated, and they develop

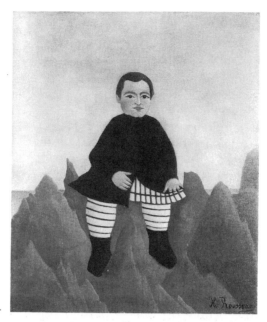

Erik Erikson believed that if people do not develop a concern for the welfare of future generations, they often "indulge themselves as if they were their own . . . one and only child." Henri Rousseau. Boy on the Rocks. *1895–97. National Gallery of Art, Washington. Chester Dale Collection.*

a fear of death. For these people there is a pervasive feeling that it is too late to begin anew, yet they cannot accept their life as it is. The stalemate of these opposing feelings produces a state of despair. For some people this feeling of despair is masked by a feeling of disgust that is frequently their reaction to events or situations in the world around them, as well as to their own life. Such despair and disgust have physiological consequences.

In the 1960s, Erikson added to his descriptions of each stage the basic virtues or personality strengths that would help to successfully resolve that stage. For generativity vs. stagnation, Erikson cites *production* and *care*, for ego integrity vs. despair, he cites *renunciation* and *wisdom*. Erikson's description of his eighth stage embodies several themes that are similar to Jung's and that are also echoed in his later theories. Key among these are the acceptance of one's own life, dealing with death, and the necessity for a spiritual view of the universe. We believe that these three points are fundamental to the maintenance of health.

The midlife crisis is a key concept in terms of this book. We believe that the reevaluation and depression that usually occur in midadulthood are actually basic tools that can help to promote change. If that change is positive, it is instrumental in producing growth and health.

The Midlife Crisis

The British psychoanalyst Elliott Jaques coined the term *midlife crisis* in 1965 in a paper appropriately called "Death and the Midlife Crisis." Interestingly, Jaques developed the concept as a result of reading the historical papers of 310 painters, writers, composers, poets, and sculptors of great renown, including Raphael, Shakespeare, Mozart, Goethe, and Michelangelo, etc. He found that these artists underwent a crisis in their creative work between the ages of 35 and 40, a crisis that expressed itself in one of three different ways. In one group, creative work stopped, either because their creative ideas dried up or because the people died. It is particularly interesting to note that the death rate for these artists showed a sudden jump between 34 and 40 years of age, attaining a rate well above the average. Among a second group, the creative work started for the first time, while in a third group, the artists' creative work showed a decisive change in quality and content.

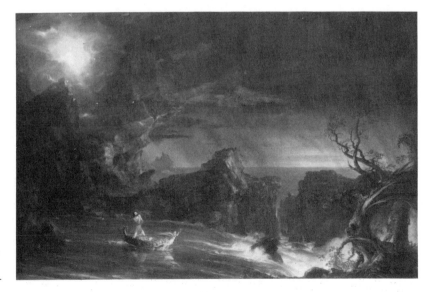

A midlife crisis can be the basis for a reevaluation that brings about change and renewed health. Thomas Cole. The Voyage of Life: Manhood. 1842. National Gallery of Art, Washington. Ailsa Mellon Bruce Fund.

Jaques theorized that youthful creativity tends to be intense, spontaneous, and spring intact from the unconscious. By contrast, creativity after the midlife crisis is shaped by an interplay between unconscious work and considered creation. The essence of creative work in mature adulthood consists of consciously reflecting on ideas, modifying them, and elaborating on them. In addition to a change in work mode, there comes a change in quality and content. The quality and content of youthful work is lyrical and descriptive. It tends to be idealistic and optimistic, embodying a belief in the inherent goodness of human nature. Middle age brings the emergence of tragic and philosophical content, evolving finally into serenity. A more contemplative pessimism arises, combined with an acceptance that goodness is accompanied by destructive forces. Jaques believes that death and human destructiveness are first taken into account by most people in middle age, and that the depression engendered by this realization must be worked through by developing a sense of constructive resignation toward the imperfections of the individual. Should they fail in this, people sometimes defend against the midlife crisis by becoming manic, hypochondriacal, obsessive, superficial, or by undergoing character deterioration.[4]

The resolution of these problems involves mental integration and often spiritual experiences as well. Dante, for example, escaped from Hell and Purgatory in the *Divine Comedy* by having a vision of supreme love and knowledge. Interestingly, a vision of unconditional love has become the healing path for many holistic physicians, including Dr. Bernie Siegel, head of ECaP (Exceptional Cancer Patients) and author of *Love, Medicine and Miracles*; Dr. Gerald Jampolsky, director of the Center for Attitudinal Healing and author of the book, *Love Is Letting Go of Fear*; and Dr. James J. Lynch, director of the Psychosomatic Medicine Clinic at University of Maryland School of Medicine and author of *The Broken Heart*. Only when people are able to integrate the harsh realities of life with goodness and love are they able to work through the depression of the midlife crisis.

Jaques believes that during the middle-age crisis people are encountering and mourning the eventual tragedy of their own personal death, emerging from this process with a greater capacity to love. At that point, the latter half of life can be lived with a knowledge and acceptance of death. As Jaques says, in successfully resolving the midlife crisis we gain a deepening of awareness, understanding, and self-realization; we attain greater wisdom, courage, and fortitude; and we develop a deeper capacity for love, affection, human insight, hopefulness, and enjoyment. Such growth is based on acceptance of our shortcomings and destructive impulses, and on a greater capacity for resignation and detachment.[5] An important part of working through the midlife crisis is the ability to accept conflict and ambivalence, and the ability to accept one's shortcomings and imperfections. From this mental perspective, a positive creativity and tone of serenity can emerge, and inner and outer worlds can mesh without friction, permitting greater productivity. Like Jung and Erikson, Jaques emphasizes the concept of inner growth through coming to terms with death and imperfection.

Life Structure and Transitions

Daniel Levinson, a psychologist at Yale, detailed his ideas on the life cycle in the popular book, *The Seasons of a Man's Life* (1978), based on his study of the biographies of working and middle-class men (Levinson did not include women in the scope of his study.) Levinson's is the most influential and controversial of recent theories dealing with the concerns of middle age and the idea of predictable transitions and crises during adult life.

The main concept of Levinson's theories concerns the *individual life structure*, which refers to the patterning of the individual's life at a given time, in a given social setting. Levinson believes that the life structure evolves through a sequence of alternating stable periods of six to eight years, and transitional periods of four to five years. During stable periods, people make life choices to attain goals, pursue related tasks, and build a life structure. During transitional periods, people reappraise their life structure, terminate facets of the existing structure, and work toward taking on the tasks of the next stage. Thus the transition periods are major developmental steps.

Early Adulthood spans the years 17–45, and includes several stages and transitions. During the *First Adult Life Structure* (22–28), the individual is exploring possibilities for adult living, and

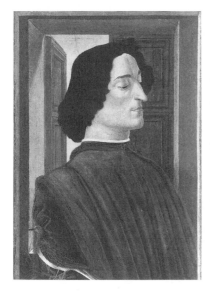 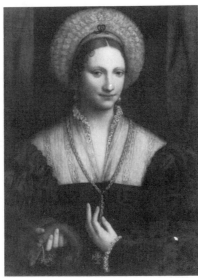

There is increasing recognition of the fact that adults pass through predictable life stages. Left: Botticelli. Giuliano de' Medici. 1478. National Gallery of Art, Washington. Samuel H. Kress Collection. Right: Bernardino Luini. Portrait of a Lady. 1520/1525. National Gallery of Art, Washington. Andrew W. Mellon Collection.

beginning to settle down and take on adult responsibilities. Some men do this slowly or tentatively, while others make strong commitments at the outset, especially in terms of marriage and occupation. During the *Age Thirty Transition* (28–32), the individual who has not worked out a defined life structure realizes the limitations of his style and seeks to take on greater order and responsibility, while the one who took on early commitments wonders whether they were premature and if they should be continued. This transitional period, like all the others, varies with the individual; it can be smooth and involve relatively minor modification, or it can present a life-crisis which requires major restructuring in work or relationships. Levinson found that most of the men in his study had a crisis in the Age Thirty Transition: divorce hit a peak, as did occupational change.

During the *Second Adult Life Structure* (32–40), a man attempts to establish a niche in society, building a strong life structure in the areas of work, family, and/or community. The goal of this period is to take on all the rights and privileges of adulthood. Toward the end of this period, around the age of 36, men enter a new phase, which Levinson calls *Becoming One's Own Man.* During this stage, the aim is to fully accomplish the goals of the settling-down period. With the increased responsibilities of this period, this accomplishment involves relinquishing to a greater degree the boy within the man. During this period, the polarity between child and adult often causes the person to get into conflicts with the people around him, and he has a sense of being controlled by other people. As a result, some men feel a need to break out. If the structure they have created is intolerable, they must dismantle it and create a new one in which they can endeavor once again to succeed at becoming their own person. Otherwise, they succumb to what has been referred to as "learned helplessness," which is a potent negative factor in terms of health.

According to Levinson, for many men a crisis in becoming one's own man is a major dilemma because if one stays in the present situation, one faces "a living death, a future without promise, a self-betrayal."[6] On the other hand, making a change at this time is very difficult because it hurts loved ones, it requires enormous time and energy to set up a new structure (8–10 years), and it often becomes entangled with the problems of the next transition.

The *Midlife Transition*, which takes place between ages 40–45, involves a major shift between Early Adulthood and Middle Adulthood. This transition is fundamental because it involves bringing out parts of the self that heretofore have been neglected and unexpressed due to the tremendous emphasis put on the outer world during a person's 30s. In the course of this transition a man comes to question the true meaning and value of the life structure he has built up. According to Levinson, 80% of the men he studied had a moderate to severe crisis at this stage, questioning nearly every aspect of their life, and needing to modify their old path. Levinson emphasizes that these are healthy problems rather than sick ones, but he admits that the transition involves a great deal of turmoil and activates many neurotic problems in men. One of the key facets of this period is the ability to see through the illusions that one has held about the world and about oneself. To make the kind of fundamental changes that are required at this stage, individuals must confront and integrate primal inner polarities and engage in a process of midlife individuation. Levinson points out that men vary in their ability to successfully resolve the Midlife Crisis.

Middle Adulthood lasts from ages 40–65. During this time a

man again makes choices and modifies his life structure. For some, there is a drastic change in job, marriage, or living site. For others, there may be less drastic changes that are nonetheless crucial. During ages 40–45 the Midlife Transition occurs, while the years from 45–50 are a period of relative stability called the *First Middle Adult Structure*. From ages 50–55 is the *Age Fifty Transition*, a transitional period comparable to the Age Thirty Transition, in which the person assesses how well the changes of the Midlife Transition have worked and modifies them if necessary. This transition will be a crisis if the person did not successfully deal with the Midlife Transition.

Between 55–60, a man again goes through a rather stable period called the *Second Middle Adult Structure*, a time in which the changes and goals of Middle Adulthood are completed. For people who successfully dealt with the Midlife Crisis, this is likely to be a period of great fulfillment as they achieve neglected dreams and work on undeveloped areas of their personality. From ages 60–65 is the *Late Adult Transition* which brings the Middle Adult years to an end and paves the way for *Late Adulthood*, which encompasses the years 65–80. During these years, men encounter increasing physical illness, deal with the loss of loved ones, and face a change in generations that signals their advancing age. The developmental task in this period is to bring youthfulness into a form that is appropriate to the tasks and realities of the later years. In addition, men must find a new balance in their relationship with society, giving up work and delving deeper into their own psyches.

Stress, Change, and Healing

All of the life cycle theories acknowledge the fact that adults, like children, go through stages that require growth and change. There is also agreement that the major change in midadulthood deals with transforming our view of life and personal fulfillment in such a way as to incorporate an understanding of our own mortality. These are inner, as opposed to outer, concerns, and they cause people to deal with parts of their personality that have often not been expressed previously. We believe that the more people fulfill their own path or destiny, the greater the satisfac-

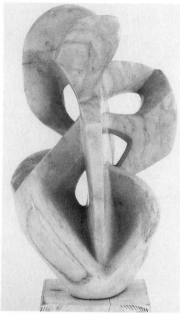

Transformation is a major goal of midadulthood. Day Schnabel. Transformations. 1956. Siena marble. 19¾" × 12 × 10½". Collection, The Whitney Museum of American Art. Purchase. 32.26.

tion in their lives and the lower the stress. As a result, health and well-being increase and disease decreases.

Canadian systems engineer John Milsum has an interesting theory that concerns they way in which stress is connected to life transitions. During periods of equilibrium, all of us feel that our world is satisfactory. Such periods are inevitably followed by periods of increasing frustration and dissatisfaction, due partly to changes in our outer world, but largely to changes in the way we view ourselves. Once our self-concept changes, we look at the world quite differently; things that were once satisfying may become less so, and new areas of interest open up. This disparity between our perceptions and our desires causes a crisis which brings on change and adaptation. Ultimately, if the changes meet our wishes, we enter a new phase of satisfaction and stability. However, if change does not occur and the disparity is not reconciled, dissatisfaction mounts, stress occurs, and we become ill. If we *do* change, growth takes place and we become healthier.

The life crises that occur between stages are painful because, not only must we adapt to the new concept we have of ourselves, we inevitably grieve for the habits and satisfactions of the old self. Milsum believes that the pain engendered by these transitions is a necessary signal from our mind-body that helps us to grow and change. From this point of view, the discomfort of each transition period is both natural and positive, in that it is essential for growth. The more we can get in tune with the changes and cycles of our inner self, the more adaptable and healthier we will be in midadulthood. Our core model holds that a sense of personal fulfillment changes our worldview and self-concept in such a way that we view life events as challenges that we can cope with, rather than stresses that we are at the mercy of. This view results in a physiological state that is healing, rather than a stressful physiological state that brings on illness.

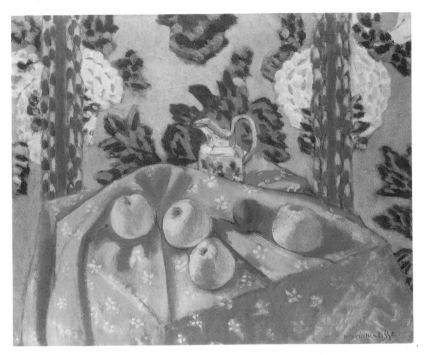

CHAPTER FIVE

Nutrition and Health

W̲e all feel better when we eat well. Our food habits have an immediate effect on our sense of well-being. Everyone knows the sluggish feeling of eating too much, the upset stomach that comes from eating greasy food, the quick-high-then-low that follows too much sugar. Likewise, we know the positive, energetic feeling we have after eating a light, nutritious meal. Over a period of weeks and months, our eating habits have even more profound effects. It is probably not too strong a statement to say that you can't feel good or be healthy if you don't eat well.

In addition to the nutritional effects of a good diet, positive feelings come from the sense of control that people experience when they consciously choose foods that they know are healthy. As we've discussed elsewhere, a sense of control is one of the

When we eat well, we feel good. Henri Matisse. Still Life: Apples on Pink Tablecloth. *1922. National Gallery of Art, Washington. Chester Dale Collection.*

most important factors in preventing and healing illness (see p. 55). A study by psychologist Kenneth Pelletier of University of California Medical School, San Francisco, found that patients who recovered from serious illnesses in spite of great odds shared certain common characteristics. One of the major factors was that the people had all altered their diet in an attempt to achieve optimal nutrition. We believe that often the mind-body effects of taking control of your diet are as important as the actual nutrients ingested.

Increasing evidence shows that certain dietary habits are closely linked to a number of major health problems, in particular, heart disease, high blood pressure, cancer, diabetes, tooth decay, diverticulitis, and of course, obesity. Nutrition is such an important factor in health that we mention it in the prevention and self-help sections of virtually every disease discussed in this book. Although the relationship between nutrition and health is very complex, there are a few modifications for the average American diet that are widely agreed upon by researchers and doctors. We are confronted by these new guidelines more and more each day. The newspapers and magazines herald the war on cholesterol; friends and colleagues order low-fat meals; and even advertising now emphasizes the healthful values of various food products. Already, many people have chosen to make positive changes in their diet. Most of these people have found that they feel better almost immediately.

Specifically, the new guidelines recommend less saturated fats and cholesterol; less red meat, and more fish and poultry; a sufficient amount of calories, but no more; less salt; more fiber; and finally, more grains, fruits, and vegetables to increase fiber and bulk without adding calories. A high intake of cholesterol and saturated fats is linked to high blood cholesterol and fat levels, which lead to atherosclerosis, heart attacks, and strokes. High fat intake is also associated with an increased incidence of cancer of the colon, breast, ovary, and prostate. Excess calories are linked with obesity, which is associated with higher incidences of adult-onset diabetes, high blood pressure, heart disease, gall bladder disease, and certain types of arthritis. High salt intake is often linked with high blood pressure. Low amounts of fiber are associated with diverticulitis, cancer of the colon, and to some extent, diabetes.

National Health Recommendations and Dietary Goals

enough calories to meet body needs but not more (fewer if overweight)
less saturated fat, cholesterol
less salt
less sugar
more whole grains, cereals
more fruits and vegetables
more fish, poultry
more peas, beans
less red meat
avoid processed foods or check ingredients carefully

Source: From the Surgeon General's Report, Healthy People.

These dietary recommendations being quite simple, and their effects on health being so direct and significant, the question becomes, why don't more people adhere to them? The answer involves complex issues relating to personal food choices and cultural dietary patterns. Personal choice relates to health *promotion*, that is, why we like to eat certain foods, and cultural patterns relate to health *prevention*, that is, which social conditions encourage us to eat certain foods.

The issues of individual choice and personal responsibility are tremendously complicated. They involve high levels of both public and professional *awareness*. Studies show that health education increases awareness, which leads to behavior changes. Presumably, because these new nutritional guidelines are beginning to be addressed by the media, the average cholesterol level in the U.S. dropped from 223 in 1974 to 211 in 1985. Heart disease rates likewise declined. Contrary to the fears of health education critics who believe that individual choice is unlikely to bring about widespread changes, it is clear that people are generally eating less fat and more carbohydrates than they were a decade ago. These are remarkable changes which will bring about a tremendous saving of lives and increased longevity. However, broader changes involving more people are needed in order to lessen the incidence of serious disease. For instance, the 1990 Health, Education, and Welfare objective for average cholesterol intake is 200, not 211; we have only come halfway in the projected drop, and even that guideline is one that many heart specialists feel is too modest. It is also distressing to note that there has not been any change in the percentage of people who are more than 20% overweight: 14% of all men in this country, 24% of all women.

The Hunter-Gatherer Diet

One of the most pertinent factors in terms of individual food choice is the type of food that we, as humans, are genetically programmed to seek. It would seem that inborn bioprograms have much to do with the "bad diet" that many of us crave. Physically and biologically, our ancestors of 1.5 million years ago were remarkably similar to ourselves, and, based on fossil find-

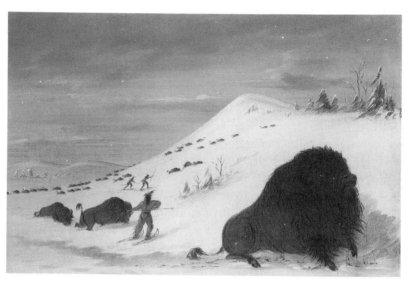

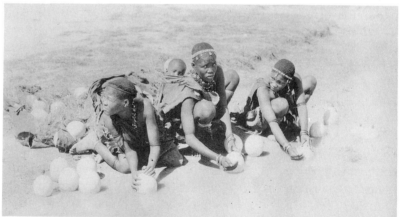

The human body is adapted to the diet that hunter-gatherers could obtain. Above: *George Catlin.* Buffalo Lancing in the Snow Drifts. *1857/1869. National Gallery of Art, Washington. Paul Mellon Collection.* Below: Filling Ostrich Eggshells with Water. *Courtesy,* The American Museum of Natural History.

ings, our ancestors of 40,000 years ago were virtually identical to us. Exciting new information about our own nutrition is coming from anthropological studies of the food habits of early humans. This information not only shows us what we are programmed to seek, it shows how our current diet is different from the one we are evolutionarily designed for. The human body is adapted for the diet that our ancestors were able to obtain. Our body is not adapted for our present diet, which is why we are succumbing to certain illnesses which are caused by what we eat. For example, it is not that fat is an unhealthy food—in fact, we could not live without it. But we're simply not equipped to handle large amounts of fat, and excessive fat intake leads to a variety of illnesses.

Anthropological studies can help us to understand why we seek in quantity foods that can be unhealthy for us. Our primate ancestors ate a diet that consisted largely of fruits and leaves; their need for calories was relatively low. As the brain of the human being evolved to be larger and larger, there was a dramatic increase in calorie needs. It has been said that the brain is "an exceptionally greedy organ." The human brain represents one-fortieth of the body's total weight, but consumes one-fifth of the body's calories. Unlike the voluntary muscles, the human brain needs energy constantly, and it cannot get sufficient energy from green leaves which are digested slowly.

What the evolving brain required was small, high-calorie packets of energy. Early humans met this need with oil-rich seeds and nuts, and protein-rich meat. This pattern has led Irven DeVore, a professor of anthropology at Harvard, to call early man "the calorie seekers." The supply of high-calorie, high-protein food was neither stable nor always readily available to early humans, and had to be shared among members of the same tribe or band. Seeds and nuts were seasonal and difficult to separate from the husk or shell. The supply of animal protein varied dramatically depending on the success of the hunter. Interestingly, anthropologists estimate that the average hunter-gatherer society got less than one-third of its food from hunting, and more than two-thirds from gathering. Anthropologists have theorized that due to the scarcity of these high-calorie packets and their importance for the development of a large brain, humans evolved to selectively favor and seek out rich, calorie-dense foods. Thus, humans seem to be genetically programmed to hunger for and enjoy the taste of a high-fat, high-protein diet.

Given the present-day availability of rich foods, this genetic programming leads to health problems. People in Western industrial countries live high on the food chain. Meat is readily available and culturally favored, as are oils, the most concentrated source of calories. Oils are a product of very affluent societies; it takes many ears of corn or large quantities of safflower seeds to press a single tablespoon of oil. Obviously, during most of our evolutionary history, such a rich diet was not possible, and it appears that the human body is often not capable of processing rich foods in the amounts that we now consume them.

Drs. Boyd Eaton and Melvin Konner of Emory Medical School in Atlanta have been studying the Paleolithic diet and its relationship to twentieth-century health. They believe that "the major chronic illnesses which afflict humans living in affluent, industrialized Western nations are largely the result of a mismatch between our genetic constitution and a variety of lifestyle factors. . . ."[1] Eaton and Konner feel that heart attacks, strokes, hypertension, adult-onset diabetes, many forms of cancer, and obesity are all caused by the incompatibility between our genetic make-up and our modern diet, exercise patterns, and exposure to alcohol and cigarette smoke.

During the majority of our evolutionary history, adults derived most of their nutrition from wild game, vegetables, fruits, and nuts. Their main beverage—water—was calorie-less. Hunter-gatherers made little use of grain, and they consumed no refined foods or food additives. They also had little salt or sugar in their diet. Interestingly, the wild game that these people ate was very different from present-day meat. It contained about the same percentage of cholesterol, but one-half of the protein, one-quarter of the calories, and one-seventh of the total fat. Not only was the fat content of meat far lower, the type of fat was different. Wild game largely contains "structural fat," fat that is integral to the structure of cell membranes. This type of fat is polyunsaturated, whereas the fat on domesticated animals that are grazed is mostly "storage fat," which is largely saturated. Saturated fats are solid at room temperature, whereas unsaturated fats are liquid. Most researchers believe that saturated fats are more directly linked to an increased incidence of heart disease.

The vegetables and fruits that we consume today are similar to those of the hunter-gatherer, but all too often they are prepared in such a way as to increase their calorie, fat, and salt load. For example, French fried potatoes have 3 times the calories of baked potatoes, 130 times the fat, and 80 times the salt. Potato chips go even further: compared to a baked potato of equal weight, potato chips have 6 times the calories, 400 times the fat, and 250 times the salt. Another significant change in our modern diet involves the processing of food. The use of refined flour and

A Hunter-Gatherer's Diet as Compared to Modern Man's

one half the fat (mostly polyunsaturated)
three times as much protein
one-sixth the salt
two times as much calcium
more potassium
four times as much vitamin C
two times as much fiber
no refined sugar
no alcohol
no tobacco

grains has lowered our fiber intake dramatically. Food processing also decreases the natural vitamin content of food. Likewise, long-distance shipping of fruits and vegetables means they are older and less nutritious by the time we eat them.

Boyd and Konner have summarized the significant nutritional differences between the late-Paleolithic and modern diets. Basically, they calculate that hunter-gatherer man ate three times as much total protein, one-half the fat (and it was much more polyunsaturated), one-sixth the salt, two times the fiber, seven times the calcium, about the same amount of carbohydrates (but theirs were unrefined, complex carbohydrates, not refined starches or sugars), and four times the Vitamin C. Based on these figures, Eaton and Konner believe that our Western diet represents "a deviation so extreme" in vertebrate experience, that our bodies now develop illnesses not seen in our distant ancestors. Eaton refers to the major present-day illnesses as "afflictions of affluence." We agree with Eaton and Konner that this information about the nutritional habits of our ancestors is very important. An understanding of our early diet explains why we find it so difficult to give up certain types of food, and can help to free us from guilt about liking "unhealthy foods," and, hopefully, motivate us to modify our own diet.

Culture and Nutrition

In addition to our individual food preferences, cultural patterns and economics can be impediments to a healthy diet. These concerns are addressed by the field of health *prevention* rather than health *promotion*. Health prevention advocates like medical sociologist John McKinlay consider socioeconomic concerns to be of even more importance than personal food choices. In the first chapter, we told the story of the heroic doctor downstream wondering who was upstream pushing people in. McKinlay considers the $161 billion food and beverage industry to be one of the "pushers," and a major manufacturer of illness.

McKinlay believes that we have completely surrendered control of our diet to private corporations, and that the food industry manipulates "our image of food away from basic staples toward synthetic and highly processed items."[2] As compared

High-Fiber Foods

FOOD	FIBER IN GMS.
apple	4
baked beans, ½ cup	9
banana	2
blackberries, ½ cup	5
bran cereal, 1 ounce	4–13
bran muffin	3
bran or wheat germ, 1 tablespoon	1
broccoli, ½ cup	2
brown rice, ½ cup	1
high-fiber cracker, 1	2–3
kidney beans, ½ cup	7
lentils, ½ cup	4
lettuce, 1 cup	1
oatmeal, 1 ounce	2
orange	3
pear	5
peas, ½ cup	4
popcorn, 3 cups	2
potato (with skin)	3.8
prunes, 5	5
psyllium seed, 1 teaspoon (e.g., *Metamucil*)	3.4
strawberries, ¾ cup	2.4
sweet potato (with skin)	3
tomatoes, ½ cup	2
white bread, 1 slice	.8
whole wheat bread, 1 slice	2.7
whole wheat spaghetti, 1 cup	4

Note: The recommended daily amount of fiber is 20–35 gms.

with only 25 years ago, people currently eat 75% less dairy products, fruits, and vegetables, and 75% more sugary snacks and soft drinks. It has been estimated that most people in the U.S. now eat more processed food than real food. McKinlay observes that "it is much cheaper to make things look and taste like the real thing than to actually provide the real thing."[3] Most of these manufactured foods are poor in nutrition. Despite well-known health risks, the food industry persists in making these products because of their popularity and high profitability.

The American food industry spends huge sums of money on advertising that is designed to convince people of the goodness and tastiness of its products, most of which nutritionists consider to be worthless or harmful. One way that processed-food manufacturers convince people to follow unhealthy behaviors is by binding their products to dominant cultural values. For example, a loving wife is shown feeding her husband a tasty, high-fat, high-cholesterol food, and the implication is that if people are loving, good, attractive, and appropriately feminine or masculine, they will buy and eat the product pictured. Fast food res-

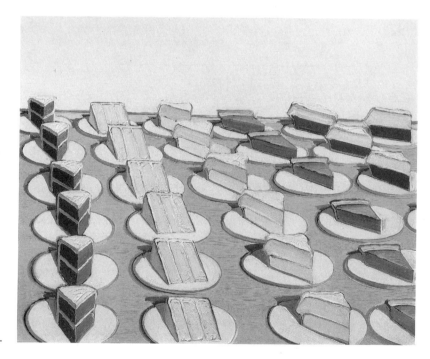

On the average, people currently eat 75 percent more sugar than they did only 25 years ago. Wayne Thiebaud. Pie Counter. 1963. Oil on canvas. 30″ × 36″. Collection, The Whitney Museum of American Art. Purchase, with funds from the Larry Aldrich Foundation Fund. 64.11.

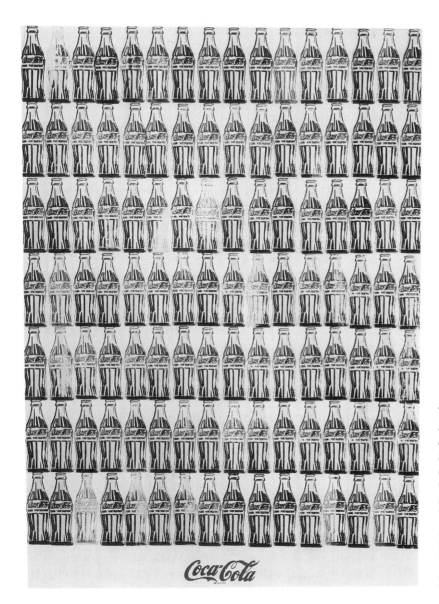

The American food industry spends millions of dollars advertising its products on the basis of image rather than content. Andy Warhol. Green Coca-Cola Bottles. *1962. Oil on canvas. 82½" × 57". Collection, The Whitney Museum of American Art. Purchase, with funds from the Friends of the Whitney Museum of American Art. 68.25.*

taurants repeatedly tie their food to positive values such as family life, relaxation, and respect for fellow human beings. Eventually, the at-risk behavior actually becomes symbolic of the positive values. Such advertising is slick, appealing, persuasive, and pervasive, bombarding us constantly, not only in readily recognizable ads, but in popular entertainment, and even on clothing with the company name on it. McKinlay points out that "many advertisements are so ingenious in their appeal, that they have entertainment value in their own right and become embodied in our national folk humor."[4] A classic example of this was the series of Wendy's commercials containing the line, "Where's the beef?"

Proponents of health prevention feel that only legislative intervention can be expected to bring about widespread change in our food habits. The Surgeon General's 1990 guidelines basically deal with health promotion and advise individual change, but they do not completely neglect the concept of health prevention through legislation. One important prevention objective is legislation requiring companies to list their products' nutritional values. Another objective is to limit the amount of salt that may be added to any processed food. Since we are programmed to seek fat, salt, and sugar, the only way we can resist the persuasive advertising and flavor of unhealthy foods is to make a conscious decision to improve our diet. The motivating factor is both to feel healthier in the present and to prevent future illness.

Diet-Related Diseases

Diet-Related Diseases

cancer of the breast
cancer of the colon
diverticulitis
heart disease
high blood pressure
irritable bowel syndrome
non-insulin-dependent
　diabetes
obesity

In order for us to actively choose a healthy diet, we have to become educated about the effects of nutrition on health, and, specifically, about what foods or eating habits are risk factors for particular diseases. Dietary information is especially important if you are at risk for a disease or if you already have a disease. In the latter case, nutritional guidelines become part of the treatment plan, not just a preventive measure. In addition to playing a significant role in a number of major diseases, nutrition also plays a role in many minor diseases. This role is described in greater detail within the discussion of specific diseases in Part II.

The most common disease in which diet plays a major role is *heart disease* or *atherosclerosis*. Many studies have linked the incidence of heart disease with dietary intake of cholesterol and saturated fat. The greatest evidence has come from epidemiological studies which show that people in countries with high cholesterol rates have high rates of heart attack. The most graphic example is a comparison between the Japanese, who have a low average cholesterol (165 mg/100 ml), versus the peo-

Cholesterol as a Risk Factor for Coronary Heart Disease		
AGE	MODERATE RISK 75TH–90TH PERCENTILE	HIGH RISK ABOVE 90TH PERCENTILE
20–29	200–220 mg/dl	above 220 mg/dl
30–39	220–240 mg/dl	above 240 mg/dl
over 40	240–260 mg/dl	above 260 mg/dl

Source: Adapted from National Institutes of Health Consensus Conference.

ple of Finland, who have a high average cholesterol (265 mg/100 ml): the Japanese heart attack rate is 94 per 100,000, while the Finnish rate is 996 per 100,000. A recent study found that for every 1% drop in blood cholesterol levels, there is a 2% drop in coronary risk. Because heart attack is the leading cause of death in the U.S., and middle-aged men are particularly at risk, reduction of cholesterol and fat intake is probably the most significant dietary change a person can make in midadulthood. (For more information on cholesterol and heart disease, see p. 260.)

The second most widespread disease affected by diet is *hypertension*, or *high blood pressure*. Untreated high blood pressure puts a person at risk for heart attack as well as stroke and kidney disease. Diet is related to hypertension through both obesity and salt intake. Hypertension can often be prevented or treated by reducing salt intake and maintaining an ideal weight. Again, most of the studies supporting these changes are epidemiological: cultures with very low salt intake have little or no incidence of high blood pressure. Studies have shown that a high salt in-

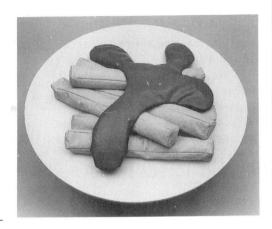

French-fried potatoes have 130 times the fat content of boiled potatoes. Claes Oldenburg. French Fries and Ketchup. 1963. Vinyl filled with kapok. 10½" × 42 × 44". Collection, The Whitney Museum of American Art. 50th Anniversary Gift of Mr. and Mrs. Robert M. Meltzer. 79.37.

Types of Fat

Saturated fats*
beef
butter
cheese
chocolate
coconut
coconut oil
egg yolk
ice cream
lard
lobster
milk
palm oil
pork
poultry
shellfish
veal
vegetable shortening (can be)

Monounsaturated fats*
avocado
cashews
olive oil
olives
peanut butter
peanut oil
peanuts

Polyunsaturated fats*
almonds
corn oil
cottonseed oil
filberts
fish
margarines †
pecans
safflower oil
soybean oil
sunflower oil

* Saturated fats raise the level of cholesterol in the blood; monounsaturated and polyunsaturated fats do not.

† Margarines may contain saturated fat depending upon what oils they are made of.

Guide to Reducing Dietary Fat and Cholesterol

- use non-fat or low-fat dairy products
- use skim-milk cheeses (ricotta, cottage, or farmer cheese)
- serve more poultry and fish, less red meat
- trim all visible fat from meat
- remove skin from poultry before cooking
- use veal instead of beef
- use lean, not prime cuts
- use lean hamburger meat
- boil, bake, or steam food rather than fry it
- broil meat on racks
- buy fish that is canned in water rather than oil
- skim fat from soups and sautéed food
- use less oil in salad dressings
- use low-fat yogurt and flavored vinegars in salad dressings
- substitute low-fat yogurt for sour cream or mayonnaise
- substitute sorbet or ice milk for ice cream
- avoid using large amounts of nuts and seeds
- avoid high-fat luncheon meats and hot dogs
- avoid or limit egg recipes
- use fewer egg yolks in recipes; add egg whites
- avoid high-fat crackers; check ingredients
- avoid crackers, cookies, tortillas, etc., made with lard
- substitute vegetable oil for lard
- substitute margarine for butter
- avoid or limit use of shellfish

take over a period of 10 days will raise blood pressure by 10 points in a susceptible person. On the other hand, reduction of salt in the diet will reduce blood pressure by 5–10 points in individuals with hypertension.

Like high salt intake, obesity correlates directly with high blood pressure in adults. Adults who are considerably overweight (20% or more) are two-and-a-half times as likely to develop hypertension in middle age. In addition, blood pressure levels routinely drop 10 points when obese people lose a significant amount of weight (see p. 278).

Probably the third most significant disease linked with diet is *Type II* or *noninsulin-dependent diabetes mellitus.* Doctors have long recognized that over 80% of the people who have this type of diabetes are overweight. Researchers now hypothesize that constant overeating produces high levels of circulating insulin which eventually leads to a decrease in the number of insulin receptors in individual cells. This decrease means that people no longer metabolize sugar as effectively. A low-calorie diet, on the other hand, results in a decrease in the amount of

Cheeses That Are High in Fat and/or Salt

CHEESE	FAT CONTENT	SALT CONTENT
blue cheese	high	very high
Camembert	medium	high
cheddar	high	medium
cream cheese	high	low
feta	medium	high
low-fat creamed cottage cheese	low	very high
low-fat processed cheese	low	high
Monterey Jack	high	medium
Muenster	high	medium
Parmesan cheese	medium	very high
processed American cheese	high	very high
processed American cheese food	medium	high
processed cheese spreads	medium	very high
provolone	medium	high
Romano	medium	high
Roquefort	high	very high
whole milk ricotta	high	low

insulin naturally produced and an increase in the amount of insulin receptors on cells (see p. 381). For this reason, dietary control is the main treatment as well as the main prevention for Type II diabetes. Studies have also shown that a high-fiber diet helps to bring diabetes under control.

As common sense would suggest, diet plays an important role in diseases of the gastrointestinal tract. *Diverticulitis* was virtually unknown before the invention of roller-milled flour, and it is still uncommon in areas where people eat a high-fiber diet. *Cancer of the colon, constipation, appendicitis,* and *irritable bowel syndrome* have all been linked to low-fiber diets as well. Although the link between cancer and diet has not been established as strongly as the link between heart disease and diet, it is still significant. The National Research Council report of 1983, called *Diet, Nutrition, and Cancer,* stated that 30%–40% of cancers in men, and up to 60% of cancers in women may be related to diet. A high-fat diet is linked to high rates of *cancer of the breast, prostate,* and *large bowel*. Interestingly, the report also gave evidence that certain foods, as well as fiber, have a protective effect against cancer. These foods include those that are high in Vitamin A, Vitamin C, and vegetables in the cruciform family (broccoli, cauliflower, brussels sprouts, cabbage, and kale).

Finally, diet plays the major role in the development of *obesity*. Obesity is a medical problem, not just a social one, because it directly leads to or aggravates a number of serious medical conditions. Among them are heart disease, adult-onset diabetes, gallstones, and osteoarthritis. Obesity is associated with high blood pressure, high blood cholesterol, and many cancers including cancer of the breast, uterus, colon, and prostate. As a result, obesity has a strongly adverse effect on longevity, an effect that becomes progressively worse as a person's weight increases (see p. 446).

All of these studies emphasize the importance of diet and also underscore what can be gained by taking diet seriously. It's important to reiterate that many of the serious diseases of adulthood can be *delayed* or completely *prevented* through changes in nutrition. Diet is also a major factor in *treating* these diseases once they have developed. A healthy diet is a less expensive and more effective strategy for staying well than relying on medical treatment to "cure" illness once it develops.

Cholesterol Content of Foods

FOOD	CHOLESTEROL IN MG
whole milk, 1 cup	34
skim milk, 1 cup	11
cheddar cheese, 1 ounce	30
ice cream, 1 cup	88
egg, 1 whole	275
butter, 1 tablespoon	33
margarine, 1 tablespoon	0
lard, ¼ pound	110
mayonnaise, 1 tablespoon	10
hot dog, 1	22
lean red meat, ¼ pound	80
chicken, 100 grams	60
fish, ¼ pound	80
lobster, ¼ pound	225
oysters, ¼ pound	225
shrimp, shelled, ¼ pound	140

Note: The recommended daily allowance of cholesterol is 300 mg.

Facts About Salt

- the sodium in salt causes cells to retain water, which leads to high blood pressure in sensitive people
- most Americans eat 4,000–8,000 mg of salt per day; for good health, the American Heart Association recommends only 2,000 mg
- under most conditions, people need only about 200 mg of salt per day
- there's enough sodium in foods naturally to meet daily requirements without adding salt

A Prescription for Diet

Because of the importance of nutritional change in terms of health promotion, several national committees have drawn up guidelines for the general public. The recommendations are sweeping. There is no doubt that if they were adhered to widely, they would have a tremendous, positive effect on health in the U.S. The most famous and widely agreed-upon recommendations, issued by the Senate Select Committee on Nutrition in 1979, are called *Dietary Goals for the United States*. This report advocates reducing fat consumption from 43% of total caloric intake to 30%, reducing saturated fat to 10% of total daily calories, reducing cholesterol to 300 mg per day, limiting salt to 5 gm per day, reducing refined sugars to 10% of total daily calories, and increasing fruit and vegetable consumption. In addition, the guidelines urge people to eat only as many calories as they ac-

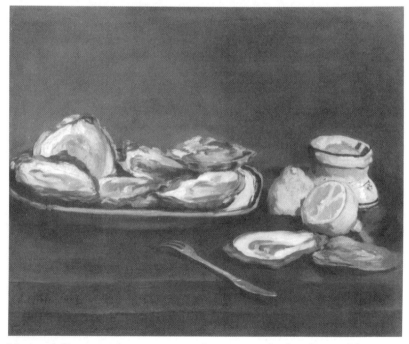

National dietary goals encourage eating more seafood and vegetables. Edouard Manet. Oysters. 1862. National Gallery of Art, Washington. Gift of the Adele R. Levy Fund, Inc.

tually need. While most diets basically agree with the national guidelines, a number go a step further than the goals set by the Senate committee in its report. For example, the most radical of these diets, the Pritikin Program, recommends getting only 5%–15% of one's daily calories from fat. As research shows a more and more direct relationship between diet and heart disease, updated guidelines suggest lower and lower figures for fat and cholesterol. If people cannot achieve a cholesterol level of under 200 with a diet of 30% fat and 300 mg of cholesterol per day, the 1987 guidelines from the National Heart, Lung, and Blood Institute recommend decreasing fat intake to 7% of total daily calories and cholesterol intake to 200 mg per day.

Most diets use several techniques to help people keep to their dietary goals. First, they suggest *keeping track of food intake, counting calories*, and *monitoring fat and salt consumption*. Although cumbersome, keeping records and calculating intake makes people much more aware of what foods they're eating and how much of them they're consuming. The positive aspect of counting calories is that as long as people stick to their limits, they can eat whatever they wish, including occasional high-calorie, fatty, or salty foods.

Secondly, to help people keep to weight-loss goals, many diets *divide food into groups*, giving people a variety of choices within each category and between categories. Generally, the categories are (1) meat, poultry, and seafood; (2) dairy products; (3) breads, cereals, and starchy foods; (4) fats; (5) fruits; and (6) nonstarchy vegetables. This system is referred to as an "exchange system." People are allowed a specific number of exchanges within the basic groups. Such a system is often used with diabetics. The third technique suggested is *restricting foods*. People are given one list of foods that should be avoided because of high amounts of sodium, fat, or cholesterol, and another list of recommended foods that are low in these nutrients.

Most diets target meat, fish, and poultry for special attention because this group, by itself, supplies almost 50% of the fat that the average person eats. Furthermore, most people are getting more protein than they actually need. Some diets emphasize seafood because it is lower in fat, contains more polyunsaturated fat, and contains special polyunsaturated fatty acids that help to reduce cholesterol. Chicken with the skin removed before cook-

High-Salt Foods to Avoid

American cheese
bacon
bouillon
corned beef
cottage cheese
dried meat or fish
frankfurters
ham
instant chocolate drinks
instant hot cereals
luncheon meats
meat tenderizers (salted)
most packaged or canned
     soups
most packaged or restaurant
     food
olives
Parmesan cheese
pickled foods
processed cheese and cheese
     products
Roquefort cheese
salted, canned meat, or fish
salted crackers
salted pretzels, chips, popcorn
salted spices (e.g., garlic salt)
sauerkraut
sausage
soy and teriyaki sauce
vegetable juices
Worcestershire sauce

Minimizing Sodium Intake

- don't add salt in cooking or at the table
- use unprocessed foods which are naturally low in salt: grains and cereals, vegetables, fruits, fish, poultry, and meat
- use dairy products that are lowest in salt: unsalted cottage cheese, Gruyere, ricotta, Swiss cheese, and unsalted margarine
- eat fresh foods, which are naturally flavorful
- avoid commercial salad dressings
- use no-salt seasonings such as citrus fruits and juices, wine, dry mustard, parsley, garlic, onions, mushrooms, green peppers, apples, and other herbs and spices
- avoid softened water (which is high in sodium)
- avoid over-the-counter and prescription drugs that contain sodium

ing or turkey with the skin removed after cooking are also low in fat. Generally, diets also recommend lowering the amount of red meat eaten because of the fat it contains, and avoiding organ meats altogether. Eggs yolks are usually limited to two per week because they are highly concentrated sources of cholesterol (see chart).

The national guidelines not only limit fat intake to 30% of the total daily calories, they advise that saturated fats be avoided or their intake lowered. The highest sources of saturated fats include meat and dairy products, cocoa, and specific vegetable oils such as palm and coconut. These vegetable oils are often used in packaged foods because of their long shelf life. Nondairy creamers, whipped toppings, crackers, commercial bakery products, and chocolate are also very high in saturated oils. Finally, many diets also recommend eating more whole grains to increase fiber and more low-fat dairy products to increase calcium.

Because Americans now eat an average of one out of three meals in restaurants, it often requires special effort to keep to the national guidelines. It is best to choose restaurants that serve low-fat foods such as broiled seafood and plain boiled vegetables. Salad should be ordered without dressing or with dressing on the side. Plain fruit is best for dessert.

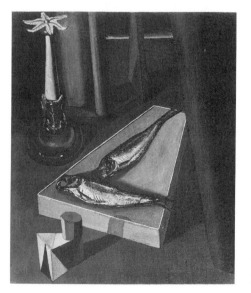

Many kinds of fish contain omega-3 fatty acids that help to lower blood cholesterol levels. Giorgio di Chirico. The Sacred Fish. 1919. Oil on canvas. 29½" × 24⅜". Collection, The Museum of Modern Art, New York. Acquired through the Lillie P. Bliss Bequest.

High-Calcium Foods

FOOD	AMOUNT	CALCIUM CONTENT
broccoli	1 stalk	160 mg
low-fat milk	1 cup	350 mg
low-fat yogurt	1 cup	452 mg
low-fat cottage cheese	1 cup	211 mg
oatmeal	¾ cup	188 mg
salmon	3 ounces	170 mg
tofu	4 ounces	150 mg

Note: The daily calcium requirement is 800 mg for men, 1,000 mg for premenopausal women, and 1,400 mg for postmenopausal women.

High-Potassium Foods

apricots
bananas
dates
figs
melons
oranges
prunes
raisins
beans
mushrooms
peas
potatoes
spinach
sweet potaotes
tomatoes
winter squash

Decreasing Dietary Sugar

• avoid cakes, candy, and cookies; instead, eat fresh fruits and low-sugar sorbets
• avoid sugared soft drinks; substitute flavored mineral waters, or a combination of juice and seltzer water
• avoid sugar in coffee or tea; substitute cinnamon or spices
• use low-sugar jams
• flavor pancakes with cinnamon, nutmeg, or vanilla extract
• dilute pancake syrup with water

To supplement the general dietary guidelines, individuals need to determine their own specific dietary goals based on their present weight as compared with their desired weight, and based on their blood cholesterol level. In addition, people need to take into consideration whether they have any existing medical condition or are at risk for a particular disease. In addition to the weight charts (see p. 442), there are two quick ways to determine if you are overweight. First, simply stand in front of a mirror without any clothes on. For most people, this exercise leaves no question as to whether or not they are overweight. Second, while lying on your back, place a long ruler lengthwise on your abdomen. If you are not overweight, the ruler should touch both your ribs and pubic bone.

Food Behaviors

Like other behaviors, food habits are deeply ingrained and require motivation and diligence to change. Behavioral medicine sheds some interesting light on people's food behaviors, and several of its strategies have been successful in helping people to lose weight and improve their nutrition. *Substitution* involves replacing a high-calorie, high-fat, salty, or sugary food with another food that is low in that ingredient. This is one of the most successful behavior changes because it merely involves modifying habits rather than eliminating them. Substitution applies to both buying and cooking patterns. *Portion control* involves reducing the number or size of food portions eaten each day. Food should be served up in the kitchen, rather than put out in bowls on the table, family style, in order to prevent people from eating seconds and thirds. Small plates are useful because psychologically they make portion sizes seem larger. Also, it's important to separate eating environments from noneating environments. Another valuable technique involves keeping a journal of what is eaten each day, what one's goals are, what techniques will be employed, and what rewards will be used for successful intervention and/or weight loss. More specific information on nutrition is given in the discussions on obesity, heart disease, hypertension, diabetes, and diverticulitis.

Without a question, dietary change is the single easiest and most far-reaching life-style improvement we can make, which is not to say that attitude change, stress reduction, exercise, and giving up smoking are not important. People inevitably make changes in their diet as health becomes a concern to them. The more we tune in to our body's signals, the better we understand the link between diet and health, and the more naturally we alter our eating habits. The cycle becomes self-perpetuating because the better we eat, the better we feel.

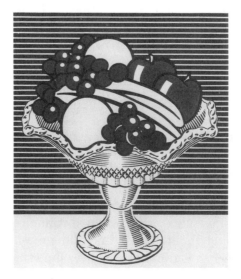

Diet is one of the most controllable factors in our life-style. Roy Lichtenstein. Still Life with Crystal Bowl. *1973. Oil and magna on canvas. 52" × 42". Collection, The Whitney Museum of American Art. Purchase, with funds from Frances and Sydney Lewis. 77.64.*

CHAPTER SIX

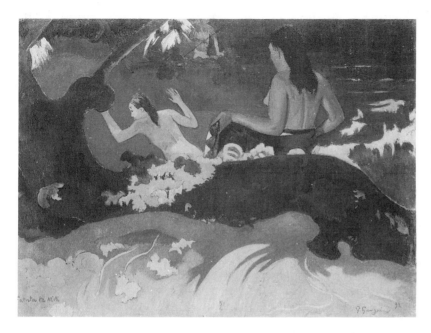

Exercise and Health

We all know how much better we feel when we are fit. People who take up a regular exercise program will tell you they look and feel better, have more energy, and feel more self-confident. When people don't exercise regularly, they can lose touch with those good feelings. People who exercise also tend to lose excess weight, and many adopt a healthier life-style in other ways, such as eating better and stopping smoking. Taken all together, increased fitness, greater energy, and more positivity add greatly to a person's sense of well-being.

An increasing number of studies shows that regular exercise is an important part of maintaining good health. Physical activity is clearly beneficial for the maintenance of the cardiovascular system, the musculoskeletal system, the autonomic nervous system, and for the mind. Frequent, vigorous exercise reduces the risk of coronary heart disease and sudden death, lowers the in-

---

Physical fitness and being in the outdoors contribute profoundly to our sense of well-being. Paul Gaugin. Fatata te Miti. 1813. National Gallery of Art, Washington. Chester Dale Collection, 1962.

cidence of diabetes, high blood pressure, and osteoporosis, helps people cope more effectively with stress, and reduces symptoms such as depression and anxiety. Because of this type of evidence, several major health organizations (the World Health Organization, the American Heart Association, the U.S. Public Health Service, and the Royal College of Physicians of London) have endorsed exercise as a means of promoting long-term health. The U.S. Public Health Service has targeted exercise as one of the most important health promotion areas.

Over the last 50 years, the average person's life-style in Western industrialized countries has become increasingly sedentary. This is especially true for adults. The majority of adults ride to work in a vehicle, sit at a desk all day, and then go home and watch television. Their only significant physical activity occurs during leisure time, if some form of exercise happens to be their choice of a leisure activity. Unfortunately, leisure activities are often sedentary.

Within the last decade or so, a trend toward regular exercise has started, but studies show that although such exercise is very visible and is given a high profile in the media, it does not actually involve a very large percentage of the people in midadulthood. Studies have shown that in terms of health, the greatest gain in the risk-benefit ratio of exercise takes place in people who are the most sedentary. Put more directly, it is important for people who engage in physical activity to increase the time they spend exercising, but it is even more beneficial for nonexercisers to begin some kind of physical activity.

The Hunter-Gatherer and Exercise

Looked at in terms of evolution, it is not surprising that exercise should have a positive effect on health. Throughout 99% of our evolution, human beings have had to be quite active. Two medical anthropologists, Drs. Boyd Eaton and Melvin Konner, have assessed the fitness or our Paleolithic ancestors, whose bone width most closely resembled that of well-conditioned modern athletes. Based on their studies, they believe that the average person today is only one-third as fit. According to Konner and Eaton, Paleolithic men and women had a "lifelong ex-

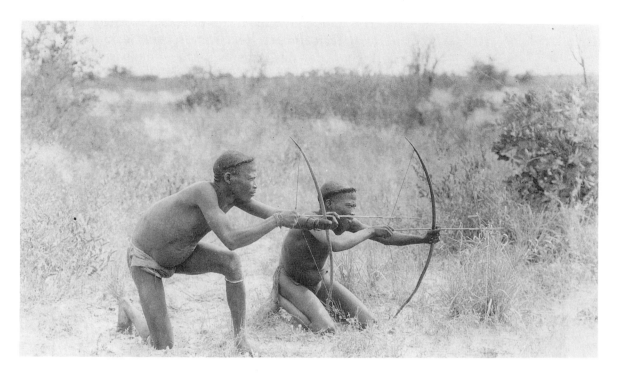

ercise program" that developed both strength and endurance, and varied with seasonal tasks. Such exercise didn't require any planning, it was simply a required part of hunting and food gathering, and as such, it was an integral part of people's lives. The necessity, variety, and change inherent in the exercise of prehistoric people prevented burnout and boredom, problems not uncommon to modern exercisers. Eaton and Konner believe that cyclical variety must be built in, in order for training to remain fresh and invigorating. They also believe that human genes are programmed so that the greatest benefit occurs when strength and endurance training occur simultaneously.

Through 99 percent of our evolutionary history, humans have had an active lifestyle. Bushmen Archers. *Courtesy, The American Museum of Natural History.*

Disease and Lack of Exercise

As compared with our prehistoric ancestors, contemporary men and women are totally unadapted for the sedentary lifestyle they lead, and it's not surprising that lack of exercise is thought to be a factor in a number of modern illnesses. In terms of death and disability, the major disease associated with lack of exercise is *heart disease*. There are several major studies that form the basis for this statement. One famous study was done by English epidemiologist J. Morris, who compared two groups of British civil servants and found that those who did *not* engage in vigorous leisure-time activity had twice the risk of heart disease. Stanford epidemiologist Dr. Ralph Paffenbarger found that among San Francisco longshoremen those men who were active had about one-half the heart attack rate of the group who were not active. In another study, Paffenbarger followed 17,000 Harvard alumni over a 10-year period. Those alumni who got moderate exercise in their leisure-time had 50% less heart attacks and sudden death than those who got little exercise. Finally, a Seattle study of leisure activity and cardiac arrests found that people who were sedentary had 2.4 times the chance of cardiac arrest.

In reviewing these and other studies, it has been theorized that a distinct threshold must be crossed in order to make exercise valuable as a preventive measure for heart disease. The threshold is estimated to be 7.5 kcal per minute, an expenditure of energy which corresponds to brisk walking, heavy gardening, or slow bicycling. However, a very recent study indicates that low-to-moderate exercise—exercise that doesn't even produce

Diseases Improved by Exercise

arthritis
heart disease
high blood pressure
low-back pain
non-insulin-dependent
  diabetes
obstructive lung disease
osteoporosis

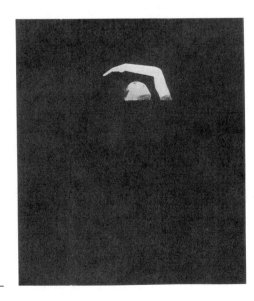

Aerobic exercise lowers the risk of heart disease. Robert Moskowitz. Swimmer. 1977. Oil and pure pigment on canvas. 90″ × 74¾″. Collection, The Whitney Museum of American Art. Gift of Jennifer Bartlett. 82.9.

physical conditioning—can still have a beneficial effect on cardiovascular health. This study found that people who walked short distances outside the house or climbed stairs were less at risk for heart disease than those who didn't.

In terms of preventing heart attacks, the protective effect of exercise is independent of other risk factors such as smoking, stress, high blood pressure, and/or obesity. In fact, the greatest effect of exercise applies to those who *are* at risk for other reasons, in particular, those who are hypertensive or obese. Exercise has also been found to be beneficial for people who have had heart attacks. Regular exercise reduces symptoms in angina patients, and it reduces the incidence of mortality from a second heart attack. All of these benefits outweigh the slightly elevated risk of cardiac arrest that accompanies vigorous exercise. For this reason, heart attack patients are monitored carefully in recovery exercise programs, and people over 40 are advised to have a physical exam before beginning a rigorous exercise program.

The second most important disease affected by exercise is *high blood pressure*. Several major studies have shown that increased physical activity is associated with a decrease in blood pressure levels. In large population studies, active people have been found to have an average diastolic blood pressure reading 2–5 mmHg lower than nonactive people. The Harvard alumni study found that those people who did not exercise were 35% more likely to have high blood pressure. Other studies have specifically dealt with the effect that beginning exercise had on blood pressure. In studies of people having either normal or elevated blood pressure, the diastolic pressure was found to drop with exercise. This effect was most pronounced among those people who had hypertension. All of this research points to the fact that regular exercise can *prevent* high blood pressure, as well as help to control it.

The third most significant disease in which exercise plays a role is *noninsulin-dependent diabetes*. Exercise not only helps in weight control, which is an important part of the diabetic regimen, it has profound and positive effects on metabolism. Studies have shown that exercise reduces blood glucose levels, increases insulin receptors within the cells, and increases the effectiveness of insulin itself. Because of these physiological effects, one would expect, and indeed does find, more diabetes in sedentary people. A study done in the South Pacific found that inactive people had a much higher incidence of diabetes than active people, regardless of obesity. Other studies have shown that there is more diabetes among urban as opposed to rural populations, and researchers have speculated that this difference may be associated with exercise patterns.

Studies have also shown that diabetics have more difficulty with glucose control when they become sedentary. The most serious complications experienced by diabetics involve an accelerated build-up of fat deposits within the large blood vessels in the legs, heart, and brain, resulting in atherosclerosis and heart disease. Exercise reduces the risk of these complications, which makes exercise even more important for a diabetic than for the average person. Exercise not only helps people with diabetes, it probably helps prevent diabetes from developing in obese people with a family history of the disease.

Recent studies have also found that exercise is important in the treatment and prevention of musculoskeletal diseases. In terms of *osteoporosis*, it has been shown that bone density is greater in active people and the incidence of fractures is lower. Several studies have demonstrated that exercise training programs specifically retard bone loss in older women, and that being bedridden or totally inactive at any age is associated with a great decrease in bone density. In addition to osteoporosis, *arthritis* and *low back pain* are often improved by exercise. There is even some evidence that exercise is beneficial for people with *obstructive lung disease* and *colon cancer*.

In addition to primary or direct preventive effects on health, exercise has secondary effects on the body's metabolism that help prevent illness by lowering the incidence of general risk factors, such as obesity, which increase the likelihood of a number of conditions. Since exercise raises resting metabolic rates and energy expenditures, people who exercise can consume about 15% more calories and still maintain a stable weight. Long-term weight control requires a balance between food intake and energy expenditure. It is interesting to note that scientists think that one of the main reasons people become obese in midadulthood is simply because they become increasingly sedentary, without lowering their food intake correspondingly.

Another secondary effect of exercise is that it raises the level

Calories Expended by Exercise

TYPE OF EXERCISE	CALORIES CONSUMED PER HOUR
biking (fast: 13 mph)	660
biking (slow: 5 mph)	210
bowling	270
driving	120
gardening	220
golf	250
hill climbing	480
horseback riding	350
light housework	180
mowing with a power mower	250
pingpong	360
racquetball	600
running (moderate: 10 mph)	900
sitting	100
sleeping	80
standing	140
swimming (moderate: 2 mph)	500
swimming (slow: ¼ mph)	300
tennis	420
volleyball	350
walking (brisk: 3¾ mph)	300
walking (slow: 2½ mph)	210

of *HDLs (high-density lipoproteins)*, one of two cholesterol-transporting substances that circulate in the blood. Whereas *LDLs (low-density lipoproteins)* carry cholesterol out to the tissues, HDLs bring cholesterol back to the liver for processing. HDLs have a protective effect on the heart because they help to dissolve the fatty plaques that form in the arteries. Exercise also lowers the triglyceride levels and eventually drops total lipid or fat levels. The effect of moderate exercise on total cholesterol levels has not yet been established.

Exercise also seems to play an important part in mental health, alleviating anxiety and symptoms of mild-to-moderate depression. Moreover, it has been found that exercisers experience improved self-confidence, increased self-esteem, and better cognitive function. For these reasons exercise is a vital adjunct to alcoholism and substance-abuse treatment programs. These psychological effects may be crucial in terms of overall health improvement. As we discussed in the chapter on stress, depression makes illness more likely. On the other hand, increased self-confidence and heightened self-esteem make illness less likely (see p. 53). Exercise has even been found to alter some aspects of coronary-prone Type A behavior (see p. 48). Furthermore, exercise changes the body's reaction to stress, which improves mental and physical health in general.

The Physical Effects of Exercise

To appreciate the full range of what exercise does to the body, we must look not only at how exercise prevents disease, but at how it makes the body healthier. Exercise consists of physical activities that expend energy through movement of the voluntary or skeletal muscles. Rhythmic contractions of large muscles require a good supply of oxygenated blood from the heart and lungs. The amount of freshly oxygenated blood that the body can easily provide is the result of long-term conditioning brought about by meeting prior demands. Thus, sedentary people are adapted to low demands on their cardiovascular system and can provide relatively little oxygenated blood to their muscles, which is the reason they can only do a small amount of work and tire

Benefits of Regular Aerobic Exercise

increased lung capacity
lower breathing rate
lower heart rate at rest
lower heart rate during exercise
increased blood volume per heartbeat
lower blood pressure
lower LDL cholesterol levels
higher HDL (protective) cholesterol levels
lower triglyceride levels
lower uric acid levels
decreased platelet stickiness
increased muscle strength
increased flexibility
increased skill
increased muscle capacity
increased insulin–receptor sensitivity
increased sense of physical well-being
increased sense of mental well-being
reduced depression and anxiety

quickly. With proper training over a period of time, sedentary people *of any age* can achieve significant improvements in their stamina and ability to do increased amounts of work. This is what makes exercisers feel better and have increased energy.

For exercise to produce a training response, it must put a stress on a given muscle, and the level of stress must slowly build up over a period of weeks and months. When a slightly increased amount of stress is put on the muscles each day, a group of physiological changes gradually occur which allow the muscles to do more work. The first result of training is an increase in the size of muscle fibers and in the blood supply to them. Like the voluntary muscles, the heart undergoes a training effect, which

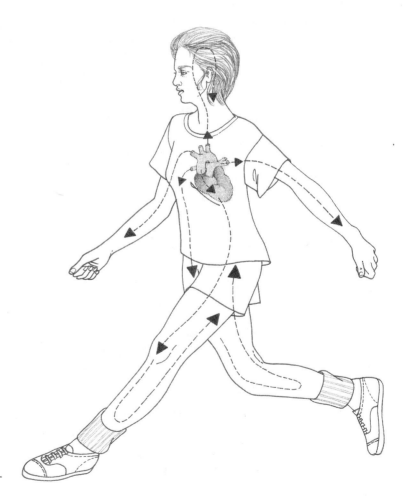

Regular strenuous exercise increases the amount the heart pumps with each beat and decreases the number of times the heart pumps at rest, sending more blood out to the body with less work.

enables it to pump an increased amount of blood with each stroke. This increase in stroke volume is the most important result of training. In addition, the body's total blood volume increases, enabling the circulatory system to carry much more oxygen at any given time.

With a month of graded exercise, the stroke volume of the heart can be increased by 10%. The stroke volume at rest in an untrained adult is 60–70 ml per beat; after a month of training, it can be raised to 66–77 ml per beat. Professional athletes can ultimately increase their stroke volume to 100 ml. As a result of increased stroke volume, people can not only do more work at any given time, but, at moments of rest and at low amounts of exertion, their heart does not have to pump as often as an untrained person's. At a submaximum workload, a trained person's heart beats 20–30 times less per minute than an untrained person's. This lower heart rate is accompanied by a lower oxygen need, and a longer rest period between beats during which the heart is able to absorb oxygen. Not only does the heart pump more efficiently, the voluntary muscles are able to take up oxygen more effectively; in turn, the mitochondria, the tiny energy factories in the muscle cells, are better able to synthesize energy. The result is that a trained person can do much more work with much less strain on the heart and muscles than can an untrained person.

Exercise also has profound effects on the body's hormone system. The hormone-releasing capacity of the pituitary and adrenal glands increases greatly with exercise, enabling a person to react more rapidly and efficiently to stress or work situations. The autonomic nervous system, the part of the nervous system that mediates a person's reaction to stress, becomes more efficient and is able to return to normal more quickly after a period of stress. These changes apply not only to physical stressors, but to mental ones as well. Both emotional tension and inactivity involve higher than normal levels of sympathetic nervous system activity. Thus sedentary people, as well as people who are under prolonged mental stress, have high blood levels of the fight-or-flight hormones. The result is that these people are constantly in a slight state of stress that causes their heart to beat a little faster and need a little more oxygen. By comparison, a person who is trained or simply relaxed goes into a relaxation state between

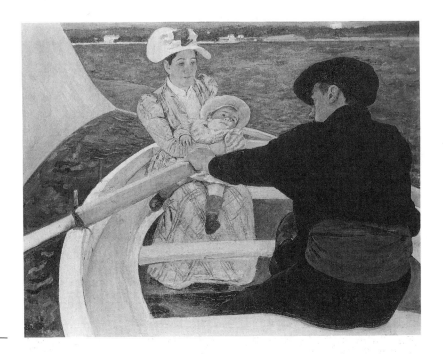

Exercise, like relaxation, helps to counter stress. Mary Cassatt. Boating Party. 1893. National Gallery of Art, Washington. Chester Dale Collection.

stresses or energy demands. It is an amazing concept that exercise can help to "tune" the body to cope with stress. And it is particularly pertinent, and important, to men and women today, whose health patterns are so greatly affected by stress. This relationship between stress and exercise points up the holistic nature of preventive medicine.

A Prescription for Physical Activity

Recent research on the relationship between exercise and health has greatly simplified the recommendations for exercise. Studies have shown how much exercise is required to achieve the minimum changes necessary for the health of the heart, lungs, and metabolic system. Currently, the consensus is that people should exercise fairly intensely two or three times a week—once at the least—for periods of at least 15–20 minutes at a time. Exhaustion should always be avoided, especially for those who are normally sedentary. As we've discussed, training only takes place if the training stimulus or stress is slightly greater than that which people are used to. Thus, any specific exercise prescription must depend on an individual's personal health, current fitness, and long-range goals. It is important to note that the goals of athletic fitness and those of health are not necessarily the same. Health goals require much lower levels of training than peak physical fitness goals, and, in fact, peak fitness goals can cause injuries and be counterproductive to health in some instances.

Only activities in which large groups of muscles are subjected to dynamic stress result in cardiovascular conditioning. Aerobic activities that have cardiovascular effects include running, cycling, swimming, rowing, cross-country skiing, climbing, and ball games such as racquetball. The most beneficial of these activities are the ones that achieve conditioning with the least short- or long-term injury to the muscles and joints. From this standpoint, the most effective activities are cycling, cross-country skiing, swimming, brisk walking, and carefully moderated long-distance running.

In terms of frequency, it has been found that the most beneficial heart-training exercise is done daily, and if that is impossible, the next best is at least three times a week. But even once a week is better than none, though the benefits are not as great. The amount of time that should be spent exercising on any given

Target Pulse Rates for Exercise

- *maximum heart rate* is determined by subtracting your age from 220
- 70%–85% of a person's maximum heart rate is the *target* for most effective aerobic training
- check pulse immediately upon ceasing exercise. Since pulse rate normally drops very quickly, count pulse for only 10 seconds, then multiply by six to determine rate

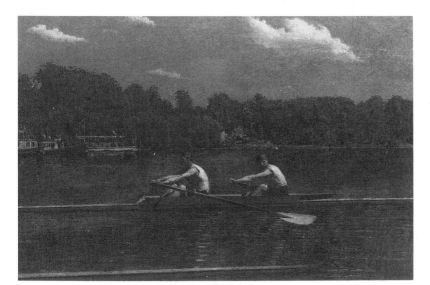

To obtain the greatest health benefits, exercise should be done on a regular basis, several times a week. Thomas Eakins. The Biglin Brothers Racing. 1873. National Gallery of Art, Washington. Gift of Mr. and Mrs. Cornelius Vanderbilt Whitney, 1953.

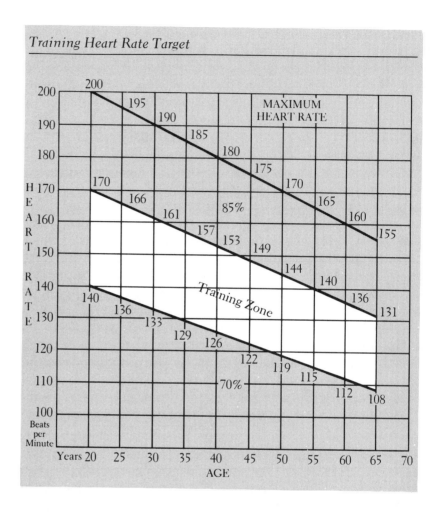

Training Heart Rate Target

occasion depends on the number of times a person exercises per week, but in general the optimum length of a session is 30–40 minutes. This amount of time is necessary to produce a significant change in the heart over a period of weeks and months. However, somewhat less time can be spent if exercise is done daily; somewhat more would be necessary if exercise is done only once a week.

To be beneficial, the intensity of the exercise has to be sufficient to produce a change, but this depends entirely upon prior conditioning. Most exercise physiologists agree that the stress should be a minimum of 50% of people's ability to bring oxygen to their muscles. The simplest way of determining this load involves measuring the pulse during exercise. The pulse is counted for 10 seconds and multiplied by six to get the number of beats per minute. Since heart rate drops quickly in a well-conditioned person, the pulse must be counted as soon as exercise is stopped. For a healthy person under 50 years of age, 50% of the maximum ability to supply oxygen to the muscles corresponds to a pulse rate of about 130 beats per minute; for healthy people over 50, the recommended pulse is 180 minus their age in years (at 60 years, the rate would be $180 - 60 = 120$).

People who are exercise beginners or out of shape should not try to reach their maximum pulse rate immediately if it causes them to become exhausted. Rather, they should start with a pulse rate of 110 beats per minute, and gradually build up to their maximum over a period of weeks. Likewise, people who are not in condition should begin with short periods of exercise, whatever they can do comfortably, punctuated by resting periods. When they become fatigued, they should stop for the day.

All exercise physiologists warn people to avoid exercising to the point of straining or becoming overly fatigued. Unfortunately, many people are impatient, competitive, or do not read their body's signs well, and they immediately go out and overexercise. Not only can this response be dangerous, it can cause people to become discouraged and give up exercise altogether. Obviously this is most important for people who have never exercised regularly but it is also important for people who have exercised routinely, but have stopped training for a time because of illness, travel, life-style changes, etc. There are three simple guidelines to determine if people are exercising too hard: (1) they develop symptoms such as tightness in the chest or lightheadedness, (2) their heart rate doesn't drop significantly within 5–10 minutes after stopping exercise, and (3) they are breathless 10 minutes after ceasing aerobic activity (see chart).

Checking the pulse is the simplest means of determining how strenuously people should exercise, but researchers have more precise and complex techniques as well. By monitoring breathing during a treadmill test, researchers can determine the exact amount of oxygen that people are using. The rate of oxygen consumption, called the VO_2 (*volume of oxygen consumed*), is the best measure of people's aerobic capacity, that is, of their

Suggestions for Increasing Daily Activity Level

- stand instead of sitting or reclining
- whenever possible, walk instead of driving
- park or get off bus several blocks from destination; walk between stores
- use stairs instead of elevators or escalators
- do your own housecleaning and yardwork
- take short walks during work breaks
- walk with your dog
- walk and talk with friends instead of sitting and talking

Advice for Exercising Safely

- get in shape slowly
- before exercising, warm up for 5–10 minutes by doing stretches, sit-ups, or slow movement
- exercise regularly: 3–5 times per week, 20–30 minutes per session, at a pulse rate that is 70%–85% of your maximum (220 minus your age), 50% if you are just starting to exercise
- after exercising, cool down for 5–10 minutes by doing slowdown activities or stretches
- stop exercising if you experience fatigue, breathlessness, or pain

Amount of Exercise Needed to Maintain Good Aerobic Condition After You Build Up to Fitness

TYPE OF EXERCISE	FREQUENCY	DISTANCE	TIME
Walking	3 times per wk.	4 miles	48–58 min.
	5 times per wk.	3 miles	36–43 min.
Running	3 times per wk.	2 miles	13–16 min.
	5 times per wk.	1.5 miles	12–15 min.
Biking	3 times per wk.	8 miles	24–32 min.
	5 times per wk.	6 miles	18–24 min.
Swimming	3 times per wk.	1,000 yards	16–25 min.
	4 times per wk.	800 yards	13–20 min.

Source: Adapted from K. Cooper, The New Aerobics.

ability to supply oxygen to the muscles. People's maximum capacity to take in oxygen is called their $VO_{2\ MAX}$. $VO_{2\ MAX}$ is a measure of people's conditioning, and increases with training. The suggested minimum target for training is 50% of $VO_{2\ MAX}$. At 80% of $VO_{2\ MAX}$, people begin to run out of air and become exhausted. Less conservative exercise physiologists recommend that healthy people train at values higher than 50%—usually 60%–75%.

Using a conditioned person to judge by, the VO_2 can become a measure of the intensity of a particular type of activity. This measure is often expressed in *metabolic units* or *METs*. One metabolic unit, 1 MET (which has a value of 3.5 ml of oxygen per kilogram of body weight per minute) is equal to oxygen consumption at rest. Moderate walking is equal to 3.5 METs, moderate jogging 10, moderate swimming 9, and average soccer playing 7–15 (see chart).

There are several general exercise guidelines that most exercise physiologists and trainers agree on. First, people should always warm up before exercising and cool down afterward. Experts commonly suggest five minutes of stretching for a warm-up, and five minutes of slow walking to cool down. The warm-up time, which is designed to minimize joint and muscle strain or injury, is especially important for people over 40 and/or for people who have not been exercising recently. The cool-down period is important to return blood from the exercising muscles to other parts of the body. Without a cool-down period, the blood tends to pool in the muscles of the legs, causing people to become dizzy and sometimes faint.

Secondly, most experts agree that people should exercise regularly at a similar time each day—at whatever time is most convenient. The lunch hour is a good time for working people to exercise—especially if they are overweight—because it minimizes overeating after exercise. While regularity is important, doctors generally advise people to forego exercise when they feel ill.

Most physiologists and trainers advise people to avoid exercising in extreme heat, especially when the humidity is also high (above 85° F and over 70% humidity). When strenuous exercise is done in such heat, a great deal of the blood goes to the capillaries near the skin to achieve cooling, and people are more likely to either run out of energy or overheat if they cannot cool sufficiently by the evaporation of sweat. When people do exercise in hot weather they should be careful to drink extra water to replace the fluid they lose and to increase their intake of salt. Experts also advise against engaging in heavy exercise at temperatures below 0° F because the body cannot warm incoming air sufficiently at these temperatures.

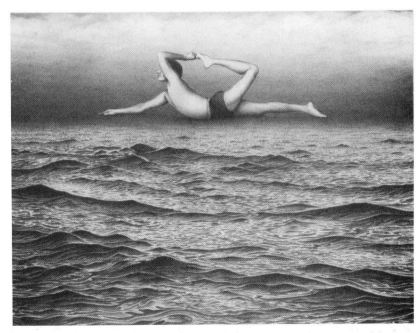

For centuries, yoga exercises have been used to integrate mind and body. Robert Moon. Swami Vishnu #5. 1970. Lithograph, 20½" × 26⁵⁄₁₆". Collection, The Museum of Modern Art, New York. John B. Turner Fund.

Finally, many doctors recommend that people who are out of shape get a general physical before beginning a training program. Doctors disagree about the exact guidelines as to who should get a physical, but most agree that people 30–40 years of age should have a regular physical and an *ECG (electrocardiogram)* if they have never had one. People who are over 40 or who have major cardiovascular risk factors such as hypertension or high cholesterol, should also have a *treadmill test* or *stress ECG*, which measures ECG during exercise, to see if there is any heart irregularity that would require moderating their exercise program. Patients with diagnosed heart disease benefit greatly from exercise programs, but they need to be evaluated carefully and follow a specially designed program.

Warm-up exercises are essential to prevent injury and promote flexibility.

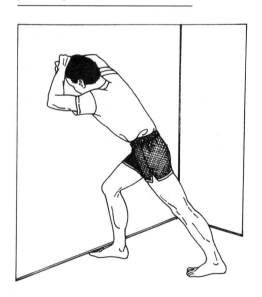 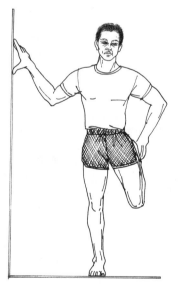 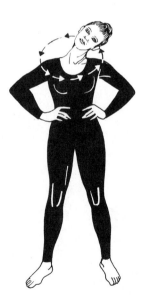

Exercise not only improves health through physical benefits, it helps to separate people from stress-producing situations at home and at work. Often being outdoors in nice surroundings, or being able to concentrate on a leisure-time activity, helps to put people in greater spiritual harmony or balance. Many people who exercise regularly find it is similar to meditation, in that it makes them calmer and leaves them in a different state of consciousness. In this state, they feel sensations of detachment from their body, a slowing of time, and a heightened ability to focus their attention. For centuries, yoga exercises have been used to help people find release from their worldly cares. Exercise helps to integrate body and mind.

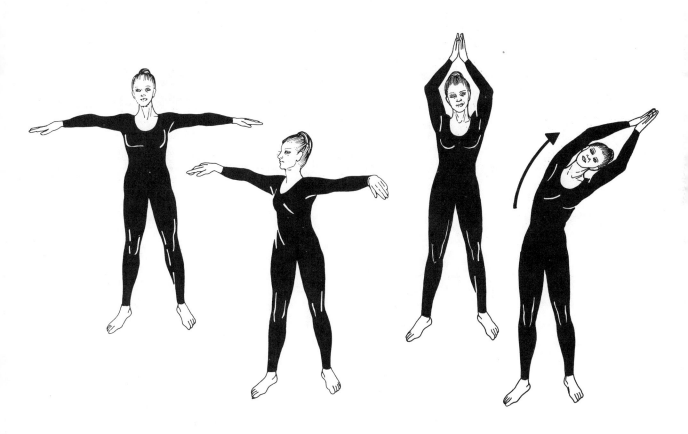

CHAPTER SEVEN

Chemicals and Health

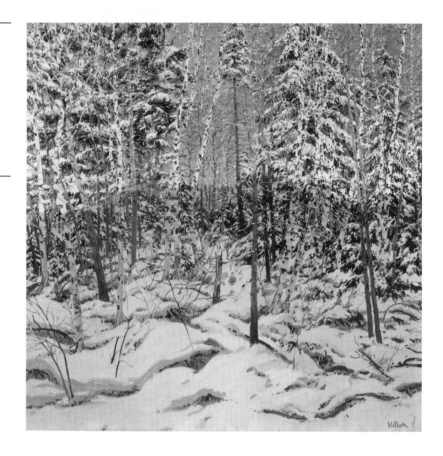

Our bodies are intimately linked to the world around us. We come into contact with all manner of substances through the air we breathe, the ground we walk on, the objects we interact with, and the substances that we ingest. Our bodies are like giant sieves; through them we are affected positively or negatively by all of the molecules around us. At the minutest level, these molecules can combine with and alter our DNA, the

Our kinship with substances in our environment makes our life possible but makes us vulnerable to dangerous chemicals. Neil Welliver. Shadow. 1977. Oil on canvas, 8' × 8'. Collection, The Museum of Modern Art, New York. Gift of Katherine Lustman-Findling, Jeffrey Lustman, Susan Lustman Katz, William Rittman, in memory of Dr. Seymour Lustman.

genetic material in our cells which guides their reproduction. This is not surprising, because we are made of the same essential elements as the substances in our environment and our molecules are joined together by the same chemical bonds. This relationship is not accidental, but a part of evolution. It is our permeability and kinship with other substances that make our life possible, that enable us to digest food and put it to use in the metabolic processes of growth, maintenance, and reproduction.

Human beings have evolved over millions of years to be able to live in harmony with and adapt to substances that were present before our existence. In the past 100 years, however, we have synthesized a vast number of new chemical substances from ancient elements, and learned to put old compounds to new uses. At present, we are exposed to a vast number of chemicals, both knowingly and unknowingly. Our voluntary exposure includes smoking and drinking, while involuntarily we may be exposed to a wide variety of harmful environmental chemicals in our air, water, and food. In many cases, these chemicals are dangerous because our bodies are not adapted to handle them, a process which takes tens of thousands of years and many mishaps. Thus it becomes critical for us to learn to identify those substances that are healthy or unhealthy for our bodies, and then to use the beneficial ones and control those that are deleterious. The number of new chemicals produced in the last several decades is so great that the task of identifying harmful and beneficial chemicals has become awesome. There are now over 4 million chemical compounds, of which 33,000 are in common use. An astounding 6,000 new chemicals are registered with the Environmental Protection Agency each week. Of these, about 700 eventually enter the marketplace in large amounts.

Chemicals can cause disease in one of two ways: (1) they can poison the body, which causes immediate illness; or (2) they can slip into the spirals of DNA molecules and alter the reproduction of cells, eventually causing illnesses such as cancer and birth defects. Poisoning, for example, includes the toxic effects of lead, pesticides, cigarettes, alcohol, and exhaust gases. The Environmental Protection Agency has named 65 substances as "priority pollutants." Of these, 33 are *proven* carcinogens, and 32 are poisons that *may prove to be* carcinogenic. People come into contact with these chemicals in a variety of ways, often

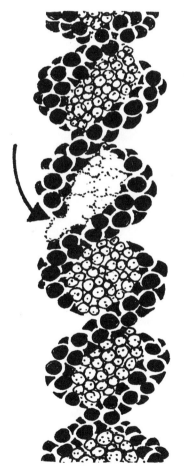

Carcinogenic chemicals can slip into the DNA within our cells and cause mutations.

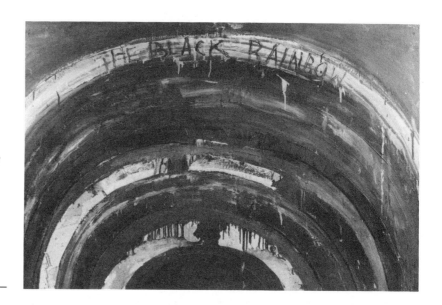

Six thousand new chemicals are registered with the Environmental Protection Agency each week. Jim Dine. Black Rainbow. 1959. Oil on cardboard, 39¾" × 59¾". Collection, The Whitney Museum of American Art. Gift of Andy Warhol.

without their knowledge. Air pollution, water pollution, food, and occupational or recreational exposure are the major sources of contact, along with smoking and alcohol. Most people don't think of smoking and alcohol in this manner, but in fact both tobacco and alcohol bring people into contact with a large number of carcinogens and cancer promoters, often on a frequent basis and in high doses.

How Chemicals Cause Cancer

The most widely known and feared disease caused by chemicals is cancer. Research over the last 20 years has focused on establishing the causal connection between chemicals and cancer, but many lay people still believe that cancer is the result of unknown causes. For some cancers, the chemical link is quite clear, as in the association between smoking and lung cancer; for other cancers, such as ovarian cancer, the link is not as direct. It is important to realize that chemicals are not the sole factor in the development of cancer. The condition of our bodies, including our genetic background, mental state, diet, and exercise patterns may or may not work to protect us.

All carcinogens basically cause cancer by the same two-step process. As a carcinogen is metabolized or broken down in the body, it creates an electron-deficient molecule that naturally seeks an electron-rich molecule within the body to bond with. DNA, the genetic material in the nucleus of every cell, happens to be electron-rich, so it readily bonds with carcinogens of all types. This first action is referred to as *initiation*, and it takes place in a single step. From a public health standpoint, it is important to note that it does not necessarily take large amounts of a carcinogen, nor persistent exposure, to cause an alteration in the genetic code of a cell. Moreover, the change is irreversible. Cancer researchers theorize that this process takes place frequently in our bodies.

After initiation occurs, one of several courses ensues. In some instances the altered genetic material is so abnormal that the cell simply dies. In other cases, the body's natural homeostatic mechanisms excise that portion of the genetic material and replace it with normal material. Probably these first two options are the most common. But, in some cases, the cell goes on to reproduce itself abnormally, and remain in a premalignant state, possibly for years. Microscopically, the cell appears different, but at this stage it is not dividing out of control.

The second stage in cancer development occurs at some undetermined time after the DNA has been altered. This stage is referred to as *promotion*. Either the same carcinogen or another substance further affects the cell, altering its enzyme activity. Over a relatively long period of time, often decades, this process, in ways still not fully understood, causes the premalignant cell to become cancerous and begin to reproduce more rapidly than normal. This second stage, promotion, can often be reversed in early stages if exposure to the chemical is stopped. Or, at a later point, the body's immune system is sometimes able to destroy the precancerous or cancerous group of cells in another two-step process. First, the body has a specific enzyme that can actually cut out or excise the abnormal parts of the DNA. Secondly, a special subset of white blood cells called killer T-lymphocytes are able to identify and destroy the cancerous cells. Both of these processes are examples of homeostatic mechanisms by which the body normally prevents and heals cancer.

Evidence That Chemicals Cause Cancer

Cancer experts now estimate that 60%–90% of all human cancer is caused by environmental chemicals, including the chemicals found in cigarette smoke, which by themselves cause a staggering 40% of all types of cancer. Two types of research have established the relationship between chemicals and cancer. In the first studies to document the link, carcinogenic chemicals that were applied directly to the skin of laboratory animals altered the DNA in their cells and caused tumors. In recent years, this type of research has been sped up by using bacteria instead of animals. Approximately 90% of all carcinogens (as established by animal studies) cause genetic mutations in bacteria, thus chemicals that alter the DNA in bacteria are suspected of being carcinogenic.

The second line of evidence linking chemicals to cancer has come from large population studies made possible by the advent of computers. Some years ago, cancer researchers began to put together maps showing the incidence of cancer in different areas of the country. These maps set forth striking pictures of cancer rates that show the incidences are distinctly higher in industrial areas. Specifically, researchers found that people who lived near chemical plants had a higher than average incidence of lung, bladder, and liver cancer; people who lived near petroleum refineries had higher incidences of lung, nasal, and skin cancer; and

Comparative Incidence of Cancer from Various Areas Throughout the World, 1985

TYPE OF CANCER	HIGH INCIDENCE AREA	TIMES	LOW INCIDENCE AREA
Colon	Luxembourg	4.6	Greece
Lung	Scotland	3	Japan
Breast	England	6	Japan
Uterus	Venezuela	4	Finland
Stomach	Japan	8	United States
Prostate	Norway	8	Japan
All sites	Luxembourg	4	Peru

Source: World Health Statistics Annual.

A Personal Cancer Plan

- Most important: STOP SMOKING (40% of all cancers).
- Avoid heavy alcohol consumption (5% of all cancers).
- Avoid long exposure to strong sunlight without protective clothing or sunscreen.
- Avoid unnecessary x-rays.
- Avoid animal fats and decrease red meats (carcinogens accumulate as you go up the food chain).
- Avoid organ meats, especially liver.
- Wash fruits and vegetables well before eating.
- Avoid foods high in preservatives, chemicals, or colorings, especially red dye #40.

- If local drinking water has many chemicals, drink bottled water that has been tested.
- If possible, do not live near a chemical plant, refinery, asbestos plant, or waste-disposal site.
- Educate yourself about any chemical you work with.
- Avoid pesticides and unnecessary chemicals in the home.
- Avoid drugs that are not absolutely necessary, especially Flagyl, Griseofulvin, Lindane (Kwell), and estrogen without progestin.
- Avoid cosmetic products with warning labels.

Source: Adapted from Samuel Epstein, The Politics of Cancer.

65 Dangerous Chemicals Targeted by the EPA

CARCINOGENS, OR SUSPECTED CARCINOGENS

Acrylonitrile
Aldrin/Dieldrin
Arsenic
Asbestos
Benzene
Benzidine
Beryllium
Cadmium
Carbon tetrachloride
Chlordane
Chlorinated ethanes
Chloroalkyl ethers (BCIE, BCEE)
Chloroform
Chromium
DDT
Dichlorobenzadine
Dichloroethylenes
2,4-Dimethylphenol
Dinitrotoluene
Diphenylhydrazines
Halomethane

Heptachlor
Hexachlorobutadiene
Hexachlorocyclohexane (BHC)
Nitrosamines
Polychlorobiphenyls (PCB)
Polynuclear aromatics
Tetrachlorodibenzo-p-dioxin
Tetrachloroethylene
Toxaphene
Trichloroethylene
Vinyl chloride

TOXINS

Acenaphthene
Acrolein
Antimony
Chloronated napthalenes
Chloronated phenols
2-Chlorophenol
Copper
Cyanide
Dichlorobenzene

2,4-Dichlorophenol
Dichloropropane
Endosulfan
Endrin
Ethylbenzene
Fluoranthene
Hexachlorocyclopentadiene
Isophorone
Lead
Mercury
Naphthalene
Nickel
Nitrobenzene
Nitrophenol
Pentachlorophenol
Phenol
Phthalate esters
Selenium
Silver
Thallium
Toluene
Zinc

Source: M. Samuels and H. Bennett, Well Body, Well Earth.

people who lived near furniture manufacturing plants had a high incidence of nasal cancer. For example, in 1970 the cancer rates for the five states with the highest incidence of cancer, all in the industrial Northeast, were 45% higher than the rates for the five rural Western states that had the lowest incidence of cancer.

When a number of population groups are studied for incidence of cancer, they show tremendous variation in the rates of different types of cancer. Worldwide rates can vary astonishingly—sometimes by as much as several hundred times. Researchers assume that the lowest rate for a particular cancer is the result of natural cell mutation, and that any increase above these baseline figures is caused by exposure to some sort of environmental chemical. This theory has been supported by immigrant or migrant studies which have found that the cancer rates of particular groups changed dramatically when these people moved to a new area and/or adopted new life-style habits.

Many carcinogens have been identified through studies in which people who were exposed to a particular chemical were compared with those who were not. The best-known of these studies concern the links between tobacco and lung cancer, and asbestos and lung cancer; subsequently, many more carcinogens have been identified by the Environmental Protection Agency. The studies have provoked tremendous controversy over what levels of a carcinogen may be deemed an acceptable risk, as compared with its economic benefit.

By examining the problems caused by a single substance, we can better understand the general problem of all chemicals. One example of the risk-benefit problem is benzene, a by-product of the petroleum industry which is used in the manufacture of pesticides, paints, plastics, rubber, and gasoline. Benzene is a ubiquitous chemical. In addition to the fact that people are exposed to it at work, it is also a common ingredient in home paint products, in food, and even in water, due to improper industrial disposal methods. In fact, 2.5% of the annual production of 260 million pounds of benzene evaporates into the atmosphere each year. There are measurable levels of benzene in the air as far as 12 miles away from plants that either use or manufacture benzene. As the most common additive in unleaded gasoline, benzene attains high levels in the air around gas stations, and is especially problematic in urban areas that have a number of

Benzene Exposure

INDUSTRY	TOTAL NUMBER OF PEOPLE EXPOSED
Petroleum refineries	6,597,000
Chemical manufacturing	9,883,000
Solvent operations	215,000
Coke ovens	16,299,000
Gasoline stations:	
Self-service	37,000,000
People living nearby	118,000,000
Auto exhausts in city air	113,690,000

Source: Adapted from Samuel Epstein, The Politics of Cancer.

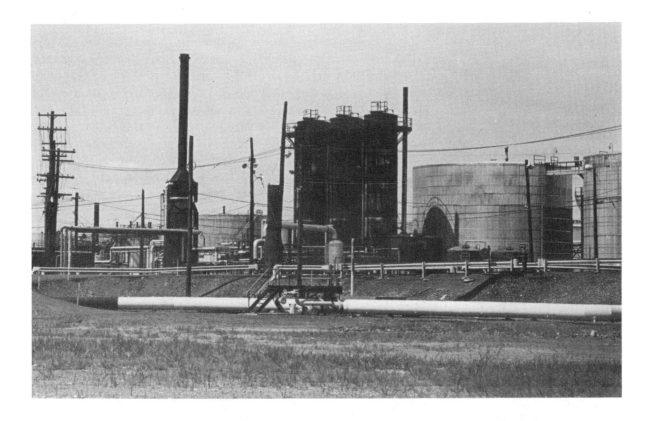

stations within a concentrated area. It has been estimated that 50% of the population is exposed to significant levels of benzene on a daily basis.

Benzene has been found to cause ear tumors, skin tumors, and leukemia in rats and mice, and it has been found that workers in a tire plant who were exposed to high levels of benzene had 10 times the leukemia rate of the general population. As a result of these studies, in 1974 the Environmental Protection Agency (EPA) and the Occupational Safety and Health Administration (OSHA) set maximum levels of benzene to which workers could be exposed. Initially, occupational exposure was set at 10 ppm (parts per million); based on later studies, this figure was lowered to 1 ppm. In 1980, the Supreme Court rejected the standard of 1 ppm, asserting there was not enough evidence to sustain it. A recent article in the New England Journal of Medicine states that special statistical analysis shows that the causal

Benzene, which is one of the most ubiquitous carcinogens, is found in unleaded gasoline, pesticides, paints, plastics, and rubber products. Oil refinery. 1984. Photograph by Michael Samuels.

relationship between benzene and leukemia can actually be projected *below* 1 ppm. The researchers estimated that for workers exposed to 10 ppm of benzene for 40 years, their risk of death from leukemia increased 154.5 times. They predict that if the average exposure were lowered to 1 ppm, the risk would drop to 1.7. An editorial in the same issue stated that studies like this "confirm the suspicion that very low levels of toxins are capable of causing serious health effects. These impressive studies should quiet the insistence that governmental efforts to control these hazards are excessive and irrational responses to chemophobic social forces."[1]

Studies such as the one on benzene are alarming because the extent of the problem is so great. Some experts now estimate that around 20% of all premature deaths could be eliminated by protecting people from a broad range of environmental hazards. The two basic ways of lowering chemical risks are health promotion, which deals with individual life-style changes, and health protection, which deals with toxic control by governmental legislation and agency guidelines. Obviously, there is only so much the individual can do to restrict the use of hazardous environmental chemicals. In the U.S., health protection responsibilities are distributed among a large number of federal regulatory agencies, the major ones being the EPA, OSHA, and the Nuclear Regulatory Commission (NRC). Air pollution, water pollution, disposal of toxic chemicals, and control of radiation come under these various agencies, but the federal government bears primary responsibility for setting and enforcing pollution standards that relate to health risks. At the present time the U.S. government is less forceful in addressing these issues than many health care researchers would like. New scientific evidence is appearing at a time of meager federal funding for occupational and environmental health and a weak federal commitment to regulation of public health hazards. Many other Western countries currently have more stringent controls over radiation and toxic chemicals than does the U.S.

Since the government is doing relatively little about environmental chemical control, it is especially important that people undertake individual health promotion efforts. John Higginson, director of the International Agency for Research on Cancer, states that a personal cancer plan can reduce a person's risk of

Occupations with Higher Than Average Risks of Cancer

OCCUPATION	HAZARDOUS SUBSTANCE	TYPE OF CANCER
Miners, textile workers, insulation workers, glass and pottery workers, chemical workers, radiologists, steel workers	Arsenic, asbestos, chromium, petroleum products, radiation	Lung
Tanners, smelters, vineyard workers, plastic workers	Arsenic, vinyl chloride	Liver
Coal and pitch workers, die users, textile workers, paint workers, leather workers	Petroleum products, coal poducts	Bladder
Explosives workers, rubber cement workers, painters, radiologists	Benzene, radiation	Bone marrow
Smelters, wood, leather, glass and pottery workers	Chromium, nickel, dust	Nasal cavity

Source: Adapted from Samuel Epstein, The Politics of Cancer.

Air Pollution Emissions in Million Metric Tons

SOURCE	TOTAL SUSPENDED PARTICULATES	SULFUR OXIDES	NITROGEN OXIDES	OZONE	CARBON MONOXIDE
Motor vehicles	1.1	0.8	9.2	11.5	85.7
Burning of fossil fuels for electricity, power, heat	4.8	22.4	13.0	1.5	1.2
Industry	5.4	4.2	0.7	10.1	8.3
Solid waste	0.4	0.0	0.1	.7	2.6
Miscellaneous, including forest fires; agricultural, refuse, and structural fires	0.7	0.0	0.1	4.5	4.9
Totals	12.4	27.4	23.1	28.3	102.7

Source: Adapted from Environmental Quality.

Carcinogens in Arts and Crafts Supplies

TYPE OF CANCER	HAZARDOUS CHEMICALS	SOURCE
Lung	Beryllium, cadmium, chromium, nickel, asbestos, arsenic	Sculpture and ceramic dust, soldering, painting, welding, etching
Liver	Beryllium, carbon tetrachloride, trichloroethylene, tetrachloroethylene	Sculpture and ceramic dust, solvents, painting, cleaning
Skin	Arsenic, arsene	Printing, etching
Nasal	Wood dust	Woodwork, sculpture
Leukemia	Benzene	Use of solvents in painting and cleaning

Source: *Samuel Epstein,* The Politics of Cancer.

getting cancer by 30%–40%, and extend the life expectancy of a 45-year-old man by 11 years. Dr. Higginson believes that personal action, whereby individuals control their own environment and that of their family, can have really significant health benefits, but he emphasizes that individual initiative does not reduce the responsibility of government to ensure public safety. Higginson has developed what he calls a "personal cancer plan" based on a number of uncomplicated life-style changes. Simply put, the object is to reduce exposure to known carcinogens whenever possible. This task involves gathering information, observing personal behavior, weighing personal risk-benefit ratios, and making appropriate life-style changes (see chart).

Smoking and Health

People seem to stop smoking for one of two basic reasons—to feel better or because they are afraid of becoming sick. Either way, as Yale surgeon Dr. Bernie Siegel observes, they have to care about themselves enough to do it.

This section perhaps should more appropriately be called "Smoking *or* Health," which was the title of a report on smoking by the Royal College of Physicians in England. Currently, the world is in the midst of an epidemic of smoking-related diseases that is as great as any infectious epidemic of the past. It is now estimated that, by itself, smoking kills around 350,000 Americans each year. If doctors, government leaders, and lay people treated this huge epidemic as they would a serious infectious disease that kills such a significant number of people annually, more funds would go into research and education, and more progress would be made.

According to a major medical textbook, "cigarette smoking is the largest preventable public health problem currently existing in the United States."[2] Similarly, a Canadian government health publication states, "Smoking is the greatest single preventable cause of disease, disability and death in our society."[3] And a World Health Organization report asserts, "Smoking-related dis-

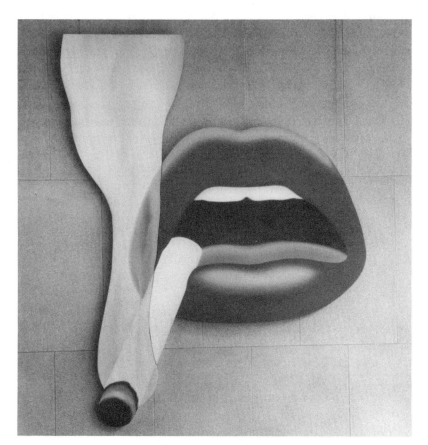

Currently, smoking is responsible for 350,000 deaths per year in the U.S. alone. Tom Wesselmann. Smoker, 1 (Mouth 12). 1967. Oil on canvas, in two parts, overall, 9′7⅞″ × 7′1″. Collection, The Museum of Modern Art, New York. Susan Morse Hilles Fund.

eases are such important causes of disability and premature death in developed countries that the control of cigarette smoking could do more to improve health and prolong life in these countries than any other single action in the whole field of preventive medicine."[4]

Part of the problem, according to many experts, is that physicians often have a complacent attitude toward smoking, which serves to placate their patients' fears and concerns, rather than encouraging them to quit. This is doubly unfortunate, because one of the most effective means of getting people to quit smoking involves serious counseling by a physician. There are many reasons why physicians, who are supposed to be healers, have traditionally not been aggressively opposed to smoking. Most physicians have never adequately been taught about the dangers of smoking, and many physicians themselves smoke. Also, the majority of physicians see their role as *treating* illness, rather than *preventing* it. Finally, physicians are not generally compensated for preventive medicine counseling.

Studies have shown that 85% of adults who smoke actually want to quit. But in order to stop smoking, people have to realize the importance and benefits of quitting. Information about the medical consequences of smoking is helpful in motivating people to quit since deep concern about lung cancer and/or heart disease is probably the major reason adults give up cigarettes. Any smoker reading this book should consider this section as advice from a physician to *give up smoking without delay*.

The most alarming smoking data deals with the smoker's increased risk of dying. Although life expectancy has improved steadily and dramatically throughout the first half of the 20th century, it showed a distinct downturn about 1950. This slowdown is largely ascribed to packaged cigarettes, which were first marketed in the 1920s and 1930s. Until that time, tobacco had mostly been smoked in pipes, and usually only by men. People sometimes assume that smoking is a "natural" pastime because tobacco is a plant that has been smoked for hundreds of years. It should be noted that most American Indians only used tobacco in small amounts during ritual ceremonies. Until the advent of flue-curing and mechanized cigarette rolling, most people neither inhaled, nor smoked in great quantity. Thus widespread heavy smoking is of comparatively recent origin.

The most impressive evidence about smoking mortality comes

from a 1964 study of British doctors, which showed that among a group of male doctors aged 35, the proportion who died before reaching age 65 was 40% for two-pack-a-day smokers, compared with 15% for nonsmokers. The study calculated that the average loss of life for a one-pack-a-day smoker is five years—or five and one-half minutes for each cigarette smoked—about the same time it takes to smoke the cigarette. New evidence doesn't refute the findings of this study; in fact, it shows the loss to be more like seven years. This average decrease in life expectancy cuts across all age groups. Not all smokers will lose seven years of life—some will lose less, but many will lose more. It is more accurate to say that one out of every three smokers will die as much as 21 years early. As depressing as these statistics are, there is good news: research has shown that if people stop smoking, their life expectancy steadily increases.

Diseases Associated with Smoking

Cigarettes affect mortality so greatly because smoking is associated with three major groups of diseases: cancer, heart disease, and lung disease. The primary illness caused by cigarette smoking is lung cancer. In addition, smoking is a major cause of cancer of the larynx, esophagus, and mouth. It is also a contributing factor in cancer of the bladder, kidney, and pancreas. But the most devastating effects of smoking are related to lung cancer, which is nothing short of an epidemic. Lung cancer is the single largest cause of cancer death in both men and women. Male smokers have twice the overall cancer death rate of men who do not smoke. For women smokers, the rate is one-third greater and increasing rapidly. Breast cancer used to be the leading cause of cancer death among women, but for the first time it was replaced by lung cancer in 1986. Rising lung cancer rates in women are thought to be due to the fact that women did not take up smoking in large numbers until the 1940s and 1950s, and the 20–25-year lag between initiation and symptoms is just beginning to show up statistically. These facts cause the advertising slogan, "You've come a long way, baby," to take on an ironic new meaning.

In 1920, lung cancer was a rare cause of death among both men and women. As of 1950 in the U.S., 20 per 100,000 males died of lung cancer. By 1965, this rate had risen to 41 per

Benefits of Quitting Smoking

more energy
less fatigue
more stamina for exercise
greater sense of taste
better sense of smell
cleaner teeth
no more stale cigarette odor on
   body, clothes
fewer colds
more money
greater sense of self-control
increased pride
less risk and fear of cancer,
   heart disease, and other
   serious diseases

Diseases Associated with Smoking

angina
asthma
bronchitis
cancer of the larynx, mouth,
   esophagus, bladder,
   pancreas
colds
emphysema
heart attacks
low–birth–weight babies
lung cancer
miscarriage
peptic ulcers
strokes

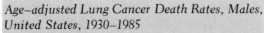

Lung Cancer Mortality by Number of Cigarettes Smoked		
NUMBER OF CIGARETES SMOKED PER DAY	MORTALITY RATIO	
	Men	Women
0	1.0	1.0
1–14	7.8	1.3
15–24	12.7	6.5
25 and above	25.0	30.0

Source: British Physicians Research Data.

100,000; and by 1975 it was 65 per 100,000. Of all lung cancer deaths, 85% are attributed to cigarettes and are therefore *preventable*. The likelihood of individuals developing lung cancer is in proportion to five factors: (1) the number of cigarettes they smoke per day, (2) the number of years they have smoked and how early they started, (3) how deeply they inhale, (4) the level of tar and nicotine in the brand of cigarette they smoke, and (5) other risk factors such as occupational exposure to asbestos. A person who smokes two packs a day has a 15–25 times greater likelihood of developing lung cancer than a nonsmoker. Approx-

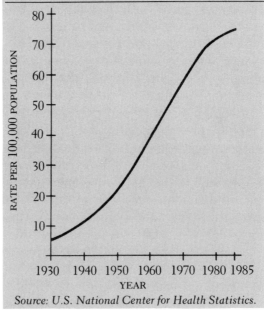

Age–adjusted Lung Cancer Death Rates, Males, United States, 1930–1985

Source: U.S. National Center for Health Statistics.

imately one-sixth of the men who smoke two packs a day will develop lung cancer. Smokers of low-tar-and-nicotine cigarettes have a slightly lower risk of lung cancer, but this is often canceled out by the fact that they smoke more cigarettes or inhale more deeply than someone who smokes regular cigarettes.

Cigarette smoking is the major cause of cancer of the larynx. This condition is much rarer than lung cancer, representing only 1% of all cancer death. Heavy smokers have 20–30 times the likelihood of developing this cancer than do nonsmokers. Laryngeal cancer develops as frequently in pipe and cigar smokers as it does in cigarette smokers—with equivalent use of tobacco. Alcohol use in conjunction with smoking more than doubles the risk of cancer of the larynx.

Cancer of the lip, tongue, salivary glands, pharynx, and esophagus is more than five times as common in cigarette smokers as it is in nonsmokers. Like cancer of the larynx, these cancers develop in pipe and cigar smokers as well, and are more common in people who drink alcohol as well as smoke. Chewing tobacco is a major cause of cancer of the cheek and gum.

Surprisingly, cancer of the kidney and bladder is three times as likely to occur in cigarette and pipe smokers as it is in nonsmokers. Occupational exposure to certain dyes, rubber products, and organic chemicals is also a factor in the development of these conditions. Cancer of the pancreas is also more likely in smokers, especially in those who drink alcohol. In addition, cancer of the colon, and especially cancer of the rectum, is more common in smokers.

It is most encouraging to note that the risk of all these forms of cancer gradually drops if people quit smoking. Within 10–15 years after quitting, people who smoked *under* a pack a day will have the same risk as someone who never smoked. A former heavy smoker—one who smoked over two packs a day—will drop their risk 10-fold. They will continue to have two to three times the risk of nonsmokers, but this is certainly much better than the 20–25-fold risk for those people who continue to smoke heavily.

The association between smoking and heart disease is as important, or more important, than the relationship between smoking and lung cancer because heart disease kills many more people annually. Cigarette smoking is a major risk factor for

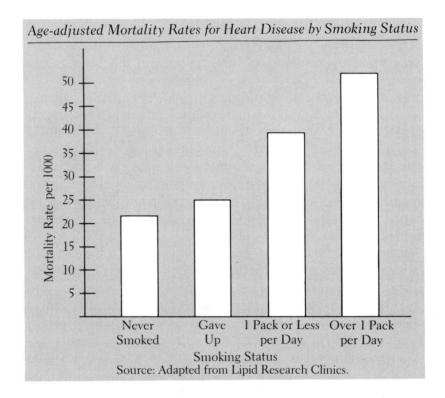

Age-adjusted Mortality Rates for Heart Disease by Smoking Status

Mortality Rate per 1000

Never Smoked · Gave Up · 1 Pack or Less per Day · Over 1 Pack per Day

Smoking Status
Source: Adapted from Lipid Research Clinics.

coronary heart disease. In fact, half of all the mortality caused by cigarettes involves some form of heart disease. Cigarette smokers have twice the risk of a heart attack as nonsmokers, especially in middle age when the coronary death rate is normally relatively low. The importance of smoking as a risk factor for heart disease is about equal to hypertension or high blood cholesterol levels. But from a public health standpoint, many more people smoke than have high blood pressure or very high cholesterol levels. Thus stopping smoking could prevent even more heart attacks per year than treating hypertension or lowering cholesterol levels. What is most disturbing is the fact that multiple heart disease risk factors are not simply additive. Thus someone who smokes, has high blood pressure, and has high cholesterol levels has seven times the risk of heart attack of someone who doesn't have these factors.

Smoking causes heart attacks by increasing the rate of atherosclerotic disease, that is, the build-up of fatty deposits in the arteries of the heart and body. It also increases heart rate and blood pressure. Due to the amount of carbon monoxide it generates, smoking decreases the oxygen-carrying capacity of the blood, thereby reducing the amount of oxygen supplied to the heart and body. As with cancer, the risk of heart attack drops dramatically when people quit smoking. After five cigarette-free years, people who smoked under a pack a day will drop to the same heart attack risk as nonsmokers. Smoking also increases the incidence of problems with heart rhythms—ventricular fibrillation in particular—and increases platelet stickiness, which is associated with blood clots. Both of these factors play a significant role in heart attacks. For unknown reasons, smoking decreases the levels of HDLs, the fraction of blood lipids that is protective against heart attacks. In addition to increasing heart attacks, smoking increases the risk of sudden death from coronary artery spasm or heart arrhythmias, aortic aneurysms (weaknesses in the wall of the aorta), and blood vessel problems of the arms and legs referred to as peripheral vascular disease. Over 90% of peripheral vascular disease takes place in smokers.

The third major illness category associated with smoking is lung disease, including smoker's cough, bronchitis, and emphysema. By the age of 60, most people who smoke have significant changes in their airways and lungs. Smoking paralyzes the cilia, the microscopic fingerlike projections that move particles and debris out of the lungs and throat. Moreover, smokers' lungs are chronically inflamed and contain unusually high numbers of white blood cells, whose function is to break down foreign particles and dead cells. Ultimately these white blood cells even break down cells in the lung itself, causing lung tissue to be less elastic, which in turn makes breathing more difficult.

Over a period of years, this inflammation of the lungs turns into *chronic bronchitis*, which produces the familiar "smoker's hack." Eventually, chronic bronchitis leads to *obstructive lung disease*, a condition in which the ability to breathe becomes limited. The same variables that affect the likelihood of lung cancer also affect the likelihood of chronic obstructive lung disease—that is, the number of cigarettes smoked, the number of years smoked, and the depth of inhalation.

Smoking carries even greater risks for women than for men. Not only is smoking during pregnancy associated with spontaneous abortion, increased prematurity, and low birth-weight ba-

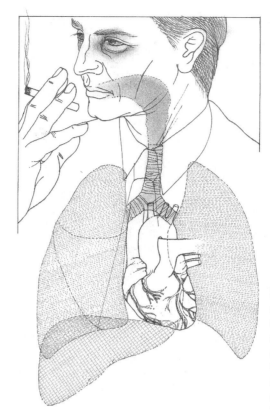

Smoking is associated with an increased risk of many cancers, including cancer of the lung, larynx, esophagus, and mouth. It is also a major factor in heart disease, emphysema, and gallbladder disease.

bies, smoking causes a dramatic increase in the risk of heart attack and stroke among women smokers who take oral contraceptives. For them, the risk of heart attack is 30 times greater than for women who neither smoke nor use oral contraceptives, and their risk of stroke is 20 times greater. Finally, smoking is also associated with higher rates of osteoporosis, a condition involving bone loss, which is much more common in women than in men.

In addition to the three major categories of disease linked to smoking, there are a number of other conditions that are adversely affected by cigarettes. For example, gum disease and loss of teeth are more common in smokers. Heartburn is more prevalent because smoking weakens the stomach sphincter, and gastric and duodenal ulcers are twice as common. Smoking is also linked to gallbladder disease.

The Physiology of Smoking

Smoking causes cancer because cigarettes contain a wide variety of toxic and carcinogenic chemicals. There are over 36,000 chemicals formed in the 950° F heat at the tip of a cigarette. Each cubic milliliter of smoke contains 5 billion microscopic particles. In terms of cancer, cigarette smoke contains three basic types of chemicals: (1) *initiators*, chemicals that alter the DNA structure, (2) *promoters*, chemicals that cause enzyme changes that allow cells to become malignant, and (3) *co-carcinogens*, chemicals that enhance the action of carcinogens. Major carcinogens in tobacco smoke include *polycyclic aromatic hydrocarbons (PAHs)*, *N-nitroso compounds*, *benzene*, and *vinyl chloride*. The best-known promoter is *formaldehyde*. In addition to chemicals that cause cancer, cigarette smoke contains a numer of chemicals that injure cilia, the airways, and the lungs. The best-known cilio-toxic agent is *cyanide*.

Carcinogenic and Toxic Substances in Cigarette Smoke			
SUBSTANCE	CONCENTRATION IN CIGARETTES (UG/CIGARETTE)	CONCENTRATION ALLOWABLE IN THE WORK PLACE (PARTS PER MILLION)	DISEASE FACTOR
Acetaldehyde	770.00	100.0	Kills cilia
Acrolein	578.00	0.1	Kills cilia
Benzene	67.00	. . .	Carcinogenic
Dimethylnitros- amine	0.08	. . .	Carcinogenic
Formaldehyde	90.00	2.0	Promotes carcinogenicity
Hydrazine	0.03	. . .	Carcinogenic
Hydrogen cyanide	240.00	10.0	Kills cilia
Nitrosopiperi- dine	0.01	. . .	Carcinogenic
Nitrosopyrroli- dine	0.1	. . .	Carcinogenic
Vinyl chloride	0.01	1.0	Carcinogenic

Source: Adapted from E. L. Wynder, "Tar and Nicotine Content of Cigarette Smoke."

Ironically, *nicotine*, the major addictive chemical in cigarettes, does not cause cancer. Nicotine is quickly and efficiently (95%) absorbed from the alveoli into the bloodstream. Within a minute of each puff, the body receives .2 mg of nicotine, and within 10 minutes—little more than it takes to smoke a cigarette—people have 40 nanograms of nicotine in their blood. Nicotine is a very potent drug that stimulates every nerve and organ in the body by causing the release of the neurotransmitters *acetylcholine* and *norepinephrine*. As a result, heart rate increases, the adrenal glands pour out hormones, and the body's metabolism is altered in a manner similar to the way it reacts to stress. One significant side effect is that the *blood platelets* become sticky, which may cause blood clotting and blockage of the coronary arteries. This process may be part of the reason smoking is linked with heart disease.

Unfortunately for smokers, nicotine is a powerfully addictive drug. A true withdrawal syndrome takes place when people give up cigarettes. The symptoms of this reaction make it difficult for people to quit. The strength of the dependence on nicotine is made fairly obvious by people's smoking habits. Very few people who smoke limit the amount that they smoke; most need a cigarette every hour or so at least. The addictive nature of smoking is attested to by the fact that most people who smoke want to stop, but find it extremely difficult.

The mood altering effects of nicotine are complex and are not well understood. Nicotine produces mental stimulation and arousal on some occasions, and relaxation on others. The mood provoked seems to depend on the situation. Interestingly, when people are angry or upset, nicotine calms them; when they are bored or fatigued, it arouses them. Thus nicotine serves to maintain a constant mood level when people are under stress. Nicotine also affects the release of *adrenaline* in the base of the brain, which causes a direct physical dependence not related to people's moods or desires. Researchers believe that nicotine causes adaptive changes at nerve synapses, which, if nicotine is suddenly removed, lead to a rebound overactivity at the junction. This heightened activity level causes a withdrawal syndrome which is very unpleasant. The specifics of nicotine withdrawal vary from person to person, but in general, withdrawal causes a group of mental symptoms, including intense craving, irritability, tension, restlessness, depression, and difficulty concentrating. In terms of physical symptoms, nicotine withdrawal causes a drop in pulse rate and blood pressure, constipation, sleep disturbance, and impaired performance at tasks.

Smoking usually starts in adolescence, and the question of whether or not to smoke has generally been decided by the age of 20. The main factors determining whether a person takes up smoking are psychosocial. Studies have shown that these factors involve a subtle relationship between the two main motivators—friends who smoke, and anticipation of adulthood—and the two main deterrents—parents' disapproval and the risk of lung cancer. Other psychosocial factors include rebellion against parents, wanting to appear tough, wanting to participate in the activities of older kids, and wanting to impress members of the opposite sex.

Interestingly, the first few cigarettes cause a number of unpleasant side effects: heart palpitations, dizziness, sweating, nausea, and even vomiting. Unfortunately for the potential smoker's health, these side effects are only temporary and people learn to control them, because they are motivated by the addictive nature of nicotine, and by peer pressure and the lure of looking adult. Once people have smoked for a while, it is thought that they continue to smoke primarily to avoid withdrawal symptoms.

During the 1970s, several significant changes took place in the smoking patterns of U.S. adolescents. The overall number of teenage smokers decreased. As of 1976, 26.8% of high school students were daily smokers; by 1985, this figure had dropped to 20%. But a higher percentage of girls took up smoking, and smoking became more prevalent among teenagers from lower socioeconomic classes.

Quitting Smoking

While quitting is clearly difficult for most smokers, it is important to realize that 30 million people have managed to stop smoking over the last 20 years. More than 90% of these people simply stopped by themselves, without the aid of any organized program. Psychologists have theorized that giving up smoking breaks down into three stages. (1) The first is a *motivational stage* in which the smokers prepare to deal with stopping. In this stage people continue to smoke, but they think seriously about the problems associated with smoking and with quitting. At present, studies show that about 85% of all smokers are continuously in Stage 1. (2) The second stage is a *behavioral stage* in which people actually give up smoking and attempt to deal with their nicotine withdrawal. People quit in a variety of ways, ranging from cold turkey to gradual behavioral procedures. Studies show that approximately 68% of those people who think about giving up actually attempt to do so. Of that group, about 50% succeed. Usually those who do succeed set goals for cutting down, targeted dates for quitting, kept track of their smoking habits, at-

---

Giving Up Smoking

If you are thinking about quitting:
- think of what you will gain by quitting: time, money, better health, increased longevity, general sense of well-being, improved physical condition for exercise, personal sense of being in control, respect of others
- realize that by quitting you will make others healthier and set a good example, especially for your children
- make a list of all the reasons why you want to quit
- set a firm target date for quitting
- try to get someone else to quit with you
- make a contract with someone about your quitting; have that person support you, monitor you

Ways to cut down before quitting totally:
- switch to a different brand that is low in tar and nicotine, or just distasteful
- smoke only half of each cigarette
- limit smoking by number or hour: postpone the first cigarette of the day, smoke only a set number of cigarettes per hour
- don't keep extra cigarettes around; purchase them by the pack
- stop carrying cigarettes; keep them in a place that is hard to get at
- stop smoking at home, at work, in public places, or in the car
- reach for gum, low-calorie foods, or water when you want a cigarette

- don't clean your ashtrays; alternatively, keep all your cigarette butts in a large glass jar

When you actually stop smoking:
- rid the house and car of all cigarettes, butts, ashtrays, lighters, and matches
- make a list of what you can buy with the money you save daily, weekly, or monthly
- keep busy
- exercise frequently
- buy something to keep your hands busy, such as paper clips, pencils, wind-up toys, or projects like knitting or needlepoint
- drink large quantities of water, seltzer, and fruit juice
- whenever you'd usually smoke, get up and walk or do something
- avoid places where people are smoking
- temporarily avoid situations and people you associate with smoking
- increase activities where you can't smoke, such as exercising, going to the movies, etc.
- do relaxation exercises to relieve tension
- use imagery exercises to strengthen your motivation and get your mind off smoking
- mark your progress—celebrate when you've been free of cigarettes for one day, one week, one month, etc.
- never think you can smoke just one cigarette— you're almost certain to start smoking again
- if you're thinking of having a cigarette, call a friend who is a "support person"

tempted to change smoking cues, took up relaxation exercises, set rewards for themselves if they did stop, and so on. (3) The third stage of quitting involves *maintenance.* The goal of this stage is to maintain a cigarette-free existence and avoid a relapse in stressful situations. In addition to using the behavioral techniques acquired in Stage 2, people at this stage come to think of themselves as nonsmokers, and learn to refuse cigarettes by replacing that urge with another thought or behavior. Most people find that turning down cigarettes is most difficult during the first three months, and progressively easier thereafter.

Alcohol and Health

Alcohol is one of the oldest mood-altering drugs known. Anthropologists believe it was probably in use long before recorded history. In early times, alcohol consumption had a religious context, and its use was limited and carefully controlled by society. The first documented sanction against alcohol was in the Code of Hammurabi in Babylonia. At the present time, however, alcohol is one of the most readily available and inexpensive over-the-counter drugs.

The 1980 Surgeon General's Report, *Healthy People,* which dealt with the current state of health in the U.S., stated, "It is difficult to overemphasize the profound and pervasive influence of alcohol abuse as a cause of death for Americans."[5] Currently more than 200,000 Americans die each year from alcohol-related causes, and about one-third of the adults in hospitals have alcohol-related conditions. It has been estimated that 20% of the national expenditure for health care deals with alcohol abuse problems. Liquor taxes contribute $50 per person per year in taxes, of which only $2 is spent on alcohol-related medical services. The health *costs* of alcohol average well over $300 per person per year.

One way of estimating the seriousness of alcohol as a problem is to look at the amount consumed. In 1983, the per capita consumption of alcoholic beverages in California was 40 gallons. This broke down to 31 gallons of beer, 6 gallons of wine, and 2.8 gallons of spirits. Data from one survey indicates that one-third of the adult U.S. population either does not drink or drinks infrequently, another one-third drinks up to three drinks a week, and another one-third drinks over four drinks a week. Researchers generally estimate that 10%–15% of the population drinks as much as 75%–80% of the alcohol. On this basis, two-thirds of the population drink a small part of the total alcohol consumed, while one-third drinks far in excess of the "average" 40 gallons.

Alcohol affects health both directly and indirectly, that is, through diseases like cirrhosis of the liver but also through accidents and violence, which people often do not attribute to alcohol. Among people between the ages of 36 and 65, three of the seven leading causes of death fall into the categories of general accidents, motor vehicle accidents, and homicides. It is estimated that alcohol is implicated in 66% of all incidents of domestic violence, in 33% of all incidents of child abuse, in 50% of all traffic fatalities, in 50% of all fire death, and in 50% of all rapes and suicides. One reliable study has shown that half of all Americans will be in an alcohol-related traffic accident in their lifetime. The same study points out that on an average weekend night, one out of every ten drivers will be driving under the influence of alcohol.

In terms of direct health problems, alcohol causes 95% of the

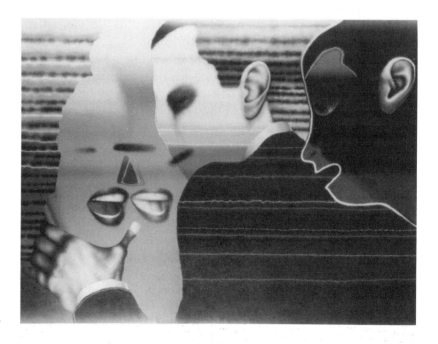

Alcohol is responsible for many deaths due to cirrhosis and is a key factor in the majority of deaths due to accidents and violence. Ed Paschke. Violencia. *1980. Collection, The Whitney Museum of American Art. Promised gift of Mr. and Mrs. Alan E. Koppel. 2.01.*

30,000 annual deaths due to cirrhosis of the liver—cirrhosis being one of the ten leading causes of death for people between the ages of 35 and 65. Alcohol use is associated with cancer of the esophagus and mouth, and it is the major cause of liver cancer. Excessive use of alcohol during pregnancy can result in fetal alcohol syndrome, a condition which can include congenital anomalies and mental retardation. Based on recent studies, heavy alchohol use is now recognized as a major contributor to heart attack and stroke. But the most prevalent severe disease related to alcohol use is alcoholism itself, which is estimated to affect at least 10 million Americans, or about 5% of the population. Together, alcoholism and alcohol abuse constitute the third leading cause of death in the U.S. One study has revealed that alcohol was the single most important factor in deaths among 50-year-old men.

Researchers are now beginning to discover the mechanisms by which alcohol causes illness. Its effect on heart attack and stroke rates is due to several factors. Alcohol, like smoking, raises blood pressure, causes blood platelets to clump, and makes arrhythmias more likely. Contrarily, there is some evidence that alcohol in moderation, that is, up to two drinks a day, increases blood levels of HDLs and therefore exerts a slight protective effect against heart attack and stroke. In terms of gastrointestinal effects, alcohol is not a direct carcinogen, but it is thought to have a drying effect that can injure mucous membranes. When the mucosal barrier's integrity is broken, nutrients leak out and carcinogens can enter the cells more readily. Finally, alcohol directly injures the liver, altering basic functions and causing excess fat to be deposited unnaturally in liver tissue.

Alcohol is readily absorbed from the stomach, quickly passes into the bloodstream, and rapidly permeates both intra- and extracellular spaces. Approximately 10% of the alcohol ingested is eliminated through the lungs and kidneys, while the other 90% is metabolized in the liver by the enzyme *alcohol dehydrogenase*. When alcohol is consumed in small amounts, it is cleared from the bloodstream relatively quickly. When it is consumed in quantities greater than it can be metabolized, the blood level of alcohol begins to rise. A 155-pound person can metabolize 9 gms of pure ethanol in about one hour, which is equal to a small glass of wine or half a beer.

Alcohol is a nervous system depressant that changes brain cell membrane permeability and causes drunkenness. *Intoxication* occurs in two stages—the *excitatory stage* and the *depressant stage*. The excitatory stage takes place when low concentrations of alcohol depress higher brain centers and act as a disinhibitor. In low doses, alcohol also acts as a relaxant, euphoriant, and anti-anxiety agent—it is this combination of psychological factors that causes most people to drink. This state is achieved with light social use that produces a *blood alcohol level (BAL)* of 50 mg per deciliter. At 100 mg per deciliter, people's balance becomes shaky and their coordination and judgment is impaired. This is the level that most states define as *driving while intoxicated (DWI)*. At blood alcohol levels above 125 mg, significant behavioral changes occur, including depression, overt aggression, and/or excessive sociability. Above 200 mg per deciliter, both the higher and lower brain centers are affected and people actually pass out. At some point above 200 mg, *alcoholic blood poisoning* takes place. This produces an alcoholic coma that requires medical treatment and can be life-threatening. To some extent, regular or heavy drinkers develop some degree of both physiological and behavioral tolerance to alcohol. To produce comparable changes, they can require almost 100 mg more than a nondrinker or infrequent drinker.

Because alcohol and its metabolic product, *acetaldehyde*, are highly toxic to the body, people develop hangovers or postintoxication symptoms that include fatigue, headache, dizziness, nausea, and neurological tremors. Alcoholics can develop *acute alcohol withdrawal syndrome*, which can include delirium tremens or withdrawal convulsions. Both of these symptoms are medical emergencies that require prompt treatment. Delirium tremens start with agitation and a tremor, and, if untreated, can proceed to hallucinations, disorientation, and even death.

Alcoholism

Scientists are beginning to learn new things about alcoholism that may help in its treatment. It is presently estimated that one-third of all drinkers will have problems with alcohol. Experts now believe that alcoholism is a multicausal disease that is due to the interaction of three influences: (1) biological or genetic

Is A.A. for You

	YES	NO
1. Have you ever tried to stop drinking for a week (or longer), only to fall short of your goal?	( )	( )
2. Do you resent the advice of others who try to get you to stop drinking?	( )	( )
3. Have you ever tried to control your drinking by switching from one alcoholic beverage to another?	( )	( )
4. Have you taken a morning drink during the past year?	( )	( )
5. Do you envy people who can drink without getting into trouble?	( )	( )
6. Has your drinking problem become progressively more serious during the past year?	( )	( )
7. Has your drinking created problems at home?	( )	( )
8. At social affairs where drinking is limited, do you try to obtain "extra" drinks?	( )	( )
9. Despite evidence to the contrary have you continued to assert that you can stop drinking "on your own" whenever you wish?	( )	( )
10. During the past year have you missed time from work as a result of drinking?	( )	( )
11. Have you ever "blacked out" (loss of memory) during your drinking?	( )	( )
12. Have you ever felt you could do more with your life if you did not drink?	( )	( )

***** WHAT'S YOUR SCORE? *****

Did you answer YES four or more times? If so, chances are you have a serious drinking problem, or may have one in the future.

Why do we say this? Only because the experience of tens of thousands of recovered alcoholics has taught us some basic truths about the symptoms of problem drinking—and about ourselves.

You are the only one who can say for certain whether Alcoholics Anonymous is for you. If the answer is Yes, we'll be glad to show you how we were able to stop drinking. If you cannot see that you have a drinking problem that is all right with us, too. All we suggest is that you keep an open mind on the subject. When, and if, you need help, we will be glad to share our fellowship with you.

ALCOHOLICS ANONYMOUS
Box 459, Grand Central Station
New York, N.Y. 10017

Source: Alcoholics Anonymous.

Signs of Excessive Alcohol Use

Symptoms
alcohol on breath
flushed face
irregular heartbeat
rapid heartbeat
night sweats
black-and-blue marks
cigarette burns
gastrointestinal bleeding
exaggerated reflexes

Laboratory findings
hypoglycemia
low magnesium
low chloride
anemia
elevated liver enzymes
clotting deficiency
ECG abnormalities

Resulting diseases
cirrhosis of the liver
gastritis
gastrointestinal bleeding
nerve disorders
seizure disorders

factors, (2) behavioral or psychological factors, and (3) environmental or social factors. Children of alcoholic parents are four times more likely than children of nonalcoholics to become alcoholic, even if they are raised by adoptive parents who are not alcoholic. Findings like this lead researchers to believe that there may be a particular gene that affects alcoholism. All alcoholics have a psychological or behavioral dependence on alcohol. Initially, alcohol provides a relief from frustration and anxiety, and a temporary euphoria. This pleasure and relief from pain creates a dependence that is the cornerstone of alcoholism. Eventually, after alcoholics develop a psychological dependence, they develop a physiological tolerance. Their liver becomes more and more efficient at breaking down alcohol, and they need more and more drinks to achieve the psychological effects they seek. Finally, a physical dependence develops, in which the nervous system actually becomes hyperexcited as a means of compensating for the depressant effects of the alcohol. Thus, when the blood level of alcohol drops, the nerves become overexcited, which produces the distressing symptoms of alcohol withdrawal. At this stage, people drink to prevent unpleasant symptoms. Experts refer to this as a secondary psychological dependence. If people are able to stop drinking, their physical dependence disappears greatly in six months, and completely in three years. Unfortunately, even a small amount of alcohol can reactivate the physical dependence.

It is known that environmental or social effects play an important role in the development of alcoholism. Family drinking habits and role models have a great effect on the drinking habits that people develop as adults. Often heavy drinking patterns start during late adolescence. At that point, depending on biological and social predisposing factors, a heavy drinker can either become a problem drinker or an alcoholic. In truth, it is difficult to distinguish an alcoholic from a problem drinker. Since both types of drinkers deny they have a problem, identification must come from the outside. Both need treatment, but in general, the alcoholic has increased evidence of physical illness and social problems related to alcohol (see questionnaire).

The goal of treating alcohol dependence is total abstinence. The three most common types of treatment are the drug *disulfiram (Antabuse)*, psychotherapy or counseling, and support

Michigan Alcoholism Screening Test (MAST)
(Including point values per various responses)

	YES	NO
0. Do you enjoy a drink now and then?	( )	( )
1. Do you feel you are a normal drinker? (By normal we mean you drink less than or as much as most other people.)	( )	(2)
2. Have you ever awakened the morning after some drinking the night before and found that you could not remember a part of the evening?	(2)	( )
3. Does your wife, husband, a parent, or other near relative ever worry or complain about your drinking?	(1)	( )
4. Can you stop drinking without a struggle after one or two drinks?	( )	(2)
5. Do you ever feel guilty about your drinking?	(1)	( )
6. Do friends or relatives think you are a normal drinker?	( )	(2)
7. Are you able to stop drinking when you want to?	( )	(2)
8. Have you ever attended a meeting of Alcoholics Anonymous (AA) for yourself?	(5)	( )
9. Have you gotten into physical fights when drinking?	(1)	( )
10. Has your drinking ever created problems between you and your wife, husband, a parent, or other relative?	(2)	( )
11. Has your wife, husband (or other family members) ever gone to anyone for help about your drinking?	(2)	( )
12. Have you ever lost friends because of your drinking?	(2)	( )
13. Have you ever gotten into trouble at work or school because of drinking?	(2)	( )
14. Have you ever lost a job because of drinking?	(2)	( )
15. Have you ever neglected your obligations, your family, or your work for two or more days in a row because you were drinking?	(2)	( )
16. Do you drink before noon fairly often?	(1)	( )
17. Have you ever been told you have liver trouble? Cirrhosis?	(2)	( )

continued

18. After heavy drinking have you ever had Delirium Tremens (D.T.s) or severe shaking, or heard voices or seen things that really weren't there? (2) ( )

19. Have you ever gone to anyone for help about your drinking? (5) ( )

20. Have you ever been in a hospital because of drinking? (5) ( )

21. Have you ever been a patient in a psychiatric hospital or on a psychiatric ward of a general hospital where drinking was part of the problem that resulted in hospitalization? (2) ( )

22. Have you ever been seen at a psychiatric or mental health clinic or gone to any doctor, social worker, or clergyman for help with any emotional problem, where drinking was part of the problem? (2) ( )

***23. Have you ever been arrested for drunk driving, driving while intoxicated or driving under the influence of alcoholic beverages? (If YES, how many times? _____) (2) ( )

***24. Have you ever been arrested, or taken into custody, even for a few hours, because of other drunk behavior? (If YES, how many times? _____) (2) ( )

** 5 points for Delirium Tremens
*** 2 points for each arrest

Scoring System: In general, five points or more would place the subject in an "alcoholic" category. Four points would be suggestive of alcoholism, three points or less would indicate the subject was not alcoholic.

Programs using the above scoring system find it very sensitive at the five point level, and it tends to find more people alcoholic than anticipated. However, it is a screening test and should be sensitive at its lower levels.

Source: ML Selzer, A Vinokur, L van Rooijen, A self-administered short Michigan alcoholism screening test (SMAST). J Stud Alcohol 36:117–126, 1975.

groups like Alcoholics Anonymous (AA). Studies show that the most successful treatment for alcoholics involves AA attendance combined with counseling by a physician. The cure rate following some form of treatment is 70%–80% for both alcoholics and problem drinkers if the condition is recognized in the early stages, and 40%–50% for those whose condition is more advanced and who already show signs of physical dependence.

Drug Abuse

In addition to cigarettes and alcohol, there are many other chemical substances that can be injurious to human health if they are used improperly. Drug abuse is an incredibly complex problem whose symptoms can range from minor physical or psychological difficulties to complete dependency and severe physiological, psychological, and social problems.

The reasons that drugs are taken include relieving pain, stress, or tension; influencing mood; enhancing social interaction; changing energy levels; or promoting sleep. Drugs are also used to satisfy curiosity, gain acceptance within a particular peer group, and to achieve altered states of consciousness. Even the term "drug abuse" is difficult to define: most broadly, it has been identified as, "the use of any substance in a manner that deviates from the accepted medical, social, or legal patterns within a given society."[6] More pointedly, drug abuse has been considered as leading to a state in which a person's health or ability to function is impaired. Only the most narrow definitions equate drug abuse with actual physical or psychological dependency. At the outset, there is no way of predicting whether or not a particular person will abuse a given substance. Both genetics and personality play a role.

Problems are most frequent with six classes of drugs: opiates, depressants, stimulants, marijuana and its derivatives, psychedelics, and inhalants. *Opiates* include heroin, morphine, meperidine (*Demerol*), pentazocine talwin, and codeine. Of these, the most common is heroin, which used to be epidemic among young urban ethnic minorities and now has spread to urban affluent adults as well, both in the U.S. and in other Western countries. It is estimated that between 5% and 10% of young city dwellers in the U.S. have used heroin at least once. Even more alarmingly, heroin addiction is actually a leading cause of death among 15–35-year-old urban males. Death can be caused by the variance in dosage, by adulterants that are used to cut heroin, by homicides and suicides that result from its use, and by infections that are associated with the unsanitary use of needles. The last problem has taken on new and frightening urgency with the spread of the AIDS virus through the use of shared needles.

Heroin use usually begins with sniffing or inhaling, which causes a sense of peace, relaxation, relief from worry, and euphoria. Although the first use may also cause nausea or anxiety, the sense of euphoria is what causes people to use it again. As with barbiturates and alcohol, repeated use produces a tolerance that necessitates larger and larger doses to produce the same effects. Eventually, most users start to inject the drug, first subcutaneously, and later intravenously. With each of the drugs classified as opiates, physical dependence ultimately develops—that is, withdrawal signs develop if the drug is not taken. These signs include anxiety, depression, tearing, perspiring, and a craving for the drug.

Depressants basically break down into several subgroups of prescription drugs, the *benzodiazepines (Valium* and *Librium),*

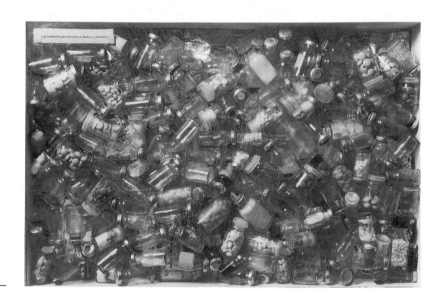

Legal, as well as illegal, drugs are the cause of drug abuse. Armand P. Arman. Valetudinarian. 1960. Assemblage of pill bottles in a white painted wooden box with glass top, 16" × 23¾" × 3⅛". Collection, The Museum of Modern Art, New York. Gift of Philip Johnson.

short-acting barbiturates (Nembutol and *Seconal),* and the *hypnotics (Doriden* and <u>*Quaalude*</u>*).* Physiologically, all these drugs are central nervous system depressants, although in small doses they may initially produce stimulation, as alcohol does in low amounts. The "high" of depressant drugs includes a peaceful feeling and/or aggression, released inhibitions, decreased anxiety, and enhanced sexual pleasure. Tolerance to the depressants develops rapidly, as does physical dependence, which is generally manifested by restlessness and anxiety, as well as various individual symptoms. Withdrawal from a serious depressant habit can be life-threatening, even more so than withdrawal from opiates.

Ironically, most addiction to depressants among adults begins with a doctor's prescription. People take the drugs intermittently to relieve anxiety or insomnia. Depressants, especially Valium, are the most widely prescribed drugs in the world. During the course of a year, one in every five women and one in every ten men in the U.S. will take Valium. Young adults can get the drugs illegally off the street. It is estimated that as many as 20% of adolescents and young adults have used depressants, often in conjunction with marijuana or alcohol.

Stimulants are a type of drug that excite the central nervous system and give the user increased energy, confidence, euphoria, and a sense of power. The most common drugs in this category include *cocaine, amphetamines,* and *methylphenidate (Ritalin).* Cocaine, which is derived from the leaves of the coca plant, has been used by Peruvian Indians for centuries. During the 1880s it was even put into "Coca-Cola," a new, "exhilarating" drink developed by pharmacist J. C. Pemberton. Although the flavor of Coca-Cola still comes from the leaves of the plant, the natural cocaine is now removed. During the late 1800s, cocaine was used as a mood elevator and as an aid in stopping nosebleeds. In the last 20 years, there has been a striking rise in the illicit use of the drug. It is estimated that over 25% of the young adult population has tried cocaine at least once. Most often cocaine is inhaled in a powder form; less commonly, it is smoked or injected. Because the price of the drug is very high, its use is greatest among affluent young adults, and it has, in fact, become synonymous with a life-style of wealth and glamour. Recently, a crystalline form called "crack" has become widely available and very inexpensive. It is considered most dangerous because it is highly addictive.

The effects of cocaine ingestion persist for approximately 20–40 minutes, and are followed by a sense of letdown. In addition to the sense of euphoria, the person high on cocaine may feel restless, irritable, and talkative. People who use the drug in quantity may develop chronic feelings of paranoia and irritability, and may use depressants such as alcohol to relieve these feelings. Physiologically, cocaine produces an increase in heart rate, blood pressure, and body temperature; relaxation of the bronchial tubes; and decreased appetite. The drug has a long list of adverse effects, the most dangerous of which are cardiac arrest, respiratory failure, tachycardia, arrhythmias, and lung damage. If sniffed regularly, cocaine can cause nasal ulcers and/or severe psychiatric symptoms. Users may experience depression, anxiety, irritability, paranoia, and compulsive or violent behavior. In rare cases, psychotic episodes or death have been brought on by as little as a single dose.

Like cocaine, amphetamines produce a sense of euphoria and increased energy. Although amphetamines used to be prescribed freely by doctors to curb appetite or elevate mood or energy levels, they are now under tighter government control. Thus most amphetamine abuse involves drugs obtained on the street. They are sometimes used, for example, by long-distance truck drivers and students cramming for exams. People who regularly use amphetamines develop tremendous tolerance to the drugs, and have to take increasing doses to get the same effects. Adverse effects include headaches, irritability, insomnia, confusion, and rebound depression. Cessation of cocaine or amphetamine use does not usually cause major physiological withdrawal symptoms, but it does involve pronounced psychological symptoms, including depression, anxiety, lassitude, and craving, all of which can make the drugs extremely difficult to give up.

Marijuana (cannabis sativa) and *hashish* are both products of the hemp plant, and have been used for thousands of years as mind-altering drugs in China, India, Japan, Assyria, and Greece. Marijuana is the most widely used illegal recreational drug in the U.S. It is estimated that two-thirds of young adults ages 18–25 have used the drug, and one-third are current users.

The effects of marijuana are felt within minutes after it is inhaled, reach a peak within one hour, and are gone within three hours. The active ingredient is delta-9-tetrahydrocannabinol, which has significant effects on a person's mood and perceptions. These effects vary widely with the dose, the user's personality, and the social setting. Reactions range from a sense of relaxation to giddy euphoria to anxiety. Perception of colors, sound, and time may also be affected. Studies show that marijuana impairs short-term memory, and sometimes affects motor coordination, including driving. First-time users report fewer effects, although they show greater motor and memory deficits. Continued use produces both physical and psychological tolerance to some degree, and cessation of regular use produces mild withdrawal symptoms of irritability and sleep disturbance.

The National Academy of Science study, "Marijuana and Health," concludes that marijuana is not completely harmless, but is not as dangerous as some people have claimed. They also state that there is no evidence that its use inevitably leads to other, more dangerous drugs. Adverse effects of regular use include respiratory symptoms such as decreased lung performance, bronchitis, and increased inflammation of the respiratory tract. There are no studies that show an increase in lung cancer rates, although cannabis smoke contains twice as much of the carcinogen benzopyrine as do cigarettes. Users can suffer unpredictable adverse psychological effects, including depression, panic, and paranoia. These feelings usually subside when the drug wears off. Chronic heavy use may cause a decrease in motivation and goal-directed activities when people are confronted with complex mental tasks. Animal studies have demonstrated decreases in immune function and fertility.

Psychedelics, a class of drugs that cause altered perceptions, have been used for thousands of years in religious rituals. Those most frequently used in the U.S. are the *indolealkylamines* (*LSD, psilocybin mushrooms,* and *DMT*), the *phenylethylamines (mescaline,* and *peyote)*, and *phencyclidine (PCP* or *angel dust)*. Of this group, LSD is the most potent; its effects include changes of perception, hallucinations, illusions, time and body-image distortions, and mood changes. Reaction to the drug is greatly influenced by the user's personality and the social setting in which the drug is taken. Adverse effects are basically

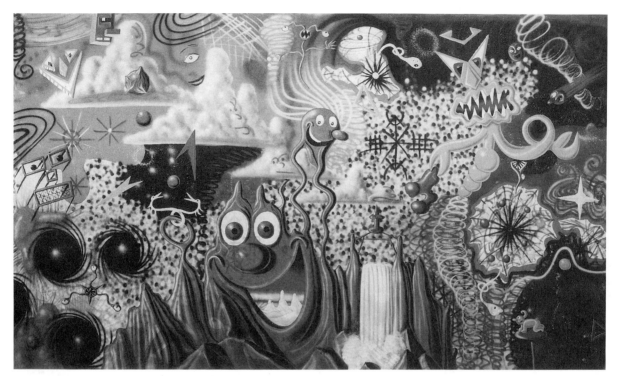

Psychedelics can radically alter a person's perceptions of reality. Kenny Scharf. When Worlds Collide. *1984. Oil, acrylic, and enamel spray paint on canvas. 122″ × 209¼″. Collection, The Whitney Museum of American Art. Purchase, with funds from Edward R. Down, Jr. and Eric Fischel.*

psychological, rather than physiological, because the drugs are generally taken in small doses. The most common results are an acute panic reaction that subsides when the drug wears off and, more severely, paranoid, psychotic, or depressive reactions that last long after the drug has worn off. Adverse effects are most common in people who are under stress or are in unsupervised settings. Angel dust has unpredictable and often unpleasant effects, and can even be fatal; it produces more dangerous symptoms than any other psychoactive substance.

Inhalants include *amyl nitrate* and *nitrous oxide*. Amyl nitrate is used for sexual enhancement, nitrous oxide for mood elevation and relaxation. Adverse effects are not all that common although amyl nitrate can produce heart palpitations and headaches.

Treatment for drug abuse is a complicated problem that depends upon the amount and type of drug(s) used and the personality of the addicted individual. Any significant drug abuse problem will need to be treated professionally, often in a residential treatment program. Professional help is most important when people have developed a physical dependence and therefore need to withdraw gradually from drugs, as in the case of addiction to opiates and depressants. Careful tapering off of the drug and/or carefully supervised use of a substitute drug (e.g., methadone) is done according to the requirements of the particular drug. Motivation is critical to the success of giving up a drug habit. When people really confront the fact that they have a problem, they usually want to stop, but need help to do so. To be successful, treatment generally involves psychological counseling and social support, as well as drug substitution in some cases.

The Living Earth

Anyone who is interested in his or her own health needs to be concerned about avoiding hazardous chemicals. Although it may be difficult to control our exposure to certain chemicals, many, such as the chemicals in cigarettes and drugs, are within the realm of our own volition. As people become better educated and experience the positive effects of other wellness-oriented

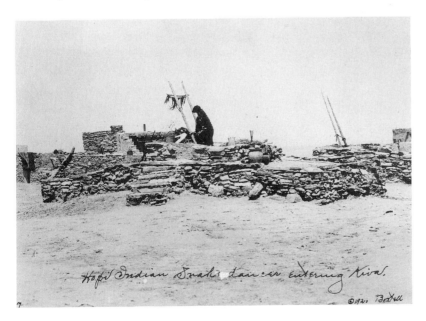

The traditional view that American Indians had of the earth was highly spiritual. Hopi Indian Snake Dancer Entering Kiva. 1920. *Library of Congress.*

life-style changes, they are more likely to make changes in habits related to smoking, alcohol, and drugs. Such changes may be easier and longer-lasting if they are undertaken to improve health and well-being, not just to prevent disease.

Any discussion of hazardous environmental chemicals inevitably brings up larger concerns about caring for the earth and for others, as well as for ourselves. In this regard, American Indian cultures have always had a highly spiritual view of the earth. In 1854, Chief Joseph Seattle made the statement: "Teach your children that the earth is our mother. Whatever befalls the earth, befalls the sons of the earth. If men spit upon the ground, they spit upon themselves. This we know. The earth does not belong to man; man belongs to the earth. This we know. All things are connected like blood which unites one family. . . . Man did not weave the web of life; he is merely a strand in it. Whatever he does to the web, he does to himself."[7] Over a hundred years later, we are just beginning to understand the ways in which we are linked to the health of the earth.

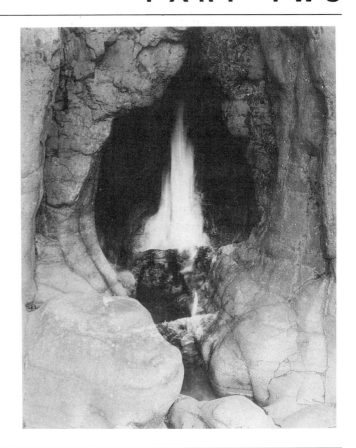

PART TWO

The Fire Inside.
Photo by Michael Samuels.

Common Illnesses
of Midadulthood

SKIN

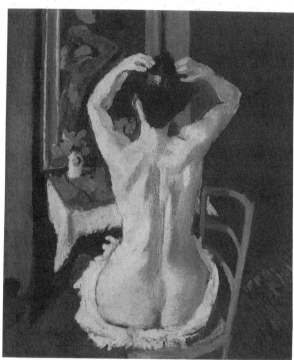

The skin is a major organ that marks the boundaries of our bodies, but does not completely separate us from the external environment. It acts as a barrier, helps regulate body temperature, produces vitamin D, and acts as a sense organ. Henri Matisse. La Coiffure. 1901. National Gallery of Art, Washington. Chester Dale Collection.

Athlete's Foot, or Tinea Pedis

Symptoms

- itching, burning, or stinging between the toes
- scales and fissures, or cracks
- small fluid-filled blisters
- raw or soft, moist, peeling areas
- occasionally a disagreeable foot odor

Description

Athlete's foot or *tinea pedis* is an extremely common fungal infection that affects the feet, most often between the third and fourth toes. Athlete's foot is caused by the *trichophyton* family of fungi—microscopic plants that, like mushrooms and yeast, do not contain chlorophyll and thus grow best in dark, moist conditions. As one dermatology text observes, athlete's foot is a penalty paid by shoe-wearing societies. Sweat between the toes has a high (alkaline) pH and serves as an ideal growth medium for fungi. In some cases the toenails become infected with the fungus, which means that the skin may be reinfected from the toenails (see p. 166). Athlete's foot is almost exclusively a disease of adult males: it is rarely seen before puberty and is uncommon in adult females. Almost all adult males carry the fungus, and 40%–80% of them show symptoms at any given time, making athlete's foot the most common skin disease between the ages of 35 and 65.

Generally athlete's foot first appears between the third and fourth toes, and, unless treated, tends to spread to the underside of the toes, then to adjacent toes, and even to the soles of the feet. Warm weather, exercise, or anything that causes the feet to sweat tends to exacerbate the condition. The itching that accompanies this complaint can be quite distracting and bothersome. In addition to the itching, people are sometimes disturbed by the odor athlete's foot causes. If cracks appear or large areas are affected, burning or pain can result, and the area can become secondarily infected from bacteria on the skin or under the nails.

Because of the prevalence of athlete's foot, many old wives' tales and misconceptions have grown up about its transmission. People warn against walking barefoot in communal showers, particularly where water collects or pools, but in fact no fungus is found in the water. Preventive foot baths and foot sprays are of unproven value, as is boiling socks or wearing only white socks. Finally, it is interesting to note that the fungus does not necessarily spread to members of the same household.

Self-Care

Self-care is very effective in treating athlete's foot. The most important principle is keeping the area between the toes dry. This is best accomplished by meticulous and careful drying of the toes after bathing, swimming, or sweating. Soft absorbent socks, made of cotton rather than wool or synthetics, should be worn and changed daily, or more often if they become damp. Sleeping without socks may prevent the feet from sweating at night. During the day, sandals, shoes that "breathe," or even no shoes should be worn. Rubber soles or shoes that cause the feet to sweat should be avoided. If fissures or cracks become severe, sports or activities that cause the feet to sweat should be avoided temporarily.

Cotton can be placed between the toes to absorb moisture and prevent rubbing. It should be replaced when it becomes damp.

It is helpful to dust the feet with a drying powder such as the nonprescription athlete's foot preparations that contain antifungal agents like *tolnaftate* or *haloprogin*. The powder should be applied in the morning and again during the day if necessary. If the powder becomes caked on, thereby trapping moisture, it should be washed off and reapplied after carefully drying the area. If powder is not removed, it can cause the skin to absorb water and become softer, which simply aggravates the problem.

During bathing, the feet should be washed with soap; then, scales and peeling skin should be gently but firmly rubbed off with a washcloth. Removing dead skin decreases the chances of trapping moisture later. Severe infections or acute episodes may require frequent bathing or soaking, as often as two or three times a day. Soaking tends to remove oil from the skin and promote dryness. *Burrow's solution*, an astringent that helps to remove crusts, can be added to the water. A cotton towel or even a hair dryer on a *cool* setting should be used to thoroughly dry the feet whenever they are bathed.

The Doctor

In order to diagnose athlete's foot, the doctor (a dermatologist, internist, or family practitioner) does a scraping to remove some scales. By adding several drops of potassium hydroxide to the scraping, the reproductive structures of any fungi become visible under the microscope. The fungus may not show up if people have used medicated powder or cream several days prior to the test; therefore, any medication should be discontinued before seeing the doctor.

In addition to recommending self-help treatments, the doctor may prescribe antifungal creams or powders such as *micanazole* or *clotri-*

mazole if the condition warrants it. In very severe cases when athlete's foot spreads beyond the skin folds, some doctors prescribe *griseofulvin*, an oral medication. This is a powerful drug that should only be used as a last resort because it has been shown to cause liver cancer in animal studies. Its immediate side effects in humans may include nausea, vomiting, diarrhea, headache, and dizziness. The drug should not be used by pregnant women, since it has caused birth defects in animals. Recurrence of infection between the toes is common and takes place rapidly.

Ruling Out Other Diseases

Unlike athlete's foot, the rash of *contact dermatitis* is found on the top of the feet (see p. 172). One form of *eczema* that appears on the feet usually occurs in adolescents or young adults and is much less scaly (see p. 177). *Atopic dermatitis* usually involves other parts of the body as well as the feet (see p. 178). *Psoriasis* can occur on the feet, but usually is found on the knees, elbows, and scalp (see p. 198). Only athlete's foot will show the presence of fungi on a potassium hydroxide smear.

Prevention

Most men carry athlete's foot fungus, so preventive steps are especially valuable for susceptible individuals. The most effective prevention is to routinely keep the feet dry. Frequent changing of socks, wearing shoes or sandals that breathe, frequent bathing, and careful drying of the feet will minimize infections and prevent relapses. Preventive measures are especially important when the weather is hot and moist or when individuals play sports. In such circumstances it may be advisable to alternate between several pairs of shoes and socks, letting each pair dry thoroughly before wearing it again.

Nail Fungus, or Tinea Unguium

Symptoms

- dull, brittle nails that break easily
- yellow discoloration of the nails
- thickening and pockmarking of the nails
- separation of the nail from the nail bed, with accumulation of debris underneath
- disintegration and loss of the end of the nail

Description

Tinea unguium is an infection of the fingernails and toenails that is caused by one of several families of fungi—microscopic plants which, like mushrooms and yeast, grow best in damp, moist conditions. Since the disease does not cause itching or pain, the main reason people seek treatment is because the nails become deformed and unsightly.

Tinea unguium is one of the most common skin conditions in midadulthood. It is unusual in children and first appears in significant numbers in the age group 25 to 35, rising steadily thereafter and reaching a peak of 70 per thousand in the age group 55 to 65, when it becomes the most common skin complaint. It affects both men and women, but is twice as common in men. Infection of the toenails is more common than infection of the fingernails, particularly in men. The infection often accompanies athlete's foot, and can be caused by the same fungi. Men frequently do not even seek treatment because they are not concerned with the appearance of their toenails. They simply accept it as a process that goes along with growing older. Women, by comparison, are more likely to be concerned about the appearance of their toenails and seek treatment. Both men and women, however, are likely to be concerned when the disease affects their fingernails. In this case, emotional distress over the way the nails look becomes more important than the medical aspects of the infection.

Tinea unguium typically begins on the side of the nail and spreads slowly across it. In the mildest form, the nail simply becomes discolored at the edge and perhaps roughened or pockmarked. This phase can last for years. Generally only one or a few nails are involved. If the disease progresses, the nail bed itself becomes involved, and starts to produce soft *keratin*, an insoluble protein, which accumulates under the nail. This provides an ideal growth medium for the fungi, which then multiply more rapidly. Ultimately, the nail can become loosened from its bed and lift up. Both the debris and the loosening become more apparent if the nail breaks and the end of the nail plate becomes visible. The soft keratin on the end of the nail plate then becomes so thick that it looks like a callus.

Self-Care

Tinea unguium can be difficult to treat, but good nail hygiene is successful in dealing with mild infections. Nails should be cut straight across and very short. Many doctors advise that the nails be trimmed or filed daily since this tends to keep the fungus from spreading. Nonprescription antifungal creams may be somewhat effective.

The Doctor

The doctor (dermatologist, internist, or family practitioner) diagnoses tinea unguium by adding potassium hydroxide to thin scrapings from a diseased part of the nail. This dissolves the nail keratin, allowing the fungus to be seen under the microscope. For mild infections involving the toenails, the doctor may simply advise home treatment. Next, the doctor may prescribe antifungal creams or ointments. In the past, these preparations have had a poor history of absorbing through the nail, but newer ones, such as *ciclopirox*, *haloprogin*, or *miconazole*, may be more effective, especially those that contain pyridone-ethanolamine salts, because those preparations penetrate the nail better than other topical agents.

For more severe infections, doctors vary in their treatment and advice. Some advise removal of the nail, either surgically under local anesthesia, or chemically through the application of a powerful solvent. It is hoped that the new nail will not be infected when it grows in. Other doctors question the effectiveness of nail removal. Many doctors prescribe oral medications such as *griseofulvin* or *ketoconazole*. Since the nails grow very slowly and take up to 6 months for new tissue to replace old, such systemic medications must be taken for up to a year to be effective. Even then, there are many treatment failures and relapses. In addition, both these oral medications are powerful and have significant side effects: griseofulvin has produced liver cancer in laboratory animals, and has caused birth defects in animals. It is also known to cause allergic reactions and gastrointestinal and neurological side effects in humans. Ketoconazole has neurological and gastrointestinal side effects, and has been associated with liver damage and death in humans.

Ruling Out Other Diseases

Tinea unguium may be confused with changes in the nail due to chemical damage from polishes or removers, or changes in the nail due to the skin condition *psoriasis* (see p. 198). Chemical damage is usually diagnosed on the basis of a history of exposure. Psoriasis is generally accompanied by a skin rash and begins at the middle rather than the edge of the nail. A positive diagnosis of tinea unguium can be made with a simple potassium hydroxide scraping.

Prevention

Good nail hygiene and prompt treatment of athlete's foot may help to prevent tinea unguium, or at least keep it under control. Some doctors feel that regular manicures may be useful because they clean the fungus out of the grooves at the side of the nails and scrape the fungus off the nail itself.

Jock Itch, or Tinea Cruris

Symptoms

- significant itching on the upper inner thighs
- spreading, red areas
- sharp boundaries that can be raised and scaly
- some areas may be moist or raw
- tiny fluid-filled blisters may be present

Description

Tinea cruris, or *jock itch*, is a skin infection found on the upper inner thighs that is caused by a type of fungus, a microscopic plant which, like mushrooms and yeast, grows best in dark, moist areas. A moderate to severe infection can cause intense itching, and raw or abraded areas can become painful enough to make walking uncomfortable.

Tinea cruris is an exceedingly common skin condition which often occurs in men, but can occur in women. The age group most commonly affected is 35 to 65, with a slight peak between

45 and 55. Heat, high humidity, and sweaty conditions predispose individuals to the disease. Tight-fitting, nonbreathing clothing that chafes, such as jockey shorts, athletic supporters, bathing suits, or bicycling pants, tends to trap moisture around the upper thighs and mechanically abrade them. Among women, panty hose, tight-fitting slacks, and tight, nonabsorbent exercise clothes are likely to favor growth of the fungus. In both men and women, the infection tends to occur more frequently among athletes and overweight people with heavy thighs. Individuals in both these groups tend to sweat more than normal and are more likely to rub their thighs together.

Generally jock itch starts in the skin folds between the leg and the trunk, spreading down onto the upper inner thigh and sometimes onto the external genitalia. In almost all cases, it occurs on both thighs. The rash spreads out in semicircular patterns with well-defined edges. The skin may be raw at the boundaries, with clear areas in the center. If not treated properly, the rash can spread over large areas of the upper thighs and become very uncomfortable.

Self-Care

Self-care is very effective in treating jock itch. The two main principles of treatment are to keep the area dry, and to prevent mechanical abrasion from clothing. Loose, absorbent, 100% cotton clothing should be worn. Clothing that touches the rash should be avoided or changed frequently. Activities that foster sweating or chafing should also be avoided.

The affected area should be bathed frequently. When soap is used, it is important to rinse it off thoroughly. The area should then be dried completely and covered with plain unscented talcum powder or cornstarch. If the powder cakes, it shows that moisture has been trapped next to the skin, and the area should be cleansed and dried again. Some doctors recommend specific antifungal powders or creams containing *tolnaftate* instead of talcum powder.

With moderate infections, it is helpful to expose the area to air, and, if possible, to sunlight, for 15 minutes to an hour, especially after bathing. In very humid weather, air conditioning can be a great help.

The Doctor

Tinea cruris is diagnosed from a skin scraping treated with potassium hydroxide to reveal the presence of the fungus. In addition to recommending self-care, the doctor (dermatologist, internist, or family practitioner) may prescribe one of several preparations. Some doctors prefer antifungal creams containing *clotrimazole* or *miconazole*; others prefer to use a solution called *Castellani paint* which contains *fuschin*. One drawback to the paint is that it stains clothing. In very severe cases, some doctors prescribe oral *griseofulvin*. This is a powerful drug with gastrointestinal and neurological side effects that should be avoided if possible because it is known to cause liver cancer in laboratory animals. Griseofulvin should not be taken by pregnant women.

Ruling Out Other Diseases

Psoriasis or *seborrheic dermatitis* can also occur on the upper thighs, but is generally associated with rashes in other areas (see p. 171 and p. 198). In the case of seborrheic dermatitis, itching is less pronounced. These diseases are ruled out by a simple potassium hydroxide smear. The doctor may also shine a *Wood's light* on the affected area. This special black light can identify a bacterial infection called *Erythrasma* that produces a similar-looking rash. A yeast infection *(Candida)* can cause a rash in the same

area but often produces small pimples outside the main boundary of the infection. Yeast can be ruled out by a smear or culture (see p. 401).

Prevention

Jock itch can be prevented and relapses avoided by eliminating chafing, wearing loose 100% cotton clothing, and keeping the thighs dry. These considerations become especially important during hot, moist weather or athletic pursuits. People who have had previous episodes of jock itch probably may be more susceptible and should be more careful. At the first sign of a problem, these people should begin aggressive home treatment.

Pale Skin Patches, or Tinea Versicolor

Symptoms

- yellowish or brownish patches on fair skin or pale patches on darker skin
- slight scaling
- mild itching
- the most common sites are chest, abdomen, and back
- patches vary widely in size and shape
- pale patches that do not tan

Description

Tinea versicolor refers to a fungal infection ("tinea") that causes patches of skin of various colors ("versicolor"). The condition is so mild that people often don't notice it or don't bother to seek treatment. Among those who do see a doctor, the chief complaint is one of aesthetics. Generally people notice patches because these areas do not tan or are slightly itchy. The infection is completely harmless, but quite common, especially among active people who perspire due to work or athletics. It is also more prevalent during warm months and in humid climates.

The patches vary widely in color from yellowish to brownish on pale skin, to whitish on darker skin. The patches also vary widely in shape and size. When areas adjoin, they can create patterns that make the infection more noticeable, especially when surrounding areas become tanned. The patches are generally found on the upper torso, but occasionally spread to the the upper arms and thighs. The infection rarely affects the face and scalp.

Self-Care

The infection tends to be chronic, but it does respond to a regimen of good skin hygiene. Affected areas should be washed frequently and dried thoroughly. Nonprescription, antifungal lotions containing selenium sulfide (*e.g.*, *Selsun Blue* or *Tinver*) should be applied for 10 minutes and then washed off. This routine should be done daily for a week. Some doctors advise leaving the lotion on overnight one time. These products may damage jewelry and are not recommended for pregnant women. Also, soaps or shampoos containing *sulfur-salicylic acid* (*e.g.*, *Sebulex*) can be used for regular bathing. Even if these remedies are effective in getting rid of the fungus, the areas involved will not tan normally for quite a while.

The Doctor

The doctor (dermatologist, internist, or family practitioner) can diagnose the condition in one of several ways. A scraping of the scales pre-pared with potassium hydroxide allows the fungus to be seen under the microscope. Under a Wood's light, the fungal patches will glow brownish-yellow in a darkened room. Often this reveals larger patches than the patient is aware of.

Because of the harmless nature of the fungus, most doctors are not concerned about treating tinea versicolor. However, there are a variety of potent medicines that will eliminate the fungus temporarily or permanently, if treatment is desired for cosmetic reasons. To eradicate the fungus entirely, doctors generally treat it aggressively for several weeks. The creams most frequently prescribed are *clotrimazole*, *haloprogin*, *tolnaftate*, and *miconazole*. An effective oral medication called *ketoconazole* is also available, but it is associated with serious liver toxicity, so its use for a medically harmless condition is questionable.

Ruling Out Other Diseases

In general, tinea versicolor can easily be differentiated from other diseases that produce patchy changes in skin color. *Seborrheic dermatitis* occurs on the face and scalp as well as the trunk (see p. 171). *Vitiligo* does not produce scales; its patches are completely white unless sunburned, and are most frequent on the elbows, knees, and hands (see p. 206). A skin scraping treated with potassium hydroxide or viewing the area with a Wood's light will make the diagnosis positive.

Prevention

Probably the best prevention involves regular bathing and keeping the skin dry. This is most important for people who are physically active during warm weather. Prompt treatment will help to keep patches from spreading.

Dandruff, Flaky Skin, or Seborrheic Dermatitis

Symptoms

- scaly patches of skin
- crusted yellowish or pinkish patches
- dandruff
- patches are most common on the scalp, eyebrows, eyelids, ears, forehead, and nose folds
- patches may be oily or dry
- patches may itch

Description

Seborrheic dermatitis is an inflammation of the skin that is very common in midadulthood and tends to be chronic or episodic. It is distinguished by oily scaling that occurs in a characteristic distribution that concentrates around the scalp, eyebrows, and face. Despite the fact that it is one of the five most common skin diseases of middle age, its cause is still unknown. There is definitely a genetic predisposition among certain groups of people. These people produce greater than average amounts of *sebum*, the oily substance made by the sebaceous glands that are located at the base of the hair follicles. The production of sebum is regulated by hormones, in particular by the male hormone *androgen*. Perspiration also seems to play a facilitating role. This is probably due to the fact that sweat or chronic moisture tends to break down the surface of the skin, especially when it is rubbed. A high-fat diet and/or stress are also thought to contribute to making the condition worse.

In its mildest form, seborrheic dermatitis occurs only on the scalp, producing dry flakes composed of *keratin*, the protein found in the dead cell layer on the top of the skin. Dandruff

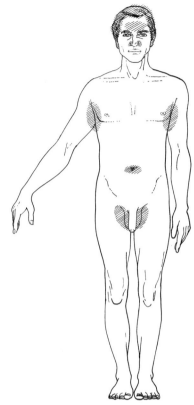

Sebhorreic dermatitis is most common in areas that have many sebaceous glands.

generally involves the entire scalp, not just small patches. If the condition becomes worse, the flakes tend to be greasy, thick, and crusty, and they may spread to the forehead, ears, back of the ears, eyebrows, and bridge of the nose. In more severe cases, the condition can spread to other parts of the body, typically the skin folds, armpits, navel, groin, and under the breasts in women. These areas have high concentrations of sebaceous glands, and they also may not be washed as thoroughly as other areas. In severe cases such as this, the skin lesions can become red, raw, and oozing. The disease tends to be episodic and sometimes clears up without treatment, although more severe cases usually require medication.

Self-Care

In mild cases, shampooing is the most important factor in home treatment. Many doctors feel that the brand name of a particular shampoo and its ingredients are less important than the regimen that is followed. The hair should be shampooed at least once a week, preferably two or three times. Nonprescription shampoos that contain *selenium sulfide* (e.g., *Selsun Blue*) are sometimes more effective than normal shampoos, and can be used regularly. *Sulfur-salicylic acid* creams or lotions (e.g., *Fostex* or *Sebulex*) are particularly useful when the scalp is oily as well as scaly.

The Doctor

The doctor (dermatologist, internist, or family practitioner) diagnoses seborrheic dermatitis based on its appearance and distribution. For severe cases of dandruff, the doctor may prescribe shampoos that contain more potent ingredients than most over-the-counter preparations. These include *Selsun* and *Neutrogena T/Gel* containing tar. A *corticosteroid* lotion may also be prescribed in more severe cases to help reduce inflammation. For skin lesions, corticosteroid creams or *coal tar* lotions can be very helpful.

Ruling Out Other Diseases

Seborrheic dermatitis is distinguished from *fungal infections* by a negative finding on a skin scraping treated with potassium hydroxide. In *psoriasis*, the lesions or scales are much thicker and are present on the knees and elbows; patches on the scalp are isolated and do not generally involve the whole scalp (see p. 198).

Prevention

Regular bathing and good skin hygiene are important in preventing seborrheic dermatitis. Also, stress reduction and a low-fat diet seem to be preventive factors (see pp. 58 and 102). Seborrheic dermatitis involving the skin folds and trunk tends to be more common among obese people, and weight reduction may be helpful in these cases.

Contact Dermatitis, Including Poison Ivy and Poison Oak

Symptoms

early signs
- red swollen patches
- raised red dots and fluid-filled blisters on the patches
- occasionally, large fluid-filled blisters
- blisters often appear in lines or squares
- rash occurs in areas where allergens have touched the skin, most often on the hands, arms, face, and legs
- itching and/or burning—often intense

later signs
- weeping or oozing from blisters
- crusts or scabs where blisters have broken
- scaling and thickening of raised areas
- scratch marks and secondary infection may be present
- continued itching

Description

Contact dermatitis is an inflammation of the skin caused by a substance that is either irritative

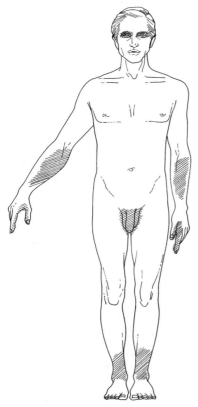

Contact dermatitis develops where allergens have touched the skin. It occurs most often on exposed areas.

recognize as foreign. Different people's bodies recognize allergic substances, or *allergens*, as foreign or "dangerous" to varying degrees. One person may not react to a particular substance at all, while another person may experience a strong allergic reaction (see p. 248). The process that causes allergic contact dermatitis is called *delayed hypersensitivity*. It takes approximately 24 to 48 hours for the lymphocytes to recognize the allergen, reproduce in large numbers, and produce an inflammation. Even the smallest amount of an allergen can cause a reaction in an allergic person, hence the term "hypersensitivity."

One of the most common examples of an allergic contact dermatitis is *poison ivy* or *poison oak*. The allergen in this case is a resin or oil called *urushiol*, which is found in the leaves and branches of poison ivy, poison oak, and poison sumac. Similar resins are found in the Japanese lacquer tree, cashew oil, the mango tree and its fruit, and the ginkgo tree.

Exposure to these oils can be direct, but the oil can also be picked up from gloves, shoes, clothing, pet's fur, tools, or furniture that has touched the plants. If the branches or leaves of the plant are burned, the oil can become airborne in the smoke. Within 48 hours after exposure to the allergen, an allergic person notices itching in the area of exposure. Next the skin swells, becomes red, and develops a rash which consists of raised red dots and fluid-filled blisters within the swollen red patches. A striking characteristic of the poison ivy rash is its tendency to appear in lines. The most common locations for the rash are the backs of the hands, the wrists, the eyelids, and the ankles. It's also not uncommon for the rash to develop in the genital area, especially in men. Oil from the plant is easily spread by hand from the original area of exposure to other sensitive areas of skin such as the eyelids or genitals.

Eventually, the blisters break, ooze, and fi-

or produces an allergic reaction. *Irritative substances* provoke an inflammation by directly damaging the top layer of skin. These substances include pesticides, industrial chemicals, petroleum products, *acids*, and *bases* such as soaps, detergents, bleaches, and cosmetics (see chart). Fiberglass and wool can also cause irritative contact dermatitis.

Allergic contact dermatitis is an immune response caused by contact with a substance that a person is allergic to. In this case the body's *T-lymphocytes*, a special type of white blood cell, multiply rapidly and cause a local inflammation in response to a particular substance that they

nally crust over. The fluid that emerges from the blisters is simply plasma; it cannot cause new areas of rash. If a person scratches the rash, which is almost irresistible, the crusts become thicker, scratch marks appear, and the open blisters may even become secondarily infected with bacteria that exists on the skin or under the nails. New blisters can occur for up to a week after exposure due to small concentrations of the oil. The duration of the infection depends upon how allergic people are and on whether they are reexposed to the allergen. At the peak of the rash, a person may become hypersensitive, experiencing a generalized itching all over the body.

Many other forms of allergic contact dermatitis are also very common. Often the allergen can be identified from the location of the rash. Nickel in costume jewelry and lingerie hooks causes rashes around the neck, wrist, earlobes, and back. Rubber allergies cause rashes on the feet, the waist, and around the breasts. Rashes on the face and eyelids are often caused by cosmetics or hair dyes. Rashes from this group of allergens appear in the area of contact, often taking on the outline of the offending object.

Self-Care

The first step in self-care is to find the source of the allergen and eliminate it. This may be obvious, or at times it may require some deduction. For example, a rash on the feet may be due to poison ivy or to a reaction to the rubber in a pair of shoes. The exact location of a rash and the circumstances under which it develops are the best clues to determining its cause. It's important to remember that there may be a lag of one to two days between exposure and appearance of the rash.

Once the allergen has been determined, the person should take care to avoid any further contact. In the case of poison ivy this means carefully washing the oil from any area that might have been exposed, paying particular attention to the fingers and nails. Soap and water or disposable wipes containing alcohol are both effective. Any kind of soap will do; time is the important factor. Once *all* the oil is washed off, the rash cannot spread. If the oil is removed

---

Self-Care for Itching

- keep cool; overheating and sweating make itching worse
- wear loose, comfortable clothes that cover the rash
- try not to scratch
- apply cool water or compresses with witch hazel or Burrow's solution (nonprescription) to the itchy area
- take cool showers and baths; Aveeno or oatmeal can be added to bath water
- a hot bath or shower will make the body release histamine, which will cause brief, intense itching, but this depletes the supply of histamine and can give up to 8 hours of relief
- apply Calamine lotion to the itchy area
- if itching is very intense, *.5% hydrocortisone cream* can be applied four to six times a day; it should not be used for long periods

---

promptly enough, it is possible to prevent the rash or lessen its severity. In the case of other allergens, the source should be removed and the area should be washed as soon as possible. All clothing and objects that may have come in contact with the allergen should also be washed. If the time of exposure cannot be established, some doctors simply recommend washing all clothing that has come in contact with the area of the rash for several days.

Mild cases of contact dermatitis can be treated at home. Once the allergen is removed, it's a case of treating the symptoms, not curing the disease. If the itching is not bothersome, no treatment is necessary. A person's subjective attitude can have a lot to do with how they react to the itching. Generally, the less thought given to the rash, the less bothersome the itching tends to be. It may help to wear cool, loose, nonirritative clothing that covers the rash. Not only does the principle of "Out of sight, out of mind" apply, but such clothing may lessen the tendency to scratch and decrease the abrasive effects when the area is scratched, thus lowering the chances of secondary infection. Fingernails should also be trimmed and washed to lessen the chances of secondary infection or spread of the allergen.

If the itching does become bothersome, there are several home remedies that are quite effective. The goal is to cool and soothe the area. Cold compresses or calamine lotion can be applied. Some doctors have found that aluminum compounds such as spray deodorants or *Burrow's solution* are especially effective. Pastes or soaking solutions can be made by cooking up corn starch and water, or by mixing *Aveeno* packets or oatmeal with water. Over-the-counter antihistamines can also be taken to help control itching, especially at night. If itching cannot be relieved using these methods, nonprescription *½%–1% corticosteroid creams* are available and can be applied 4–6 times a day. These creams are not always effective, and some of the steroid is absorbed through the skin. Long-term use should be avoided to prevent serious systemic side effects such as suppression of the adrenal glands.

The Doctor

Often the doctor (a dermatologist, internist, or family practitioner) can diagnose allergic contact dermatitis by looking at the rash and reviewing the history of the illness. In cases where the allergen is unknown, the doctor can do *patch testing*, which involves applying small amounts of common allergens on the skin and checking to see if they produce a reaction in 24–48 hours.

If the rash is severe or very uncomfortable, the doctor may prescribe a strong corticosteroid cream or oral steroids, such as *prednisone*. Because steroids are a potent medicine with side effects, many doctors only prescribe oral steroids if a person has had a severe allergic reaction in the past, or has significant swelling around the eyes, genitals, or mouth. The dosage of steroids must be tapered off gradually to avoid a rebound effect when they are discontinued. Many doctors also prescribe an *antihistamine* to help control itching. It is generally taken at night because it tends to make people drowsy and because it helps prevent people from scratching the affected areas in their sleep. An antibiotic may also be given if the rash is pustular or if the doctor believes that *staph bacteria* are delaying the rash's healing.

Ruling Out Other Diseases

The major disease that contact dermatitis should be differentiated from is *eczema* (see p. 177). Factors that help to distinguish between the two diseases are the pattern and location of the rash, as well as the history of exposure. Contact dermatitis is actually an eczema-type rash (raised red dots and blisters), but it is caused by an external agent, whereas eczema is set off within the body. Contact dermatitis occurs in lines and squares; eczema in larger, round patches. Eczema tends to occur on the scalp, neck, and skin folds such as the elbows and knees; often it is bilateral. Another disease which can be confused with contact dermatitis is *scabies* (see p. 194), a rash caused by mites under the skin. Scabies is characterized by short lines of blisters and pimples, and itches most at night.

Prevention

Once the cause of a contact dermatitis is determined, prevention becomes a matter of avoiding contact with the allergen. In the case of poison ivy or poison oak, this means learning to identify the plant and eliminating it from areas near the house. Household pets should be kept from running loose, or should be kept outside the house. Prompt washing, even using alcohol-based wipes during the course of a hike, can sometimes prevent the rash. Studies have shown that, contrary to folk belief, ingesting poison ivy does not make a person immune. In the case of other types of allergens, the offending object should be discarded and replaced with a nonallergenic substitute. For people with pronounced allergic reactions, many doctors recommend eliminating strong-scented soaps, hair dyes, or cosmetics, and wearing cotton clothing that does not have any exposed rubber.

Eczema, or Atopic Dermatitis

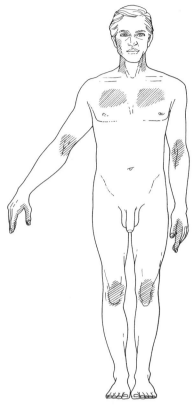

Eczema is an intensely itchy rash that causes areas of the skin to become thickened.

Symptoms

early signs
- red swollen patches
- raised red dots and fluid-filled blisters on the patches
- most often on the face, neck, upper body, hands, inner elbows, and behind the knees
- severe itching and burning

later signs
- weeping or oozing from blisters
- crusts or scabs where blisters have broken
- scratch marks and secondary areas of infection may be present
- continued severe itching
- rash areas become thickened and leathery, sometimes darkening
- skin lines become exaggerated

Description

The term *eczema*, which comes from the Greek word for "boil out," applies to a group of skin diseases tht cause characteristic, intensely itchy rashes. The rashes consist of inflamed areas with red dots and tiny blisters which eventually lead to thick, red, leathery patches. Eczema (or dermatitis) has been used to describe more skin conditions than any other term. The term covers, or includes, *atopic dermatitis*, *hand eczema*, *lichen simplex* or *neurodermatitis*, and *xerotic eczema* or *winter itch*. Although the rash is virtually the same in all these conditions, their locations, causes, and outcomes are varied enough to justify using different names to define them.

Approximately 3% of all Americans have some form of eczema. It is thought to be the result of an inherited sensitivity to skin trauma and a low threshold of tolerance to itching. When people with eczema scratch their skin, the skin weeps, thickens, and hardens more than normally. Research shows that there are specific chemical differences between normal and eczemous skin, including a greater sensitivity to stress hormones in the latter. Whereas *contact dermatitis* represents a reaction of normal skin to an allergic or irritative substance, eczema represents a reaction of sensitive skin to trauma or abrasion.

Lichen simplex, or neurodermatitis: This is a condition in which a thick, well-delineated area develops on the back of the neck, wrists, inside of the wrists, forearms, inner thighs, inner elbows, or backs of the knees. It is caused by repeatedly rubbing and scratching the skin in a particular area in response to itching. Lichen simplex is most common among women over 40 and is often found in people who have atopic dermatitis (see below). Interestingly, one person in five has the kind of skin that will thicken in this manner when scratched repeatedly.

Hand eczema, or housewife's eczema: This is a common skin disease that is associated with dryness, redness, and peeling on the backs of the hands, fingers, and palms. Many factors contribute to its development, including prolonged exposure to detergents or soaps; slight allergic reactions to handling food in the kitchen; a sensitivity to rubber gloves, plastics, or dyes; and exposure to cold weather, which causes chapping.

Atopic dermatitis: This condition involves a low threshold of tolerance to itching and is associated with a family history of allergy, including asthma, eczema, hay fever, etc. It has been described as an "itch that rashes, rather than a rash that itches." Atopic dermatitis often develops in infancy, although it can first appear in adulthood. In adults, the rash typically occurs on the insides of the elbows, backs of the knees, neck, forehead, and hands. There are several theories about its cause. One theory holds that it is due to an inborn characteristic that makes a person's nervous system react differently. A second theory speculates that it is basically an allergic reaction. And a third emphasizes the role of stress and personality as causal factors.

Xerotic eczema, or "winter itch" or "winter dry skin": Patches of skin become dry and eventually become red and scaly. In some cases the skin becomes shiny and crackly like porcelain. It is most common on the arms and legs, especially the shins. It is associated with hot, dry air in overheated rooms, and with overbathing.

Self-Care

For all forms of eczema, the basis of home treatment is good skin care. Irritative chemicals, soaps, detergents, and fabrics such as wool or synthetics should be avoided. In particular, excessive exposure to soap and water tends to dry the skin and make it more vulnerable. Special soaps such as Alpha-keri, Neutrogena, Dove, or Basis may be less irritating. Oil can be added to the bath water, and/or moisturizing oils or creams can be applied after showering. The absorption of these creams and oils can be increased by covering the affected area with gauze pads or cotton gloves. Plastic wrap can even be put over the cream for short periods.

Some doctors advise patients to eliminate common allergenic foods from their diet and to make efforts to lower daily stress in their lives. Scratching or rubbing of affected areas should be strenuously avoided because it only makes the rash worse and can exacerbate the itching. Itching can be difficult to control once it starts. Cool compresses may be soothing. Eczema tends to be chronic, flaring up or subsiding depending on exacerbating factors. Thus it is very important to try to identify underlying factors, whether they be stress, diet, or allergenic substances that come in contact with the skin.

The Doctor

Eczema is usually treated by a dermatologist, although it may be diagnosed by an internist or family practitioner. Eczema is basically diagnosed from the appearance of the rash and its history. The doctor will recommend basic self-help measures and, if necessary, prescribe *corticosteroid* or *coal tar* creams to reduce the body's inflammatory reaction. In more severe cases, the doctor may also recommend the use of *Cetaphil lotion* for cleansing, instead of soap and water, since soap tends to be irritating and drying to sensitive skin. In addition, oral antibiotics and a topical corticosteroid solution may be prescribed. For long-term use, corticosteroid ointments or creams are often prescribed in a two-day on, two-day off regimen. In severe cases, many doctors prescribe *prednisone*, an oral steroid, for one to two weeks. Its use is limited because it is a powerful drug with potentially serious side effects, including suppression of the adrenal glands. Doctors may also prescribe an *antihistamine* to help control itching. It is generally taken at night because it tends to make people drowsy and it helps prevent people from scratching affected areas in their sleep. An antibiotic may also be given if the rash is pustular or if the doctor believes that *staph bacteria* are delaying the rash's healing.

Ruling Out Other Diseases

Fungal infections (see p. 164) are ruled out by preparing a skin scraping with potassium hydroxide and examining it under the microscope. *Contact dermatitis* (see p. 172) causes an eczema-like rash, but the inflamed areas are generally linear or square, not circular.

Prevention

As in many chronic diseases, prevention is really the best treatment. The basic principles are to keep the skin moist and to avoid irritation. Flare-ups are often precipitated by changes in temperature and humidity. Especially in winter, individuals with eczema should minimize bathing and use of soap, and increase their use of oils and creams. The cool moist air found near the ocean or in the mountains is most beneficial. When a temporary change in climate is not possible, a humidifier or air conditioner may help to alleviate itching and prevent recurrences.

Activities that produce perspiration should be limited if a flare-up seems likely, because sweat itself is irritating. If people can't avoid such activity, they should bathe and apply oil afterward. Perfumed soaps and cosmetics and scratchy clothing should generally be avoided. During flare-ups, swimming in pools and freshwater lakes should be avoided because it tends to dry out the skin. Salt water, by comparison, may have a beneficial effect. Finally, some doctors feel that emotional stress is the single most important factor in triggering flare-ups. Relaxation exercises and relaxing activities are recommended (see p. 60).

Acne

Symptoms

- whiteheads or pimples (raised dots filled with pus)
- red raised dots
- blackheads
- cysts (deep, fluid-filled sacs)
- hard, red, raised lumps
- most commonly on the face, neck, back, shoulders, and upper arms
- occasionally, pitting and scarring

Description

Acne, an inflammatory condition of the hair follicle ducts resulting from plugged oil glands, is the most common of all skin diseases. Acne first occurs during puberty when its incidence is fairly universal. Contrary to popular opinion, it is not just a disease of adolescence, but remains quite common into people's 60s.

The disease occurs in areas of the body that have high numbers of sebaceous glands. These glands produce a fatty substance, called *sebum*, which lubricates the skin. The sebaceous glands drain into the hair follicles, and sebum emerges alongside the hair shaft. These glands are stimulated by the male hormone *androgen*. In men, androgen is not only responsible for secondary male sexual characteristics, it contributes to muscle and bone growth. In women, the adrenal glands produce small amounts of androgen that are likewise necessary for growth and bone development. The sebaceous glands are dormant during early childhood, but undergo a huge initial spurt during puberty and remain active until menopause in women, and well into the 70s in men.

Cells in the base of the sebaceous glands pro-liferate continually, pushing older cells upward. These cells produce a fatty substance, then explode and die. Sebum is a mixture of the fatty substance and dead cells. In acne, the sebum becomes plugged up in the hair follicles, causing them to widen and swell. Two problems can result: one is a *blackhead*, which is simply a plug of sebum visible at the widened, open mouth of a hair follicle; the other is a *whitehead*, which is a closed hair follicle behind which the sebum has built up until it ruptures the bottom of the follicle. When this happens, bacteria that are naturally present in the follicle multiply and convert triglycerides into free fatty acids, which are irritative, and the follicle becomes inflamed and infected. In the initial stage, acne consists of oily skin, blackheads, and whiteheads. If the bacteria continue to multiply inside the plugged ducts, the infected areas enlarge, resulting in larger pus-filled pimples, tiny hard lumps, and fluid-filled cysts.

Mild acne occurs most commonly on the chin, cheeks, and forehead. Generally the pimples leave no mark when they heal. In more se-

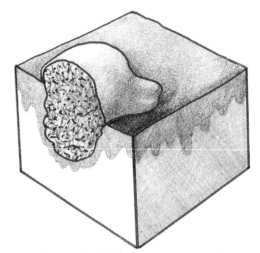

Acne pustules *are fluid-filled sacs that contain bacteria and white blood cells.*

vere cases, the neck, back, shoulders and upper arms may be involved. In these cases the pimples tend to last longer and become more infected, which can lead to pitting and scarring that persists after the pimples have healed.

Many factors contribute to acne. It has been recognized for years that genetic background plays a role. Individuals whose parents have had acne are more likely to develop it themselves. Diet used to be regarded as a major factor; people were told to avoid chocolate and greasy foods. More recent studies have shown that chocolate has no effect on pimple formation, and the whole issue of diet is often downplayed now, although some doctors still believe diet plays a role in some people and will therefore do a diet history and may suggest food allergy testing. Emotions are another factor associated with acne. Stress is definitely associated with flare-ups, presumably because it affects the body's hormone levels.

Self-Care

Mild acne responds well to a consistent self-care regimen. The basic principle is to keep the skin clean. Cleanliness involves removing excess oil, keeping the follicle openings unplugged, and lowering the number of bacteria naturally present on the skin. There is a vast array of antibacterial cleansing preparations, including creams, soaps, washes, and gels. Doctors currently disagree as to whether or not inflamed areas should be scrubbed vigorously, as was recommended in the past. Some continue to advise it; others feel it may contribute to the inflammation and simply advise frequent washing. All doctors advise washing with *hot* water to help open plugged follicles. As in any infection, hot moist towels or compresses help to bring white blood cells into the areas to fight the infection. Some doctors recommend using a special tool called a *comedo extractor* to pop out blackheads after washing. If the hands are used, they should be clean. It is never advisable to repeatedly pick at or squeeze pimples.

There are many topical acne preparations designed to be applied after washing. These medications contain chemicals such as *benzoyl peroxide*, *salicylic acid*, and *resorcinol*. These agents promote drying and peeling, which tends to heal the acne. If benzoyl peroxide preparations are used, they should be applied thinly, once or twice a day, 15 minutes after washing, to avoid irritation. Individuals may respond differently to various preparations, so if one doesn't seem to be effective, another should be tried.

Ultraviolet light seems to have a beneficial effect on acne pimples, probably because it also causes dryness and peeling. Sunlight is best and

---

Self-Care for People with Acne

- wash face gently with antibacterial soap 1–2 times a day
- do *not* scrub face with wash cloth or brush
- avoid using oils, oil-based makeup, or suntan lotion on face
- keep hair clean
- do not scratch or squeeze pimples excessively
- avoid foods that make your acne worse
- if *benzoyl peroxide* preparations are used, in order to avoid irritation, they should be applied thinly and evenly, 1–2 times a day, 15 minutes after washing (because they are irritating to moist skin). These preparations should be applied in sufficient quantity so that the skin feels dry and tight but does not turn red or become irritated.
- if *tretinoin (e.g., Retin-A)* is used, it should be applied thinly and evenly to dry skin once a day or every other day until the skin becomes slightly red, but should be stopped or used less frequently if the skin becomes irritated. Care should be taken with sun exposure because some people become sun sensitive when using this medication; sunscreens can be used in conjunction with tretinoin.

safest, but tanning lights may be useful if the eyes are protected and care is taken not to burn the skin. Used properly, sun blocking lotions will prevent burning. Doctors advise gradually increasing exposure until the skin becomes slightly pink.

The Doctor

It is important to seek treatment for moderate-to-severe acne, to prevent both physical scarring and emotional distress. The doctor (usually a dermatologist) can prescribe stronger antibacterial cleansing agents that contain *benzoyl peroxide* (e.g., *Desquam-X wash* and *Benzac W wash*), as well as creams and gels containing *retinoic acid* (*Retin-A*), a form of Vitamin A that causes significant redness and peeling, and thus helps the sebum to slide out of hair follicles, rather than to become blocked. The redness and peeling can be severe if these medications are not started slowly. Retinoic acid is a strong medicine that should not be used during pregnancy. It also should not be used in conjunction with sunlamp treatments, when people are sunburned, or when they must spend long periods in the sun, as it may increase sunburn sensitivity and the likelihood of skin cancer.

In addition to topical preparations, oral antibiotics have long been effective in treating moderate-to-severe acne. Antibiotics kill the bacteria on the skin that cause inflammation and infection. This treatment was a breakthrough in preventing significant acne scarring. Depending on the severity of the case, the doctor may prescribe an antibiotic intermittently or for long periods of time. Two antibiotics are commonly used and are reported to have surprisingly few side effects even with long-term use: *tetracycline* (500–1000 mg per day initially; reduced to 250–500 for long-term therapy) and *minocycline* (200 mg per day). Neither should be used during pregnancy because they cause discoloration of the developing baby's teeth. Both antibiotics also occasionally cause nausea, diarrhea, or the overgrowth of *candida* yeast (see p. 398).

Recently a new oral medicine, *Isotretinoin*, has been used to treat severe cystic acne only. This drug is a form of Vitamin A which inhibits sebaceous gland activity. Although it has been used with success, it is a powerful drug with significant side effects. Patients taking the drug have been known to experience dryness of the skin and mucous membranes, itching, swollen lips, and nosebleeds. Some patients also have more serious side effects. Isotretinoin is absolutely contraindicated during pregnancy because it has caused malformations in developing fetuses. If women of childbearing age take this drug at all, they should be on a reliable form of birth control. Should a woman accidentally take the drug during pregnancy, a therapeutic abortion will be discussed. Because of the significant adverse effects of this drug, its use generally is reserved for people with very severe acne that has not responded to other forms of therapy.

In addition to treating acne episodes, dermatologists have several methods of dealing with the scarring sometimes caused by acne. The most common treatment is *dermabrasion*, in which the scarred skin is frozen and the top layer of skin is sanded or brushed off.

Ruling Out Other Diseases

Several chemically induced forms of acne can result from industrial exposure to *chlorinated hydrocarbons*, such as cutting oil, or from taking drugs that contain large quantities of iodine or bromine. This type of acne can be ruled out by the patient's history.

Prevention

Because acne tends to be a chronic condition, prevention becomes very important, particularly among susceptible individuals or people with a family history of the disease. A thorough, regular schedule of cleansing the skin is the key to avoiding or minimizing outbreaks. Oily creams and cosmetics should be avoided because they tend to plug the pores. Repeated scratching or squeezing of acne pimples tends to promote infection and may make scarring worse. Avoiding fatty foods may help in some people. Stress-reduction techniques may also help to minimize outbreaks (see p. 58). Finally, regular exposure to sunlight also seems to be helpful in preventing acne flare-ups.

Skin Tumors: Benign and Malignant

Symptoms

benign characteristics
- small skin growths that are flat or raised
- flesh-colored, tan, dark brown, or black in color
- fast or slow-growing
- located anywhere on the body, in areas exposed to the sun, or not
- soft to hard consistency, fluid-filled or not
- possibly have wrinkles or skin lines
- regular in shape, often domelike or round

possible malignant characteristics
- uneven coloration
- blue-black, red and white, or translucent in color
- sudden increase in size or steady, fixed growth
- no skin markings or wrinkles
- irregular shape
- raw or bleeding areas that don't heal, particularly in the center

Description

Skin tumors develop from cells that no longer conform to normal growth patterns. They can originate in the top layer of skin (the *epidermis*), the middle layer (the *dermis*), or any of the specialized skin cells, such as the *melanocytes* which give the skin its color. Generally benign tumors are like the cells they arise from and do not spread or continue to grow at a faster rate than normal. Malignant or cancerous cells undergo more profound change as they develop, and become unlike their parent cell. They continue to multiply indefinitely and may spread to other areas.

Although it is not known what causes cells to begin reproducing at a faster rate, two major factors are associated with such a change in growth patterns. First, a tendency toward certain types of skin growths is hereditary. Secondly, exposure to certain environmental factors is known to be associated with particular tumors, either benign or malignant. Sunlight is the most important of these predisposing factors. Ultraviolet rays in sunlight can change the reproductive information in the DNA of a cell's nucleus and cause the cell to grow in an altered fashion. Many types of skin tumors are most prevalent on the head, neck, and arms, areas of the body that are constantly exposed to sunlight. In terms of

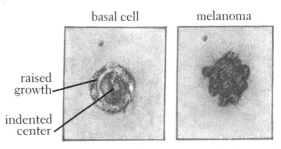

Two important types of skin cancer are the basal cell carcinoma (left), *a raised growth with an indented center, and the* melanoma, *which appears as a dark lump with an irregular border* (right).

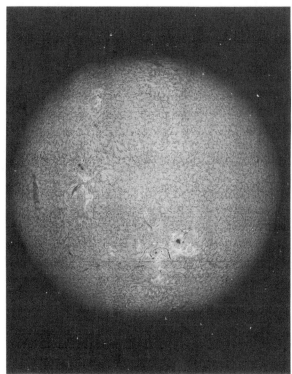

Prolonged exposure to the sun is the cause of the majority of skin tumors. Photograph of the sun taken with a red hydrogen line. Mt. Wilson and Palomar Observatories.

benign tumors require no treatment unless a person is concerned about the way they look. Because malignant skin tumors continue to grow, they have to be removed, even though such tumors are rarely life-threatening. Melanomas, on the other hand, will spread to other parts of the body if left untreated.

Benign skin tumors: There are many types of benign skin tumors, the most common being *melanocytic nevii*, which are often called *moles* or *beauty marks*. A few are present at birth, but most appear gradually over the next 20 years of life. By adulthood, the average person has 40 of them. Interestingly, melanocytic nevii tend to disappear with age, and few are seen in people over 80. These growths, which can occur anywhere on the body, may be flat or raised, and vary widely in color and surface texture, but typically they are oval-shaped, have well-defined borders, and exhibit skin wrinkles. Infrequently, one of these growths can turn into a malignant melanoma. Thus, if one suddenly changes in size, shape, color, becomes raw, or starts bleeding, it should be evaluated by a dermatologist.

The second most common benign tumors are *seborrheic keratoses*. These are sometimes re-

geography, skin tumors tend to be more frequent in regions close to the equator, especially among people who work outdoors and among those with very fair skin.

As a group, skin tumors, both those that are benign and those that are malignant, are the second most common type of skin disease, following fungal infections, in the age range 35–65. Benign tumors peak at age 45–55, whereas the incidence of malignant tumors, although much smaller, continues to rise with age. Statistically, few skin tumors are found to be malignant in people under 40. Evaluating benign tumors is a large part of any dermatological practice. Many

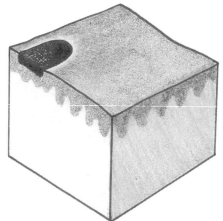

A macule is an area of skin that has changed color.

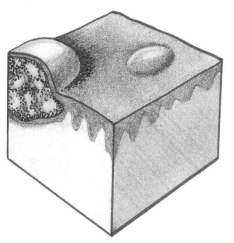

A nodule *is a solid lump of cells.*

ferred to as "barnacles of old age" because they look as if they had been stuck on the skin. Seborrheic keratoses are sharply defined growths, from flesh-colored to brown, with a velvety or warty surface. There is generally more than one, and they occur most frequently on the chest, back, and abdomen, although they are occasionally seen on the face and arms. They grow slowly and can have greasy scales on them. They are not dangerous and normally increase in size and number slowly over a period of years.

In addition to moles and seborrheic keratoses, there are a number of other kinds of benign tumors. *Sebaceous cysts* or *wens* are fluid-filled sacs which contain a soft yellow liquid. They develop when a hair follicle becomes plugged, possibly due to acne. They are found mostly on the face and chest. A *lipoma* is a soft, compressible collection of fat that looks like a lump under the skin. Lipomas occur most often in middle age and are frequently found on the buttocks, thighs, arms, back and neck. *Skin tags* or *acrochordons* are small soft growths on the surface of the skin that are suspended by a stalk. They are most commonly found on the eyelids, neck, armpits, and groin, and can occur in numbers.

Premalignant tumors: Actinic keratoses or *senile (solar) keratoses* are small, premalignant tumors that become increasingly common after the age of 35. They are caused by exposure to sunlight or ultraviolet radiation and are found on exposed areas of the skin; in particular, the face, lips, backs of the hands and arms, and back of the neck. They generally occur in groups and look like raised, red or brown patches covered with a rough scale. Often the skin around them is dry, wrinkled, and leathery, a condition referred to as *sailor's* or *farmer's skin*. Senile keratoses are most common in fair-skinned people who experience prolonged exposure to the sun. If allowed to go untreated, about 25% of these tumors will gradually enlarge and turn into *squamous cell carcinomas.* Although the latter tumors are malignant, they don't usually spread to other areas and are easily treated. Signs of malignant change include increasing redness, inflammation, rawness, and bleeding.

Malignant tumors or *skin cancer:* By far the most common type of skin cancer is *basal cell carcinoma.* It arises in the basal cells which produce new cells in the epidermis, the top layer of skin. Basal cell carcinoma is uncommon among blacks and Asians; it is most common among people of Northern European background who have blue eyes, fair skin, and blond hair. Like many other skin tumors, it occurs more frequently in people who spend long hours in the sun in warm climates. This type of tumor is also more common in men than in women, and occurs in steadily increasing numbers after the age of 35. A basal cell carcinoma starts as a small translucent, reddish area that shows tiny underlying blood vessels. The surface is generally shiny and no longer shows normal wrinkles or skin markings. Growth is slow, but eventually the center develops a depression, then becomes raw and bleeds. This condition is referred to as a *rodent ulcer.* Most of these tumors occur on the face, 90% between the forehead and the upper lip. If neglected, basal cell carcinomas will continue to grow and will eventually destroy underlying structures, but they will not *metastasize* or spread to other areas of the body.

The second most common skin cancer is *squamous cell carcinoma*. It arises in epidermal cells which naturally become progressively hardened with the protein keratin before being sloughed off. Like basal cell carcinoma, this form of skin cancer is caused by sun exposure and occurs most often in fair-skinned people. Generally, squamous cell carcinomas arise rapidly from the premalignant tumors called *actinic keratoses*. They appear in exposed areas as inflamed, raw, bleeding lumps. The tumor has been described as resembling a wart with an eroded top that is situated on a swollen base. This kind of skin cancer has a low tendency to metastasize, that is, spread to other areas, but if untreated it will damage underlying tissues. The average age of incidence for squamous cell carcinoma is 60.

A dangerous but uncommon type of skin cancer is the *malignant melanoma* which arises in the melanocytes, the pigment-producing cells in the top layer of skin. It is much less common than basal or squamous cell carcinoma. Melanomas are most frequent after the age of 50, although in recent years they are increasingly being found in younger people. Like other malignant skin tumors, melanomas are most prevalent among fair-skinned people with a history of exposure to the sun. They can appear anywhere on the body, but are most common on the head, neck, trunk, legs, and forearms. Melanomas may arise by themselves or may develop from preexisting pigmented moles. They appear as darkly pigmented lumps with an irregular border. Generally they have a dormant period of months to years during which they do not invade lower skin levels or spread to other parts of the body. As they grow, melanomas often become

varied in color and their borders become irregular. Occasionally they develop satellite tumors nearby. Eventually they may ulcerate and bleed. Unlike other skin cancers, if left untreated melanomas will spread widely throughout the body, and they can be fatal.

It is reassuring to note that most skin cancers are not life-threatening. The overwhelming majority of skin tumors are not malignant, and even the great majority of malignant ones do not metastasize.

Self-Care

In general, benign skin tumors do not require any care unless they are unsightly, grow, are in areas where they become irritated, or they develop possible malignant symptoms. Self-care largely consists of self-awareness with regard to particular kinds of pigmented areas and lumps, and seeking a doctor's opinion if any of them develop malignant characteristics.

The Doctor

Dermatologists—doctors who specialize in skin diseases—can diagnose most skin tumors by their characteristic appearance. Generally dermatologists do not remove benign tumors unless they are visually unappealing or are located in areas where they are likely to be irritated and become abraded. Seborrheic keratoses are often scraped off under local anesthesia, and sebaceous cysts are drained if they become large. Actinic keratoses may be either removed surgically or with a chemical because they have a tendency to become malignant. If a tumor appears to be malignant or there is some question as to whether it is, it will be *biopsied*, that is, removed and examined under a microscope. In the event that a tumor is malignant, not only the tumor but an area around it will be *excised* or removed to prevent spreading. In the case of a melanoma, further treatment depends on how the tumor is *graded*, which is determined by how large it is and how far it has spread. With a small, shallow melanoma, the cure rate is excellent (almost 100% if the tumor has not gone below the *epidermis*, the top layer of skin); as melanomas become larger and deeper, the cure rate drops significantly. This is the reason that doctors urge people to seek treatment promptly if they notice any significant change in a mole or skin growth.

Ruling Out Other Diseases

The main issue with this group of skin conditions is differentiating the less common malignant tumors from the more frequent benign ones. Since the distinction can be a fine one, it's important that any tumor that has malignant characteristics be examined by a dermatologist. In terms of other skin diseases, seborrheic keratoses look something like warts, but the growths have more the appearance of being "stuck on." Warts are less waxy-looking and have a rougher surface.

Prevention

The most important principle of prevention in terms of the majority of skin tumors is avoiding prolonged exposure to the sun, particularly at midday when the ultraviolet rays are strongest, and especially in the tropical climates. Limiting sun exposure is most important for fair-skinned, blue-eyed people who burn easily, and for people who live in the tropics. Doctors recommend wearing broad-brimmed hats, long-sleeved shirts, and gloves if a person works out of doors or has a history of skin tumors. They also suggest that people apply *sunscreen* to exposed areas of skin. These preparations contain *PABA* (*para-aminobenzoic acid*), a chemical that absorbs the specific ultraviolet rays that cause

sunburn and skin cancer. Because skin tumors are the second most common skin condition from ages 35–65, and skin cancer is the most common malignancy, most dermatologists recommend that people routinely apply sunscreen with a *skin protection factor (SPF) of 15* whenever they are in bright, hot sun for any length of time. People with fairer skin should use an even higher SPF. Of all malignancies, skin cancer is the most preventable.

Herpes Simplex: Cold Sores or Fever Blisters, and Genital Herpes

Symptoms

- small fluid-filled blisters on top of a red base
- groups of blisters
- commonly occur around the mouth or genital area
- ulcers or sores that remain after blisters pop
- nearby lymph nodes are often swollen as well
- sores can be itchy, tender, painful

Description

Herpes simplex is a skin infection caused by one of two types of viruses. These viruses are microscopic living entities that are made up of pure DNA, or genetic information, loosely encased in a protein membrane. Like all viruses, *herpes simplex virus (HSV) type 1* and *type 2* are parasites that can only reproduce inside of living cells from which they get the basic materials for growth. HSV type 1 affects the area around the mouth, while HSV type 2 affects the area around the genitals. Both are spread from person to person, type 2 by intimate sexual contact, type 1 by oral secretions.

The initial occurrence of herpes simplex is referred to as the *primary infection*. Type 1 most often occurs in infants and children; over 90% of all people contract type 1 by the age of five. Type 1 sometimes causes no symptoms, or it may cause painful skin sores inside the mouth or on the lips or cheeks. In addition, people may experience tiredness, fever, and swollen lymph nodes in the neck. Adults may also experience a sore throat or headache.

Primary genital herpes is most commonly seen in adolescents and adults because it is only spread by sexual contact. As of 1980, one study showed its incidence at 128 per 100,000 people, which was approximately ten times the rate seen in 1970. Characteristic blisters, which are often painful, develop on the vagina, vulva, perineum, penis, or buttocks. Like type 1, the primary infection for type 2 may be accompanied by tiredness and fever, as well as nearby swollen lymph nodes (in the groin).

With either type 1 or 2, the primary infection disappears within two weeks, but some viruses remain in the ganglia of nearby nerve cells, where they exist in a latent state. At this point, the infected person will have no sores or blisters, and no virus on the skin. However, 20%–40% of people who have a primary infection of type 1 and 60% of people with type 2 will experience at least one *recurrent infection*. Recurrences may then taper off; over 50% of people with genital herpes will not have any more recurrences after seven years.

The number and timing of recurrent infections is unpredictable, but they generally involve a milder rash, less pain, and virtually no systemic symptoms. Recurrent infections often seem to be triggered by various factors such as colds, fever, exhaustion, stress, menstrual periods, sun, and wind. The initial symptoms will

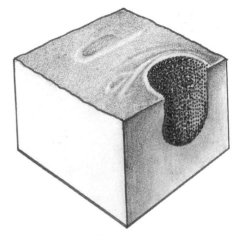

Herpes ulcers *are small eroded areas that penetrate through the top layer of skin.*

be tenderness, itching, or burning that lasts for several hours to a day. These early symptoms, called the *prodromal phase*, are followed by the appearance of the characteristic blisters. These blisters pop, form ulcers, and crust over after several days, eventually disappearing within seven to ten days. The most common sites for recurrent infections of type 1 are the lower lip, nose, and cheeks. Recurrent infections of type 2 affect the same areas as the primary infection.

Doctors believe that type 2 virus is largely transmissible just before and during the *active phase* when a person has the blisters. The infection goes away by itself and is not dangerous to healthy adults; however, the disease is painful (initially) and emotionally stressful. Also, at present, genital herpes carries a definite sexual stigma. The problems associated with genital herpes have led to the formation of a nationwide self-help group called HELP (check local listing in larger cities) which offers emotional support to people with genital herpes.

For women, genital herpes can have special consequences because the virus can be dangerous to newborns. If a pregnant woman has an active infection at the time of delivery, her baby can be exposed to the virus during passage through the birth canal. A recent study found that 2 out of 35 infants (8%) who were exposed to the virus in this way developed the infection. In the rare instance that the baby develops a systemic infection, the disease can be life-threatening. Currently, women who have a history of genital herpes are followed closely in the final weeks of pregnancy. If cultures indicate the presence of live virus in the vagina around the time that a woman goes into labor, she will be delivered by cesarean section to avoid having the baby pass through the birth canal. A cesarean may not be performed if the mother's bag of waters has broken some hours before the baby can be delivered surgically, since the baby is then considered to have already been exposed to the virus. A newborn is thought to be at greater risk if the mother is experiencing an initial infection, rather than a recurrence. Finally, women who get genital herpes may have a higher risk of cancer of the cervix. Women with cervical cancer have been found to be more likely to have antibodies to type 2, indicating previous exposure. However, these statistics do not constitute a proven cause, and their importance is unknown (see p. 418).

Self-Care

Both primary and recurrent infections of herpes type 1 and 2 go away by themselves within several weeks. The principle of self-care is to make a person more comfortable during the active phase. Ice packs tend to lessen itching and discomfort. When the sores are inside the mouth, popsicles or cold liquids are soothing. A number of nonprescription preparations are sold to make type 1 lesions feel better (e.g., *Orabase, Blistex, Campho-Phenique,* and mouthwash). *Styptic pencils,* which are generally used to stop bleeding from shaving nicks, sometimes help

---

Self-Care for People with Herpes

Prevention:
- avoid sexual contact from the first sign of tingling until sores are healed (unless the sores can be covered with a condom)
- avoid kissing or sharing food utensils when you have mouth sores
- wash hands after touching sores
- don't share towels while sores are present
- women who have herpes should get yearly Pap smears

Treatment:
- sit in a warm bath for 15 minutes two to three times a day (Epsom salts or Burrow's solution may be added to the water); pat lesions dry with a towel or use a hair dryer set on warm
- apply ice packs to the genital area for 5–10 minutes at a time to relieve itching and inflammation
- wear loose cotton underwear and loose pants or skirts to avoid perspiring or abrading the inflamed area; avoid pantyhose
- to decrease pain on urination, urinate in the shower or squirt tepid water over the genital area while urinating
- take aspirin or acetaminophen to relieve discomfort caused by the sores

---

make external lesions go away more rapidly, as does *zinc sulfate lotion,* which is available without prescription.

There are several home remedies for treating genital lesions. Warm baths definitely make people more comfortable and may even inactivate the virus on the skin. One of the reasons baths are effective is that they are relaxing, which is important since stress affects how uncomfortable a person is, as well as playing a role in triggering recurrent episodes. *Ether, 70% alcohol solution, calamine lotion,* and *talcum powder* or *cornstarch* all have a drying effect on external lesions and may make them less bothersome. A

Mayo Clinic study has shown that frequency of recurrence and symptoms may be reduced by eating foods that contain the amino acid l-lysine, such as dairy products, potatoes, and brewer's yeast. Unfortunately there is still no completely effective home treatment for either cold sores or genital herpes.

The Doctor

A doctor (dermatologist, internist, or family practitioner) can diagnose both type 1 and 2 herpes by the way the sores look and by several laboratory tests, including a smear, a culture, and an *antibody titer*, a blood test which demonstrates the presence of antibodies if a person has ever been exposed to the virus. Other than confirming the diagnosis, the doctor usually only recommends self-care.

There are several new drugs that are effective against herpes, but currently they are only recommended for primary infections, in particular for individuals whose immune systems are suppressed. The most popular drug, *acyclovir*, is not approved for treatment or prevention of recurrent episodes of herpes for several reasons: 1) it doesn't lessen the spread of the virus; 2) it tends to cause resistant strains of the virus; and 3) in animal studies it has been found to change the genetic structure of cells. For this reason, the drug should not be used by pregnant women.

Ruling Out Other Diseases

Because it also has a crusting phase, *impetigo* (see p. 203) is sometimes confused with herpes, but impetigo produces a characteristic straw-colored fluid and crusts, and it generally affects different sites. Genital herpes is sometimes mistaken for *primary syphilis*. To rule out syphilis, a *dark field* microscopic examination of fluid from a blister is done to determine if syphilis organisms are present.

Prevention

It is virtually impossible to prevent herpes type 1 because it is so widespread throughout the population. However, it may be wise to avoid kissing or sharing food utensils with individuals who have active cold sores. In addition, people exposed to herpes should wash their hands before touching their eyes or mucous membranes.

Genital herpes can be prevented by temporarily avoiding intimate sexual contact with a person who has active lesions. It is probably safe to have intercourse if *condoms* cover the sores completely and prevent direct contact with them. Those who have a history of herpes may be able to minimize recurrent episodes by avoiding the specific situations that seem to trigger them. Relaxation exercises are particularly important for people who find that episodes tend to be set off by stress (see p. 60). At the start of prodromal symptoms such as itching, pain, burning, or tingling, sexual activity should be curtailed to avoid infecting others. *Neonatal herpes* can be prevented by careful management at the end of pregnancy.

Hives, or Urticaria

Symptoms

- wheals—whitish or reddish raised patches surrounded by a red halo
- occasionally, red dots or pimples
- patches that come and go fleetingly
- intense itching, stinging, or prickling

Description

Hives is a skin disease in which areas of skin react to external stimuli by temporarily swelling up. The swelling results when special skin cells

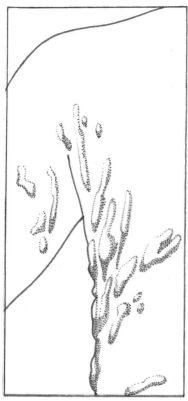

Hives are an allergic skin reaction that can be caused by foods, insect bites, or drugs.

clude sudden exposure to cold, heat, sunlight, or water, as well as exercise, injury, emotional stress, and insect stings.

Shortly after exposure to the triggering factor, the susceptible individual experiences itching and possibly numbness in the affected area. These feelings are probably due to the sudden release of histamine. In a short time, the fluid released under the top layer of skin produces *wheals*, raised reddish or whitish patches of skin that generally have a red halo and sometimes red pimples. Wheals develop very suddenly and usually disappear within a day, though they can recur. During this time they often change tremendously in appearance, varying even over the course of a few minutes. Any part of the body can be affected, but the most common sites are the lips, eyelids, cheeks, palms, soles, and areas where clothing presses against the skin. Occasionally, the mucous membranes can be involved, including the mouth, larynx, and intestines. In the uncommon situation that a person with hives has trouble breathing, the situation is a MEDICAL EMERGENCY and a doctor should be seen immediately (see p. 475).

called *mast cells* release several chemicals, including *histamine* which causes cells in the *dermis*, the middle skin layer, to release their cellular fluid. Hives are triggered by two basic causes—an allergic reaction to a particular substance or an unusual response to a physical factor. Allergic reactions can be caused by a variety of foods, drugs, and chemicals (see chart). Foods most frequently associated with hives are shellfish, strawberries, chocolate, nuts, and tomatoes. The most common drugs causing hives are penicillin, aspirin, sulfonamides, and narcotics. Chemicals that have been known to cause hives include food additives, dyes, and cosmetics. Physical causes, which are less common, in-

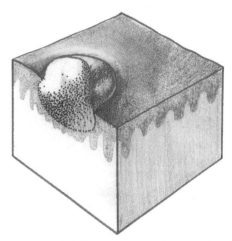

Bullae—fluid-filled sacs, ½ cm or larger—develop under the skin in people with hives.

Self-Care

There are two aspects involved in self-care for hives: finding the cause, and treating the symptoms. To determine the cause or causes, people often have to keep a detailed diary, listing the foods, drugs, chemicals, and physical stimuli they were in contact with shortly before each episode of hives. The accompanying charts provide a brief checklist. If people develop hives fairly often, they can generally pinpoint what triggers the reaction. If individuals suspect a food but are not certain which one it is, they can try an *elimination diet* in which only nonallergenic foods are eaten and common allergic foods are reintroduced one at a time (see chart). If no specific cause can be isolated, people can try eliminating all forms of aspirin, both in drugs and that which occurs naturally in certain foods. Interestingly, the majority of hive reactions occur only once, often making it impossible to determine the cause.

The main point of home treatment is to relieve the itching, which can be intense. Nonprescription *antihistamines* may be effective, but they often cause sleepiness and can interfere with driving. Cold compresses, cool showers, and *colloidal baths* using *Aveeno*, oatmeal, or cornstarch (1 cup per tubful of water) are alternative aids to help relieve itching, as are calamine lotion and lotions containing menthol or phenol.

Foods That Commonly Cause Allergic Reactions
Citrus—oranges, lemons, grapefruit
Cola—chocolate, cola
Fish—flounder, halibut
Food dyes, aspirin, preservatives (benzoic acid)
Gourds—melons, cucumber, squash
Grains—wheat, corn, rye, oats, rice
Legumes—peanuts, peas, alfalfa, clover, licorice
Meat—cow, goat, sheep, and or their milk
Poultry—turkey, chicken, duck and/or their eggs

The Doctor

In the rare event that a person experiences difficulty breathing during the course of an outbreak of hives, the situation is a MEDICAL EMERGENCY. The doctor will treat the reaction with a shot of *epinephrine* which acts rapidly to reduce swelling in the larynx (see p. 475).

Generally, the doctor (an allergist, dermatologist, internist, or family practitioner) will assist in determining the cause of hives by having the person keep a diary, and, if necessary, by having them follow an elimination diet or no-aspirin diet. If home remedies are not sufficient, the doctor will prescribe strong antihistamines, most commonly *hydroxyzine (Atarax or Vistaril)* or *diphenhydraminl hydrochloride (Benadryl)*. In recent years, doctors have become less enthusiastic about antihistamines because they only seem effective in about a third of all cases, and they generally produce drowsiness. For a moderate-to-severe episode of hives, the doctor may prescribe *steroids* (e.g., *prednisone*) or *epinephrine* along with an antihistamine.

Ruling Out Other Diseases

Occasionally, if hives have pimples on the wheals, the condition may be confused with *contact dermatitis* (see p. 172). Hives, however, are fleeting and leave no trace, whereas contact dermatitis generally produces blisters that weep and crust. Bacterial infections can look like hives, but they are hot and painful rather than itchy, and don't clear up as rapidly.

Prevention

The main principle of prevention is avoiding the causal agent, whether it's a food, drug, chemical, or physical factor. Also, there is a definite emotional component, as evidenced by the fact that placebos (inactive drugs) can actually give people relief from hives. Relaxation exercises may be helpful if the hives appear to be stress-related (see p. 60). For a general discussion on preventing allergies, see *Allergies*. Over several years, the condition often disappears by itself.

Insect Bites: Lice, Scabies, Chiggers, Ticks, Fleas, Bedbugs

Symptoms

general
- itching
- raised red papules
- scratch marks
- occasionally, fluid-filled blisters
- occasionally, pus-filled pimples (secondary infection)

specific
- head lice: white egg cases near the base of hair shafts
    tiny white lice on skin or clothes
- pubic lice: brown dots at the base of pubic hairs
- scabies: itching at night
    lines of red dots, often on the sides of fingers or the abdomen
- chiggers: red dots, especially around the beltline, neck, or cuffs
    small red mites on the skin
- ticks: dark oval insect with head burrowed in the skin
- fleas: small dark insects that jump and are hard to kill
    clusters of red papules, often on the ankles, legs
- bedbugs: nighttime biting and itching
    dark bugs seen in bedding

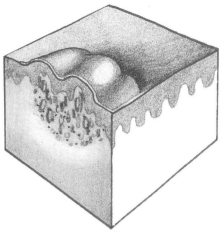

A papule *is a small, raised area on the skin.*

Description

Many insects cause minor but annoying rashes on humans as well as animals. The insects bite because they derive their nutrition from blood. When they bite, their saliva gets under the skin, and chemicals in the saliva that are slightly toxic cause an irritative or allergic reaction. Raised red areas occur where the body naturally releases *histamine*, a chemical that causes local inflammation and swelling. Such swelling helps to protect the body by keeping the reaction confined to a local area. Once the body has learned to recognize and make antibodies against a particular substance, a slight allergic reaction also occurs. The itching that generally develops causes people to scratch at the bites, which can become secondarily infected from bacteria that are naturally found under the fingernails and on the skin. Thus the typical rash not only has raised red areas called *papules*, it may even show scratch marks, tiny allergic blisters, and small infected pimples. The location and grouping of the rash depend upon the particular insect. Many of the insects in this group used to be associated with poor living conditions and lack of cleanliness, but now they seem to affect families of all classes and living standards.

Lice, or pediculosis: There are three types of lice that affect distinct areas of the body: *head*, *body*, and *pubic* lice. All three are so tiny they are difficult to see without a magnifying glass, but their *egg cases* are not. The egg cases, or

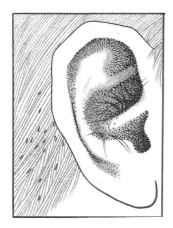

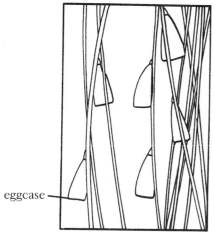

eggcase —

Head lice are not visible to the naked eye, but their egg cases can be seen on the hairshafts around the ears and back of the scalp.

nits, are pearly white, oval bodies about the size of the head of a pin. When an insect lays eggs, it attaches its egg case to the base of a hair shaft; as the hair grows, the case moves away from the skin at about the rate of a ½ millimeter a day. Egg cases are best spotted in bright sunlight or very strong artificial light. The insects themselves are rarely seen because they are very mobile, secretive, and short-lived. On the average, only 15–20 lice are active at any one time.

The most common sites for *head lice* and their egg cases are around the ears and the hairline at the back of the head. *Body lice* and their nits may be found on the hair shafts of the shoulders, trunk, and buttocks, but are most commonly found in the seams of clothing where they live between feedings. *Pubic lice*, or *crabs*, generally live in the shafts of hair in the pubic or perianal area, but they have also been found on the hair shafts of the eyebrows, eyelashes, and armpits.

Scabies: This condition is caused by a microscopic mite. The male mite lives on the surface of the skin, but the female actually burrows just under the skin's surface and makes tunnels in which it lays eggs. The combination of characteristic scabies tunnels, pustules, and associated red lines are most commonly found on the sides of the fingers, between the toes, at the base of the palms, on the upper arms and elbows, and on the abdomen. They can also be found around the armpit, beltline, nipple, or penis. Scabies cause intense itching, especially at night. Generally the itching does not become severe until several weeks after the infestation begins, by which time a person has become allergic to the mite or its products.

Chiggers, or red bugs: These are the *larvae* of tiny mites, larvae being a developmental stage that is a forerunner of the adult. The larvae live outdoors on foliage in grassy or shrubby areas, especially where there are blackberry bushes. In the United States they are primarily found in rural areas of the South and are most prevalent in summer and fall. When people walk through chigger-infested areas, the larvae attach themselves to clothing and eventually bite the skin. The areas most commonly bitten are the wrists, ankles, and beltline. Red papules appear within several hours after the bite. Sometimes the tiny reddish body of a chigger can be seen in the center of the bite, although they drop off in a short time. The rash from chigger bites itches intensely and may burn at the same time.

Ticks: These are smooth, dark, shiny grayish-brown insects about ⅛ of an inch in size. They live on tall grass, but when a warm-blooded creature goes by, they launch themselves in that direction and attach themselves wherever they land. The tick burrows its front pincers and head under the skin, and feasts on blood for days, causing its body to swell and become firm. Generally a person does not notice when the tick first attaches itself, but often chemicals in the saliva soon cause the area to become tender and painful. People have described the sensation as feeling somewhat like a bruise. Occasionally the tick is discovered accidentally and is initially mistaken for an irritated mole. It is important to remove ticks because in some parts of the country they carry serious diseases, including Lyme disease and Rocky Mountain spotted fever.

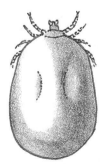

Ticks can be removed with gentle, steady traction.

Fleas: These insects do not live on people; they simply "visit" them for a bite. They actually live on dogs and cats, or in carpets, upholstered furniture, bedding, or cracks, where they lay their eggs and grow. The adult flea has Olympic jumping ability and can hurl itself long distances, often landing on people's ankles or lower legs. People who haven't been exposed to fleas can become allergic to them when they are first sensitized to the saliva. When this happens, blisters and hives develop alongside the flea bites. Such allergic reactions seem to spontaneously disappear after a year or two of exposure to fleas, and at that point, the bites themselves may not even be noticeable. This pattern is most common in areas where fleas live year-round without going into a dormant phase.

Bedbugs: These are relatively large (¼ inch), reddish-brown bugs that live in bedding, upholstered furniture, and cracks in the wall. They feed at night, jumping onto the skin briefly, and making two or three bites in a small area before jumping off. The sites most commonly bitten are the face, ankles, and buttocks. Generally people aren't even awakened, but first become aware of the bites when they see the red papules. The bugs themselves are often difficult to see because they avoid light. The can sometimes be seen by pulling back the bedcovers abruptly.

Self-Help

Self-help for insect bites has three basic principles. *1) Kill or remove the bug(s).* Simple washing with soap and water is actually somewhat effective in removing insects, and helps to prevent secondary infection, but specific preparations are listed below for the various conditions. *2) Remove the insects from the environment or clothing.* Bed linen and clothing should be laundered in hot water, dried in a hot dryer (at 140 degrees) for 20 minutes, and/or dry-cleaned.

These procedures kill both the insects and the eggs. Articles that cannot be washed or dried, such as pillows or hats, should be sealed in plastic bags for four weeks, which is enough time for the eggs to hatch and die. For insects such as fleas, the upholstered furniture, rugs, and floors should be thoroughly vacuumed. In some cases, insecticide powders, bombs, or foggers may be necessary to rid the house of insects. If combs and brushes are affected, they should be boiled or soaked in a *Lysol* solution for an hour. Generally home treatment is all that's necessary for insect problems. Most often treatment fails because it is inadequate or reinfestation occurs, not because the remedy is ineffective. It's important that all linens, clothing, and furniture be treated *at the same time* as the infested person. 3) *Treat the rash and relieve the itching.* To control the itching, cool soaks, starch or baking soda baths, calamine lotion, and even antihistamines are useful (see chart p. 175).

Lice: There are a number of *synergized pyrethrins* (e.g., A-200, RID) available over the counter which are effective against lice, and easy to use. These preparations consist of a combination of *piperonyl butoxide* and pyrethrins, which are a natural pesticide derived from the chrysanthemum plant. The solution should be applied undiluted (except on the eyelashes and eyebrows), left on for 10 minutes, and then washed off. If necessary, the treatment can be repeated in a week. After the application, the dead nits can be removed with a fine-tooth comb or tweezers. This is easiest if the hair is wet or oiled. To treat lice on the eyelashes and eyebrows, *petroleum jelly* should be carefully applied twice a day for 8 days, or these areas can be washed with baby shampoo. For all types of lice, bed linens and clothing, including hats, should be washed in hot water, put in a hot dryer, or dry cleaned in order to prevent reinfection. Articles that cannot be cleaned should be sealed in a plastic bag for a month.

Scabies: Benzyl benzoate lotion is an effective nonprescription product for killing scabies. It should be applied over the whole body (except for the face and genitals), left on for 24 hours, and then washed off. If necessary, the treatment can be repeated in a week. The old home treatment of covering the body with a mixture of *powdered sulphur* and *petroleum jelly* is effective, but messy and smelly. For this reason, the mixture is applied at night and washed off in the morning for three successive days. Washing and drying all clothing and towels at high heat is very important to prevent reinfection with scabies.

Chiggers: If any chiggers remain attached to the skin, they can be removed with a pyrinate product such as RID or A-200. Since the chigger larvae generally drop off by themselves, the basic problem is treating the itching and burning sensation they cause. The itching can be treated with any of the common home treatments (see above).

Ticks: There are a number of effective ways to remove ticks. The most popular is constant gentle traction with tweezers, either pulling the tick straight out or "unscrewing" it with a rotating motion. Other methods include applying petroleum jelly, oil, or alcohol, which should cause the tick to back out within an hour or so. A hot match tip or caustic substances are also home remedies, but unless used carefully they can hurt the skin. The goal is to get the tick out with its head intact, because the bite will then heal more quickly and there's less chance of a secondary infection or the spread of tick-carried disease. In addition, clothing and the rest of the body should be checked for other ticks.

Fleas: To deal with a flea problem, the house and any pets must be treated at the same time as the infested person. For a moderate-to-severe infestation, foggers or bombs are the most effective method to clear the house. If possible, the less toxic, *pyrethrin-based* products should be used. In households that have pets, fleas are often a continuous problem, but they can be kept to a reasonable level with frequent vacuuming and regular bathing or dusting of the animals. Care should be taken to avoid having children come into contact with flea collars, powders, or sprays.

Bedbugs: To eliminate bedbugs, all bed linens should be carefully dry-cleaned, or laundered and dried at high temperatures. For moderate-to-severe infections, it is generally suggested that the mattress, frame, and immediate area be sprayed with some insecticide, preferably a less toxic, pyrethrin-based product. *Malathion* is also effective, but it is dangerous and should not be used around children. For severe infestations, the safest solution may be a new mattress.

The Doctor

If home treatment fails, doctors do have prescription medications to treat insect infestation, but many of them are significantly more toxic than over-the-counter preparations and not that much more effective. *Lindane* products (e.g., *Kwell* and *Scabene*) are the most commonly prescribed medicines for lice, scabies, and persistent cases of chiggers. Lindane, which is absorbed through the skin, is a toxic substance with occasional serious nervous-system side effects, including headaches and even seizures. It is especially toxic to young children and pregnant women. Overuse and repeated use is not advised even in adults. If used, the directions for lindane products should be followed very carefully. *Eurax*, another product used to treat sca-

bies, is effective and helps to relieve the itching. It is nontoxic, but should not be used near the eyes or mouth because it is irritative.

Ruling Out Other Diseases

Insect bites vary in how difficult they are to diagnose. Generally the diagnosis is made from the history, the account of when the bite was first noticed. In the case of scabies, the doctor can actually scrape the mite out of its tunnels and identify it under the microscope. If there is a question about lice, the doctor can diagnose them by spotting the egg cases.

Prevention

With all types of lice, scabies, fleas, and bedbugs, prevention or avoiding reinfestation is a matter of minimizing initial exposure and treating the condition promptly and thoroughly. It's important to make sure that all family members or friends are checked and treated at the same time if they also are affected. This is especially important in the case of head lice or pubic lice. Clothing, bed linens, and the environment must be cleared of the insects at the same time.

Chiggers and ticks are an outdoor problem that only affects certain areas. These areas should be avoided, or protective measures should be taken when they are visited. Long-sleeved shirts and long pants should be worn and the cuffs should be tied or tucked in. Powdered sulphur or insect repellents can be applied as a preventive measure. Hikers or people who work in grassy, shrubby, tick-infested areas should routinely check for ticks when they get home.

Psoriasis

Symptoms

- bright red, round or oval patches with sharp raised borders
- silvery white scales, which can flake off .
- common sites: elbows, knees, base of spine, palms, or skin folds such as armpit or groin
- dimpled fingernails
- occasionally, associated with arthritis

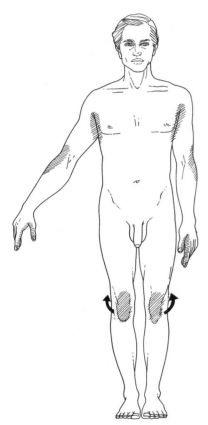

In psoriasis, the top layer of skin overproduces cells, creating thick, silvery scales in characteristic areas.

Description

Psoriasis is a chronic skin disease of unknown origin that affects an estimated 2% of the population of the United States, being equally common among men and women. It has long been observed that a tendency toward psoriasis is inherited. Although the first symptoms can occur even in infancy, the average age of onset is about 30. By far the greatest number of people seeking treatment are between the ages of 35 and 65.

Psoriasis has a characteristic rash of bright red, raised areas that are generally oval or round in shape and have sharply demarcated borders. Dry silvery scales cover the red patches, and when these scales are rubbed off, they expose tiny areas that bleed. Psoriasis often has an unpredictable course. Although it tends to be chronic, it sometimes worsens or disappears for varying periods of time. It is rare for psoriasis to be cured completely, but it can be controlled and recurrences can be minimized.

Although the cause of psoriasis is unknown, much has been learned about the physiology of the disease. In healthy skin, it takes 28 days for cells in the top layer, the epidermis, to multiply, rise to the surface, and be shed. Where there are patches of psoriasis, the entire process takes place in 7 days. In other words, the skin is "overproducing," making more cells than are needed. The result is thick silvery scales wherever psoriasis is present. In addition, there is an enlargement of tiny blood vessels in the middle layer, the dermis, which is the cause of bleeding when the scales are rubbed off. Often the rash begins or spreads when areas of skin are injured by mechanical or chemical abrasion, sunburn, or injury. This reaction is so characteristic it has been named the *Koebner phenomenon*.

There are several varieties of psoriasis, the most common being *plaque* or *nummular psoriasis*, which affects the elbows, knees, scalp,

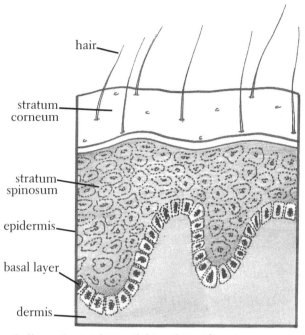

hair

stratum corneum

stratum spinosum

epidermis

basal layer

dermis

Cells in the top layer of skin, the epidermis, *grow from the bottom, move upward, die, and are shed.*

ciple of self-care is to keep the skin healthy and prevent it from being traumatized. Protective lotions that minimize itching, petroleum jelly, and nonprescription starch baths and tar shampoos all exert a beneficial effect (see p. 175) and lessen the chances of injuring the skin through scratching. Rash areas should be bathed daily and *gently* scrubbed with a soft, soapy brush. Rashes on the scalp can be washed with regular shampoo and rubbed with mineral oil or nonprescription skin-moistening oils. Moistening creams and ointments soften and lubricate dry patches and aid healing. When the rash is on the palms, cotton make-up gloves can be worn over cream to keep it from being wiped off and to increase absorption. In other areas, plastic wrap can be put over the cream for short periods to increase its absorption. Both plastic wrap and rubber gloves for cleaning should only be worn for short periods since they eventually cause sweating which depletes the skin of moisture. *Moderate* exposure to the sun or a sunlamp is also beneficial.

and back. A less common type is called *inverse psoriasis.* It affects the skin folds under the arms, around the groin, between the buttocks, and under the breasts. In nummular psoriasis the patches may or may not itch, but in inverse psoriasis, itching is likely to be intense. Other less common types of psoriasis affect the palms or are associated with pus-filled pimples. Any of the various types of psoriasis may be associated with tiny pits or spots on the nails, or with arthritic pain in the joints, especially in the fingers. For unknown reasons, arthritis occurs much more often among people with psoriasis than among the general population.

Self-Care

Mild psoriasis can be effectively controlled with home treatment. The most important prin-

The Doctor

When psoriasis becomes chronic or severe, it should be treated by a doctor. Dermatologists have several regimens that are quite effective in improving or controlling episodes of psoriasis. *Corticosteroid ointments or creams* can be prescribed to reduce inflammation. These medications vary in strength, and will be prescribed according to the seriousness of the rash. Some ointments (e.g., *Diprolene*) are strong enough that doctors generally prescribe them for only two to three weeks and monitor their use. Another treatment program involves applying *coal tar ointments* to affected areas, then washing the ointment off and exposing the areas to ultraviolet light for short periods of time. In severe cases, this may be done on a daily basis. Occasionally in very severe cases, doctors prescribe powerful systemic drugs, such as *aromatic retinoids* (e.g., *Etretinate*), which can have serious side effects and are therefore only used under close medical supervision. *Etretinate* should never be used during pregnancy.

Ruling Out Other Diseases

The red scaly patches of psoriasis are generally so characteristic that there is little question about their diagnosis. Occasionally, a fungal infection may look like psoriasis, but it can be ruled out by preparing a skin scraping with potassium hydroxide and viewing it under the microscope (see p. 165). When psoriasis occurs in skin folds, it can be difficult to distinguish from *seborrheic dermatitis*, but generally, the scales in seborrheic dermatitis are moister and yellower and are more likely to occur on the scalp, face, and chest (see p. 171).

Prevention

Because psoriasis is a chronic, somewhat hereditary disease of unknown origin, prevention is mostly a matter of minimizing spread and avoiding recurrences. It is important for people with a history of psoriasis to set up a consistent pattern of good skin care, paying close attention to individual exacerbating factors and being especially vigilant whenever the disease seems to be in a period of flare-up. Scratching of affected areas should definitely be avoided; for that reason nails should be kept short and efforts should be made to minimize itching. Also, work habits that cause constant rubbing of affected areas should be altered. In addition, reducing stress can play a beneficial role (see p. 58). It is not surprising that psoriasis is known to improve when people go on vacation. Sunny climates—deserts in particular—also seem to have a positive effect. When psoriasis affects skin fold areas, weight reduction may prove valuable.

Warts

Symptoms

- a raised area with a rough, brown or tan surface
- flat and calloused, or moist and soft appearance
- single or numerous
- may hang by a stalk
- frequently found on the the hands, feet, knees, face, or genitals
- may itch or be tender

Description

Warts are an extremely common skin lesion caused by a *papilloma virus*, a small DNA virus that grows slowly, spreads to other cells, and causes them to multiply. Over 30 different types of papilloma virus have been identified. The incubation period for the virus is 1–20 months. Many people carry the virus on their skin or mucous membranes, but do not develop warts. Once a wart appears, its course is unpredictable: it may remain unchanged, grow and spread, or disappear by itself. Studies have shown that people can develop antibodies to the papilloma virus. This response appears to be strongest in individuals whose warts recede naturally, and weakest in individuals whose warts spread or remain unchanged.

There are several different kinds of warts. *Common warts* first appear as a tiny bump, enlarge up to ½ centimeter, and develop a characteristic rough, calloused, folded appearance. Generally they are brown in color. Common warts are most often found on the hands and fingers, around the nails, on the feet and knees, and on the face. *Plantar warts* are flat, calloused warts found on the weight-bearing parts of the foot. They are often tender because they press on nearby nerves. Sometimes they appear to have tiny black specks under the surface; these are actually tiny capillaries within the base of the wart. Both common and plantar warts can spread to other areas of the body by contact, and can spread within an area. Some doctors believe that warts can even spread from person to person in a limited fashion, but this is generally not accepted. Often there is a history of a skin injury in the area where a wart develops.

Genital or *venereal warts* are soft, moist, cauliflower-like growths that are reddish in color. They are found where skin and mucous membranes meet around the vulva, cervix, penis, or anus. These warts do not spread to other areas of skin and may be caused by other kinds of viruses than the ones that cause common or plantar warts. Genital warts spread locally and can be spread to other people by means of sexual contact. According to one study, the transmission rate was 64%, with an incubation time of four to six weeks.

The significance of internal venereal warts in women may be greater than previously thought. Recently, two types of papilloma virus, HPV 16 and HPV 18, which cause genital warts on the cervix, have been linked to cervical cancer. These two viruses have actually been found in cancer cells, and the warts themselves are often seen near the site of a cervical cancer. The exact connection between these viruses and cervical cancer has not yet been worked out. External genital warts, those found on the vulva, are caused by the papilloma virus HPV 6. This virus has not been linked to cervical cancer.

Self-Care

Approximately 66% of all warts go away within two years without any treatment. Because so many warts clear up by themselves, many forms of home treatment *appear* to be ef-

fective. Probably for this reason, over a thousand types of home remedies have been chronicled in medical annals.

In general, treatment of common and plantar warts tends to be most effective if it is instituted soon after the wart is discovered, before a number of them develop. Nonprescription *salicylic acid plasters* or drops such as *Vergo* or *Compound W* have proven very effective when applied daily until the wart is gone. Every day or two, the dissolving tissue on top should be removed and new drops or plaster applied. Sometimes soaking the wart in water makes it easier to remove the dead tissue. Studies have shown that salicylic acid treatment actually cures 70% of common warts and 80% of plantar warts.

Some of the most remarkable types of wart treatment involve hypnosis or suggestion, also referred to as "hexing" or "witching." Numerous studies have demonstrated that if a person *believes* a wart will disappear, it often disappears rapidly without a trace. Doctors have used this knowledge for years by hypnotizing people or painting colored water on the wart and then telling them the wart will go away. People can apply the same principle themselves by actively visualizing the wart disappearing (see p. 67). Apparently, positive suggestion works by raising a person's antibody response to the papilloma virus. Cancer researcher Lewis Thomas has pointed out that this example of curing a viral cell overgrowth with the mind is more astonishing than most of the medical discoveries reported in the press.

The Doctor

Dermatologists have developed many methods for treating warts with chemicals or surgery. For common and plantar warts, physicians sometimes prescribe a mixture of *salicylic acid* and *lactic acid* that is stronger than the nonprescription remedies. These preparations come in liquid or plaster form and are applied daily until the wart is gone. More powerful liquids such as *trichloroacetic acid* or *nitric acid* may be applied by the doctor in the office. A relatively new treatment for warts involves sensitizing the immune system to *dinitrochlorobenzene* and then painting it on the warts at weekly intervals until they go away.

Surgical treatments involve scraping the wart off under local anesthetic, freezing the wart with *liquid nitrogen*, burning the wart with an electric needle, or vaporizing the wart with a *carbon dioxide laser*. Generally, all these forms of treatment are effective, although a certain percentage of warts stubbornly return despite treatment. One of the most important considerations in treating any exposed wart is to avoid producing scars. This is especially important when a person has a number of warts. Because warts are completely harmless and often eventually go away by themselves, the scarring caused by treatment can be worse than the illness.

Doctors treat venereal warts with a caustic liquid containing *podophyllin*. Petroleum jelly is usually painted around the warts to protect the surrounding skin. The medication is left on for one to four hours, then carefully washed off with soap and water. The treatment is generally successful, but does produce local inflammation that is painful for several days. The medication is so powerful that it should be used with caution.

Ruling Out Other Diseases

Most warts can easily be diagnosed by their rough, cauliflower-like surface, but occasionally they may be confused with *seborrheic keratoses* which tend to look waxier and appear as if stuck on (see p. 184).

Prevention

Because common and plantar warts are caused by a virus, it may be possible to prevent their spread by avoiding contact with the virus. Although warts do not spread easily, new ones do appear, especially in areas where the skin has been injured or scratched. To prevent developing additional warts, individuals should avoid scratching the wart and should keep the area clean. Prompt treatment of warts is important in preventing spread.

Because venereal warts are readily spread through sexual contact, people should avoid intimate contact with infected individuals until they have been treated. Condoms probably offer some protection, provided they completely cover the warts.

Bacterial Skin Infections, Including Impetigo, Boils, Folliculitis, and Cellulitis

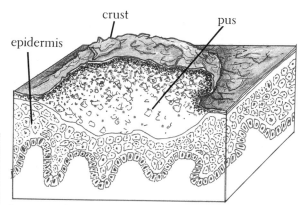

Impetigo is a superficial skin infection caused by a bacterium.

Symptoms

impetigo
- raised pus-filled pimples of varying size
- fluid-filled pimples
- gummy, honey-colored crusts
- commonly occurs on the face, especially around nose; in skin folds
- itching

folliculitis
- small pus-filled pimples around hair follicles
- burning and itching
- pain when the hair shaft is moved
- commonly occurs on the face, armpit, groin, and buttocks

boils
- swollen red area, approximately 1 cm wide, around a hair follicle
- extremely tender and painful
- can be warm to the touch
- forms a pus-filled whitehead after several days

cellulitis
- hot, red, swollen area
- tenderness
- red streak from the inflamed area
- nearby lymph nodes tender

Description

The human skin is normally home to literally millions of *bacteria*. Four million are found on the hands alone, living in colonies of 1,500–10,000. Generally these bacteria cause no prob-

lem, but under certain circumstances, some overgrow where the skin is broken or when new bacteria simply invade and cause infection. Just two of the many types of bacteria cause most skin infections: *staphylococci* (staph) and *beta-hemolytic streptococci* (strep). Between 15% and 50% of people normally have staph present somewhere on their skin, most commonly around the nose, perineum, or hairy areas of the body. Staph generally invades through hair shafts, most often at spots where the skin has been injured and is moist. Thus staph infections are most common in hairy areas such as the face (in men), arms, armpits, buttocks, and groin. Even after an infection has subsided, bacteria may continue to live in the lower layers of the skin for months or even years with no further signs. Strep is usually found on the skin, and in the throat and respiratory passages. It readily enters through abrasions in the skin and multiplies in the epidermis, just under the dry dead cells on the surface. Because it does not pass through hair follicles, it can cause infection anywhere on the body—not just in hairy areas.

Several common skin infections are caused by either staph or strep. *Impetigo* is a skin infection most often caused by strep. It begins with a small red, itchy area which soon develops one or more

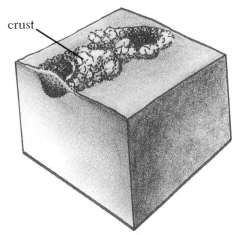

crust

Impetigo has crusts that are made up of clotted, dried blood cells and plasma.

tiny fluid-filled vesicles or pimples. Eventually these pimples burst, exuding a pusy, yellowish-brown fluid that dries into characteristic honey-colored crusts. Impetigo most frequently occurs around the nose, upper lip, or in the skin folds of the arms and legs. It is more common and more contagious among children; among adults, it is less frequent and not as easily transmitted. Often it is found in areas where other skin infections or lesions, such as insect bites, have been scratched, thereby breaking the skin. Impetigo has been called a "soap-and-water disease" because it can be transmitted under the fingernails and it tends to be most common in situations in which washing and bathing are limited. In rare cases, untreated impetigo can not only spread, but cause *glomerulonephritis*, a disease that involves the kidneys.

Folliculitis or *barber's itch* is an infection of the hair follicles generally caused by staph. It consists of a reddened, swollen pimple around a hair shaft or over a hair follicle. Generally this pimple or group of pimples develops a whitehead filled with pus. The infection most often takes place on the thigh, face, armpit, or groin. When infection occurs on men's faces, it can be spread by shaving. Lack of cleanliness is a promoting factor. If the infection spreads all the way down into the bottom of a hair follicle and out into surrounding tissue, a *boil* or *furuncle* can form. Should the infection spread among several adjacent hair follicles, a larger boil, called an *abcess* or *carbuncle*, will develop. At this point the swollen area will be a centimeter or more in diameter, red, and extremely tender. Within several days to several weeks, the infection will become pus-filled, then soften, rupture, and drain.

A deeper, more serious skin infection caused by strep is called *cellulitis*. It involves a hot, red swollen area that has a diffuse border. It may or may not have a pimple on the surface, but it is very tender to the touch. Because it involves underlying tissues, this infection can spread through the lymph channels to a nearby *lymph node*. When this occurs, a red streak will be visible on the surface of the skin, and the node will be tender. Cellulitis most often develops from an infected wound. If the infection becomes systemic, the individual will develop a fever and chills, and will feel tired. Cellulitis can become serious and should be treated promptly with antibiotics.

Self-Care

The main principle of self-care is washing with soap and water to remove bacteria from the skin. Healthy skin has a dry layer on the surface that acts as a barrier to potentially harmful bacteria. Under normal circumstances, healthy skin also has a negative charge, as do most bacteria, so they tend to repel each other. But when skin becomes infected or bacteria start to overgrow, the skin loses it negative charge and/or its dry protective layer. Washing with soap and water returns the skin to its negative charge and tends to dry it out, making it more difficult for bacteria to grow.

Mild cases of impetigo or folliculitis respond well to home treatment. The area around the infection should be scrubbed briskly with a brush or washcloth to remove the scab, since bacteria tend to collect under it. When the crusts stubbornly adhere to the skin, soaking with warm soapy water will soften them and make them easier to get off. Scrubbing should be repeated several times a day until the infection clears. Swabbing with hydrogen peroxide will also help to kill staph bacteria. Although some studies question the value of *anti-infective creams* or *ointments* (e.g., *Bacitracin*), they are recommended by most doctors. These creams should be rubbed on the infected area after each washing, and the area should be covered to help prevent the infection from spreading.

Small, uncomplicated boils also respond well to home treatment. Hot, moist compresses or soaks should be applied to the area several times a day for at least 10–15 minutes at a time. The area should then be wiped with *hydrogen peroxide*. Moist heat increases blood flow to the area, bringing in additional white blood cells to fight the infection and remove pus and toxic materials that build up in the area. Moist heat also helps bring the boil to a head, thereby speeding up the natural course by which it ruptures and drains externally. By promoting both internal and external drainage, compresses or soaks also help to relieve pain and tenderness in the area of the swelling.

The Doctor

If an infection spreads, causes a fever, develops a red streak, or simply doesn't heal, it should be seen by a doctor (dermatologist, internist, or family practitioner). A large boil should be treated promptly. For moderate infections that are spreading or not healing, the doctor will prescribe stronger antibiotic creams containing *polymyxin B, tetracycline,* or *erythromycin*. The doctor may also prescribe oral *penicillin* or *erythromycin* in addition to, or instead of, an antibiotic cream. If necessary, the doctor will do a culture to determine what bacteria is causing the infection. The culture will only be valid if use of antibiotic cream is stopped one to two days prior to seeing the doctor.

In treating a large boil, the doctor may open the pustule if it has come to a head. If the boil has already ruptured or is opened, the doctor will culture the discharge to determine which antibiotic will be most effective in fighting the infection. For a large boil or cellulitis, the doctor will start antibiotics immediately and then switch them if the culture indicates that the bacteria would be more sensitive to another medication.

Ruling Out Other Diseases

Occasionally an impetigo infection may look like *herpes simplex* (see p. 187) or *contact dermatitis* (see p. 172). Herpes sores generally do not have either pus or honey-colored crusts, and tend to burn more. Contact dermatitis generally itches more than impetigo and lacks crusts unless it becomes secondarily infected with strep or staph bacteria. Folliculitis sometimes looks like *acne*, but acne is usually accompanied by blackheads and is found on the face, neck, and back. Boils and cellulitis are obvious because of their tenderness, redness, and heat.

Prevention

Impetigo and folliculitis are best prevented by good hygiene. Frequent bathing with soap and water lowers the bacteria count on the skin and stops small infections before they progress. Washcloths, scrub brushes, and loofah sponges help to mechanically remove bacteria. People who have had recurrent skin infections should pay particular attention to washing areas previously infected. Cleanliness becomes especially important whenever the skin is cut, abraded, or subject to some other kind of skin condition such as insect bites, eczema, or poison ivy, that itch and often promote scratching. Washing efforts should also be redoubled if a member of the family has a skin infection; and that person should not share towels, linens, or articles of clothing until the infection has cleared up.

Light Skin Patches, or Vitiligo

Symptoms

- well-outlined areas of white skin
- possibly white hair in these areas
- often, patches are symmetrical
- commonly seen on face, chest, hands, elbows, knees, groin
- patches sunburn easily

Description

Vitiligo is a relatively common skin condition in which areas of skin lose their color because the *melanocytes*, the cells which normally produce pigmentation, disappear. The condition is essentially harmless, except in terms of cosmetic considerations and sunburning. Although vitiligo can occur in childhood, it increases steadily in frequency between 40–60 years of age.

Approximately 1% of the population has these white patches, and of those people, about a quarter have a family history of vitiligo. Vitiligo is thought to be due to an autoimmune mechanism in which the body rejects its own melanocytes in certain areas. The great majority of people with vitiligo are otherwise healthy, al-

though individuals who have thyroid disease or adult-onset diabetes are more prone to develop vitiligo.

Once a patch appears, it may remain unchanged, it may slowly enlarge, or new areas may appear. Initially the patch may be only slightly lighter than the surrounding skin, but eventually it tends to lose all pigmentation so that there is a marked contrast, especially in dark-skinned people. The borders of the patches remain sharply demarcated even as the areas spread. Generally patches are symmetrical on either side of the body. The most common sites affected are exposed areas, skin folds, and body openings, including the face, hands, armpits, groin, mouth, ears, navel, genitals, elbows, and knees. Because these areas lack pigmentation, they sunburn easily and need extra protection from the sun. Partial repigmentation often occurs in spotty areas, especially around hair follicles. Infrequently, complete repigmentation may occur.

Self-Help

No home treatment presently exists for vitiligo, nor is it necessary for small patches. The only concern is cosmetic. Moderate exposure to the sun may help, but care should be taken that the areas do not burn. Patches tend to stand out just as much when they are sunburned. Sunscreen lotions with a high sun protection factor (SPF) should be applied. A waterproof cosmetic preparation such as *Covermark* may be useful in certain situations, especially if the face is involved.

The Doctor

Doctors (dermatologists) can prescribe medicines to treat vitiligo, but the drugs work slowly and are not always successful. The most common treatment involves application of ultraviolet light and a drug called *methoxsalen*, which is a photosensitizer. It is the opposite of a sunscreen lotion, and causes the skin to absorb more ultraviolet rays than normal. Doctors believe that in cases that are successfully treated, melanocytes from nearby hair follicles repopulate the skin in the whitened areas. Methoxsalen treatment is questionable on two grounds: first, the treatment is long, tedious, and often not effective; second, the drug is powerful and can have significant side effects, including severe skin and eye burns. More importantly, the drug is known to be an animal carcinogen and has caused both *basal cell carcinoma* and *malignant melanoma* in humans.

Some doctors prescribe *steroid creams* for vitiligo, again with questionable results. Finally, for cases in which cosmetic considerations are a real concern, doctors sometimes bleach the surrounding skin to make the contrast less noticeable, or even tattoo the pale areas with a color that matches the normal skin.

Ruling Out Other Diseases

Lightened patches of skin can be caused by *tinea versicolor*, a fungal infection, but in that case they are only partially de-colored (see p. 169). Tinea versicolor, which is most common on the torso, also causes itching and produces small scales over the affected area. A doctor rules out tinea versicolor by treating a small scraping with potassium hydroxide and examining it under the microscope for the presence of fungal spores.

Prevention

There is no known prevention for vitiligo, but fortunately it is not serious except in a cosmetic sense.

HEAD

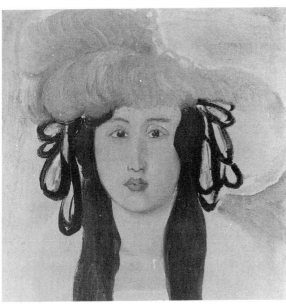

The head is the master control area of the body, containing the brain, eyes, and ears, as well as the entrances to the respiratory and gastrointestinal systems. Henri Matisse. The Plumed Hat. *1832. National Gallery of Art, Washington. Chester Dale Collection, 1962.*

Common Cold, or Upper Respiratory Infection

Symptoms

- runny nose
- sneezing and/or nasal stuffiness
- tiredness
- fever
- headache
- coughing
- sore throat
- laryngitis

Description

The common cold is a viral infection of the cells that line the nose and throat. Worldwide, the cold is the most frequent illness people have, representing 60% of *all* illnesses. One large-scale study found that people have an average of 5.6 colds per year, adults having relatively fewer colds than children (four versus seven to eight). Women tended to have more colds than men, presumably because they are more involved in caring for sick children. The study also showed that the incidence of colds rose as family size increased, with preschoolers infecting the family most often, school-age children next, and adults least. Once one person develops a cold, there is a 25%–40% chance that another household member will catch it. Finally, it is interesting to note that colds are no respecters of season, although in temperate climates they are less common in the warmer months.

There are over 100 different viruses that cause the common cold, of which the *rhinovirus group* is probably the source of 15%–40% of all colds. This group is made up of at least 90 individual viruses, each of which sets up its own immune response in the body. The second most common viral group is the *coronavirus*, which consists of three separate viruses and accounts for 10%–20% of all colds. For unknown reasons, the rhinovirus is most common in the fall and spring, while the coronavirus is most common in the winter.

Cold viruses are simple microorganisms consisting of a protein coat surrounding pure RNA that contains the same type of genetic material that directs protein synthesis in the body's cells. Once a virus enters an epithelial cell in the lining of the nose or throat, it uses the cell's materials to replicate itself. In an 8–12-hour-period the virus replicates many times, kills the host cell, and spills out literally thousands of new viruses, which immediately infect neighboring cells. During this period, the infected person is unaware that anything unusual is happening. By the second or third day, the number of infected cells reaches a peak, often producing a million viruses per milliliter of nasal secretions.

The body reacts to the virus almost immediately by initiating a multifaceted response to fight the infection. The immune system learns to identify the invading virus and begins to manufacture antibodies specifically designed to kill the virus. At the same time, immune cells release *interferon*, a natural antiviral agent, and *pyrogen*, a chemical that causes body temperature to rise. Interferon and pyrogen are proteins produced by the special white blood cells called *lymphocytes*. Interferon interferes with the viruses' ability to replicate. Pyrogen actually causes a change in the body's thermostat in the brain's *hypothalamus*, increasing heat production and decreasing heat loss. An increase in temperature makes it more difficult for the virus

to live. Other cells release *histamine*, a chemical that causes nearby blood vessels to open up, thereby bringing additional blood to the area, which in turn helps to raise the temperature in the infected area and brings in more white blood cells to kill the virus. Histamine also causes local swelling. This swelling, in conjunction with cell damage and increased blood flow, makes nasal passages stuffy. The presence of dead cells, extra plasma or body fluid, and the virus itself, increases the production of mucus.

Ironically, most of a cold's symptoms are caused by the body's defense against the virus. The initial symptoms of tingling or burning in the nose are probably caused by the body's release of histamine. Stuffiness and/or runny nose, coughing, and sneezing are caused by the body's systematic efforts to kill the virus and flush out the dead virus and cells. A sore throat develops when the virus affects cells in the throat as well as the nose. Typically, the common cold causes local symptoms, as opposed to general ones like high fever and muscle aches. It's important to realize that when you feel the sensations of a cold, your body has already begun to heal itself.

The average common cold lasts about nine days. Generally, the *incubation period* before symptoms become apparent averages two days. Thereafter people may have symptoms for as few as three to four days or as many as seven to ten days. The first sign of a cold is often a mild sore throat or slight scratchiness of the throat. People coming down with a cold frequently find they are more sensitive to drafts (hence the name "cold"), and naturally try to keep warmer than usual. These early symptoms are generally followed by nasal stuffiness, a runny nose, burning eyes, a headache, and/or sneezing. All of these symptoms may be accompanied by a slight fever, muscle aches, and tiredness, but a high fever and pronounced muscle aches are more characteristic of the *flu (influenza)* (see p. 215).

Within a day, the cold usually goes into its

second phase. Nasal secretions become thick and abundant, an annoying dry cough may develop, and there is a feeling of fullness in the head. Over the next several days, mucus becomes thicker and greener in color, and the Eustachian tubes leading to the ears may become swollen and blocked. In an uncomplicated cold, the muscle aches, fever, and tiredness generally disappear after the fourth or fifth day, but the head-cold symptoms tend to persist for several more days until the body heals itself completely.

Sometimes toward the end of a cold, a secondary bacterial infection may develop. This occurs because the mucous membranes are raw and irritated from the virus, and bacteria in the area can easily multiply. If a secondary infection develops, the mucus tends to become even thicker and greener than usual, and coughing is likely to bring up phlegm. Usually a cold disappears by itself within a week or so, but occasionally the viral infection spreads, and specific complications arise, such as a *sinus infection*, an *ear infection*, or *bronchitis* (see p. 226, 221, and 304).

How the common cold spreads from one person to another has been the subject of much conjecture, superstition, and study. In recent years scientists have refuted most theories and discovered some startling new facts. Doctors Jack Gwaltney and Owen Hendley of the University of Virginia have found that colds basically spread by hand-to-hand contact. Previously it was believed that the virus was spread by people coming into contact with airborne droplets produced by the infected person's sneezing and coughing. In fact, Gwaltney and Hendley found that coughing and sneezing don't spread nasal secretions, rather they spread saliva, which contains relatively little of the virus. What does spread the virus is direct contact: people with a cold touch their nose and the infection is transferred to their fingers; then they touch an object or a person's hands, and the virus is passed to the other person. The virus stays alive for several hours on the skin or other objects. After picking up the virus the other person must touch their fingers to the mucous membranes of their own nose in order to complete the transfer. In the course of their study, Gwaltney and Hendley found that people often do touch their nose and "inoculate" themselves in this way. These researchers found that only 5% of people caught colds from coughing or sneezing, while 75% picked up the virus from hand-to-hand contact. Backing this up, Dr. Eliot Dick, another researcher, found that it is very difficult to spread colds by kissing, even when it is quite intimate and passionate. Finally, researchers have found that, when the air is dry, people are twice as likely to develop a cold in the presence of a virus. It is thought that the immune response of the nasal cells is lowered when they are dried out.

Studies have shown that psychological stress is also associated with getting a cold. Richard Totman of the Common Cold Research Unit in Salisbury, England, has found clear evidence of the psychosomatic component of colds. In his study, introverts and loners developed significantly worse symptoms and higher levels of virus after being exposed than did people who were extroverts. People who had had a number of recent life changes and limited their activities because of this also had greater numbers of virus. These results correlate with many other studies that have shown that stress lowers the body's immune response in general (see p. 46).

In a classic study done at the University of Illinois in 1960, Dr. George Jackson found even more remarkable links between colds and psychological factors. At the time of his study, it was not certain which viruses caused colds or how viruses were spread. In order to shed light on this area, Jackson randomly put either small amounts of salt water or nasal secretions with cold viruses in the nasal passages of volunteers. Among those who received drops containing the virus, 33% actually developed symptoms. Thus

Jackson proved that colds could be spread by introducing the virus directly, but, of equal importance, he found that many people in the control group became sick even though they were only given salt water. The study showed a direct relationship between the number of colds these people reported annually and their likelihood of "catching a cold" following the administration of the saline drops. Jackson concluded that reporting symptoms was not necessarily synonymous with harboring the virus. In other words, people who thought of themselves as sickly were more likely to develop symptoms whether or not they came in contact with the virus. People who did not think of themselves as sickly often didn't report symptoms even when they were harboring the virus. In addition to these startling findings, the results also debunked a number of old wives' tales. Jackson proved that chilling, fatigue, and sleep deprivation had no affect on catching a cold. Among women, he found that susceptibility was greater during ovulation and directly before menstruation, but was lower during menstruation.

Self-Care

Self-care is the only treatment necessary for a common uncomplicated cold in a healthy person. It's important to remember that all treatment of a viral cold is symptomatic; nothing "cures" a cold other than the body's own immune system. Many traditional treatments are effective, though some are not. The first principle of self-care is *rest*. This means not going to work, even staying in bed if a person feels bad enough. Resting not only allows the body to build up energy to fight the infection, it reduces stress, which tends to hinder the immune response.

The most bothersome symptoms of a cold are generally *nasal congestion* and a *runny nose*. Sometimes the tip of the nose becomes red and sore from wiping, or the lips become dry and chapped when stuffiness necessitates breathing

---

Self-Care for Colds and Flu

Helping your body heal itself

REST: sleep as much as possible, or engage in quiet peaceful activities such as listening to the radio, watching TV, or reading. Don't do anything strenuous.
FOOD: eat what you like; drink plenty of water, juice, or soda.
ATTITUDE: adopt a relaxed, positive attitude about suspending normal activities and about getting well.
DRUGS: take vitamin C and zinc supplements if desired.

Relieving symptoms

FEVER: do nothing unless you're really uncomfortable. Remove clothing or sponge off when hot; wrap up when chilled. If necessary, take aspirin or acetaminophen to lower fever.
NASAL CONGESTION: drink hot liquids, use a vaporizer, take hot showers. Use nose drops or decongestants for a short time if necessary.
SORE THROAT: drink cool drinks or herb tea with honey; suck on cough drops.
COUGH: drink plenty of fluids, run a vaporizer or humidifier, take hot showers. Take cough suppressants at night if a nonproductive cough keeps you awake.

---

through the mouth. Both a sore nose and chapped lips can be relieved with various ointments containing petroleum jelly. Hot showers and humidifiers help to clear congestion. Hot liquids, including herb teas and soups, have been shown to loosen nasal mucus, and they probably help to keep the nasal membranes from drying out. Cold researcher Dr. Marvin Sackner did a study rating several different liquids and found that chicken soup gave the most relief of cold symptoms, followed by hot water, and last, cold liquids. It is interesting to note that chicken soup was first prescribed for a cold by Moses Maimonides, a rabbi and doctor, in 12th-century Egypt.

When nondrug treatments are not effective and a person is very bothered by cold symptoms, an over-the-counter decongestant containing *pseudoephedrine* (e.g., *Sudafed*) will help to relieve congestion by causing the blood vessels in the nose to constrict. Since increased blood flow is important to bring in white blood cells and raise body temperature, decongestants may slow healing even though they relieve symptoms. If a runny nose is very bothersome, it can be treated with mild *antihistamines* (e.g., *chlorpheniramine* is used in *Chlor-Trimeton*). Antihistamines not only dry up nasal secretions, they cause a dry mouth and drowsiness, and should not be taken when a person has to drive. If taken continuously for more than three to four days, both decongestants and antihistamines can cause rebound effects; that is, the return of symptoms that are greater than the initial ones. Even nasal sprays can cause rebound effects.

The second most common symptom of a cold is a *sore throat*. Gargling with salt water and drinking warm liquids such as soup or herb tea with honey are standard remedies to soothe a sore throat. Many people also find hard candies or lozenges to be soothing. Both honey and candy moisten and coat the throat and relieve burning. Some medicated lozenges such as *Cepastat* now contain a mild anesthetic called *phenol/menthol*). Sometimes a sore throat is accompanied by *laryngitis*, an inflammation of the vocal cords. Laryngitis is helped by resting the vocal cords, stopping smoking, inhaling moist air, and applying hot compresses to the neck.

Headaches, bodyaches, and fever frequently accompany a common cold. Rest and relaxation help to ease aches and pains, and are also indicated for fever. Since a slight fever helps to prevent the virus from multiplying, it's probably better not to treat the fever unless it causes a great deal of discomfort. The standard drugs for both fever and aches are *aspirin* or *acetaminophen* (e.g., *Tylenol, Panadol*, or *Datril*). Because of an association with *Reye's syndrome*, a rare and potentially fatal childhood complication of viral infections and influenza, aspirin and aspirin compounds should not be taken for cold symptoms by children under 18. Aspirin has also been found to lower interferon levels and increase the amount of virus in nasal secretions in both adults and children, possibly causing a delaying effect on healing.

A *cough*, which is another specific symptom of a cold, is the body's way of bringing up phlegm and preventing the cold from spreading down into the respiratory system. Drinking quantities of liquids, using a humidifier or vaporizer, and breathing moist air in the shower help to keep mucus thin and easy to raise. Tea with honey or cough lozenges help to ease a dry cough. *Cough suppressants*, which commonly contain *dextromethorphan*, should not be taken if the cough is bringing up phlegm, but they can be useful when a dry cough prevents a person from sleeping. Smoking is especially bad when a person has a cold. Smoking actually paralyzes the *cilia*, the tiny hairlike projections in the nose, throat, and bronchial tubes that help to raise mucus. Smoking not only slows the body's ability to heal a cold, it increases the chances of developing bronchitis. If people can't give up smoking completely, they should at least cut back radically until their cold is over.

Most cold experts don't advise taking cold preparations that contain a combination of ingredients to attack all phases of the cold. There are several reasons for this. First, the specific medications may not be in the proper amounts to adequately treat a certain symptom. Second, some of the ingredients may not be necessary if a particular symptom is not present, and a person may experience unnecessary side effects. Third, mixed preparations are generally more expensive than single components. Finally, a number of preparations contain *caffeine* to counteract the side effects of antihistamines and to provide a feeling of energy, which can be problematic because it may interfere with a person getting adequate sleep or rest.

Since 1969, when Nobel Prize winner Linus Pauling wrote his book on Vitamin C and the common cold, *Vitamin C* has become the nation's most popular cold remedy. Although Vitamin C has many ardent proponents, scientific studies have not tended to bear out its effectiveness. No study has shown that it prevents colds, and only one study found it shortened the average span of a cold (by one day). Present knowledge does not warrant routine use of large doses of Vitamin C for colds. Since cold symptoms are known to be strongly influenced by psychological factors, it is possible that people's belief in Vitamin C may have a positive effect on their cold symptoms. In any event, in the doses generally recommended Vitamin C is not toxic and does not do any harm.

Possibly of more interest is a study on *zinc*. Dr. Donald Davis of the University of Texas found that when zinc was dissolved in the mouth, it shortened the average length of a cold by seven days. *Zinc gluconate* tablets are so distasteful that many people will not use them, but palatable zinc tablets are beginning to appear on the market. Before zinc tablets are put into widespread use, more studies are needed to demonstrate their effectiveness.

The newest drug to be studied for the common cold is *interferon*, a natural antiviral agent that can now be manufactured in bulk through genetic engineering. Studies have found that interferon nasal spray prevents person-to-person spread of certain types of cold viruses (rhinovirus in particular) and shortens the symptoms of colds that are already in progress. But its use is not entirely without problems. Interferon itself causes nasal stuffiness and, quite often, bloody mucus. Due to these side effects and the fact that interferon isn't effective for many types of colds, its use is still experimental.

The Doctor

Generally the doctor is not needed to treat the common cold. In fact, many doctors advise their patients to stay home so they can rest and not spread the cold further. But due to complications that can develop from a common cold, there are times when a doctor visit is recommended. These include: significant ear or chest discomfort; a cough that raises foul-smelling, thick, green, or blood-tinged phlegm; a fever over 103°F; wheezing or shortness of breath; a *very* sore throat with a temperature above 101°F; and persistence of cold symptoms for longer than two weeks. People who have lung conditions such as asthma or emphysema, as well as other serious underlying conditions, might also be advised to see their doctor for a bad cold.

The doctor will examine a person's ears, nose, throat, and chest to rule out various complications. Provided none are found, the doctor will simply recommend the treatments suggested under self-care. Unless there is evidence of a secondary bacterial infection, the doctor will *not* prescribe antibiotics, because they are not effective against viruses. Not only are antibiotics useless against the common cold, they can cause problems. Occasionally, antibiotics cause the emergence of resistant strains of bacteria that are present in low numbers. Moreover, doctors are rightfully conservative about prescribing antibiotics because of the small percentage of people who become allergic to penicillin, the most commonly-used antibiotic. Finally, some women develop a vaginal *yeast infection (candida)* following a course of antibiotics (see p. 398).

Ruling Out Other Diseases

There are several bacterial and viral diseases that have symptoms similar to those of the common cold. These diseases include mild *flu* (see p. 215), mild *strep throat* (see p. 219), and even mild or early cases of *chickenpox* and *measles*. Distinguishing these diseases from the common cold is often impossible without viral cultures, which are expensive and time-consuming, or a strep culture, which is relatively fast and inexpensive. Since all the symptoms are treated similarly, it's not necessary to distinguish one disease from another unless the person becomes sicker.

Hay fever (see p. 247) also produces some of the symptoms of a common cold, but it doesn't usually produce a sore throat, and the person's eyes tend to be itchy as well. Generally people with hay fever have noticeably worse symptoms during pollen season and have a previous history of allergy.

Prevention

Since the primary means of spreading the common cold is hand-to-hand contact followed by "self-inoculation," there is much that can be done to prevent transmission. Hand washing and disinfecting household surfaces are the major means of prevention. When one person has a cold, everyone in the household should wash his or her hands with soap and water more frequently than normal. It is especially important that sick people wash their hands after blowing their nose. Tissues should be used instead of handkerchiefs, because the latter simply harbor the virus. Likewise, people who are well should wash their hands after touching or caring for the sick person. To prevent infecting themselves, people should specifically avoid touching their nose or eyes until they are able to wash their own hands. The more often people wash their hands, the more likely they are to prevent the cold from spreading.

A study by Dr. Jack Gwaltney has shown that spraying infected household surfaces with a disinfectant containing *phenylphenol* (e.g., *Lysol*) reduces the presence of virus from 42% to 8%. It also lowers the rate of people picking up the virus on surfaces from 60% to 21%. As compulsive as such cleanliness may seem, it appears to be effective and certainly makes sense in large families or group-living situations—or in the presence of someone who is especially susceptible because of other underlying disease. Because of the ease of hand-to-surface spread of the virus, sick people should avoid preparing food for household members and should use only their own cups and utensils.

Perhaps the most important and most overlooked way to minimize the spread of colds is to have people with colds *stay at home* until they are better. In this regard, it is important to note that the third day of the cold is the time of maximum shedding of virus. Often adults convince themselves that they are indispensable to their job, that they can "power through" a cold, or that they're no longer infectious. But in fact it's a person's right to stay home, and it's simply common courtesy for people to keep their colds to themselves. They'll probably more than make up for lost time once they're feeling better, and co-workers will appreciate not having to catch the cold.

In a more general way, prevention is bound up with the condition of the "host." When their immune system is strong, people are not as likely to catch colds or flu. Eating well, exercising regularly, and effectively coping with and reducing stress all serve to optimize the body's defenses against infectious disease. Likewise, positive attitudes tend to improve health (see p. 51).

Influenza, or Flu

Symptoms
- sudden onset of fever and chills
- muscle aches in the limbs and back
- joint aches
- tiredness
- headache
- lack of appetite
- dry cough
- sore throat
- runny nose
- hoarseness
- aching, burning eyes and sensitivity to light
- dizziness
- nausea

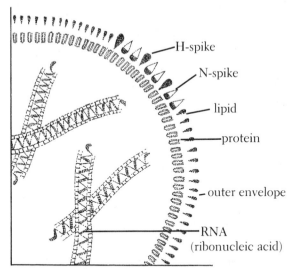

Influenza virus, which contain genes of RNA (ribonucleic acid), are surrounded by an envelope that consists of lipids and protein. The H-spike on the envelope enables the virus to bind to cells; the N-spike helps to release the virus from cells and spread the infection.

Description

Influenza is an infection caused by influenza A or B virus, which produce a relatively specific set of symptoms. Generally the flu occurs in outbreaks or epidemics every winter. Although mild cases can be confused with the common cold, the flu can usually be differentiated by its relatively sudden onset and by the fact that its general or systemic, symptoms are much stronger than its upper respiratory symptoms.

Of all the organisms causing human illness, influenza viruses are one of the most flexible and successful. Both influenza A and B are simple microorganisms made up of pure RNA, which is similar to the genetic material in the nuclei of our own cells that controls the manufacture of proteins. Influenza virus is covered with two types of surface projections: H-spikes that bind the virus to cells in the respiratory tract, and N-spikes that help to spread the virus to other cells. Once the human body learns to recognize either

spike of the virus, it begins to produce antibodies to neutralize the virus. Normally, antibodies produce immunity to a specific type of virus: that being the case, it would seem that people would become immune to the flu after one infection, as they do with measles or chickenpox, which are also viral illnesses. Unfortunately for humans, influenza virus has managed to outwit our immune system by developing the ability to slightly alter its spikes, thereby presenting the appearance of a new virus to the body's immune system. This unusual ability is referred to as *antigenic drift*. Hundreds of variants of the basic A and B subtypes of influenza have developed over influenza's 400-year history, and researchers now label each new arrival by the subtype, the place and year of identification, and the type of H- and N-spike (e.g., A/Texas/77/H3N2).

When two or more different viruses affect a

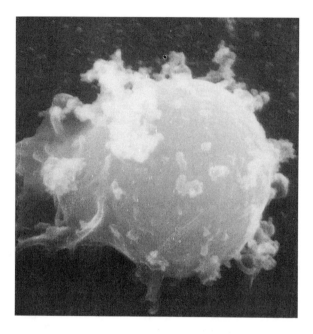

The white blood cells fight a flu by manufacturing antibodies designed to kill the specific virus. Scan electron micrograph. Magnification: 14,000 X.

cell, the situation becomes even more problematic because the viruses are capable of exchanging genetic information between them to develop a totally new H- or N-spike. In this situation, the immune system has to begin anew to recognize the virus and produce new antibodies to fight it. This ability to further tax the human immune system is called *antigenic shift*. When such a shift takes place, the new influenza variant can literally sweep around the whole world in what epidemiologists refer to as a *pandemic*. An influenza pandemic that began in the Kweichow province of China in February 1957 was documented to have spread throughout the world in less than a year. Once a pandemic has taken place, there is widespread immunity to that particular form of the virus, but over the next few years antigenic drift leads to minor changes in the virus and produces smaller and

smaller epidemics in local areas. Ultimately, antigenic shift produces another major change in the virus and a new pandemic occurs. In recent years it has been observed that pandemics take place on the average of every ten years, and major epidemics every two to three years.

Influenza epidemics tend to follow a characteristic pattern. An epidemic begins with a few sporadic cases, usually in children, increases dramatically in number, and reaches a peak in around six weeks, then gradually tapers off after ten weeks. By the time the epidemic is over, approximately 10%–20% of the local population will have been affected. Among children and older people, the incidence is often much higher. As opposed to influenzas, the common cold does not tend to take place in epidemic clusters, but occurs much more evenly throughout the year, being somewhat more frequent in the colder months.

The physiology of influenza resembles that of the cold in some respects, but differs in others. In both cases, the virus invades the cells lining the nose and throat. Within a period of four to six hours, the influenza virus replicates itself thousands of times, and infected cells die and burst open, spilling enormous amounts of new virus which immediately attack neighboring cells. People generally do not notice any symptoms for 18–72 hours after initial exposure. By this time they are already beginning to shed the virus and can infect other people. It takes another one to two days for the body to begin to produce its own *interferon* in large amounts. In about the same time, the body also begins to produce *antibodies* to the virus in both nasal secretions and the blood. Unlike the common cold, the flu is known to be spread by airborne droplets produced by coughing and sneezing, as well as by hand-to-mouth contact.

The progression of symptoms resulting from the flu virus usually follows a characteristic pattern that is quite different from that of a cold.

The flu commonly comes on so abruptly that people can often identify the moment they first feel ill. They are suddenly taken with chills and shivering, rapidly followed by tiredness, headache, and muscle aches in the limbs and back. Eye symptoms may include tearing and burning, heaviness or achiness in response to movement, and sensitivity to light. The initial symptoms are generally accompanied by a rising fever. As a group, the symptoms are disabling enough to require a person to give up normal activities and go to bed.

As the flu progresses, people experience a runny nose, a sore throat, hoarseness, and a dry but uncomfortable cough. Unlike a cold, the most disturbing symptoms are not upper respiratory in nature, but more generalized aches and pains that are enough to cause a normally healthy person to feel quite miserable. Muscle aches can even cause individuals to have difficulty sleeping, although it's unlikely they will feel good enough to do anything else. General muscle aches may be accompanied by joint pain, dizziness when getting up from a sitting or prone position, and nausea. Even if people are not nauseous with the flu, they rarely feel like eating.

A fever is one of the body's natural defenses against a virus. With the flu, people typically run a relatively high fever—above 101°F—for several days, often peaking on the first and third days. Although the fever usually lasts an average of three days, it can persist for as long as five days. During this time the fever may remain constant, or it may fluctuate, particularly if medication is taken to lower it. Once the fever breaks, people usually notice that their aches and pains improve. For the last few days of the flu, the respiratory symptoms become the most pronounced—especially the cough—and many people complain of aching when they cough. Although people often recover rapidly after the fifth day, they may find they continue to be tired

for several more days, and their cough may persist for up to one to two more weeks.

Although almost no healthy people develop complications, people who are very old or who have debilitating diseases can actually become extremely ill with the flu. A small percentage of elderly people with heart disease, lung disease, kidney disease, or diabetes develop a serious case of *pneumonia* (see p. 307). It is pneumonia that causes the deaths that are associated with flu epidemics. On the other hand, people often have such mild flus that they simply think they have a cold. Some researchers believe that many so-called "winter colds" are actually Type B influenzas.

Self-Care

An uncomplicated flu in a healthy person does not require a doctor and is best treated with self-help. *Bed rest* is advisable with the flu because of associated aches and fever. In fact, muscle aches, dizziness, and weakness can be so pronounced that people who have the flu require real "nursing" care from other members of the household. Flu sufferers should be encouraged to drink large amounts of clear fluids and eat small amounts of bland, nongreasy foods (e.g., soup, toast, and crackers) to keep up their strength. Even reading or watching television may be too strenuous in the first several days if people have a high fever or their eyes ache.

If a person does not have a high fever, a warm bath may be relaxing and serve to soothe muscle aches. A gentle massage can also help to relieve muscle aches. For adults, *aspirin* is the most effective over-the-counter preparation for relieving muscle aches and joint aches, but it can upset the stomach, especially if a person is nauseated. Aspirin should not be taken by children under the age of 18 because of the possibility of developing a rare and potentially fatal complication of the flu called *Reye's syndrome*. Acet-

aminophen (e.g., *Tylenol*) can also be taken, although it does not tend to be quite as effective for muscle and joint discomfort. Some people find that an over-the-counter sleeping preparation helps them rest if they are having trouble sleeping and simpler measures haven't worked. If nausea is significant, it may be relieved by over-the-counter *antacids* (e.g., *Pepto-Bismol*). Specific treatments for coughs, stuffiness, runny nose, sore throat, and headache are dealt with in the Self-Care section under Common Cold (see p. 211).

The Doctor

The doctor is not required for uncomplicated cases of influenza, but should be seen if a person has a continued high fever and a cough which begins to produce thick, foul-smelling, greenish or rust-colored phlegm. Chest symptoms such as difficult breathing, chest pain, or significant coughing may be signs of pneumonia and should be reported to the doctor. In general, elderly people, pregnant women, and people with heart or lung diseases should consult their doctors whenever they have the flu. The doctor will listen to the person's chest with a stethoscope to determine if sounds of lung congestion are present. If there is any question of pneumonia, a chest x-ray and a sputum culture will be done.

An antiviral agent called *amantadine (Symmetrel)* is available by prescription, but it is not widely used in the U.S. It is thought to prevent spread of the virus's RNA into other cells. This medication has been found to shorten flu symptoms by several days, especially when it is started soon after symptoms begin. Although some doctors believe the medicine is safe and effective, others believe its side effects and possible dangers outweigh its usefulness in healthy people. (Its major use is in treating the tremor of Parkinson's disease because it increases the release of dopamine, a chemical that helps facilitate nerve

transmission.) Amantadine's mild side effects include insomnia, jitteriness, anxiety, and difficulty concentrating; its more serious side effects can include hallucinations and convulsions. Also, the drug has been shown to cause birth defects in animals.

Ruling Out Other Diseases

A mild case of the flu resembles the common cold. There is no particular reason to distinguish one from the other because they are basically treated the same way.

Once viral blood titers have been done on a few people to establish the presence of a new epidemic of influenza, doctors can be reasonably sure that people with the characteristic symptoms have the flu.

Prevention

People can help prevent the flu from spreading by staying home when they are sick and by being diligent about normal hygiene. Frequent hand washing is advisable and it's important that sick people avoid handling food (see p. 214). Unlike the common cold, however, airborne droplets dispersed through coughing or sneezing can spread the flu.

Researchers have developed a fairly effective vaccine that makes use of attenuated, or weakened, virus from influenza A and B. The vaccine is actually updated yearly in order to be effective against those strains of the flu that have caused recent epidemics elsewhere and are expected to be the most prevalent in the U.S. in the following year. The annual vaccines are thought to be 70%–80% effective against the flu; their immunity is believed to last from several months to a year. Approximately 1%–2% of people who are vaccinated experience slight fever and aches; 25% have a sore arm from the shot. The U.S. Public Health Service recommends yearly vaccination in the fall for people with heart and lung problems or debilitating diseases. Many doctors generally advise an annual shot for people over 65 since they are more likely to have other diseases. When immunization is not feasible, the Public Health Service suggests that people at risk use the drug amantadine as a means of preventing the flu when an epidemic is in progress.

Strep Throat, Acute Pharyngitis, and Tonsillitis

Symptoms

- sudden onset of a severe sore throat
- pain on swallowing
- fever and/or chills
- headache and/or muscle aches
- tender, enlarged lymph nodes in the neck
- swollen tonsils
- tiredness
- lack of appetite
- occasionally, nausea

Description

Sore throats are the third leading reason for doctor visits in the U.S. Basically they are either due to viruses that cause the common cold (80%–85%), or to bacteria (15%–20%)—most commonly, *beta-hemolytic group A streptococci*. A viral sore throat is self-limiting and simply requires good self-care. Generally strep throat is too, but it is treated by the doctor to prevent more severe illness that is infrequently associated with strep. A throat culture is needed to diagnose strep because a history and physical exam are often not sufficient to distinguish it from a viral infection.

With a *strep throat*, the pharynx (back of the throat) or tonsils are infected with strep bacteria. This condition, which is most common among children, generally occurs in epidemics during the winter months in families or in situations of close contact such as those that exist in schools, military bases, and other group-living environments. As far back as 1895, strep was recognized as the cause of sudden, severe sore throats, as well as the less frequent *scarlet fever*, a skin rash that sometimes accompanied a severe sore throat. Later it was recognized that two other important illnesses occasionally followed a bout with strep throat: *acute rheumatic fever* and *acute glomerulonephritis*. Acute glomerulonephritis is an inflammation of the kidneys that generally heals without a problem, but which in very rare instances causes permanent damage. Rheumatic fever, which is by far the more serious of the two illnesses, is an inflammatory disease that affects the joints and the heart, often causing severe impairment of the heart valves.

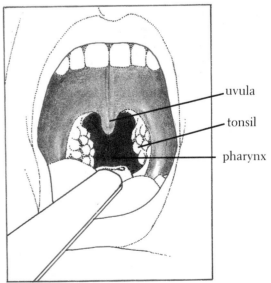

uvula

tonsil

pharynx

With strep throat, the tonsils are red, swollen, and often pus-covered.

Before the widespread introduction of antibiotics after World War II, and even today in underdeveloped countries, rheumatic fever was the major cause of heart disease in people under 50. The damage done to the heart valves by rheumatic fever can lead to chronic disability and even death. Antibiotic treatment of strep throat does not prevent glomerulonephritis, but it does prevent rheumatic fever.

The greatest percentage of rheumatic fever cases occur in children 5–15 years of age, while adults over 35 rarely develop it. Throughout the 1970s and 1980s, rheumatic fever rates dropped precipitously from 3,000 or more per 100,000 strep throats to less than .2 cases per 100,000 strep throats. Thus rheumatic fever has gone from a virtual epidemic to a disappearing disease. With the declining incidence of rheumatic fever, and its virtual absence in people over 35, there is a significant debate over how to treat severe sore throats in adults. Doctors question the value of expensive lab tests and penicillin treatment, however a recent comission has concluded that antibiotics have been the major cause of the decline in rheumatic fever, and that penicillin treatment for children must be continued to keep down the incidence of the disease.

Strep throat is spread to others by tiny airborne droplets produced by coughing and by hand-to-hand contact. Typically the incubation period is two to four days, at which point a person experiences a sudden onset of a sore throat, with pain on swallowing. It is also common for a person to have a fever, headache, muscle aches, enlarged lymph nodes in the neck, tiredness, and lack of appetite. Generally the symptoms are at their worst on the first day, and lessen on subsequent days. In years past, the symptoms used to be very pronounced, but recently they have been appearing in milder and milder form, apparently because the bacteria are gradually becoming less virulent. Often, not all of the usual symptoms are present. With the lessening of strep throat symptoms, especially among adults, it is becoming harder and harder to identify the disease from clinical symptoms. If no complications develop, a strep throat disappears within three to seven days without antibiotics, and slightly faster with antibiotics. The complications that most commonly follow untreated strep throat are sinus and ear infections.

Self-Care

Experts now agree that self-care is sufficient for an adult with a sore throat unless he or she has a high fever and feels very ill. Throat lozenges, warm beverages such as tea with honey, and gargling with salt water can all help to lessen the discomfort of a sore throat (see p. 211).

The Doctor

Since 1986, experts have been advising that adults consult their doctors when they have a fever over 101°F, have difficulty swallowing, and generally feel very ill. Because of the controversy surrounding the treatment of sore throats, doctors vary widely in how they handle them. The trend is for doctors to do a lab test on anyone who they suspect has a strep throat and on people with a personal or family history of rheumatic fever. With adults, doctors will test anyone with a high fever, swollen pus-covered tonsils, and big lymph nodes. In the middle of a strep epidemic, doctors are more likely to culture all severe sore throats.

At present, there are two types of lab tests used to diagnose strep—a culture, or the newer antibody test. A culture involves swabbing the back of the throat and tonsil area to obtain a sample of mucus which is then touched to a growing medium and incubated overnight to see if strep bacteria grow. With the antibody test the swab is mixed with reagents and the results are known within a matter of minutes. Generally, the two-day delay in getting the results of a culture does not affect prevention of rheumatic fever, but people with a personal or family history of rheumatic fever should begin treatment immediately. Likewise, most doctors will treat very sick children immediately. If the culture comes back negative, therapy may be discontinued, although some doctors will suggest taking the antibiotic for five days anyway to prevent resistant strains of the bacteria from developing.

If test results are positive, the doctor will prescribe oral *penicillin* G or *penicillin* V for 10 days, or give a single long-acting penicillin shot. People who are allergic to penicillin will be given *erythromycin* for 10 days. A full 10-day course of antibiotics must be taken to eradicate all the bacteria, which is necessary in order to prevent rheumatic fever.

Some doctors don't culture or treat adults at all as a rule. It is no longer common practice to culture or treat asymptomatic family members, to repeat treatment on asymptomatic people with positive follow-up cultures, or even to do follow-up cultures.

Ruling Out Other Diseases

Strep throat is very difficult to distinguish from a sore throat caused by a *cold virus* (see p. 208). The only certain way to diagnose strep is with a lab test or throat culture. Cold symptoms like a runny nose or cough make it more likely that a sore throat is viral in nature. On the other hand, a sore throat in the middle of a strep epidemic is more likely to be strep. *Infectious mononucleosis (mono)* can also cause a sore throat and enlarged lymph nodes in the early stages, but generally is accompanied by more pronounced tiredness, lack of appetite, headache, and muscle aches. If mono is suspected or is going around, a *monospot* blood test can be done to rule it out.

Prevention

Since strep throat is spread by airborne droplets and hand-to-hand contact, it's important that infectious people cover their mouth when they cough and wash their hands before handling food, etc. Caretakers and visitors should also be more attentive than usual to hand washing.

Middle Ear Infection, or Acute Otitis Media

Symptoms

- earache or pain following a cold
- feeling of fullness or blockage in the ear
- some degree of hearing loss
- occasionally fluid loss from the outer ear
- fever

Description

Acute otitis media is an infection of the middle ear caused by a variety of viruses and bacteria, including the common cold viruses and *streptococcus pneumoniae, betahemolytic group A streptococcus,* and *staphylococcus.* Middle ear infections, which are much less common among adults than they are among children, are generally a complication that follows a cold or strep throat. The bacteria or virus growing in the nose or throat spread up the Eustachian tubes to one or both ears (see illustration). Swelling caused by local inflammation blocks the Eustachian tubes, trapping both germs and fluid from the inflammation in the space around the middle ear. This situation provides an ideal environment for virus or bacteria to multiply. Increasing numbers of bacteria or virus, coupled with fluid

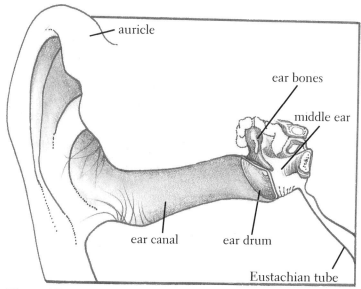

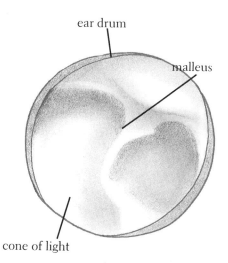

The middle ear is an air-filled chamber surrounded by the eardrum and the bones of the skull. When examined with an otoscope, a healthy eardrum reflects light in a characteristic manner.

blockage, can put extreme pressure on the sensitive nerve endings in the middle ear, causing great pain. Occasionally, if the pressure is sufficient, the eardrum may spontaneously rupture and leak fluid into the outer ear. This will relieve the pressure, and the drum will eventually heal by itself.

An ear infection usually begins several days after the onset of a common cold or strep throat. Often the first symptom is fullness in the Eustachian tubes and middle ear. With mild viral infections, the symptoms may not become any more pronounced, but with more severe viral infections or bacterial infections, the feeling of blockage may progress to the point of significant pain, accompanied by a fever and/or chills. As fluid builds up behind the drum, the person will notice a distinct loss in hearing, which gradually returns as the fluid in the middle ear is resorbed over the course of a week or so.

Self-Care

Self-care is all that's necessary for mild viral ear infections. A procedure called the *valsalva maneuver* will help to open the Eustachian tubes and let air into the middle ear, thereby promoting drainage. The maneuver is accomplished by gently but firmly blowing through the nose while holding both nostrils closed. Since air cannot escape from the nose, it is forced up the Eustachian tubes, breaking the vacuum that has sealed the middle ear. This maneuver can be repeated frequently, as often as necessary, and is especially useful after arising.

Sniffing should be avoided because it drops the pressure in the Eustachian tubes and tends to block them. *Oral decongestants* (e.g., *Sudafed*) or decongestant nose drops help to keep down swelling in the Eustachian tubes and may prevent them from becoming blocked. Often a heating pad or hot water bottle and pain medication such as *acetaminophen* (e.g., *Tylenol*) will help to relieve more severe pain. A humidifier helps to keep mucus thin and encourages drainage during an ear infection.

The Doctor

The doctor should be seen if fullness in the middle ear progresses to severe pain. Since there is no way to culture fluid from the middle ear without puncturing the drum, treatment is based on visual examination of the eardrum with an *otoscope*. If earwax blocks the drum, the doctor will scrape or flush it out. If the drum is red and bulging, as opposed to the normal shiny and white, the doctor will prescribe a broad-spectrum antibiotic, usually *ampicillin* or *amoxicillin*. Treatment with antibiotics prevents the infection from spreading to the mastoid bone behind the ear, a serious complication that is now rare but which occurred fairly often in the days before antibiotics. In addition to antibiotics, the doctor will prescribe a decongestant and recommend the valsalva maneuver (see Self-Care).

If significant ear pain persists after one to two days of medication, the doctor should be seen again. If fluid is still building up behind the eardrum, a doctor who specializes in conditions of the ear, nose, and throat might decide to make a tiny cut in the drum and allow the fluid to drain out naturally or remove it with suction. This procedure is uncomfortable, but it does relieve the pressure.

Ruling Out Other Diseases

Two other conditions can cause ear pain after a cold: an *external ear infection* (see below), or viral blisters on the outside of the eardrum. Either of these can be diagnosed visually when the doctor examines the outer ear with an otoscope. Another condition which can be confused with an ear infection is *temporomandibular joint syndrome (TMJ)*, a situation in which muscle tension causes unilateral or bilateral pain in the temple and jaw, which can radiate to the ear.

Prevention

Prompt treatment of a common cold or a strep throat probably helps to prevent acute otitis media. Use of the valsalva maneuver whenever the ears feel blocked and/or occasional use of decongestants helps to keep the Eustachian tubes open; these remedies are especially useful for people who seem prone to ear infections. Also, some people prone to ear infections find that cold, windy weather can precipitate earaches, so they keep their ears covered in bad weather.

Swimmer's Ear, External Ear Infection, or External Otitis

Symptoms

- itching or tickling in the ear canal
- pain in the ear canal which can be severe, particularly when the earlobe is pulled
- watery fluid or pus draining from the ear
- crusting or scaling in the ear canal
- a feeling of fullness in the ear
- some loss of hearing

Description

External otitis is an infection of the skin lining the external canal leading to the eardrum. It is generally caused by a bacteria called *Pseudomonas aeruginosa*. The most common form of the condition, *swimmer's ear*, is precipitated by water trapped in the ear canal. Convolutions in the canal can make it difficult to drain moisture that collects during swimming or bathing. The canal does not tend to dry by itself, particularly in humid weather. Normally, oil glands in the lining of the canal secrete a protective, antibacterial coating of earwax (cerumen), but if water

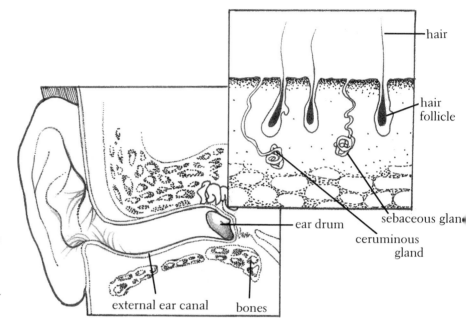

Glands in the lining of the external ear canal produce wax that protects the canal against water. However, if water becomes trapped in the canal, the lining swells and it can then become raw and infected.

remains in the canal, the top layer of skin eventually absorbs the water, swells, and becomes raw. A moist, abraded area provides an ideal place for the growth of bacteria. Swelling blocks the canal and further hinders drainage. The potential for external ear infections is accentuated if plugs of earwax accumulate in the canal, or if people scratch the canal or clean their ears too frequently or vigorously.

The first symptom of an external otitis is itching, which is caused by inflammation of the top layer of skin lining the canal. As the skin becomes more and more inflamed, the itching intensifies and finally becomes painful when swelling puts pressure on sensitive nerve endings in the narrow space between the ear canal and surrounding bone. If the inflammation becomes severe, the pain can become intense and constant. The pain is often sharpest when people chew or touch their earlobe. The raw skin lining the canal produces a watery discharge which develops pus when white blood cells come in to fight the infection and clear away dead cells.

Swelling and blockage in the canal produce a feeling of fullness and a temporary, partial loss of hearing.

Self-Care

Prompt treatment is important because external otitis can get worse or persist for long periods of time. The basic goal of self-care is to clean and dry the canal without further damaging the top layer of skin. An effective way to dry the canals is to use a hair dryer set on warm and held about 10 inches away from the skin, so as not to burn it. In the early stages, when itching is the only symptom, the canal can be gently flushed with an ear syringe filled with a 3% saline solution (1 T salt to 1 qt. water) and then with a 10% alcohol solution to promote drying. If this produces little or no discomfort, a few drops of 70% alcohol can be put in the ear once a day or after bathing, until the itching stops. Nonprescription eardrops, which are 97% alcohol, can also be used after showering. If the infection is painful, dry heat can be applied to the outer ear with a heating pad or hot water bottle three times a day for 20 minutes at a time.

The Doctor

A doctor should be seen if the ear becomes painful or the itching becomes severe or persists for more than five days. To diagnose external otitis, the doctor simply examines the canal with an otoscope. If necessary, the doctor will flush out the ear canal to remove excess wax, then dry the lining with a cotton-tipped applicator. The doctor will prescribe *Burrow's solution* or antibiotic ear drops containing *penicillin, polymyxin, neomycin,* and *bacitracin.* If the canal is sufficiently swollen, the drops may initially be applied to a piece of cotton, and the cotton gently placed in the ear canal. Additional drops should be added once or twice a day as the cotton dries. As swelling in the canal subsides, the cotton ball will fall out of its own accord, and then drops can be put directly in the ear. In addition to an antibiotic, some doctors prescribe *corticosteroid drops* (e.g., *Cortisporin Otic Suspension*) to reduce swelling in the canal. If necessary, the doctor will prescribe pain medication, even *codeine* if the pain is very intense.

Ruling Out Other Diseases

Otitis media, a middle ear infection, can also produce pain and occasionally discharge from the ear (see page 221). The doctor rules out a middle ear infection by examining the eardrum with an otoscope. Visual inspection will also serve to rule out the possibility of a boil caused by *staphylococcus,* or a skin condition such as *eczema* (see page 177) or *contact dermatitis* (see p. 172). In the case of a skin condition, scaling and flaking will usually extend beyond the ear canal to the earlobe or scalp. Ear pain can also be caused by *temporomandibular joint syndrome (TMJ),* a condition in which muscle tension causes unilateral or bilateral pain in the temple and jaw that can radiate to the ear.

Prevention

Much can be done to prevent external otitis. Preventive measures are particularly important for people who have a history of external ear infections. Earplugs may be beneficial for swimmers who are at risk. Care should always be taken to see that no water remains in the canal after swimming or bathing. Hopping or shaking the head helps to get water around the convolutions in the ear canal. Several drops of 97% alcohol can be applied to help dry the canal after swimming or bathing.

Cotton swabs and long pointed objects should not be used to clean the ears. If wax does not work its way out naturally, the canal should be gently irrigated with an ear syringe or a water jet machine (e.g., *Water-Pic*) set on the lowest level, using warm water or a dilute salt solution. Other effective remedies for removing wax include *baby oil drops* and *3% hydrogen peroxide drops.* Over-the-counter wax dissolvers should be used with care because they contain enzymes that can actually irritate the lining of the ear canal.

External ear infections respond best to early treatment, before the canal becomes swollen and the bacteria have started to multiply. Alcohol drops should be applied at the first sign of itching.

Sinus Infection, or Acute Sinusitis

Symptoms

- pain in the forehead or cheeks
- headache
- pain in the nose
- stuffy or blocked nose
- copious, green, foul-smelling mucus
- temporary loss of smell
- cheeks and forehead tender to the touch
- occasionally, swelling of the skin over the sinuses
- occasionally, fever
- toothache in the upper jaw or a feeling of the teeth being "longer than normal"

Description

Acute sinusitis is an infection of the sinus cavities caused by one of several bacteria or viruses. Generally it follows a common cold, but it can also occur after swimming or diving, a tooth extraction, or an allergy attack. The sinuses consist of eight air chambers that lie within the facial bones, above and to the side of the nose (see illustration). The sinuses drain into the nose and are lined with mucous membrane that is continuous with that of the nasal passages. Interestingly, the purpose of the sinuses has yet to be established, although researchers currently speculate that the sinuses provide a constant supply of fresh mucus to the back of the nose.

The largest of the sinuses are the *maxillary sinuses*, which lie in the cheekbones to either side of the nose. The sockets of the upper molars project into these sinus cavities. Next in size are the *frontal sinuses*, which lie above and behind the eyebrows. These cavities are not present at prominent during puberty when secondary sexual characteristics develop. The last two pairs are much smaller. The *ethmoid sinuses* are a group of small air sacs that lie behind the bridge of the nose; behind these are the *sphenoid sinuses*.

Because the lining of all the sinuses connects to that of the nasal passages, any infection in the nose can readily spread to the sinuses. In fact, 20% of sinus infections are caused by either *rhinovirus* or influenza virus, which are the causes of most colds and flus. The other 80% are caused by bacteria, largely *streptococcus pneumoniae* or *haemophilus influenzae*, which sometimes proliferate when resistance is lowered by a viral cold. When the sinuses become inflamed, the membrane lining the sinus cavities swells and can block drainage into the nasal passages. After one to two days, virus or bacteria begin to grow in the fluid that is trapped in the sinuses.

Typically, about seven to ten days into a cold, the watery nasal discharge becomes thick and pussy rather than abating. The nose continues to be blocked, sometimes even causing the sense of smell to diminish. Swelling in the sinus cavities causes pressure to build and pain begins. With the most common sinus infection, which affects the maxillary sinuses, the pain is located behind the cheeks. Maxillary sinusitis can also cause pain in the upper forward molars and bicuspids, or a sensation of the teeth being "long." When the frontal sinuses are affected, pain occurs above the eyebrows and can even affect the eyes. Typically this kind of headache starts in midmorning and ends by midafternoon. If the deeper sinuses are affected, they may produce a vague, deep-seated pain between and behind the eyes which may become worse when the eyes are moved. Often people simply experience a sinusitis attack as a headache. Unlike other types of headaches, those caused by sinus infections frequently start on one side of the face, are not

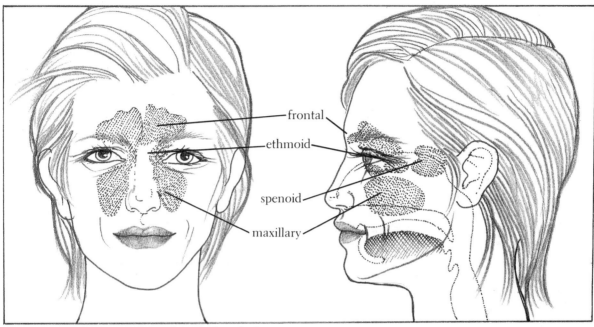

frontal
ethmoid
spenoid
maxillary

The sinuses, which are air chambers within the bones of the face, drain into the nose. The mucous membranes that line the nose are continuous with those that line the sinuses.

improved by closing the eyes and resting, and are accentuated by jarring movements or bending the head forward.

In some cases the skin over the affected sinuses becomes swollen and feels thick and tender to the touch. If the infection is significant, it may even produce a fever and chills. Sinus infections usually heal by themselves in a week or so.

Self-Care

For most sinus infections, self-care is adequate. Moisture from a humidifier, a vaporizer, a shower, or even a sinkful of hot water helps to thin and dissolve the mucus that is preventing the sinuses from draining. By comparison, dry air tends to paralyze the cilia, the microscopic hairlike projections that line the mucous membranes and normally move the mucus down into the nose. Drinking plenty of water also helps thin the mucus. Applying heat to the face, either with a heating pad or with warm, wet towels increases blood circulation and often helps to relieve discomfort. Some people find that mentholated ointments used for colds and muscle aches bring heat to the area and break up the congestion. Care should be taken not to get these preparations near the eyes.

Over-the-counter nasal decongestants containing *ephedrine sulfate*, *pseudoephedrine hydrochloride* or *phenylpropanolamine* can give temporary relief by reducing swelling and allowing the sinuses to drain. These drugs are very useful at the onset of a sinus infection. However, they should not be overused or taken for long periods of time because they also decrease blood flow to the area. Some doctors feel that decongestant nose drops are helpful, but if they are taken for more than three days, they will cause a

Self-Care for Sinus Infections

- use a vaporizer or humidifier
- take hot, steamy showers
- drink plenty of fluids
- apply hot compresses or a heating pad to the affected area
- use decongestant tablets or nose drops if necessary

rebound congestion when they are stopped. To relieve the headache that accompanies a sinus infection, adults can take either *aspirin* or *acetaminophen* (e.g., *Tylenol*); children under 18 should not take aspirin-containing compounds because of the chance of Reye's syndrome, a rare disease that can be fatal. Self-care recommendations for the common cold also apply in treatment of a sinus infection (see p. 211).

The Doctor

People should see a doctor (internist, family practitioner, or ear, nose, and throat specialist) if a sinus infection is accompanied by a persistent fever, or if the infection does not get better with self-care after a week or two. The specific cause of a sinus infection is difficult to determine because nasal cultures do not necessarily reveal the organisms present in the sinus cavities. If the doctor suspects a bacterial infection, he or she will prescribe a broad-spectrum antibiotic such as *amoxicillin* or *ampicillin*. Possible indications of a bacterial infection are a high fever and a thick, pussy discharge from the sinuses. Most doctors will recommend an oral decongestant or nose drops whether or not they suspect a bacterial infection.

An ear, nose, and throat specialist will often transilluminate the sinuses by putting a bright hooded light inside the person's mouth or near the sinuses. When the room is dark, light will be transmitted through the sinuses if they are not blocked. For a severe or persistent infection, a specialist may flush out the sinuses with warm saline to promote drainage.

Ruling Out Other Diseases

A *toothache* produces pronounced swelling and the pain tends to localize to a particular tooth. To distinguish a sinus infection from a toothache, dentists will sometimes have people bounce sharply on their heels. If this action produces a sharp pain that radiates up into the head, the problem is likely to be a sinus infection. *Tension headaches* (see p. 238) are more likely to affect both sides of the head and are often worst at night. They are also less affected by bending over, and are more likely to improve when a person rests with eyes closed.

Prevention

Prompt treatment of a cold or flu may help to prevent sinusitis from developing, especially in people who are prone to sinus infections. It's important to prevent the sinuses from becoming really blocked by encouraging good drainage with warm, moist air or hot, wet compresses. Some people also find that when they have a head cold, it helps to promote drainage if they sleep with their head slightly elevated.

Pinkeye, or Conjunctivitis

Symptoms

- sensation of something in the eye
- burning or scratchy sensation in the eye
- eye itches
- eye appears bloodshot
- lining of eyelid appears red
- pussy or clear discharge from the eye
- tearing from the eye
- eyelashes or lids may be stuck together
- eyelids may droop and feel heavy

Description

Conjunctivitis is an infection or an irritation of the mucous membrane that lines the eyelids and the white part of the eye. It is the most common eye disease in developed countries. A number of things can cause conjunctivitis, including bacterial infections, viral infections, allergic reactions, and irritation due to smog, smoke, or other chemicals.

The main symptom of conjunctivitis is a feeling of something in the eye, accompanied by itching or burning. The infectious or irritating agent hurts the mucous membrane of the eye, causing swelling and a general widening of tiny blood vessels in the area, which produces the sensations described, as well as a bloodshot appearance. White blood cells that come in to protect the area join with tears and mucous to produce a discharge that makes the eyelids and eyelashes gummy and can actually cause them to stick together.

Most cases of conjunctivitis heal on their own within 10–14 days. The structure and physiology of the eye naturally encourage healing; tears continuously bathe the eye with a fluid that contains antibodies and antibacterial and antiviral substances. Moreover, the eyes are constantly cooled by evaporation, a process that discourages the growth of bacteria and virus.

The most common type of conjunctivitis is a *bacterial infection* caused by *Streptococcus pneumoniae, Haemophilus influenzae,* or *Staphylococcus aureus.* Generally the infection starts in one eye, but spreads rapidly to the other. The discharge in a bacterial infection is usually thick, pussy, and copious, and the eyelids often stick together during sleep. The lining of the eyelids tends to be very red and is occasionally swollen. A bacterial infection can be a complication of a cold or it can develop independently.

Viral infections of the eye are also common, especially in the summer, but they have slightly different characteristics. Generally they are caused by *adenovirus type 3,* which also causes a fever, sore throat, and tiredness. In this case, the discharge tends to be thin and watery, rather than pussy, and it is often accompanied by profuse tearing.

Allergic conjunctivitis, such as is associated with hay fever, tends to be milder but itchier than the infectious varieties. The various types of *irritative conjunctivitis* characteristically produce very bloodshot eyes with little discharge. Chemicals that frequently cause irritative conjunctivitis are found in soaps, hairsprays, makeup, deodorants, fertilizers, air pollution, swimming pool chlorine, and cigarette smoke.

Self-Care

All forms of conjunctivitis tend to be self-limiting, although moderate or severe bacterial ones respond more quickly when treated with antibiotics (see next section, *The Doctor*). Home treatment is effective for viral and allergic conjunctivitis, and usually also for irritative types. The eyes should be washed gently with water or a mild saltwater solution (1 T salt to 1 qt. water) or a nonprescription preparation such as *Artifi-*

cial Tears. All of these fluids will help soothe the eyes and wash out irritants, virus, or bacteria. *Murine* and *Visine* are not recommended for this use because they contain a vasoconstricting agent that makes the blood vessels of the eye narrow. If the eyes are glued shut in the morning, a warm moist washcloth should be applied for several minutes until the eyes can be opened.

The Doctor

The doctor should be seen for a conjunctivitis that has a copious pussy discharge. He or she will examine the eyes and prescribe antibiotic eye drops or ointment to kill the bacteria and speed healing. These preparations contain *sulfonamides* and/or *neomycin with polymyxin and/or bacitracin*. Drops should be warmed slightly to make their application more comfortable and applied hourly because normal tears quickly wash the drops out. Antibiotic ointments last up to four to six hours, but they tend to make vision a little blurry.

Ruling Out Other Diseases

A doctor should be seen immediately if a person has acute eye pain, significant sensitivity to light, impairment of vision that does not disappear after blinking, or pupils that don't react to light in the normal manner. These symptoms, which generally occur in one eye only, can be signs of *uveitis (infection of the iris)*, *corneal ulceration (infection)*, or *acute glaucoma* (see p. 233), which are MEDICAL EMERGENCIES that can rapidly damage the eye if left untreated. A corneal infection causes markedly blurred vision, pain, and light sensitivity. It most commonly develops after an injury and is often accompanied by a clear discharge. An infection of the iris also causes acute pain, blurred vision, and light sensitivity, but it usually does not produce any discharge. Acute glaucoma has no discharge, but is characterized by a sudden onset

of severe pain and blurred vision. Like the other conditions, it produces a reddened, bloodshot eye. Although uncommon, these conditions should be ruled out by a doctor's exam and lab tests if a diagnosis of conjunctivitis is not certain. Injury to the eye, either physical or chemical, can also produce some of the same signs as conjunctivitis, but it is preceded by a traumatic event (see p. 478).

Prevention

Both bacterial and viral forms of conjunctivitis spread readily with hand-to-eye contact. To prevent spread, people who have an infection should use their own towels, washcloth, and pillowcase, and everyone in the household should take special care with handwashing. Allergic and chemical forms of conjunctivitis can be prevented by avoiding the irritating substances (see p. 247).

Eyelid Infections, Including Sties and Blepharitis

Symptoms

- a red swollen area on the margin of the eyelid
- pronounced pain and tenderness
- burning, itching, or irritation of the eyelid
- scales or granulations on the eyelashes
- red-rimmed eyelids

Description

A number of conditions affect the skin and the glands on the edge of the eyelid. Several different kinds of glands within the eyelid contribute to making tears and perspiration. Tears, which bathe the eye constantly, are actually a complex substance that consists of three layers. The top layer, which lessens the evaporation of tears, is a one-molecule-thick, oily substance produced by the eyelid's *meibomian glands*. The middle and thickest layer of tears is salt water which is produced by the *lacrimal glands*. The third layer, *mucus*, which is produced by the mucous membrane lining the eyelid, is a wetting agent that helps the tears to spread readily across the eye. In addition, the *zeis glands* in the eyelid produce a substance that oils the skin, and the *moll glands* produce sweat.

Any of the glands that line the eyelid can become infected with *staphylococcus* bacteria, producing a tiny abcess that contains pus. When the superficial zeis or moll glands become infected, the condition is referred to as an *external hordeolum*, or *sty*. An infection of the deeper meibomian glands is called an *internal hordeolum*. In either case, a red, swollen area develops on the eyelid. Often these abscesses are very painful because they stretch a small area which has many pain nerves.

Staphylococcus bacteria can also cause infections in the lid margins themselves, producing an inflammation and a characteristic scaling or granulation along the eyelashes. This condition, which is referred to as *marginal blepharitis*, can also be caused by excess production of oil by the zeis glands. Blepharitis causes red-rimmed eyes that itch or burn. With the staph type, there are dry scales, tiny red raw areas along the margins, and loss of eyelashes. The seborrheic type produces oily scales and may be associated with scaling or excess oil production on the scalp, eyebrows, and ears. (See p. 171). Most commonly, blepharitis is a mixture of the two types. Often blepharitis is accompanied by sties, which can also be caused by staph on the eyelids.

Self-Care

Generally, both sties and blepharitis respond well to home treatment. The treatment for sties is basically the same as for any other skin infection: warm soaks with a moist clean washcloth for 10–15 minutes three to four times a day. Within a day or two, an abscess will usually come to a point and drain, either externally or internally, or it will disappear spontaneously.

Blepharitis usually clears up gradually in response to regular gentle washing with soap or shampoo, especially antidandruff or baby shampoos which are available over the counter. The eyes should be closed tightly and the eyelid margins rubbed each day with a soapy washcloth. The scales can also be carefully rubbed off with a cotton-tipped applicator and water.

The Doctor

If a sty is very bothersome or doesn't respond to home treatment within several days, the doctor should be seen. The doctor will prescribe an *antibiotic ophthalmic ointment* which will help speed healing. If the sty is large and pointed, the doctor may drain it to give relief, but this is generally not necessary.

The doctor should be seen for blepharitis when the lids are very inflamed or raw, or when home treatment fails and the itching becomes uncomfortable. If the infection appears to be bacterial, the doctor will also prescribe antibiotic ophthalmic ointment.

Ruling Out Other Diseases

A sty looks something like a *chalazion*, which is an inflammation of the meibomian gland, but a chalazion is simply swollen; it is not red, hot, or tender. Although a chalazion does not require treatment, it will not disappear by itself. If it becomes large or annoying, it can be removed surgically.

If the whole eye swells, the cause may be *orbital cellulitis*. With orbital cellulitis, the eye and the eyelids swell severely, and fever and significant pain are present as well. This condition is a MEDICAL EMERGENCY which requires immediate treatment with oral antibiotics.

Prevention

Daily face washing can prevent bacterial infections of the eyelids and keep seborrheic blepharitis under control. Cleanliness is particularly important if people are prone to these conditions or if a household member has any kind of staph infection.

Glaucoma

Symptoms

- no signs or symptoms in early stages.
- possible family history
- slow loss of peripheral vision over a period of years
- blurred vision and halos around lights in late stages

Description

Glaucoma refers to a group of diseases all of which are characterized by a rise in fluid pressure within both eyes. If the pressure remains high for a long enough time, the optic nerves and nerve fibers in the retinas at the back of the eyes undergo irreversible damage that ultimately leads to partial or total loss of sight in one or both eyes.

Glaucoma is not an uncommon illness—it affects approximately 1%–2% of all people over the age of 35. Of the estimated 2,000,000 cases of glaucoma in the U.S., 25% remain undetected. Some 50,000 individuals in this country are blind because of glaucoma. Although glaucoma is not *preventable*, it is *treatable*. The great majority of people blinded by glaucoma could have had their sight saved if their condition had been discovered in the early stages.

The eye has two liquid-filled chambers, a small one in front of the lens, and a larger one behind it (see illustration). The rear chamber is filled with a clear gelatinous substance that allows light to pass through and hit the retina. The front chamber is filled with a fluid called the *aqueous humor*, which is produced by the *ciliary body*, a small organ that lies to the side of and behind the lens. The aqueous humor flows between the ligaments of the lens into the front chamber, then passes through a filter to either side of the eye, called the *trabecular meshwork*, and ultimately drains through tiny canals into the veins around the eye. This cycle goes on at a slow, constant rate. Normally, if pressure begins to build up in the front chamber, more canals open to drain off fluid at the edge of the eye.

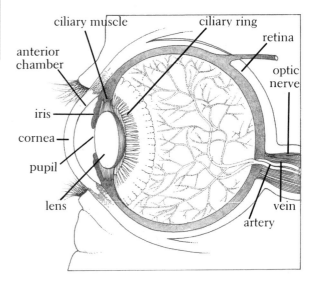

The eye is a complex structure which transmits light rays through a lens that focuses the rays on light-sensitive cells in the retina at the back of the eye.

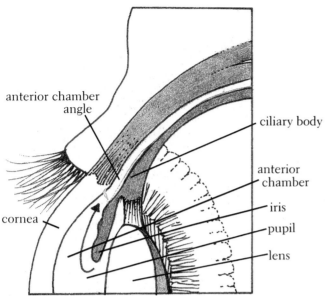

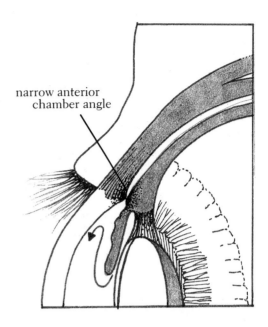

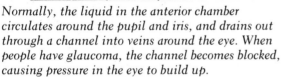

Normally, the liquid in the anterior chamber circulates around the pupil and iris, and drains out through a channel into veins around the eye. When people have glaucoma, the channel becomes blocked, causing pressure in the eye to build up.

When a person has *open angle glaucoma,* which accounts for over 90% of all cases, the trabecular meshwork slowly degenerates, blocking the drainage of aqueous humor, which is continously produced. As a result, the pressure within the eye rises. If this intraocular pressure remains elevated long enough, the optic nerve deteriorates and finally the light-sensing cells and nerve fibers in the retina are destroyed. Unfortunately, this form of glaucoma has no early symptoms, although it does tend to occur in some families. By the time a person notices any decrease in vision, permanent damage has already been done. However, open-angle glaucoma can be picked up in the early stages by an eye doctor or ophthalmologist, during a routine eye exam, before any damage to the eye has taken place.

Another form of glaucoma, which is very rare, is called *angle-closure glaucoma* or *acute glaucoma.* Unlike open-angle glaucoma, this type develops very suddenly and has noticeable symptoms. Angle-closure glaucoma is a MEDICAL EMERGENCY because permanent damage to the eye can occur within 24–48 hours. Symptoms include a sudden onset of blurred vision and excruciating eye pain, which are caused by an abrupt blockage of the aqueous humor before it even reaches the trabecular meshwork. Acute glaucoma only occurs in individuals in whom the *anterior chamber angle,* the area leading to the trabecular meshwork, is unusually narrow (see illustration). This congenital narrowing can be seen by an ophthalmologist during an eye exam.

Self-Care

No type of glaucoma can be treated at home.

The Doctor

An eye doctor, or *ophthalmologist*, can diagnose glaucoma by examining the eyes. Open-angle glaucoma is diagnosed by a test called *tonometry* which measures the pressure in the eye. The most common form of *tonometry*, called *applanation tonometry*, involves blowing a puff of air at the eye and measuring how much force is necessary to flatten the eye. The second method involves putting a drop of local anesthetic on the eye and then briefly placing a small device against the cornea to measure how much force it takes to flatten the eye.

The normal pressure of the eye is 12–20 millimeters Hg of pressure. A reading in the 20–30 range can simply be caused by a normal fluctuation in pressure, but the test should be repeated several times to determine if the pressure is constant at that level. If glaucoma is suspected, the doctor will perform a more complete checkup that includes testing for peripheral vision, and visually examining the optic nerve and retina for damage. Also, a test called *gonioscopy* may be done to measure the width of the anterior chamber angle with a high magnification viewer.

Constant elevated pressure confirms the diagnosis of open-angle glaucoma and is treated with drugs called *miotics* that increase the efficiency of the drainage channels. The most commonly prescribed drug is *pilocarpine drops* which are put in the eyes five times a day. *Epinephrine drops* are frequently used instead; they are applied one to two times a day. Other types of medication that are sometimes used slow the production of aqueous humor. These drugs include *carbonic anhydrase inhibitors* (e.g., *acetazolamide*) and *beta-adrenergic blockers* (e.g., *timolol*). If drug therapy does not prove to be effective, there are several surgical procedures that can be done to increase drainage.

In cases of acute glaucoma, the ophthalmologist lowers the intraocular pressure with drugs and then surgically widens the anterior chamber angle.

Ruling Out Other Diseases

Open-angle glaucoma is not confused with any other diseases. Acute angle glaucoma can be visually differentiated from *uveitis* (see p. 230), an inflammation of the iris that is treated with antibiotics.

Prevention

Early diagnosis and treatment of glaucoma can prevent damage to the eyes. Ophthalmologists recommend that everyone over the age of 20 have a *routine tonometric exam* every three years. Individuals who have a family history of glaucoma should have the exam done annually. A person who develops glaucoma at the age of 40 will be blind by the age of 60 if the condition is not diagnosed and treated. With diagnosis, treatment, and good follow-up, eyesight can be preserved. Glaucoma is the *most preventable* cause of blindness.

Difficulty with Near Vision, or Presbyopia

Symptoms

- difficulty in reading, especially fine print
- headaches
- visual fatigue
- tendency for printed matter to be sharper when held at arm's length

Description

Several factors contribute to how sharply an image is focused on the retina at the back of the

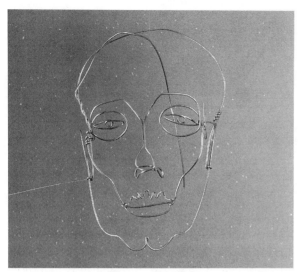

In midadulthood, the lens of the eye becomes less flexible and therefore less able to focus sharply on near objects. As a result, many people then need bifocals or reading glasses. Alexander Calder. Portrait of a Man. 1929–30. Brass-wire construction, 12⅞" × 8¾" × 13½". Collection, The Museum of Modern Art, New York. Gift of the artist.

eye. One is the ability of the lens to bend light rays so that they come to a focal point on the retina. Another is the ability of the lens to change its shape in order to focus sharply on objects that are varying distances away. With age, the lens gradually loses its ability to change shape, and focusing on near objects becomes difficult. This condition is referred to as *presbyopia*.

When light rays pass from one medium to another, for instance, from air into water or through a glass lens, the rays are bent. Basically the lens of the eye does the same thing to incoming light. The eye has a *double convex lens*; that is, the lens bulges outward in both the front and the back. This type of lens tends to bend incoming parallel rays together at a point on the retina called the *fovea*. The fovea is a 1-millimeter area in the center of the retina that is specially adapted for sharp vision. It consists only of *cones*, nerve receptors which register an image very clearly in good light and connect directly to the brain.

If incoming light rays are focused directly on the fovea when the lens is in a resting state, vision is said to be normal or 20/20. However, if the rays come together in front of the fovea, a person is said to be *nearsighted* or *myopic*. After incoming light rays have converged inside the eye, they tend to spread out again. Thus, in a nearsighted person, the image that actually lands on the retina is slightly out of focus. Nearsighted people can't see distant objects clearly, but by squinting, which causes the lens to bulge more, they can bring near objects into sharp focus. For nearsighted people, eyeglasses with a *concave* (thinner in the middle), or inward-bend-

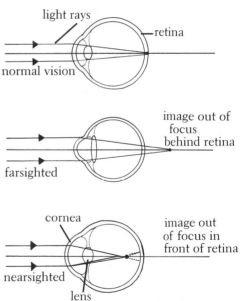

When vision is normal, an image focuses directly on the retina and appears to be sharp. If people are nearsighted, the image falls in front of the retina; if people are farsighted, the image is in focus behind the retina. When images fall in front of, or behind, the retina, they appear blurry.

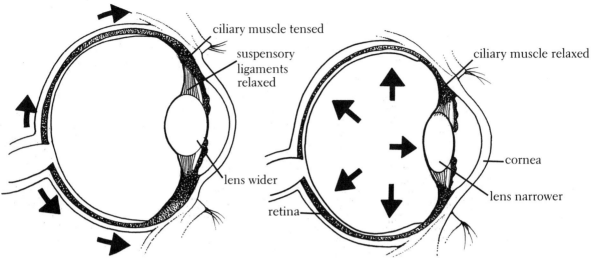

The ciliary muscles of the eye adjust the shape of the lens by tensing. When the lens is round, near objects are in focus; when the lens is flat, distant objects are in focus.

ing lens, can adjust incoming rays so that they will actually converge on the fovea.

If incoming light rays come together behind the fovea, a person is said to be *farsighted* or *hyperoptic*. In these people the eyeball does not grow as fast as normal, so the eye tends to be narrower from front to back, causing an image to be in focus behind the retina. Farsighted people can adjust the lens of the eye to see distant objects sharply, but sometimes have difficulty making sufficient adjustment to see very close objects clearly. Farsighted people are more prone to eyestrain because they must use more energy to constantly adjust the lens to bring near objects into focus. Farsightedness can be corrected with a *convex* (thicker in the middle) or outward-curving lens that causes incoming light rays to converge closer to the lens.

In actuality, most people do not have perfect 20/20 vision. The reason individuals are farsighted or nearsighted has to do with the shape and size of the eyeball, which is largely determined by genetics. In nearsighted people, the eyeball grows unusually large, especially during adolescence. As a result, the eyeball is so long in relation to the bending powers of the lens that the focal point falls short of the fovea.

Whether nearsighted, farsighted, or 20/20, everybody has to adjust the lenses of their eyes in order to focus clearly on objects that are closer than 18 feet (6 meters). This is due to the fact that light rays coming from objects this close are not parallel, but are divergent (see illustration). Unless the lens curves more to compensate, these rays would meet at a point behind the retina. The process by which the shape of the lens is changed to focus an image sharply on the retina is called *accommodation*. It takes place when the *ciliary muscle* that surrounds the lens contracts, which in turn decreases the tension on tissues that usually keep the lens somewhat flattened. When these tissues relax, the lens pops back into its usual round shape. Normally, this complex action takes place automatically and is unnoticed.

The lens of the eye is made of a soft pliable material composed of sugar, protein, and collagen. With age, this material gradually tends to harden and become more and more resistant to changing shape. In childhood the lens has tremendous powers of accommodation, but by the age of 15 a measurable decrease has already taken place, although a person will not be aware of it. By their early 40s, however, most people begin to notice that words are no longer in sharp focus at the normal reading distance. In order to focus sharply, they have to hold their reading matter farther and farther away. When people find that their arms have become "too short" for comfortable reading, they generally see an eye doctor about a corrective prescription.

Other symptoms of decreasing accommodation are eyestrain or tiredness after doing close work. People who are nearsighted and already wear glasses begin to find themselves taking their glasses *off* in order to read more comfortably. Most people also notice that distant objects are initially blurred when they look up from close work. This effect is due to the fact that the lens no longer changes shape quickly in response to the ciliary muscle relaxing. On the average, lack of accommodation becomes a problem for both nearsighted and farsighted people in their early 40s.

Self-Care

Although reading or *magnifying glasses* are widely sold without prescription, it is better for people to have their eyes checked by a professional—an ophthalmologist or optometrist. Not only can the acuity, or sharpness, of the two eyes vary, too strong a magnification can accentuate problems of accommodation. Finally, anyone over 40 should have a glaucoma test.

The Doctor

An ophthalmologist will do a routine examination of the eyes, including a glaucoma check and a *refraction* to determine the visual acuity of the eyes. If both individual and doctor agree that corrective lenses are in order, the doctor will issue a prescription.

A wide variety of glasses are available. Far-

sighted people can often just use reading glasses for close work, although they may eventually need bifocals or a separate pair of glasses for distance. Nearsighted people will need either two pairs of glasses (one for reading, one for distance) or bifocals. People who wear contact lenses generally get reading glasses to wear in addition to their contact lenses, although some people prefer to have two pair of contacts.

Traditionally, bifocal lenses have been split with a distance prescription on the top and a reading prescription on the bottom, or they have a reading prescription inset in the bottom half of the lens. More recently, lenses have become available that are ground with a continuous range from distance to reading and without a line between them. This kind of lens actually has a midrange that functions like a *multifocal* or *trifocal* for work that is at arm's length.

Switching between distance and reading glasses can be a nuisance, and most people who need both eventually do get bifocals. Wearing bifocals requires an initial adjustment that may involve several days to several weeks, so people have to be motivated to make the change. Since bifocals require looking through the upper part of the lens to view distant objects, and looking through the lower part of the lens for reading and close work, people have to move their head more and position their eyes appropriately to achieve sharp focus. Initially, if people look directly at their feet with bifocals, they have an unsteady sensation and feel that the ground is "coming up at them." This effect is most noticeable in going down steps and disappears within a few weeks. In the interim, people should descend steps slowly and use the railing to steady themselves.

Ruling Out Other Diseases

Provided people have normal distance vision, and a gradual decrease in the sharpness of near vision, there are no diseases that have to be distinguished from *presbyopia*. *Cataracts* cause a gradual loss of both near and far vision, and generally do not cause problems before the age of 60 although they can be detected earlier by visual examination. *Sudden loss* of vision, near or far, can be a sign of serious eye disease and should be evaluated immediately by an ophthalmologist. *Acute uveitis* (an infection of the iris), *corneal ulcers* (see p. 230), *acute glaucoma* (sudden high pressure) (see p. 233), a *detached retina* (see p. 382), or an *injury to the eye* (see p. 478) are all medical emergencies that can cause sudden loss of vision in one or both eyes.

Prevention

Presbyopia is considered to be part of the normal aging process. Ophthalmologists currently do not believe it can be prevented by either eye exercises or dietary changes, although they do suggest resting the eyes and avoiding eye fatigue by not focusing on the same view for too long at one time.

Headache: Tension Headaches, Migraines, and Cluster Headaches

Symptoms

tension headache
- steady, nonpulsing headache
- tightness at the temples or back of the head
- bandlike pain around the head
- cramping sensations in the neck and upper back
- pain on one or both sides of the head
- commonly occurs in the morning or evening
- difficulty falling asleep
- depression, low appetite, diminished sexual drive

migraine headache
- pain on one or both sides of the head
- throbbing or pulsating headache
- pain above the eyebrows
- often, nausea, vomiting, and sensitivity to light
- occasionally, numbness in the hand of the unaffected side
- attacks may last one to two days
- may be preceded by blind spots or light flashes
- often familial

cluster headache
- excruciating, burning, one-sided pain
- pain mostly around the eye socket
- flushing, tearing, and/or runny nose on the affected side.
- commonly occurs at night during sleep
- attacks last 10–60 minutes
- attacks occur in groups over a period of several weeks.

Description

Headache, which is one of the most common complaints of our times, ranks ninth in reasons for visits to a doctor. However, the great majority of headaches are fleeting and most people never even consult their doctor about them. Of the three main causes of headache, the most common is muscle contraction, which accounts for the majority of ordinary *tension headaches*, as well as the majority of severe headaches that are seen by a doctor. The second most common cause of headache is abnormal dilation of blood vessels in the base of the brain, which is the

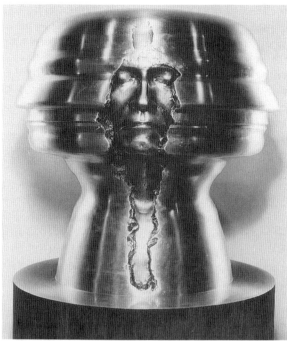

Emotional factors are a key aspect of muscle tension headaches. Harold Tovish. Vortex. 1966. Bronze and enameled aluminum. 66″ × 18″. Collection, The Whitney Museum of American Art. Purchase, with funds from an anonymous donor. 66.132.

cause of *migraines* and *cluster headaches*. The third cause of headache, which is actually uncommon, is organic disease of the skull, which includes *sinus infection, meningitis,* and even more rarely, *tumors.*

The head and brain, being the most evolved structures in the human body, seem to be exquisitely sensitive to stress and tension. Anatomically, the reason headaches are so painful is that the head has an unusually high number of pain nerve receptors as compared with the rest of the body. The scalp, the muscles in the head and neck, the arteries in the head, and the lining of the brain are all richly supplied with pain nerves. Moreover, the fact that people often become anxious about headaches tends to increase their

perception of the pain. One of the most respected medical books on headaches, by Seymour Diamond, M.D., notes that it is uncommon for severe headache to be caused by organic disease. Most often headaches are caused by stress, or as Diamond observes, frequently they represent an inability in some way "to deal with the uncertainties of life." Diamond further suggests that headaches symbolize being out of step with oneself, but this is not to say that headaches are imaginary or that they are not accompanied by physiological changes.

Tension headaches: Muscle tension is such a pervasive element in everyday life that it is no surprise that tension headaches are the most common form of headache. The great majority of tension headaches are brief, occasional, and go away within several hours by themselves, or respond to mild, over-the-counter pain relievers. In general, people do not worry much about this kind of headache as long as they are mild or infrequent. Doctors believe that these headaches are caused by fatigue and/or stress. *Temporomandibular joint (TMJ) syndrome* is a variant of a tension headache. With this condition there is unilateral or bilateral pain and tenderness in the temples, which can radiate to the jaw. TMJ syndrome is sometimes caused by tooth grinding, and often the pain becomes worse with chewing. Like other types of tension headaches, these are thought to be caused by stress and muscle tension.

Sometimes tension headaches can be severe enough or frequent enough to arouse concern and send people to the doctor. With a severe tension headache, people feel a steady, nonpulsing ache, most commonly situated in the forehead, temples, or back of the head. People often describe the pain as a bandlike or viselike feeling of tightness or pressure. Tension headache sufferers also notice that their neck and shoulders frequently feel tight, cramped, and painful. The

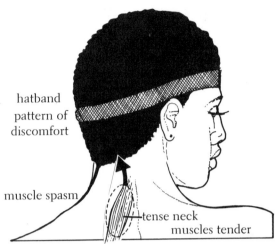

Muscle contraction headaches, or tension headaches, often produce a hatband pattern of pain circling the head; they may involve muscle spasms and tender areas over the neck and shoulders.

pain may be so intense that brushing their hair becomes uncomfortable.

Unlike the other forms of headache, a severe tension headache may be steady and unrelenting over a period of days, weeks, or even months. Some people who suffer from chronic tension headaches find the pain occurs most often or is most intense between 4–8 in the morning and 4–8 in the evening. Frequently people notice that the pain comes on during or after tension-producing episodes in their life. Unlike other types of headaches, tension headaches tend to occur on both sides of the head, are less commonly associated with nausea and vomiting, and rarely wake people up from sleep. Tension headaches are somewhat more common in women.

Emotional factors have been found to be important contributors to muscle tension headaches. Several studies have shown that people who suffer from severe or chronic tension headaches often experience conflict in areas of their lives such as marriage, family, or job. The ma-jority of people who experience conflict also feel some degree of depression, which shows up as sleep difficulties, poor appetite, diminished interest in sex, and/or feelings of being low or "blue." People with chronic tension headaches may also exhibit other physical symptoms of emotional upset such as dizziness, heart palpitations, and constipation.

In recent years doctors have gained a greater understanding of how life stresses cause tension headaches. When anxiety is perceived in the brain, nerve impulses are sent to the muscle bundles in the neck and shoulders, causing them to tense. Normally, after *motor nerve cells* fire and a muscle contracts, the nerve cells stop sending impulses, and the muscle then relaxes. But when a person is anxious, the cerebrum directs the motor nerve cells to continue to fire impulses, and the muscles continue to tense. Contraction causes the muscles of the neck and shoulders to bulge, which puts pressure on nearby nerves and cuts down on blood flow. Due to a lack of oxygen, the muscles at the back of the neck, jaw, and temple accumulate metabolic waste products, which produces pain. Studies have also shown that the pain threshold in people who have severe tension headaches and in people who are depressed is lower than normal. These people have abnormally low amounts of *serotonin*, a brain transmitter that causes the body to release its own natural pain relievers called *endorphins*.

Migraine headaches: Migraines are a common form of headache suffered by 8–12 million Americans. The name "migraine" refers to the fact that the initial pain is usually one-sided; the word originally comes from the Greek word for "half a head." Migraines occur periodically in single attacks. They generally begin as a dull ache around the forehead and temples, progress to a throbbing or pulsating ache, and finally develop into a constant steady pain. Approximately

70% of the time, they remain confined to one side of the head, although they sometimes involve both sides. Attacks vary in length from four hours to one or two days, and vary in frequency from once a year to once every few days, the average being two to four per month.

A *common migraine*, such as described above, comes on with no warning signs and may be associated with nausea and vomiting, cold hands and feet, and sensitivity to light and noise. Occasionally abnormal water retention may cause a person to experience slight bodily swelling, an effect that can make the skin feel "thick" and cause abdominal distention and a slight gain in weight. A *classical migraine* resembles a common migraine, but is associated with a specific group of symptoms that regularly precede an attack. About 35% of all migraine sufferers experience classical, as opposed to common, migraines. The hallmark of a classical migraine is a group of neurological symptoms that take place for a half hour immediately before the headache, and cease before the pain begins. These symptoms, which are referred to as the *aura* or *prodromal stage*, include seeing blind spots, zigzag lines called *fortification spectra*, or bright flashing lights. Other prodromal symptoms are *visual* or *auditory hallucinations* or *distortions*, and numbness of the mouth or the hand on the side opposite the headache. The shrinking and expanding figures described by Lewis Carroll in *Alice in Wonderland* were visual hallucinations that Carroll experienced before one of his migraine attacks. Less common neurological prodroma include dizziness, double vision, lack of balance, and difficulty speaking. For some people, a migraine attack is signaled by mood changes, irritability, restlessness, depression, or unusual hunger or thirst occurring the day before the attack. Variants of migraine symptoms include pupillary changes, temporary drooping of an eyelid, and eye movement problems. Migraines can also be associated

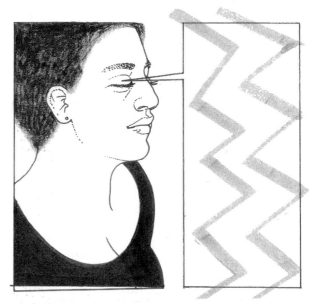

For about a half-hour prior to an attack, migraine sufferers often experience a visual aura consisting of blind spots or zigzag lines.

with a continuous aura, speech problems, even paralysis of one side of the body. Post-headache symptoms include fatigue, tenderness of the scalp, and pain when the head is moved.

Both common and classical migraines are slightly more frequent among women than men. Most commonly, the attacks initially take place when people are in their 20s and 30s, occur with wide variation in frequency, and eventually tend to decrease with age. Although no gene or mode of inheritance has been established proving genetic transmission, 70% of migraine sufferers have a family history of the condition.

Some researchers believe that there is a migraine personality that applies to many people who have migraines. Migraine sufferers often tend to be set in their ways and may experience anger that they have difficulty expressing in response to circumstances that require significant change and flexibility. Often, migraine sufferers are found to be perfectionists or driven people.

As all migraine sufferers know, a number of factors are associated with, or play a role in, precipitating an attack. The stress of adapting to life changes such as switching jobs or moving is known to trigger migraines. Attacks tend to be more common on weekends and holidays, and may correlate with a change in sleep patterns. Among women, there seems to be a strong connection with hormonal cycles, attacks being more likely to occur around the time of the menstrual period. Often the attacks disappear during pregnancy, yet they are sometimes made worse by birth control pills. Attacks may tend to increase around the time of menopause, and may be exacerbated by *postmenopausal estrogen therapy*.

Among both men and women, diet is another significant causal factor (see chart). Migraine attacks are triggered in some people by eating foods that contain *tyramine*, a protein that causes dilation of blood vessels and release of the stress-response hormone *norepinephrine*. Tyramine is found in aged cheeses, pickled herring, chicken livers, and the pods of peas, lima beans, and navy beans. Other vasodilators that sometimes cause attacks are *alcohol* (in particular, wines that contain large amounts of *histamines*); the food preservative *sodium nitrite*; and the flavor enhancer *MSG (monosodium glutamate)*. It has also been observed that attacks may be brought on by *low* or *high blood sugar levels*, which can be caused by either skipping meals or by eating large amounts of sugar or carbohydrates at one sitting.

Much new information has been uncovered about migraine headaches in the last decade. Understanding the physiology of migraine attacks can be very helpful in dealing with attacks and working to prevent them. Research has shown that the brain has two types of blood supply: large arteries that supply the base of the brain, and smaller arteries that lead to the rest

Foods to Be Avoided by the Headache Patient

alcoholic beverages
avocado
banana (only half per day)
ripened cheeses:
   Brie
   Camembert
   Cheddar
   Gruyere
chocolate
citrus (only one per day)
coffeecakes made with yeast
cured meats
donuts
excessive caffeine
fermented foods
herring
MSG
nuts
onions
peanut butter
pickled foods
pizza
pork (only twice a week)
sour cream
vinegar (except white vinegar)
yogurt

of the brain. This double system of blood flow helps to ensure that the brain gets enough blood in emergencies. The large arteries, which are referred to as the *innervated vascular system*, are under the control of the *autonomic nervous system*, the part of the nervous system that regulates involuntary body functions and responds to stress. The large arteries are very responsive to *catecholamines*, or stress hormones (such as norepinephrine), while the smaller arteries, which are in direct contact with brain tissue, widen in response to high levels of carbon dioxide in the blood. Any stress or stimulus that arouses the autonomic nervous system for fight-or-flight reduces blood flow in the large arteries leading to the base of the brain, resulting in an initial drop in blood flow and oxygen to the entire brain. Low levels of oxygen in the brain are thought to be responsible for the aura or prodromal symptoms that precede a classical migraine attack. In response to the sudden low levels of oxygen, the smaller arteries in the brain suddenly widen, causing a rush of blood that results in the release of *histamine* and other chemicals that are responsible for the body's inflammatory processes. These chemicals cause an influx of white blood cells and cellular fluid which cause the brain to swell. At the same time, a decrease in the body's natural opiates called *endorphins* causes an individual's pain threshold to drop markedly. These three factors—increased blood flow, swelling, and a drop in endorphins—cause the pounding migraine headache. However, the factor that actually triggers the headache is whatever event alerts the autonomic nervous system and causes the decrease in blood flow to the base of the brain.

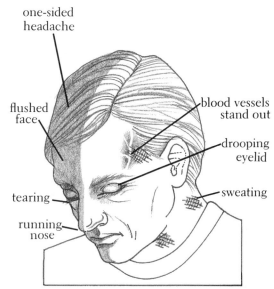

Cluster headaches are severe, short-lived, one-sided headaches that occur in groups over a period of days, weeks, or months. Several specific symptoms may accompany a cluster headache.

Cluster headaches: Cluster headaches consist of a series of short-lived, but extremely severe headaches that occur periodically in groups. Like migraines, they are caused by changes in the vascular supply to the brain, whereas tension headaches are caused by muscle contraction. Cluster headaches last from a few minutes to a few hours, the average being about 30 minutes in length. A single attack is always confined to one side of the head, although opposite sides may be affected in separate attacks. Occasionally a cluster headache starts as a knifelike pain behind the nostrils or eye then spreads to the forehead. Cluster headaches produce a burning pain that is so severe that sufferers may pace about restlessly, or even hit their head in an attempt to stop or alter the pain.

There are several specific physical symptoms that may accompany a cluster headache. On the affected side, symptoms include a tearing eye and runny nose. On the unaffected side, a group of symptoms called *Horner's syndrome* may occur, including constriction of the pupil, a feeling of retraction in the eye itself, a drooping eyelid, and flushing. Common cluster headache variants include unusual location or frequency, or brief bursts of jabbing head pains.

Individual headaches occur from once to several times a day over a period of days, weeks, or months. Quite often the headaches begin at night, waking a person up from sleep. Occasionally they occur at the same time each night. Cluster headaches appear most commonly in the spring or fall, the average cluster lasting one to two months. At the end of a cluster, the headaches disappear for months or years.

Cluster headaches are five times more common in men than women and the majority of people who have them are between 20 and 40 years of age. Generally there is no family history. A significant number of people who suffer from cluster headaches are smokers, but cigarettes do not appear to actually trigger attacks. Also, the incidence of peptic ulcer is higher than average among cluster headache sufferers. Alcohol or *vasodilating* drugs such as *nitroglycerin* frequently precipitate attacks in the midst of a cluster of headaches, although alcohol does not seem to have this effect between clusters.

The physiology of cluster headaches is still not well understood. Like migraines, they are thought to be associated with changes in blood flow to the brain, but the specific changes are not known. One study has shown that blood flow is different on the affected side during an attack. The same study found that the blood vessels on the headache and nonheadache side differed in the way that they dilated in reaction to oxygen. Some researchers speculate that cluster headaches may be produced by irritation of an autonomic nervous system ganglion.

Self-Care

Most tension headaches, and many migraine and cluster headaches, are amenable to self-treatment, especially if people learn to become aware of the early symptoms of an attack. Relaxation and biofeedback techniques for headache are being prescribed increasingly by physicians, and the same principles and exercises can be used as part of a self-care regimen. All three types of headache are all strongly affected by stress and the reactions of the autonomic nervous system (see section on *Prevention*).

In the early 1970s, two discoveries were made concerning the effectiveness of relaxation as a treatment. First, it was found that deep relaxation of the muscles in the head and neck relieved muscle tension headaches. Second, it was ob-

served that when migraine patients imagined that their hands were warm, their headaches often disappeared. Researchers believe that visualizing warm hands tends to shunt blood away from the brain and lower the heart rate, both of which lessen autonomic nervous system activity.

Visualizing the hands being warm helps to break an unconscious, reflexive headache response pattern that many migraine sufferers actually become conditioned to. Headache clinics advise migraine sufferers to do relaxation exercises and to visualize warmth in their hands at the first sign of a migraine aura or prodrome because it has been found that muscle tension headaches often accompany the onset of a migraine attack. Patients are told to concentrate on the neck, shoulders, and jaw, especially if they tend to clench their teeth (see charts, and sections on stress and relaxation, p. 58 and 60). In addition, massaging the neck may bring relief.

The great majority of headaches that are not severe—whether they be tension, migraine, or cluster—are often helped by over-the-counter preparations containing aspirin or acetaminophen. Many people believe aspirin is more effective because it lowers the level of the body's *prostaglandins*, substances that cause blood vessels to contract and that lower a person's pain threshold.

The Doctor

Severe, persistent headaches that do not respond readily to self-care should be seen by a general practitioner or internist, who can make a referral to a neurologist for a more complete work-up if necessary. The doctor diagnoses the type of headache through a careful history, a general physical, and a basic neurological exam testing for normal reflexes, muscle strength, balance, and eye movements. Lab tests such as skull x-rays and CT scans are generally not done because they're expensive and rarely are necessary to make a diagnosis.

Tension headaches: Frequent, severe muscle contraction headaches that persistently fail to respond to home treatment are often treated with *antidepressant* or *antianxiety drugs*. It is thought that these drugs are effective because of the relationship between tension headaches and stress, or depression. The most commonly used antidepressants include *amitriptyline hydrochloride (Elavil)*, *imipramine hydrochloride (Tofranil)*, and *nortriptyline hydrochloride (Aventyl HCl)*. Antidepressants are usually given in the evening because of their sedative side effects. Other side effects include dry mouth, nausea, and dizziness. Generally, a drug is started at a low dose, and the dosage is increased if necessary. Full effectiveness may not be achieved for several weeks. The most common antianxiety drug prescribed for tension headaches is *diazepam (Valium)*. Treatment for two to four weeks with one of these drugs will often break up a cycle of anxiety or tension, giving prolonged relief even after the drug is discontinued. Since the antidepressant and antianxiety drugs can cause physical dependency, they should be carefully monitored by a doctor, and used only after other therapies have been tried. Some doctors do not prescribe these drugs at all because of the high potential for addiction.

Some doctors recommend *psychotherapy* in addition to drugs in order to deal with the underlying conditions that are causing the headaches. Doctors may also recommend *physiotherapy*, including massage and postural alignment. Physical exam sometimes reveals that headache sufferers have tiny, extremely painful nodules within the muscles of the neck and shoulders. Massage can often break up these nodules and relieve the headaches.

Migraine headaches: Doctors use several types of drugs to treat migraine headaches. If attacks are infrequent, *abortive drugs* are prescribed to stop headaches as they begin; if attacks are frequent, *preventive drugs* are given to avoid the onset of headaches. By far the most common of the abortive drugs is *ergotamine tartrate (Gynergen)*, which is often given in a combination form with caffeine *(Cafergot)*. A number of other combinations are available. All of these drugs are *vasoconstrictors* that counteract the dilation of the arteries going to the brain, in particular, the *carotid arteries* in the neck. These drugs should be taken as soon as the onset of symptoms is noticed. Since ergotamine preparations can have serious effects on blood pressure and the nervous system, they cannot be taken again for half an hour. They should never be taken by women who are pregnant or might be pregnant, because they cause uterine contractions. Because these drugs are not well-absorbed from the stomach, they are available in *sublingual* (under the tongue), *inhalant*, *suppository*, and *injectable* forms.

If migraine attacks are frequent, preventive drugs may be prescribed. The most common are *propranolol (Inderal)*, *amitriptyline (Elavil)*, and *cyproheptadine (Periactin)*. Individual migraine sufferers often find that one drug is effective, while another is not. Since a number of drugs are available, and new preventive drugs with different mechanisms of action are being developed all the time, the doctor may try one drug after another in an attempt to break the attacks. Once a medication proves to be effective, it can often be tapered off over a period of several months.

Cluster headaches: Because cluster headaches are vascular in nature like migraines, they are treated somewhat similarly. But abortive drugs tend to be less effective with cluster headaches because this type of headache, or even the whole cluster of attacks, may subside before the drug begins to work. Men can be given *ergonovine* or *methyl ergonovine (Methergine)*, but these drugs cannot be used with premenopausal women because they can cause contractions in pregnant women. *Sansert* is only prescribed for brief periods because it has adverse reactions when taken continuously on a longterm basis. For particularly resistant clusters, a 10–day course of a diminishing dose of *prednisone* is used. It has been found that breathing pure oxygen for 15 minutes will often stop a cluster attack. Preventive drugs (see above) are used once a cluster has started, and discontinued when the cluster ends. In some cases, *lithium carbonate* helps people with cluster headaches. It is taken for two weeks, then gradually withdrawn. Cluster headaches are often difficult to prevent, and, unlike standard migraines, referral to a neurologist or other doctor specializing in headache is often necessary.

Because the powerful drugs used to treat various kinds of headaches are not always effective and may have significant side effects, doctors have begun to treat headaches using nondrug therapies such as biofeedback, relaxation, and imagery (see p. 60), massage, conditioning, and acupuncture. Tension headaches have been very successfully treated with *electromyographic biofeedback*, in which a deepening sound indicates when muscles of the neck, shoulder, and face are relaxing. The same relaxation exercises are also practiced two times a day at home without the machine. The goal is ultimately for the patient to be able to achieve relaxation without the machine's feedback. Migraine headaches are treated with a temperature biofeedback signal monitor that beeps when the temperature of the hands goes up (see section on *Self-Care*). These machines may be used with a therapist, or rented and used at home. Eventually, the patient learns to achieve the desired temperature rise without the machine. In a large study dealing with all three types of headache, it was found

that after biofeedback training, 40% of the people experienced permanent relief, while another 32% had temporary improvement.

Ruling Out Other Diseases

There are a number of causes of headache other than muscle tension, migraine, or cluster headache. Even in these conditions, headache is rarely a sign of serious illness. The so-called "Chinese restaurant syndrome," caused by MSG, is a headache accompanied by tightening sensations in the head and face, and possible light-headedness. Mild headaches that begin in the eyes may be caused by *farsightedness* or *presbyopia* (see p. 234), or *astigmatism*, another cause of focusing difficulties. An ear infection can also cause a headache (see p. 221). Acute or chronic sinus infections cause headaches that are generally localized over the affected sinus, and are often accompanied by fever or a runny nose (see p. 226). Dental problems can cause referred pain in other parts of the head, as well as in the teeth. A sudden severe headache confined to one eye can be caused in rare instances by *acute glaucoma*, which is a MEDICAL EMERGENCY that should be treated immediately by an eye doctor.

Severe high blood pressure can also cause headaches, especially in the morning. A sudden, severe headache accompanied by a fever, a stiff neck, and possible confusion and vomiting can be caused by *meningitis*, an infection of the lining of the spinal cord. A headache virtually always follows trauma to the head and can last for several hours to several days. If the person loses consciousness after the injury, even briefly, or the headache is accompanied by drowsiness, confusion, abnormal pupil changes, or muscle weakness, a doctor should be seen immediately (see p. 472). By far the rarest cause of headaches is a brain tumor. Newly occurring headaches that get worse with time, or chronic headaches that change radically, especially if they are associated with vision problems, convulsions, mental changes, muscle weakness, or paralysis should be seen promptly by a neurologist.

Prevention

The frequency and severity of all types of headache are greatly lessened by reducing stress. Dealing with marital problems, job pressures, or family difficulties directly affects the underlying causes of many headaches, especially those resulting from muscle tension (see p. 58). Massage, manipulation, hot pads, and hot baths can often relax the muscles of the neck and shoulders and help to prevent tension headaches. Migraine attacks can sometimes be lessened by avoiding changes in sleeping and eating patterns, and by avoiding foods that dilate the blood vessels (see chart) or that seem to trigger attacks. Cluster headaches are often prevented by avoiding alcohol during the period of the attacks. In severe cases, preventive drugs can be taken to stop cluster or migraine attacks (see section on *The Doctor*).

Hay Fever, Grass or Pollen Allergies, or Allergic Rhinitis

Symptoms

- stuffy nose
- watery, runny nose
- attacks of sneezing
- itching eyes, nose, or throat
- tearing, and possibly sore eyelids
- seasonal or chronic occurence of symptoms

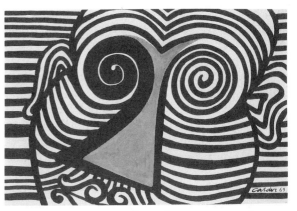

In an allergic person, cells in the mucous membrane lining the nose produce histamine in response to pollen or other allergens. The release of histamine causes sneezing, stuffiness, and a running nose. Alexander Calder. Slanting Red Nose. 1969. *Gouache, 29½″ × 43¼″. Collection,* The Museum of Modern Art, *New York. Gift of Mr. and Mrs. Klaus G. Perls.*

Description

Allergic rhinitis is an allergic reaction of the nasal lining to inhaled particles, which is caused by a genetically determined sensitivity to grass and tree pollens, household dust, molds, or animal dander. The condition may be seasonal or perennial depending upon the particular *allergen*, that is, the pollen or dust that causes an allergic reaction. Allergies are so common that they affect 17% of the population of the U.S.; approximately 15 million Americans have allergic rhinitis, 9 million have asthma (and may or may not have allergic rhinitis in addition), and some 11 million have eczema, or food or insect hypersensitivities.

Generally, the onset of allergic rhinitis occurs in childhood or adolescence, although occasionally it begins in midadulthood. Once it develops, the condition tends to persist, varying in intensity depending on the individual, the given year, and the locale. However, there is a definite percentage of people whose symptoms eventually disappear entirely. Allergic rhinitis has no serious medical consequences, but it can involve a considerable amount of discomfort, annoyance, and lost work time.

The nasal passages have many functions, including warming, humidifying, and filtering incoming air, and fighting germs. Special immune cells within the mucous membrane have the capacity to make large amounts of specific antibodies so as to protect the body against viruses and bacteria. Directly beneath the mucous membranes of the nose lie a rich network of tiny blood vessels which serve to warm and moisten incoming air. These blood vessels dilate and contract in response to the autonomic nervous system.

Incoming particles are effectively trapped by tiny hairs in the nose. Once trapped, these particles are slowly moved by the *cilia*, microscopic hairs that cover the mucous membranes, to the back of the throat where they are removed by swallowing. Normally this process causes no allergic reaction, but when a person is allergic to a particular substance or substances, a whole different set of responses takes place within the nasal passages. Understanding the physiology of the allergic reaction can be very useful in terms of treatment and prevention of attacks.

When an *allergen* is inhaled by an allergic person, it dissolves into the top layer of the mucous membrane in a normal fashion, but then nearby *mast cells* begin to produce *IgE antibodies* against the particular allergen. This process may go on over a period of several years without causing any symptoms. During this time, a high percentage of the mast cells in the nasal passages become sensitized to the allergen and become capable of rapidly producing large amounts of antibodies specific to that allergen. Ultimately each particle of allergen is "caught" by two antibodies and attached to a mast cell in the nasal

lining. In response to this clumping mechanism, the mast cell secretes powerful chemicals that cause local inflammation and tissue destruction. One of these chemicals, *histamine*, produces blood vessel dilation and fluid release from cells, which leads to swelling, sneezing, stuffiness and a runny nose. Allergic rhinitis is categorized into two distinct groups, seasonal and nonseasonal. Although their physiology is the same, they have different symptoms and causes.

Seasonal allergies: Seasonal allergic rhinitis, which occurs during approximately the same months each year, is caused by specific pollens and mold spores. The pollens responsible for seasonal symptoms include the abundant, lightweight pollens from weeds, grasses, and trees that rely on the wind for cross-pollination.

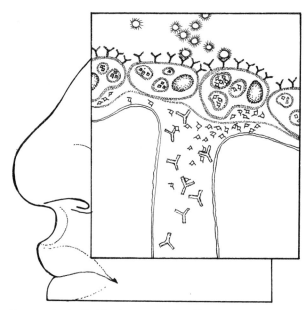

In certain individuals, ragweed pollen triggers an allergic reaction in the mast cells in the lining of the nose. If allergic individuals have been desensitized through allergy shots, IgG antibodies block the reaction.

Larger pollens, produced by flowers and polli-nated by insects, never become airborne, and consequently only cause problems when they are touched or smelled. A single plant or tree, on the other hand, can liberate literally millions of pollen grains annually. Most wind-borne pollen falls within 10–15 feet of the plant, but approximately 10% of lightweight pollens get into moving air layers and are dispersed over long distances. Although people most often are affected by pollen that falls nearby, they can actually develop symptoms from large fields of a particular plant that are over 10 miles away.

Since the timing of the pollinating season for each type of plant is relatively constant for a given area, allergy sufferers generally are affected during the same months every year.

Highly allergic individuals develop symptoms as soon as a particular pollen appears, become progressively more affected as the pollen concentration peaks about midseason, and then become better as the season comes to an end. Some people's symptoms disappear quite abruptly; other people experience gradually diminishing symptoms over a period of weeks. These latter individuals are considered to have a "primed nose" that, late in the season, temporarily reacts to additional substances that wouldn't even cause a reaction at the season's start.

People with seasonal allergies often find their symptoms are worst in the morning. Normally, within one to three hours after sunrise, the temperature rises, the humidity drops as the dew evaporates, and the wind picks up. When tem-

---

Seasonal Plants and Grasses That Cause Allergies

East Coast
Trees—February–June
 Elm—March–April
 Maple, poplar, birch—March–May
 Oak, walnut, hickory—April–June
Grass—mid-May–mid-July
Weeds, ragweed—August–October

Southeast
Trees—February–May
 Pecan, gum, maples, oak—March–May
Grass, Bermuda grass—March–September
Ragweed—August–October

Central Plains
Trees—January–May
 Ash, oak—January–May
 Walnut, mulberry, pecan—March–May
Grass—Same as East and South
Weeds, ragweed—August–October

Rocky Mountains
Trees—January–June
 Elm—February–April
 Alder—March–April
 Poplar—April–May
Grass—May–July (decrease with altitude)
Weeds—few above 5,000 feet

Southwest
Trees—February–April
 Ash, poplar, cypress, mesquite
Grass—all warm months
Weeds, ragweed—July–October

California
Trees—January–April
 Alder, acacia, poplar
Grass—March–November
Weeds, ragweed—July–October

Northwest Coast
Trees—January–June
 Alder, willow, ash—February–April
 Birch, poplar, elm—March–June
Grass—May–August
Weeds, ragweed—August–September (low
 amounts—almost ragweed-free)

perature, moisture, and wind speed reach a certain critical point, plants release their ripe pollen. Hot, dry winds are generally bad for allergy sufferers, while rain, particularly small drops, tends to clear the air and lessen symptoms.

Approximately 75% of seasonal allergy sufferers are alergic to *ragweed pollen*, the plant which causes the longest and most severe symptoms in the East and Midwest of the U.S. In these areas, ragweed pollinates from the second or third week in August through the beginning of October. Another variety, Western ragweed, causes symptoms in the late summer and early fall in the Pacific states. Approximately 40% of all people with seasonal allergies react to various grass pollens, including *Kentucky bluegrass*, *timothy*, and *rye* or *orchard grass*. Grasses pollinate between May and early July in the East and Midwest. Around 10% of allergy sufferers are allergic to tree pollens, including *ash*, *elm* and *oak*. These trees pollinate in the early spring—April, May, and June in the Northeast, and earlier in the South.

In addition to pollens, airborne *mold spores* also cause seasonal allergies. Molds grow indoors as well as outdoors, and are especially common in damp areas such as basements, closets, and bedding. Although molds can grow all year round, they proliferate best when the weather is warm and damp. Thus in the East and Midwest, mold spores generally first appear in significant numbers in the spring, are worst in the summer, and drop off in the fall. In the West, mold problems are worst during rainy winter months. Unlike the lightweight pollens, mold counts go up in humid weather.

Perennial allergies: With the second type of allergy, *perennial* or *nonseasonal allergic rhinitis*, people experience symptoms throughout the year. These individuals are often allergic to a wide variety of substances, including house dust, animal dander (hair, dried saliva, and dry skin cells), feathers, and mold. Occasionally, people are allergic to specific substances found in the workplace, such as flour, sawdust, or detergent powders. House dust is actually a complex substance that contains varying amounts of cloth fibers, human and animal skin cells, remnants of foods, molds, bacteria, and insect parts, including microscopic dead house mites. Many doctors believe that house mites are the most allergic component of house dust. Generally there are over 2,000 mites per gram of dust.

Perennial allergies do not vary much by the season, although affected individuals may have fewer symptoms in the summer when they are outdoors a great deal. Individual rooms and houses vary greatly in the amount of mold, animal dander, fibers, and food particles they harbor. Symptoms worsen in the presence of high concentrations of allergens or when allergens are stirred up by cleaning.

The primary symptoms for both seasonal and perennial allergic rhinitis are sneezing, stuffy or runny nose, and itchy eyes. The symptoms of seasonal allergies tend to be more pronounced because the specific allergens often occur in higher concentrations at certain times of the year. Also, seasonal allergy sufferers tend to look at and treat their symptoms differently.

With seasonal allergies, sneezes often occur in groups or paroxysms of 10–20 sneezes, especially in the morning when allergen counts rise. Often sneezing is preceded by a slight itching in the nose. The paroxysms can be so prolonged and so strenuous that they actually cause fatigue. Typically, the nasal discharge is thin, watery, copious, and fairly constant. At times, the discharge itself and wiping the nose irritate the skin on the nose and upper lip. Not uncommonly, stuffiness is intermittent at the beginning of the season, but becomes relatively continuous as the season goes on. Such stuffiness can result in headache or earache due to blocked sinuses or Eustachian tubes. Stuffiness can also lead to a diminished sense of smell, taste, or hearing. Along with nasal symptoms, seasonal allergies may cause pronounced eye symptoms, including itching, tearing, light sensitivity, and fatigue. Occasionally the allergic reaction even causes an itchy throat, a nonproductive cough, and/or tightness of the chest, but generally nasal itchiness and stuffiness are the major symptoms. Frequently the local symptoms are accompanied by feelings of weakness, tiredness, irritability, and depression.

People with perennial allergies often have less severe symptoms, but the symptoms tend to be more constant. These individuals have chronically blocked noses, which are often interpreted as sinus conditions or continuous colds. In addition to a constant stuffy nose, people with seasonal allergies usually have itchiness in their nose or eyes, and other symptoms such as tearing, loss of smell, headache, blocked ears, or decreased hearing.

Self-Care

The main principle of self-care is to *avoid* the specific allergens that cause an allergic reaction. Avoidance treats the cause of the allergy, not just the symptoms. A single allergen that is readily identified and eliminated, such as pet hair or feathers, is relatively easy to manage. Unfortunately, most cases of allergic rhinitis are not so simple to deal with, either because they involve multiple allergens or because the allergens are the type that become airborne. Even so, the goal is to keep exposure to a minimum.

Self-care involves a general *antidust program* to make the house as allergen-free as possible, but should concentrate on making one room, usually the bedroom, a "safe haven." The extent of the program depends on how severe a person's allergy is. Feather pillows should be removed, or, like the mattress and box spring, covered with plastic. Upholstered furniture should be covered, removed or cleaned frequently. Wall-to-wall carpet, bedspreads, bed pads, and dust-collecting objects should be removed. Heating ducts should be covered with a filter. In addition, the room should ideally be air-conditioned and equipped with a high-efficiency particulate air cleaner (HEPA) or an electrostatic dust precipitator. If individuals are allergic to animal dander, household pets should be kept outdoors. Allergic individuals should have someone else do household cleaning or wear a mask if they do it themselves (see chart).

If people are allergic to mold, they should use a dehumidifier. Bathrooms, damp closets, the

---

Allergy-Proofing the House

- concentrate on areas used most—bedroom, family room
- do not allow smoking in the house
- remove stuffed furniture, carpets, carpet pads, curtains
- use only washable, synthetic curtains and throw rugs
- use washable, synthetic bedding—avoid flannel, wool, down
- encase box spring and mattress in plastic; seal zippered end with tape
- empty closets of infrequently used cotton and wool clothing
- eliminate dustcatchers such as venetian blinds, books, piles of paper, knickknacks
- have rooms vacuumed frequently by someone other than the allergic person; have the dust bag emptied often; use water vacuum if possible
- seal off heating ducts with plastic and tape; use electric heaters and mattress pads
- put clothes dryer in garage if possible
- remove outdoor flowering plants that are hung near windows
- use electrostatic dust precipitators
- carry a synthetic pillow when traveling
- keep pets outdoors at night and during the day if necessary

inside of garbage cans, and any other areas where mold tends to grow should be cleaned frequently with an antiseptic solution. Running a heater or electric light in damp areas will tend to discourage the growth of mold. Often old foam rubber cushions and pillows harbor mold spores; Dacron stuffing will not. People who are allergic to mold should avoid working in damp barns or basements, or handling moldy hay or dead leaves. Individuals with mold allergies should also avoid foods such as beer, wine, melons, mushrooms, and cheeses that are high in mold content.

Avoidance of outdoor allergens is often very difficult for people with seasonal allergies. Local sources of pollens such as ragweed should be eliminated near the house. This action can be very beneficial since most pollens fall close to the plant they come from. A severely allergic individual should avoid hiking or working outdoors during the pollen season, and should close house and car windows and use air conditioning if possible. Electrostatic air filters are also strongly recommended because they are very effective at removing pollen as well as mold spores. People with severe seasonal allergies are wise to plan their vacations and weekends so as to avoid areas of high pollen concentration. People with severe allergies might even consider moving to low pollen areas, provided job opportunities are favorable and family ties are not too strong. However, some doctors feel that a move only provides temporary improvement, because people often become allergic to substances in their new environment.

The Doctor

To diagnose an allergy, the doctor (an allergist, internist, or family practitioner) does a careful history and skin testing. The history concentrates on the timing of symptoms and the locales that produce them. Skin testing involves "challenging" the skin with a small amount of various suspected allergens either by pricking or scratching the skin, or by injecting the substance under the skin. If a person is allergic to a particular substance, within 20 minutes a red raised area, called a *wheal*, will develop. Instead of a skin test, an allergy may be diagnosed by a *radioallergosorbent test (RAST)*, in which allergens are added to a blood sample to see if antibodies are produced.

Treatment for allergies includes three basic procedures: 1) avoidance of the allergen; 2) drugs to control the symptoms; and possibly 3) allergy shots to desensitize the individual. Avoidance of the allergen is discussed in Self-Care. Symptomatic treatment with drugs commonly involves the use of *antihistamines*. Unfortunately, these drugs are not completely effective, and their side effects are sometimes significant. Antihistamines work by binding to cells in the lining of the nose, which prevents the body's histamine molecules from binding to those sites and producing an allergic reaction. Antihistamines are most effective if they are taken before an allergic reaction starts, and if they are taken on a regular basis.

There are several families of antihistamines that vary in their efficacy and side effects, but they all tend to become less effective over time. Doctors often prescribe different antihistamines to see which works best and to combat the tendency toward diminished effectiveness which occurs when the drugs are taken long-term. The most common and significant side effect is drowsiness; others include stomach upset, dizziness, and dryness of the mouth. The three most common families of antihistamines are the *alkylamines* (e.g., *Dimetane* or *Chlor-Trimeton*), *ethanolamines* (e.g., *Benadryl*), and *ethylenediamines* (e.g., *Pyribenzamine*). The alkylamines are generally the most popular because they have the least number of side effects—especially drowsiness—whereas the ethanolamines cause significant drowsiness, and the ethylenedi-amines cause moderate drowsiness and upset stomach. A new antihistamine called *terfenadine* (e.g., *Seldane*) does not cause drowsiness because it isn't absorbed from the bloodstream into the brain. It does, however, cross the placenta and appear in breast milk, so it should not be taken by pregnant and nursing mothers unless absolutely necessary.

In addition to antihistamines, allergic rhinitis is sometimes treated with *sympathomimetic agents*, drugs that constrict the blood vessels. These drugs are applied locally as drops or sprays. They work well against stuffiness and nasal congestion, but can only be used for a few days at a time because longer use is followed by a rebound effect in which the nasal membranes become even more congested. When these agents are given in tablet form, they tend to produce nervousness and insomnia, which somewhat counteracts the drowsiness that can occur if a person is also taking antihistamines.

Other sprays or drops that are sometimes prescribed for severe nasal symptoms are *corticosteroids*, which block the inflammatory reaction, in particular the swelling and fluid discharge. The corticosteroids that are prescribed for allergies are ones that are rapidly metabolized by the body. The most common of these drugs is *beclomethasone dipropionate inhaler* (e.g., *Becklovent*) which is most often used for severe hay fever that doesn't respond to antihistamines. In general, steroids are avoided in the treatment of allergic rhinitis because they can produce dangerous systemic effects, including suppression of the adrenal glands.

Immunotherapy or *desensitization* is a long and therefore expensive process that is designed to decrease a person's reaction to a particular allergen or allergens. Allergy shots do not "cure" a person's allergies, they just gradually decrease a person's symptoms so that they are more easily controlled by medication. Studies show that

shots are beneficial for 70% –90% of individuals with allergic rhinitis. Immunotherapy is generally reserved for people who have significant symptoms that are not helped by a careful program of avoidance and drug therapy. Most often, these are people with severe perennial allergic rhinitis or people who are allergic to a number of pollens with overlapping seasons. Immunotherapy is most effective against pollens, grasses, trees, and house dust. It is not generally effective with allergies to animals.

Desensitization begins with a careful history and skin testing to positively identify which allergens an individual reacts to. Thereafter the person is given a weekly shot of gradually increasing amounts of the allergen(s). The individual is also taught to watch carefully for any signs of a significant local or systemic reaction, because the shots can occasionally produce *anaphylactic shock*, which is a MEDICAL EMERGENCY (see p. 475). The local reaction should not be larger than 2 centimeters or produce swelling for more than 24 hours. Signs of a systemic reaction include a generalized rash, hives, a runny nose, or difficulty breathing. The amount of allergen given is generally based on the individual's sensitivity. The maximum amount given is just below what produces a significant local reaction; it is increased gradually until a high dose is achieved. This dosage is given at two-to-six-week intervals for a period of three to five years. When treatment is effective, individuals notice some decrease in symptoms after six to twelve months, although gradual improvement is usually noticed throughout the process. Treatment is usually stopped when no further improvement occurs. After three to five years of treatment, 33% of people treated with immunotherapy show significant improvement for ten to twenty years, 33% show improvement for five years, and 33% need longer therapy to achieve control. For many people, shots are a way to prevent the yearly recurrence of symptoms.

Ruling Out Other Diseases

A history and skin testing will differentiate allergic rhinitis from rhinitis caused by other conditions such as repeated *colds, tonsillitis,* and *sinus infections,* (see p. 208, 219, and 226). Generally, colds and tonsillitis are accompanied by fever and a thicker nasal discharge, as well as a sore throat. They are also not as seasonal in occurrence. Sinus infections tend to produce a thicker mucus, and may produce pain over the affected sinuses. An uncommon cause of allergy symptoms is *vasomotor rhinitis,* a condition which is thought to be caused by an autonomic nervous system imbalance. It is often triggered by physical or psychological factors such as stress, smoke, or drafts. The symptoms respond poorly to antihistamine therapy, somewhat better to nasal steroid sprays.

Prevention

The genetic tendency toward allergic sensitivity is inherited. There is some thought that avoiding allergic substances, especially certain foods, in the first year of life may lessen the likelihood of priming a person's immune system. Once a person has allergies, avoidance or immunotherapy can lessen attacks. Some allergists also feel that avoiding allergenic foods (see p. 192) and minimizing stress (see p. 58) can significantly lower allergy symptoms. In large, double-blind studies done to test the efficacy of immunotherapy, it was found that, compared to the group that received allergy shots, 10%–56% of the control group were helped as much by *placebo* shots that contained no allergens. These results point up how important a factor a person's attitude and mental state is in regard to allergy symptoms.

Introduction to Cardiovascular Disease: Causes and Prevention of Atherosclerosis

Cardiovascular disease is the major cause of death and disability in the U.S. after the age of 35. The basis of most cardiovascular disease is *atherosclerosis*, a process that causes the walls of the midsized arteries to thicken and harden; the resulting disease is called *coronary artery disease (CAD)*. The affected areas, known as *atheromatous plaques*, narrow or block the inside of the artery, reducing the flow of blood. Decreased blood flow to the heart is the cause of a large proportion of both *heart attacks* and *angina*— that is, chest pain caused by insufficient oxygen to the heart. Decreased blood flow to the brain is the cause of most *strokes*.

Atherosclerosis is a slow, insidious process that starts as early as the first or second decade of life, and often progresses without any symptoms until a heart attack, angina episode, or stroke occurs. In the U.S., almost 35 million people—approximately 15% of the population— have heart disease, and more than 6 million of them have overt signs of heart disease, such as chest pain or shortness of breath. There are 1.5 million heart attacks and 500,000 strokes each year in this country. In 1981, heart disease accounted for almost half of the 2 million total deaths in the U.S., killing more people than all forms of cancer combined. One of the largest

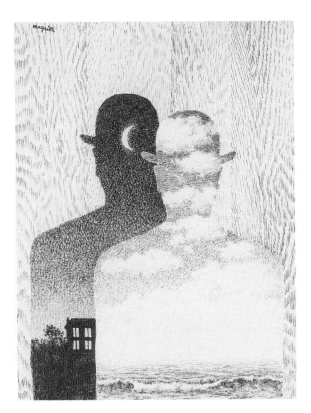

The chest contains the heart and lungs, and is the center of the circulatory and respiratory systems. Rene Magritte. The Thought Which Sees. 1965. Graphite, 15¾" × 11⅝". Collection, The Museum of Modern Art, New York. Gift of Mr. and Mrs. Charles B. Benenson.

255

studies ever done on coronary artery disease found that heart disease occurred in 1 out of every 8 men aged 40–44, 1 out of every 6 men aged 45–49, 1 out of every 5 men aged 50–54, and 1 out of every 4 men who were 55 years or older. Among women the figures were much lower: only 1 out of every 17 women under the age of 60 developed heart disease.

Over the last few years, studies have conclusively shown that the process of atherosclerosis is largely preventable. The most effective tools for prevention involve life-style changes that deal with smoking, diet, exercise, and stress. Current estimates are that with simple changes (see p. 260) people can rapidly decrease their own risk of heart disease by as much as 50%.

The Anatomy and Physiology of Atherosclerosis

In the last few years, research on the anatomy and physiology of atherosclerosis has shown clearly how risk factors such as a high-fat diet and cigarette smoking create damage at a cellular level. Most remarkably, the latest experiments show that *early plaque formation is actually reversible*, making life-style changes all the more important no matter what a person's age.

The physiology of heart disease can be described with a fairly simple model. Every artery has three layers. The inside layer, called the *intima*, is in direct contact with the blood. Endo-

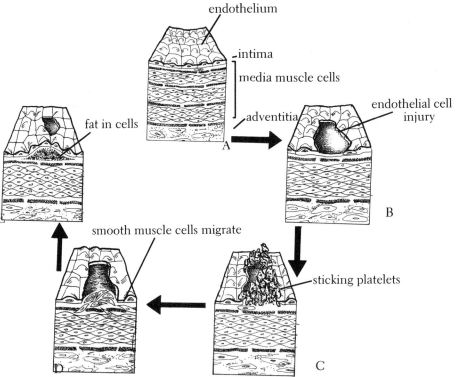

An atherosclerotic plaque can develop in a healthy artery (a) when the inside lining becomes injured or abraded (b). Blood platelets adhere to the abraded area and are joined by more and more platelets (c). Then smooth muscle cells migrate into the area (d) and attract lipid (fat) cells (e), which cause the center of the plaque to die.

thelial cells that line the intima normally form a barrier that prevents certain substances in the blood from passing into the arterial walls. Beneath the endothelial cells is a thin layer of elastic fibers. The middle layer of the artery, the *media*, is made up of smooth muscle cells surrounded by elastic collagen fibers that enable the artery to widen or constrict. The outer layer of the artery is made up of connective tissue which gives the arteries strength. It is the outer layer that contains the artery's own blood supply as well as the nerves from the autonomic nervous system that control dilation and constriction.

The process of atherosclerosis, which involves a progressive clogging of the arteries, is thought to begin with an injury to the endothelial lining. A number of factors can cause injury to the lining of the arteries. First, if blood pressure is high, the sheer force of blood flow can be damaging when vessels clamp down or spasm under stress, or even when the blood forms eddy currents in certain areas. Second, if certain kinds of fat constantly circulate in the blood at high levels, they can damage the lining of the arteries. Third, injury to the endothelial cells can be caused by large amounts of *carbon monoxide*, a gas present in high levels in the blood of cigarette smokers.

Like rocks in a streambed, the injured cells alter the flow of blood, causing cells to be torn from the artery walls, which eventually exposes large areas of the thin elastic membrane underneath. Once the epithelial cells are injured, their ability to function as a barrier is lost, and substances from the blood can enter the walls of the arteries. Normally *platelets*, a type of blood cell that helps stop bleeding, do not stick to the walls of the arteries, but when the walls have been injured, platelets begin to adhere to the underlying elastic cells and project out into the center of the artery. Once platelets stick together, they normally break open, releasing various chemicals. In terms of heart disease, the most impor-

tant of these chemicals is *platelet-derived growth factor hormone*, a substance that causes the smooth muscle cells in the middle layer to grow more rapidly, penetrating the elastic fibers in the inside layer, and forming an unnatural dome on top of the elastic layer. This dome or growth of smooth muscle cells eventually protrudes into the central core of the artery, further diminishing the flow of blood.

The development of lumps of smooth muscle cells in arterial walls is the first pathological step in the process of atherosclerosis. The second fundamental step occurs in response to the lumps. Under normal conditions, molecules of fat and cholesterol circulate in the blood without penetrating artery walls, but once the inside endothelial layer is broken, two things happen: fat molecules actually stick to the exposed elastic layer, clumping in between the smooth muscle cells that have formed domes; more importantly, the smooth muscle cells themselves have receptors that absorb and bind large numbers of fat globules. The result is that the domes balloon as they fill up with fat and project farther and farther into the center of the artery.

Normally, after endothelial cells are injured, they rapidly regrow, repairing the break in the artery wall. But if such injuries are continuous or repetitive, the body's natural healing ability is eventually overwhelmed. The likelihood of this situation is particularly great if there is a high level of fat constantly circulating in the blood. Fat molecules not only create a pattern of continual injury, the globules of fat in the smooth muscle cells prevent the endothelial layer from healing.

During childhood, certain areas of the arteries become thicker than others, a process that seems to be fairly universal. Onto these thickened areas, fat accumulates and forms fatty streaks. By the third decade of life, such soft yellow streaks are very common in the arteries. Although these streaks can disappear, they are thought to be the precursors for *atherosclerotic plaques* or domes, whose pathology was described above.

As plaques enlarge, they accumulate more and more smooth muscle cells, elastic fibers, and lipid (fat) deposits. Within the center of the plaques, calcium crystals begin to form. Ultimately, cells within the large plaques die off for lack of adequate blood supply, creating a mixture of dead cells and crystals in the center, covered by a cap of smooth muscle cells and elastic fibers. At this stage the plaques become clinically significant. They now project so far into the arteries that they block blood flow enough to produce angina or a heart attack. Moreover, the plaques can now rupture at any time, releasing the fats, dead cells, and calcium crystals into the bloodstream. The debris from this kind of rupture can cause an artery to spasm, can cause an *embolus* or bloodclot that moves through the bloodstream and then blocks an artery, or it can attract platelets and create a *thrombus* or clot at the point of rupture. A thrombus is present in 90% of acute heart attacks.

Risk Factors for Cardiovascular Disease

Since the 1940s researchers have known that coronary heart disease is associated with certain factors that do not occur randomly in the population. Over the years, a large body of evidence has accumulated that shows conclusively that certain factors put people at high risk for coronary disease. The evidence is of three types: cellular and animal studies, genetic studies, and epidemiological studies dealing with large cross-sections of the population.

Cell studies have shown that smooth muscle cells that are grown in the laboratory proliferate rapidly in the presence of added fat. Animal studies have shown that rhesus monkeys develop plaques similar to human atherosclerosis when fed peanut or coconut oil in quantities sufficient to raise their blood cholesterol levels. Studies show that individuals who have *inherited hypercholesterolemia*, a genetic inability to process fat effectively, have very high cholesterol levels and develop coronary disease during early adulthood.

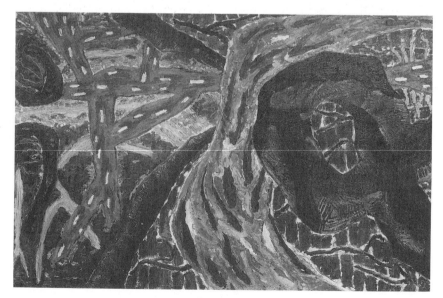

The walls of the arteries thicken and become clogged with plaque in response to a high-fat diet, smoking, high blood pressure, and stress. Gregory Amenoff. Gordian Knot. 1985. Oil on canvas. 105" × 160". Collection, The Whitney Museum of American Art. Purchase, with funds from the Louis and Bessie Adler Foundation, Inc., Seymour M. Kline, President. 85.12.

Deaths Due to Heart Disease in Different Countries *	
COUNTRY	PERCENTAGE
Finland	42%
Scotland	40%
Australia	40%
Norway	39%
U.S.A.	39%
England and Wales	38%
Israel	34%
West Germany	26%
Italy	18%
Japan	7%

* Percentage of deaths per 100,000 men, aged 55–65.

By far the greatest amount of evidence about cardiovascular disease comes from epidemiological studies. Cross-cultural studies show vast differences in coronary disease rates in different countries. In no country where people have a low average cholesterol level is there a high rate of heart disease. Conversely, in every country where people have a high average cholesterol rate there is also a high rate of heart disease. Finland and all the English-speaking countries have high rates of coronary heart disease, followed by the rest of the Western nations. In comparison, atherosclerotic heart disease is still relatively uncommon in Japan and very low in nonindustrialized nations. Although the rate is now rising in response to a more fatty diet, researchers believe these low rates are a direct reflection of the small amount of dairy products and red meat consumed by the average person in these non-Western countries. Significantly, studies have shown that when individuals move from a country with low rates of heart disease to one with high rates, their risk of heart disease increases as they adopt the food habits of their new country.

The most impressive and sobering research on heart disease involves long-term studies of large groups of people who show no evidence of heart disease at the start of the study. The participants are monitored at various intervals for weight, blood pressure, cholesterol levels, smoking habits, and basic diet. These studies are considered "natural experiments" because no attempt is made to alter people's life-style, even though they are followed closely. Such experiments are called *prospective studies*. The most famous of many such research projects, the Framingham Study, has followed 5,127 men and women from 1949 to the present, as well as many others for shorter periods. Another type of study compares two groups of randomly assigned people—one of which makes no life changes, the second of which makes specific changes. These studies are called *double-blind intervention studies*. The most significant of this type of

Risk Factors for Heart Disease
family history of heart disease
heavy drinking
high blood pressure
high cholesterol level
high salt intake
high stress
lack of exercise
male gender
obesity
smoking

study, The Lipid Research Clinic's Coronary Primary Prevention Trial, found a 19% reduction in fatal and nonfatal heart disease as a result of a 9% decrease in cholesterol levels.

Both prospective and intervention studies incontrovertibly demonstrate that a number of factors put people at increased risk for coronary disease. Of these, the three most important are a high serum cholesterol level, cigarette smoking, and high blood pressure. Two out of three heart attacks and angina episodes that occur take place in individuals who are subject to one

Coronary Artery Disease
Mortality Rates

NUMBER OF RISK FACTORS *	MORTALITY RATE **
0	13
1	23
2	44
3	82

* Risk factors: smoking, high blood pressure, high cholesterol levels.
** Per 1,000 men, aged 30–59.
Source: Adapted from Circulation.

of these factors. While each one of these factors is very significant by itself, the presence of more than one risk factor is especially hazardous (see chart).

Fat and cholesterol: One of the most clearly demonstrated risks for heart disease is the presence of high levels of fat in the bloodstream. The amount of fat in the blood is basically determined by the amount of fat in the diet. The Japanese, who eat a relatively low-fat diet, have an average cholesterol level of 165 mg/100 ml and a very low rate of heart disease (94 heart attacks per 100,000 people per year). Conversely, the Finns, who eat a very high-fat diet, have the highest rate of heart disease in the world (996 heart attacks per 100,000 people per year) and an average cholesterol level of 265 mg/100 ml. Fat levels in the blood are also affected by one's inborn capacity to process fat, but this factor affects far less people than does diet.

To better understand how fat levels affect coronary risk, and to be able to assess your own risk, it's helpful to understand how fat is transported in the blood. Fat is actually carried in the bloodstream in combination with proteins; the resulting complexes are called *lipoproteins*. Digested fat is picked up in the intestines in the form of *triglycerides* and carried to the liver, where it is metabolized into *very low-density lipoproteins,* or *VLDLs*. Neither triglycerides nor VLDLs

have been demonstrated to be a great risk factor for heart disease. VLDLs are subsequently broken down in blood plasma to *low-density lipoproteins* or *LDLs*, which are the component of fat in the blood that are most closely linked to coronary heart disease. LDLs, which are 50% cholesterol, are designed to transport cholesterol to cells for the production of certain hormones and for the storage of energy in liver cells.

Another byproduct of fat metabolism is *high-density lipoproteins,* or *HDLs*, which are thought to be made in the liver. Unlike the LDLs, which are related to atherosclerosis, HDLs actually prevent heart disease. They are *inverse risk factors* or *protective factors;* that is, the higher the HDL level, the lower the risk of heart disease. The role of HDLs is to pick up fat and carry it back to the liver. HDLs can be viewed as a clean-up squad that clears fat out of the cells. High levels of HDLs are associated with exercise and a low-fat diet, while low levels are associated with a high-fat diet, obesity, and smoking.

The higher a person's total cholesterol level, the greater his or her risk of heart disease. This is especially true at the high end of the scale. When cholesterol levels are very low, there is almost no heart disease. The question becomes, what is a safe or acceptable level? Ten years ago, it was thought that only the highest levels of cholesterol, 265–300 mg/100 ml, were important enough to treat. These figures were arbitrarily chosen and comprised the 5%–10% of the population *most* at risk. Cholesterol figures in this range did represent a significant number of people with heart disease, including 50% of the heart attacks, but they did not represent *all* the people at risk. As doctors and lay people alike have become better educated about diet and risk, there has been a tendency to treat cholesterol levels between 200 and 265, since half of all heart attacks occur in people with levels under 265. Currently, doctors not only take into account a person's total cholesterol, they look at

Distribution of Low-Density and High-Density Lipoproteins by Age and Sex

AGE	PERCENTILE BASED ON LDL/HDL LEVELS			
Men	5%	50%	75%	95%
30–34	80/30	125/30	145/45	185/60
35–39	80/30	135/30	155/45	190/60
40–44	85/25	135/30	155/45	185/65
45–69*	90/30	145/30	165/50	205/70
Women	5%	50%	75%	95%
30–34	70/35	110/40	125/55	160/80
35–39	75/35	120/40	140/55	170/80
40–44	75/35	125/40	145/60	175/90
45–49	80/35	130/40	150/60	185/85
50–54	90/35	140/40	160/60	200/90
55 and over	95/35	150/40	170/60	215/95

Note: *The higher the LDLs, the greater the coronary risk; whereas the lower the HDLs, the greater the coronary risk. In terms of the ratio of total cholesterol to HDLs, 3.5 to 1 is considered a low risk coronary factor, 3.5–4.5 to 1 is considered a moderate risk, and 4.5–5 to 1 is considered a high risk.*
* *The figures are not further broken down by age because they are very similar.*
Source: *R. Levy,* Symposium on Initial Hypertensive Therapy.

the ratio of total cholesterol to HDLs as an indicator of risk. A ratio of 3.5 to 1 is considered low risk, 3.4–4.5 to 1 is considered moderate risk, and anything over 4.5 to 1 is considered to be high risk.

In reviewing all the coronary data in 1984, the National Institutes of Health report noted that an increased risk of developing premature heart disease is associated with cholesterol levels of 200–230. Figures in this range used to be considered "normal," and unfortunately they are common—currently *over* 50% of all the adults in the U.S. fall within this range. The good news is that for every 1% drop in blood cholesterol levels, there is a 2% reduction in coronary risk. The National Institutes of Health (NIH) report recommends "aggressive treatment" for middle-aged adults who have cholesterol levels over 260 and "moderate treatment" for those over 240. Aggressive treatment initially calls for strict di-

etary therapy. If this fails to lower blood cholesterol, even stricter dietary changes are recommended, and finally cholesterol-lowering drugs may be prescribed. The report suggests that all Americans, especially those over 30, maintain a cholesterol level under 200. More radical experts suggest that an individual's cholesterol should be no more than 100 plus his or her age.

NIH has a simple set of guidelines for a *moderate-fat, moderate-cholesterol diet*. They advise that no more than 30% of a person's calorie intake should be in the form of fat, as opposed to carbohydrate or protein. Less than 10% of this fat should be saturated—that is, from animal sources. Moreover, the report recommends that total cholesterol intake be kept under 250–300 mg/day, as opposed to the current average of 500 mg/day, since the body makes virtually all the cholesterol it needs. Plaque formation begins so

Distribution of Cholesterol Levels by Age and Sex

AGE	PERCENTILE BY BLOOD CHOLESTEROL LEVEL				
Men	5%	25%	50%	75%	90%
30–34	142	171	190	213	237
35–39	147	176	195	222	248
40–44	150	179	204	229	251
45–49	163	188	210	235	258
50–54	157	189	211	237	263
55–59	161	188	214	236	260
60–64	163	191	215	237	262
Women	5%	25%	50%	75%	90%
30–34	133	158	178	199	215
35–39	139	165	186	209	233
40–44	146	172	193	220	241
45–49	148	182	204	231	256
50–54	163	188	214	240	267
55–59	167	201	229	251	278
60–64	172	207	226	251	282

Moderate risk *for heart disease involves the 75th–90th percentiles of total cholesterol.* High risk *is greater than the 90th percentile.*
Source: Adapted from Lipid Research Clinics Population Studies Data Book.

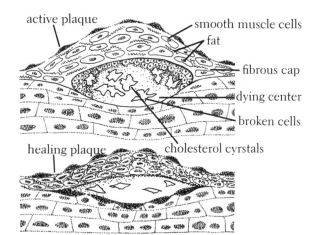

Animal studies show that atherosclerotic plaques can actually heal: the dead tissue and fat in the center is removed by the body and the fibrous cap shrinks. This is a positive image for people to visualize.

early in life that NIH recommends these dietary limits for anyone over the age of 2 years! For people who do not respond to this diet or who require more aggressive therapy, NIH recommends a *low-fat, low cholesterol diet* which involves only 20%–25% of total calories as fat, only 6%–8% of total calories as saturated fat, and less than 150–200 mg of cholesterol per day. People who are most at risk—those with preexisting heart disease, and especially those who've had coronary bypass surgery—should use aggressive measures to lower their blood cholesterol (see p. 102).

New animal studies show that dietary therapy can definitely stop the progress of atherosclerosis and may even reverse the process. One study found that animals fed a high-fat, high-cholesterol diet developed significant plaque formation

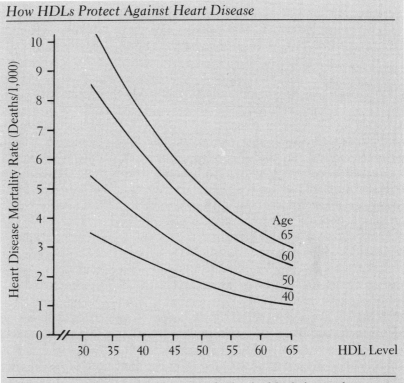

Coronary heart disease mortality rates by level of high-density lipoprotein (HDL) cholesterol in United States white males. From the Lipid Research Clinics population.

within a year, but subsequently, the animals put back on a low-fat diet showed cessation of plaque formation and even regression of disease. After a time, plaques actually shrank, had a lower lipid and cholesterol content, and involved less collagen and elastic cells from deeper layers. Most importantly, the large fat-filled centers of the plaques disappeared, and breaks in the surface endothelium healed. These results are tremendously encouraging for people who have high cholesterol levels and/or a history of heart disease in their family.

Smoking and cardiovascular disease: Smoking is another major risk factor for heart disease.

The U.S. Surgeon General's office has declared that smoking is the single most preventable cause of heart disease, accounting for 30% of all the coronary deaths in this country each year. Smokers have a 70% higher heart disease mortality than nonsmokers. Heavy smokers, people who smoke more than two packs per day, have two to three times the mortality rates of nonsmokers. Low-tar and -nicotine cigarettes do not lessen these risks because people tend to inhale them more deeply.

The mortality figures are much worse for smokers who are otherwise at risk for heart disease because of higher cholesterol levels, obesity, or high blood pressure. In combination, smoking and oral contraceptives act synergistically to raise the risk of heart disease. Women on oral contraceptives who smoke have 10 times the risk of heart disease as women who neither smoke nor take the pill. On the positive side, people who give up cigarettes lose their added risk of heart disease within several years.

High blood pressure and cardiovascular disease: High blood pressure, or *hypertension,* is also a risk factor for coronary disease because it increases the likelihood of damaging artery walls. As with cholesterol, the higher the figures, the greater a person's risk. A *diastolic* pressure of over 95 and/or a *systolic* pressure of over 160 is associated with two or three times the risk of heart disease (see p. 275). Lowering blood pressure reduces the mortality associated with all forms of heart disease.

Stress and cardiovascular disease: The physiological effects of tension and stress (see p. 42) on heart disease are well known. Over the last ten years, doctors and psychologists have studied a number of psychological factors—dissatisfaction, personal loss, stress, and life changes—in terms of how they affect heart disease. Pioneering work on stress and heart disease was first done by Doctors Meyer Friedman and Ray Rosenman who concluded from their studies that a certain type of behavior, which they labeled *Type A behavior,* is as significant a risk factor for heart disease as diet, smoking, or high blood pressure. Friedman defined Type A behavior as acting *aggressively* in a *chronic, incessant* struggle to get more done in less and less time, even against the efforts of other things or opposing people. He characterized Type A people as frequently hard-driving and competitive, with a tremendous sense of time urgency. Often, they do two things at once—like filing things while they talk on the phone. Although they may appear secure, they have a hidden lack of self-esteem;

they lack security in their status and engage in solitary self-harassment, comparing themselves unfavorably with others or criticizing themselves for not having accomplished their goals. Type A people have a tremendous amount of aggression and hostility; this hostility is free-floating and is even expressed in regard to trivial matters. Type As are constantly engaged in a fight with some person or with time. Characteristically, they not only must win in situations, they must dominate. Recent studies have shown that hostility is a more important part of the Type A personality than is time urgency.

The most significant evidence supporting Type A behavior comes from a large prospective study called *The Western Collaborative Group Study.* The study divided up its subjects into two groups based on a personality assessment: Type A and non-Type A. Follow-up reports at four, six, and eight years showed that those in the Type A group had a rate of new heart disease that was 1.7–4.5 times greater than that of the non-Type A group. Not all subsequent studies have shown a correlation between Type A behavior and coronary disease; thus many cardiologists view the data with some caution, considering Type A behavior to be a less important risk factor than high blood pressure, smoking, and high cholesterol levels.

Research indicates that stress's effect on the body's hormones may be responsible for the development of coronary artery disease. Studies have shown that Type A people have higher than normal levels of *norepinephrine,* the "fight-or-flight" hormone, and ACTH *(adrenocorticotropic hormone),* the hormone that regulates the adrenal hormones. Norepinephrine constricts blood vessels and causes overenergetic heart contractions, raising blood pressure, which is more likely to cause damage to artery walls and may cause pieces of plaque to break off. Friedman also believes that norepinephrine lowers the liver's ability to remove fat from the blood.

Animal studies show that animals put under high stress have higher levels of norepinephrine and ACTH, and are thus more likely to develop heart disease. Other research has found that animals under stress also have higher levels of fat and cholesterol in their blood.

It is well known that emotion affects heart rate and function through the autonomic nervous system, in much the same way as exercise. Both exercise and emotional excitement cause increases in blood pressure, heart rate, oxygen consumption, and resistance to arterial blood flow. It is also well known that emotional stress and anxiety cause *arrhythmias* or irregular heartbeat patterns, which can be dangerous for a person who has heart disease (see p. 291).

Recently Friedman concluded a large study called The Recurrent Coronary Prevention Project. The study followed two groups of patients who had had an initial heart attack. Half the patients were given normal cardiac counseling that included information on diet and exercise; the other half were given regular cardiac counseling and a course in changing Type A behavior. In the latter group, 43% of the people were able to reduce their Type A behavior significantly, whereas no change was seen in the control group. More importantly, the rate of second heart attacks was only 7% in the altered Type A group, while it was 14% in the control group. These results show not only that Type A behavior can be changed, but that it can be changed within a matter of months to years. Further research now underway should determine whether personality counseling can reduce the incidence of initial heart attacks.

Although it has always been controversial, the concept of Type A is now undergoing even more scrutiny. Many cardiology researchers feel that there is a strong link between behavior and coronary disease, and believe that those people at risk tend to react to stress with excessive physiological changes. However, many researchers are shifting away from viewing Type A as the core of the coronary-prone personality. Instead they are looking more closely at personality characteristics such as depression, hostility, self-absorbedness, intimacy, and coherence.

A new study has found that among Type A personalities who survive a heart attack, subsequent mortality was actually lower among Type A people than among non-Type A people. Researchers speculate that this may be due to better coping ability among the Type A people once they become ill. This makes sense in light of the fact that control and self-efficacy are generally associated with longevity. This study points again to the complex interrelationships between stress, personality, and heart disease.

Obesity and cardiovascular disease: Obesity (see p. 441) appears to be associated with heart disease, although it is a secondary risk factor; that is, obesity is usually associated with primary risk factors such as a high fat intake and sedentary lifestyle. Excessive weight is definitely a long-term *predictor* of coronary disease, especially in the under-50 age group. Obesity may simply act as a mediator for other risk factors. When people lose weight, for instance, their cholesterol levels drop, their HDL levels rise, and their blood pressure decreases. Interestingly, researchers have found that the highest rates of heart disease in obese people are found in men with large abdomens, which is sometimes referred to as *abdominal obesity* or *middle-aged spread*. Whatever the fine points of the relationship between obesity and other risk factors, there is no question that cardiologists urge people to lose weight to lower their coronary risk.

Exercise and cardiovascular disease: Many studies have dealt with the role that exercise (see p. 109) or a nonsedentary life-style play in deterring the development of atherosclerosis. The

Framingham study showed a definite drop in the rate of heart attack, sudden death, and angina in those people who exercised regularly or were physically active. But rather than being a primary factor in itself, exercise may only affect other risk factors. For example, exercise is associated with higher levels of HDLs, the fat component that has a protective effect against heart disease. Currently, most investigators now believe that lack of exercise, although harmful, is not as important a risk factor as is smoking, high fat intake, or high blood pressure.

Preventive Cardiology

More and more doctors now focus on *preventive cardiology* as a means of prolonging life, improving the quality of life, and saving millions of lives. Positive changes are already taking place in national heart disease patterns. This trend had its beginnings in the 1950s, but most of the change has taken place since 1970. In that period there have been dramatic changes in heart disease rates in the U.S.: the *age-adjusted cardiovascular mortality rate* has dropped by a remarkable 40% and overall life expectancy has increased by two years. No one factor is the cause of these very significant figures. Obviously, advances in medical and surgical treatment have played a role in these changes, but the major factor is thought to be a *voluntary* change in lifestyle due to awareness of various risk factors.

In great part due to their own efforts, Americans have made tremendous progress in the prevention of heart disease. First, they have decreased cigarette smoking by 30%. Second, over three times as many people are presently being diagnosed and treated for high blood pressure as before 1970. Third, many people have significantly altered their dietary habits. In the last 20 years, Americans have decreased their consumption of high-fat foods—milk and cream by 24%, butter by 33%, eggs by 12%, and animal fat by 40%. The average cholesterol intake has dropped from 800 mg/day to 500 mg/day, resulting in a drop in average cholesterol from 265 in the 1950s, to 240 in the 1970s, to 205 in the 1980s. It is believed that this cholesterol drop alone is responsible for a significant percentage of the decline in heart attacks. Experts feel that a combination of stopping smoking, treating high blood pressure, and lowering dietary fat and cholesterol, coupled with losing weight, exercising, and reducing stress can make further significant progress in eliminating the major cause of death in the U.S.

Given the current frequency of heart disease in this country, and given the fact that heart disease takes decades to develop, many researchers presume that most Americans have some degree of narrowing of the arteries, even though they have no overt symptoms.

In 1988, researchers released the results of a major double-blind study which dealt with the effect of aspirin on preventing cardiovascular disease. In the study, 22,000 U.S. physicians were randomly assigned to one of two groups. Members of the first group were given 1 aspirin tablet (325 mg) every other day, while members of the control group were given a placebo. After 57 months, statistics showed that there were 47% fewer heart attacks among the group taking aspirin. The effects of aspirin are due to the fact that it prevents platelets from clumping, which decreases the likelihood of a blood clot forming in the arteries. At the present time, it is unclear whether aspirin should be recommended to everyone on a regular basis, or be specifically prescribed for people at high risk. Also, researchers emphasize that aspirin does not eliminate the need for other life-style changes that reduce the likelihood of heart disease.

An important study in progress by Dr. Dean Ornish, a preventive cardiology researcher, underlines the value of life-style changes in preventing, and even reversing, heart disease. Ornish is studying a group of patients with heart disease symptoms and demonstrated narrowing of the coronary arteries. These people have been randomly assigned either to a control group which is given conventional medical treatment, or to an experimental group which is given an intensive program involving life-style changes in addition to medical therapy. The life-style changes are far-reaching. The people in the experimental group do yoga stretching exercises, meditation, and imagery for 1½ hours a day; eat a vegetarian diet that has only 8% of its calories in fat; and walk or do other physical exercise for one hour a day. In addition, the experimental group meets two evenings a week as a support group to discuss common problems and concerns. In only one year, members of the experimental group decreased the narrowing in their coronary arteries by an average of 4%, while members of the control group showed a 5% increase in the narrowing of their arteries. Thus, among the control group, heart disease is progressing, while among the experimental group, heart disease is slowly being "cured" through life-style changes.

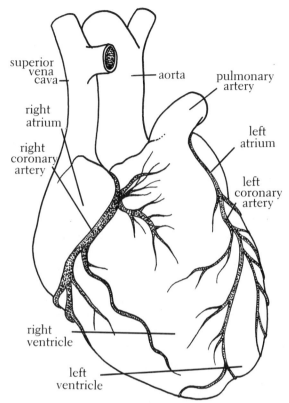

The coronary arteries supply oxygenated blood to the heart muscle itself. In people who have angina, one or more of the main coronary arteries is blocked, reducing the flow of blood.

Angina Pectoris

Symptoms

- squeezing, pressure, tightness, or pain deep within the chest
- pain usually in the middle of the chest or slightly to the left
- pain comes on with exertion and stops with rest
- pain is usually short-lived
- attack is commonly accompanied by anxiety

Description

Angina pectoris is a condition that involves chest pain caused by an insufficient supply of oxygen to the heart. Like all muscles, the heart needs oxygen to contract. When its workload increases, a muscle needs more oxygen. Thus the heart needs more oxygen when it beats faster or pumps harder with exertion or emotion, or when it beats against resistance in the arteries due to high blood pressure or cold temperatures. Generally angina is caused by atherosclerotic plaques in the *coronary arteries* of the heart. There are three main coronary arteries, any or all of which can become blocked. Testing shows that an equal number of people with angina have one, two, or three blocked arteries. Angina pain is usually experienced during strenuous activity if the blockage is above 70%, but often symptoms are not experienced until the blockage is nearly complete (see Anatomy and Physiology of Atherosclerosis, p. 256). The situation in which people have significant blockage of the coronary arteries but don't experience chest pain is referred to as *silent heart disease*.

The classic symptoms of chest pain attacks were first reported by an English doctor, William Heberden, in 1768. He referred to the condition as "angina," which comes from the Latin word for "strangling." Patients typically refer to the pain of angina as a sensation of pressure that is viselike, heavy, suffocating, squeezing, burning,

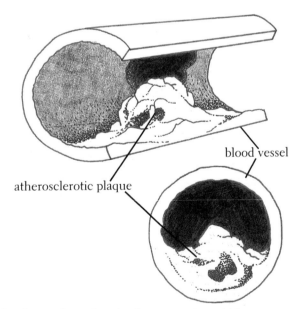

In time, atherosclerotic plaques can become large enough to cause angina, a heart attack, or a stroke.

atherosclerotic plaque

blood vessel

Common Triggers for Angina Attacks

• exertion
• strong emotion
• heavy eating
• exposure to cold temperatures

choking, or tight. It is characterized as a deep, generalized aching that cannot be pinpointed, as opposed to a sharp, localized pain. Angina pain is generally felt directly behind the sternum (breastbone) or slightly to the left. Occasionally the pain radiates to the neck and inner surface of the left arm. Even less frequently, the pain is sometimes felt in the jaw or right arm.

Angina pain commonly comes on with exertion such as climbing stairs or walking up hills. It can also be brought on by physical work in the cold, by eating a large meal, or by significant emotional stress or upset. Other activities that frequently provoke angina pain are walking against the wind, hammering overhead, walking after a large meal, and becoming emotionally upset in the midst of physical activity such as a tennis game.

The pain usually comes on gradually, reaches a maximum within minutes, forcing people to stop their activity, and then subsides within several minutes after resting. Many times, people with angina can predict quite accurately the type and amount of an activity that will bring on the pain. The amount of exertion required to precipitate an attack is usually lower in the cold, during emotional disturbances, and after meals when blood is shunted to the digestive system. Generally, attacks provoked by exercise are relatively brief, lasting less than three to five minutes, whereas attacks that follow a meal can last for up to 30 minutes. Deep or sharp chest pain that lasts less than a minute or for hours, or that can be pinpointed with one finger is generally not caused by angina (see p. 274).

The angina condition described above is referred to as *stable angina*. It is by far the most common type of angina. The course of stable angina is unpredictable, but most people live with it for years. The frequency of attacks varies tremendously. Attacks can occur fairly steadily, or, less commonly, the disease can go into remission for years. The long-term prognosis ultimately depends upon how many arteries are blocked and how occluded they are. Usually, angina attacks themselves are not fatal. However, each year 1%–15% of people with stable angina experience a heart attack or a heart spasm caused by an occlusion, a coronary spasm, or an arrhythmia, that results in sudden death.

There are several other less common varieties of angina which are more dangerous than stable angina. *Unstable angina* is a condition in which attacks are intermediate between stable angina and a heart attack. In this type of angina, attacks suddenly become more and more frequent and are precipitated by less and less effort, finally resulting in pain that may last a long time, or occur at rest. Unstable angina can be a medical emergency if blood flow to the heart is reduced so much that the risk of a heart attack is increased. Another type of angina, called *variant angina*, is caused by coronary artery spasm as opposed to atherosclerotic narrowing of the arteries. This condition, which is not provoked by exertion or emotion, is characterized by pain at rest.

Self-Care

Although stable angina is serious enough to necessitate medical evaluation and management, much can be done to lessen the number and duration of attacks. First, any patient who smokes cigarettes should stop. Smoking increases both heart rate and blood pressure, and constricts coronary blood vessels—all of which help to bring on attacks. Smoking also raises the blood level of carbon dioxide and lowers the

level of oxygen; this is obviously undesirable since angina attacks are caused by a lack of oxygen. Finally, smoking may precipitate *arrhythmias*, a disturbance of heart rate or rhythm that results in palpitation. In particular, smoking may cause *ventricular premature beats (VPBs)*, a type of arrhythmia associated with increased death from heart attacks or spasms in people with heart disease (see p. 286).

Secondly, people with angina should moderate or avoid the physical activities that bring on their attacks. In particular, sudden bursts of activity should be avoided because they require a great increase in the work of the heart. This does not mean that people with angina should give up all activity. Some activities can be done with little or no change; some require a person to slow down or take occasional brief rests. Other activities may require more radical change or modification. For example, a golfer may have to use a cart rather than walk the course. People with angina are advised to treat an anginal episode as a warning signal from their heart to slow down. Frequent episodes should be avoided because they are stressful to the heart, but occasional episodes are probably not harmful—in fact, they help people define their limits by trial-and-error. Often angina patients have a tendency to limit their activities more than necessary, which may be counterproductive since the heart needs a moderate amount of exercise to remain in good condition.

More and more commonly, doctors are recommending that angina patients follow a *carefully graded exercise program*. It should be emphasized that regular aerobic programs are not suitable because they can be too strenuous, but specially-designed, medically-supervised aerobic programs can actually improve cardiopulmonary function. As a result, a person will be able to do a given amount of work with a lower heart rate and blood pressure than someone who does not exercise. Since angina patients who are in good condition need less oxygen during exertion, they can do more work without precipitating an attack. One study of a medically supervised bicycle program found that angina patients were not only able to do more work after training, they actually delivered more oxygen to the heart muscle. The most common exercise program currently prescribed by doctors involves a graduated walking regimen that is done on level ground in moderate temperatures. Walking should always be slow enough that it does not bring on an episode. Moreover, people with angina should never try to "walk through" an episode of chest pain. The long-range goal is to achieve a rate of 1 mile in 15–20 minutes after a month of training. Thereafter, people can extend the distance or decrease their time according to what they feel comfortable with. There have been no studies yet dealing with the effects of exercise programs on longevity for angina patients, but there is no doubt that regular exercise makes these people feel better. Graded exercise may build up collateral circulation, or even help to reduce the plaque in the arteries. It will definitely help to reduce depression and anxiety, as well as increase both physical and mental strength and well-being.

Doctors also advise angina patients to go on the low-fat version of the American Heart Association Diet (see p. 102), and to lose weight if they are obese (see p. 441). By keeping the fat level in their blood low, angina patients may stop the progression of fatty deposits that block their arteries; moreover, new evidence suggests they may even shrink the plaques in their arteries. This is of great importance because an angina patient's likelihood of a heart attack or heart spasm is largely based on the number of coronary arteries that are blocked and the degree of blockage. Under a heavy fat load, the atherosclerotic process can only worsen.

Although they are not fragile, angina patients are generally encouraged not to become really exhausted and to schedule regular rest periods. They are also advised to deal with stress and avoid becoming overly upset since emotional agitation and stress increase the oxygen needs of the heart. People can develop more control over their thoughts through meditation, and can learn to change their personality characteristics

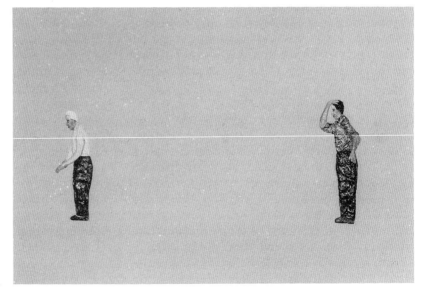

Emotional stress increases the oxygen needs of the heart and can cause arrhythmias. Nicholas Africano. An Argument. 1977. Acrylic, oil, and wax on canvas. 69″ × 85½″. Collection, The Whitney Museum of American Art. Purchase, with funds from Mr. and Mrs. William A. Marsteller. 77.68.

through behavior modification techniques (see p. 60 and 265). Relaxation and visualization exercises can help people to lower both their blood pressure and heart rate, and to deal with stress. Dr. Dean Ornish, a preventive cardiology researcher, believes that dealing with stress is the most important factor in reversing coronary artery disease. He is currently using meditation, relaxation, and imagery in conjunction with diet and exercise, in a program to reverse symptomatic heart disease (see p. 266).

The Doctor

Angina can be treated by a family practitioner, an internist, or a cardiologist—a doctor who specializes in heart problems. The diagnosis of angina is made largely on the basis of the patient's history. There are many causes of chest pain, but angina generally has a characteristic history of squeezing pain under the breastbone which appears on exertion and disappears with rest. An *electrocardiogram (ECG)*, which graphically reveals the patterns of electrical activity produced by the heart, is routinely done. A *resting ECG* is normal in at least 25%–50% of all people with angina, but shows *nonspecific* changes in the others. Unless people show signs of significant heart disease, they will then undergo an *exercise-stress test* in which an ECG is performed while their heartbeat is elevated by walking on a treadmill or riding a stationary bicycle. During this test, people are subjected to a gradually increasing workload while their blood pressure and heart rate are continuously monitored. Changes in one particular segment of the electrocardiogram are strongly indicative of angina, but the exercise-stress test does have a small but significant number of false-positive and false-negative results. Thus stress test results are always evaluated in light of the person's history.

If the doctor strongly suspects angina, but the ECG results are unclear, *radioisotope imaging* may be done. This is also done to delineate the extent of the narrowing of the coronary arteries. At the peak of exercise, a small amount of radioactive isotope *thallium-201* is injected into the bloodstream. This substance is taken up by the heart muscle in varying amounts depending upon how much blood is reaching each area of the heart. A reduced uptake in any area usually indicates coronary artery narrowing or blockage. Another heart scan test involves the use of the radioisotope *technetium-99m*, which is taken up by red blood cells. This test not only shows the walls of the heart beating, it enables doctors to measure the amount of blood pumped by the heart.

There are three aspects to the treatment of stable angina: risk factors are corrected, life-style adjustments are made, and drugs are prescribed. Correction of risk factors and life-style adjustments are covered in the Self-Care discussion above and in the Introduction to Cardiovascular Disease (see p. 255). The major angina drug, *nitroglycerin*, has been used for almost a hundred years. The drug is so specific for angina pain that it is considered to have some diagnostic value. Nitroglycerin relaxes smooth muscle, including the muscle in the walls of the arteries and veins, which opens up the blood vessels and reduces the amount the heart has to pump. This also makes it easier for the heart to pump because the pressure in the vessels beyond the heart is lower too. Decreasing the work of the heart lowers its demand for oxygen.

At the onset of chest pain, or prior to exertion or a situation known to produce an attack, a nitroglycerin tablet is placed under the tongue. A second pill should be taken if the first one fails to work. Relief should be experienced in under three minutes. If resting and taking two to three pills does not relieve the pain, the doctor should be called. It is not uncommon for nitroglycerin to cause some side effects including headache, flushing, dizziness, and faintness upon standing up. To be effective, the pills must be less than 6–12 months old and must be kept out of the light. In recent years nitroglycerin has become available in longer-acting, steady release forms such as ointments, skin patches, and tablets. These forms are generally used for people who need frequent medication or are engaged in symptom-producing activities such as walking uphill.

Several drugs are prescribed to prevent angina attacks. One family of drugs called *beta-adrenergic blocking agents* (e.g., *propranolol*) helps to lower the number of angina attacks that patients experience. These drugs, which are taken daily, specifically lower heart rate and blood pressure in response to exercise. They do so by blocking the receptors in the heart which normally pick up the stress hormones that mediate the fight-or-flight response (see p. 42). As a result, the heart needs less oxygen. The beta blockers are contraindicated for people with asthma or diabetes. Another group of drugs taken daily to prevent angina attacks are the *calcium channel blocking agents*. These drugs lower the heart's uptake of calcium, which promotes dilation of the coronary arteries and improves coronary blood flow. Patients with severe angina may be treated with a combination of nitroglycerin, beta blockers, and calcium channel blockers. The two blocking agents are believed to be responsible for extending the life expectancy of angina patients.

The doctor may advise further testing for one of several reasons. If angina patients on medication have attacks during ordinary activity or even at rest, if they appear to have unstable angina, or if they are suspected of having advanced life-threatening coronary disease, a more involved test called a *coronary arteriogram*, or *cardiac catheterization*, is done. The purpose of this test is to determine more precisely the location and degree of narrowing in the coronary arteries

in order to evaluate people for corrective procedures such as *coronary angioplasty* or *coronary bypass surgery*. Coronary arteriography involves passing a thin tube into the opening of the coronary arteries, then injecting a dye that is visible on x-ray. While ECG's and heart scans are noninvasive tests that pose no danger to the patient, coronary arteriography has a low but definite risk—at 0.2% risk of causing a heart attack or stroke, and a 0.1% risk of death. This risk is considered acceptable because the people who need arteriography generally face a greater risk from their own heart disease.

The first successful coronary artery bypass surgery was performed in the mid-1960s by Dr. Michael DeBakey. The procedure involves removing a vein from the patient's leg, or an artery from the chest, and inserting it as a *bypass* or *shunt* in the blood supply to the heart. The new blood vessel connects the aorta with the coro-

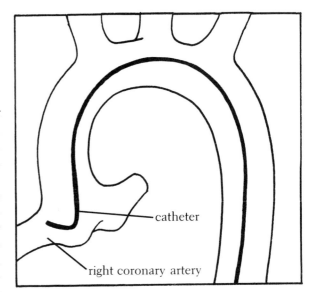

Coronary arteriography involves passing a thin tube into the coronary arteries in order to inject a dye that shows which arteries are blocked.

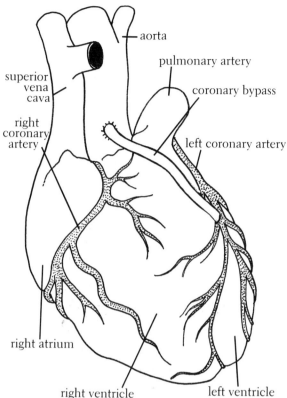

superior vena cava

aorta

pulmonary artery

coronary bypass

right coronary artery

left coronary artery

right atrium

right ventricle

left ventricle

A coronary artery bypass is an operation in which a blood vessel is inserted as a bypass between the aorta and the coronary artery past the point where the artery is blocked; its purpose is to increase the supply of oxygenated blood supplied to that area of the heart.

and safer, and the operative mortality has fallen to 1%–2% in many centers. This risk factor is considered acceptable for patients with severe angina because they have a significantly greater risk of dying from a heart attack within a year.

The indications for bypass surgery have changed over the years. The main criterion for surgery remains significant pain or disability that does not respond to drug therapy. Such a description inevitably involves both medical judgment by the doctor and a life-style judgment by the patient. Arteriography and radioisotope imaging are an essential part of the physician's judgment because they help to precisely determine the location and extent of the blockage.

Currently, bypass surgery is reserved for people who have greater than 70% narrowing of one or more coronary arteries. Surgery is usually successful in relieving symptoms, but studies have shown that the operation only extends longevity in people who have major blockage of the left main coronary artery, a particularly dangerous site for blockage. A large collaborative study done by the National Heart, Lung, and Blood Institute found that people with mild or moderate angina who did not have left coronary blockage had no significant increase in survival difference based on medical or surgical treatment. The controversy is whether people who lack significant left coronary blockage but have moderate-to-severe angina should undergo the operation, based on the expectation of pronounced relief of symptoms, but no increase in life expectancy. Some studies indicate that people with severe 3-vessel disease may have a somewhat increased life expectancy, but not all studies support this conclusion. Currently, most people who undergo bypass surgery do have significant pain and disability, but do not have left coronary disease.

The great majority of people who have bypass surgery experience *symptomatic relief*. It is not known exactly how much of the relief is due to

nary artery beyond the point of blockage. The inserted vessel delivers freshly-oxygenated blood to areas of the heart that were previously oxygen-starved. The operation is very successful in relieving angina pain; 75%–95% of patients report complete or marked relief of angina symptoms. For this reason, the operation is now the most widely performed cardiac operation, and is one of the most common major operations in the U.S. In 1979, 24,000 bypass operations were done; in 1981 the number had risen to 159,000. Over the years, the operation has become safer increased blood flow, and how much is due to the placebo effect of major surgery, which is a significant factor. The operation does not cure the underlying disease, even though it does relieve symptoms. In a number of people, symptoms reoccur in the years after the operation, as a result of ongoing atherosclerotic disease. Some of these people even require repeat bypass surgery.

For many angina patients, bypass surgery remains a choice rather than a necessity. For these people, a low-fat diet that is strictly adhered to, and a serious graded exercise program constitute a reasonable option to surgery. Such a treatment regimen may affect the disease as well as the symptoms. Moreover, current evidence shows that a high-fat diet in post-bypass patients definitely increases the likelihood of blocking the graft, so doctors prescribe a similar routine *after* surgery anyway. While some cardiologists encourage patients to try life-style changes before suggesting surgery, others do not. Many cardiologists believe that surgery remains the best option for a great many patients with angina.

In recent years, a procedure has been developed which does not involve major surgery, called *pericutaneous transluminal coronary angioplasty.* In this procedure, which is somewhat like arteriography, a thin tube is advanced into the coronary arteries under local anesthesia. The tube, or catheter, contains an inflatable balloon at the tip. When expanded at a point of blockage, the balloon opens up the artery by compressing the plaque against the artery wall. In 1987, approximately 150,000 coronary angioplasties were performed in the U.S. A recent study showed that the success rate in relieving blockage was 90% as of 1986. The procedure does have some risk; there is a 1%–2% mortality risk, as well as a 5% risk of inducing a mild heart attack and a 4% risk of requiring emergency bypass surgery. Studies show that there is a definite rate of reblockage, which runs about 15%. Approximately 13% required a second angioplasty procedure.

Initially, angioplasty was largely recommended for people with narrowing in only one coronary artery. As more experience has been gained with the procedure, it is increasingly being used for people with narrowing of more than one coronary artery, and for people with poor pumping in the left ventricle.

Ruling Out Other Diseases

Although angina has a characteristic history, it is often difficult to differentiate it from chest pain due to numerous other causes. A very common cause of chest pain is actually the fear of heart attacks, which is sometimes called a *psychophysiologic cardiovascular reaction.* Such attacks are characterized by a dull, aching chest pain that lasts for hours to days and is not relieved by resting. These pains can also be knife-like and only last for a matter of seconds. Also, if people become emotionally upset, they may experience heart *palpitations* (skipped heartbeats) and difficulty breathing due to *hyperventilation* (too rapid breathing).

Another nonserious cause of chest pain is *anterior chest wall syndrome,* in which pain is associated with tenderness of the chest muscles or ribs. This pain, which is caused by inflammation of the cartilage or the bone-muscle attachments of the chest wall, can be elicited by pressing on these areas. *Lung infection* can also cause chest pain (see p. 307). In this case, the pain becomes more intense with coughing or deep breathing. In some people, *bursitis* can cause arm and chest pain that may be confused with angina pain (see p. 310). However, in this case the pain is intensified by certain arm movements. A number of gastrointestinal conditions can cause burning pain under the sternum. These include *inflammation of the esophagus, hiatus hernia, ulcers,* or a *gallbladder attack* (see pp. 377, 353, and 372). In all these gastrointestinal conditions, symptoms are related to food intake rather than exertion, and are relieved by antacids.

The most serious cause of chest pain that must be ruled out is a *heart attack.* (see p. 284). In this case, the pain is not relieved by resting, lasts longer than angina pain, and is not relieved by nitroglycerin. It is often accompanied by sweating, shortness of breath, nausea, and/or an irregular pulse. In some cases, these symptoms may not be severe or may not be typical. For this reason, heart attacks are sometimes misdiagnosed by the patient, and treatment may be delayed. Delay only increases the risk of heart damage and death, so the doctor or rescue squad should always be called if a heart attack is even suspected (see p. 286).

Prevention

Coronary artery disease is largely—if not totally—preventable. A complete discussion of risk factors and prevention is included in the *Introduction to Cardiovascular Disease* (see p. 284).

High Blood Pressure, or Hypertension

Symptoms

commonly
• no symptoms

occasionally
• headaches
• light-headedness
• ringing in the ears
• feeling of fullness in the head
• loss of energy

Description

One of the leading texts on heart disease states simply that in modern societies, hypertension is the leading cause of death and disability among adults. Mild or moderate high blood pressure has no symptoms and is not incapacitating, thus many people do not view it as a "disease" in the conventional sense, even though it is potentially more dangerous than most other illnesses. Hypertension puts people at risk for several other very serious conditions: heart disease, stroke, and kidney disease. These three diseases kill over half the people in the United States.

Mild or moderate hypertension can go unnoticed for years unless a person has regular blood pressure checks. Estimates are that as many as 20% of Americans have unrecognized or inadequately treated hypertension. Over the years, untreated hypertension causes significant damage. One long-term study of people with *untreated* mild-to-moderate high blood pressure showed that within 7–10 years, 53% developed an enlarged heart, congestive heart failure, stroke, or kidney disease, and that 29% developed coronary artery disease.

The pressure of the blood in the arteries is determined by three major factors: (1) *cardiac output*; that is, how forcefully the heart pumps with each stroke, (2) *peripheral vascular resistance*; that is, how much resistance the blood encounters from the arteries, and (3) the *total fluid volume* of the blood. Actually, understanding these factors is a matter of common sense. Given a pump and a sealed group of tubes, the pressure will go up if the pump works harder, if the tubes are narrowed, or if more fluid is forced into the system.

Unlike a standard pump and tubes, the body has a very complicated set of sensors whose job is to regulate the blood pressure so that the brain will constantly receive enough blood to function effectively, but not so much as to damage blood vessels or other structures. Blood pressure varies according to physical activity, position, time of day, and emotional stress. Moreover, within a group of people, blood pressure levels will vary somewhat even though the people are doing the same task.

Sensors in the cartoid arteries in the neck continuously register blood pressure and relay the information to the brain via the sympathetic portion of the autonomic nervous system. When blood pressure is too low, the heart is directed to speed up and the blood vessels receive signals causing them to close down slightly. The same sympathetic nerves and neurotransmitters that release epinephrine and norepinephrine in a stressful situation are responsible for raising blood pressure. Thus psychological stress is one mechanism that can elevate blood pressure. Each sympathetic nerve ending consists of a tiny bulb which releases norepinephrine, the major neurotransmitter. This hormone crosses over to muscle cells in the heart or blood vessel walls where it is picked up by special receptors that cause the cells to contract or relax.

Many factors affect peripheral resistance. The arteries contract and the heart speeds up in response to sympathetic arousal and stress hormones. Slight steady elevations in blood pressure for any reason cause a gradual process of thickening, abrasion, and reduced elasticity within the blood vessels. Abraded areas are ready sites for the deposition of cholesterol plaques. Narrowed arteries and plaque buildup are the cause of angina, heart attacks, and strokes.

In addition to the natural pressure sensors by which fast, temporary changes in blood pressure are made, the body adjusts blood pressure over a longer time by raising or lowering blood volume. In response to elevated pressures, the kidneys lower total blood volume by releasing more salt and water into the urine. Salt intake strongly affects people's water retention: the more salt ingested, the more water is held in the blood rather than released in the urine. The kidney also produces a hormone called *renin*, which activates a hormone called *angiotensin II*, a potent blood vessel constrictor that causes an almost instantaneous rise in blood pressure.

The exact cause of high blood pressure in most people has still not been determined by scientists. This is not altogether surprising considering the number of factors involved and the complexity of their interaction. The common type of high blood pressure is referred to as *essential hypertension*. Some scientists theorize that essential hypertension is caused by excess autonomic nervous system arousal (stress); some feel that the peripheral arteries are extrasensitive to autonomic nervous system control or angiotensin II. Other scientists feel that high blood pressure is directly related to the amount of salt ingested. Still others believe that essential hypertension is caused by the heart pumping too much blood. Finally, there are scientists who feel that hypertension is caused by irregularities in the production of hormones, especially *aldosterone*, an adrenal hormone that decreases the kidney's output of salt and water.

Doctors debate about the optimum range of blood pressure that will decrease the risk of disease or damage. Currently, high blood pressure is defined as the level above which blood vessel damage will occur, and is estimated to be about 160/95 millimeters of mercury. The first figure represents the *systolic pressure*—that is, the pressure in the arteries when the heart is actively pumping; the second figure represents the *diastolic pressure*—the pressure in the arteries when the heart is resting between beats.

In Western cultures, high blood pressure is very common. Over 60 million Americans, or about 40% of the adult population have high blood pressure. Among people over 35, hypertension is the leading reason for doctor visits, and the number one reason for prescribing medicine. In Western cultures, from the age of 40 upward, blood pressure generally rises in direct proportion to age, increasing by an average of ½–1 mm of mercury per year. Although some adults initially have low values and have a below-average increase, others begin at the high end of

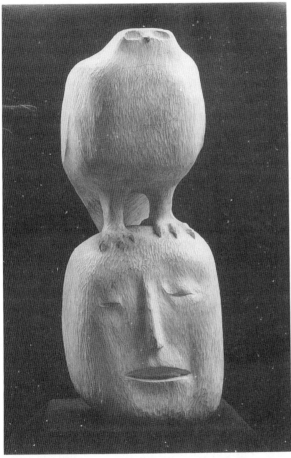

Stressful situations stimulate the sympathetic nervous system and cause blood pressure to go up; chronic stress is thought to be a contributing factor in hypertension. Leonard Baskin. Oppressed Man. 1960. Painted pine. 31″ × 13″ × 11½″. Collection, The Whitney Museum of American Art. Purchase. 60.30.

normal and experience higher than average increases year by year. People in their 30s and 40s who have high normal values or *borderline high blood pressure* have a definite likelihood of developing hypertension. Another potential indicator of problems is occasional high readings in middle age, which are referred to as *labile high blood pressure.*

Hypertension occurs much more commonly among individuals who have a family history of high blood pressure. This genetic factor has been studied, but its significance remains unclear because of the difficulty in separating out other factors such as diet and stress. In addition to a genetic factor, there also appears to be something of a racial susceptibility, in that adult blacks of African origin, as well as Asians, experience higher frequencies of hypertension than do Caucasians.

. Blood pressure has also been found to correlate somewhat with levels of stress (see p. 48). Studies have shown that high blood pressure can be brought on in animals by a variety of stressful factors, including overcrowding, competition for food, and noxious stimuli. Among humans, blood pressure has been found to increase in response to military combat, high-pressure jobs, being fired, and poverty. Cross-cultural studies have shown that in stable, traditional cultures, people's blood pressure values tend to be low and do not rise with age. When these same cultures become Westernized, blood pressure values take on a more Western pattern.

In explaining how stress causes high blood pressure, scientists theorize that some people have hypersensitive autonomic nervous systems, most likely due to genetics. In these people, stress causes intermittent increases in cardiac output and blood pressure. As a result of these occasional changes, the blood vessel walls become thickened and less elastic, eventually resulting in a permanent state of high blood pressure. Cardiologist Robert Eliot has referred to these people as "hot reactors." He believes that by learning to change their behavior and reducing their reaction to stress, these people can lower their blood pressure.

There is a great deal of evidence that salt has a significant effect on blood pressure. Cultures that have very low-salt diets have *no* incidence of hypertension, and no rise in blood pressure values with advancing age. If people from these cultures adopt a normal Western diet that is generally high in salt, they tend to develop Western blood pressure rates. Conversely, doctors have found that if hypertension patients with high-salt diets eliminate most salt from their diet, their blood pressure drops to normal values. Other studies show that as little as 10 days of a high-salt diet can raise the blood pressure of susceptible people by an average of 10 points.

Similar to stress, there is probably a genetic susceptibility to salt-caused hypertension. People with borderline high blood pressure or whose parents were hypertensive are likely to show a rise in pressure in correlation to their salt intake, whereas there are some people with normal blood pressure values who don't show a rise with increasing salt intake until the salt level is huge. These so-called "resistant" people have kidneys that are better able to excrete salt.

Several other factors affect blood pressure and are considered to be risk factors for hypertension. Obesity correlates with high blood pressure in children as well as adults. Obese people over 40 are 1½ times as likely to have high blood pressure as those who are not overweight. Further, it has been shown that blood pressure drops steadily as obese people lose weight. The reason for this link between weight and hypertension is not known. It may be due to greater cardiac output, increased blood volume, or higher insulin levels. To a lesser degree, alcohol consumption (2 oz or more per day) and cigarette smoking are also associated with increased blood pressure.

Many studies have demonstrated the importance of treating high blood pressure. Both the 1967 Veterans' Administration Study and the Hypertension-Stroke Study demonstrated dramatic reductions in death and organ damage among people with a diastolic pressure of over 105 who received treatment. An Australian study showed a 20% reduction in risk of cardiovascular disease and death among people treated for a diastolic pressure of over 95. The 1979 Hypertension Detection and Follow-up Program that dealt with 11,000 patients showed a 17% overall reduction in mortality in the group that were aggressively treated for a diastolic pressure of over 90. In particular, there was a 20% reduction in mortality among the group that had mild high blood pressure (90–105), with a 45% drop in deaths from strokes and heart attacks. Based on the results of this study, a national advisory panel for the first time recommended treating all patients with a diastolic pressure of over 90.

In 1985, the Medical Research Council Working Party tried to determine specifically whether or not drug treatment of diastolic pressures between 90 and 109 was really necessary. Among the 17,000 participants treated, the number of strokes was significantly reduced, but the number of heart attacks was not. In fact, the number of heart attacks was slightly greater. Since heart attacks outnumbered strokes 7 to 1, the overall mortality of the treated group was relatively unaffected. Diuretics and beta blockers, the drugs commonly used for hypertension, raise blood cholesterol levels. Doctors believe that elevated cholesterol levels *increase* high blood pressure levels in a linear fashion. Thus the treatment of *mild* high blood pressure has now shifted away from simple drug treatment to a concerted effort to reduce all of a person's risk factors after careful evaluation. However, the value of drug treatment for a person with a diastolic pressure of over 105 remains unquestioned.

No matter what a person's specific blood pressure reading is, the probability of heart disease and stroke depends on his or her other risk factors as well. Each positive risk factor in addition to high blood pressure increases a person's likelihood of problems. Cholesterol is probably the most significant risk, and the risk rises as cholesterol values rise. For people 30–39 years of age, a cholesterol level of over 220 is considered a moderate risk; for 40 years and up, 240 is a moderate risk. People with high blood pressure are at greater risk at any given cholesterol value. Generally, people with high blood pressure also have elevated cholesterol values.

Other important risk factors for people with hypertension are age and sex. The younger a person is when high blood pressure develops, the greater the risk. Women, for unknown reasons, are at much less risk than men. Blacks and Asians are more at risk than Caucasians. Finally, smokers are more at risk than nonsmokers.

Self-Care

Self-care plays an important role in the treatment of hypertension, especially mild hypertension, for which it is the cornerstone of treatment. Doctors refer to it as "nonpharmacological" treatment. The main aspects of non-drug therapy include life-style changes that deal with diet, stress reduction, and exercise. For people with borderline or mild high blood pressure, nonpharmacological therapy may be all that is needed. Just because drugs are not involved does not make the treatment any less effective or less important. While nondrug therapies do not have the side effects of drugs, they do seem to be more difficult to adhere to. For people with higher blood pressure or a number of risk factors, self-care is an important adjunct to treatment with drugs.

The first dietary change suggested for people with high blood pressure is salt reduction. For

---

Self-Care for High Blood Pressure

- eat a low-salt, low-cholesterol diet
- maintain a reasonable weight
- do aerobic exercise three to five times a week
- learn ways to cope effectively with stress
- stop smoking
- meditate or do relaxation exercises daily
- motivate life-style changes by learning about the dangers of high blood pressure
- take medication regularly if prescribed by a doctor

---

most hypertensives, the lower their salt intake, the lower the blood pressure will be. Reduction of salt intake to 100 mEq/day (see p. 102) will drop diastolic pressure 3–5 mm by itself. A more severe reduction to 70 mEq/day may reduce diastolic pressure as much as 10 mm or more, and has been found to be as effective as drug treatment. It's important for people who are put on a low-salt diet to realize that the average American salt intake is enormous and that even a good-sized reduction generally does not really constitute a low-salt diet. Although many people initially find it hard to restrict salt, most find that within several months they no longer miss their high-salt diet.

The second dietary change recommended for people with high blood pressure is a reduction in calorie and cholesterol intake (see p. 100). The value of a low-fat diet is that it reduces the most significant heart disease risk factor that can accompany high blood pressure. The weight loss that results from a low-calorie/low-cholesterol diet can be very effective in lowering blood pressure, especially in people who are significantly overweight. One study found that a significant weight loss in obese people dropped diastolic pressures by an average of 10 mm.

Several other dietary regimens proposed for hypertensives are more controversial. Studies have shown that increasing either potassium, calcium, or magnesium, or reducing fat, resulted in lower blood pressure readings. There are several diets based on the principle of increasing potassium while decreasing salt at the same time. Decreasing alcohol consumption to under 2 oz a day is thought to drop blood pressure values by about 2 points as well.

A number of studies have shown that various stress reduction techniques can reduce blood pressure (see p. 60). The decreases ranged from a diastolic drop of 4 mm with meditation, to 8 mm with breath awareness meditation, to 10 mm with progressive muscle relaxation, to 9–16 mm with a combination of meditation and biofeedback.

One of the least studied life-style changes as related to hypertension involves regular vigorous exercise (see p. 107). One study found that walking or jogging twice a week for 30 minutes dropped blood pressure an average of 12 points. Other studies have not all shown consistent results. Even if regular exercise does not lower blood pressure directly, it has other beneficial results that make it valuable as therapy for people who are hypertensive. Positive changes include weight loss, stress reduction, lowering overall cholesterol, and raising HDLs, the protective component of cholesterol (see p. 260).

The Doctor

High blood pressure is treated by an internist, a family practitioner, or a *cardiologist*, a doctor who specializes in heart problems. It is diagnosed with a remarkably simple device, the *sphygmomanometer*, or *blood pressure cuff*. To measure blood pressure, the cuff is temporarily inflated enough to compress the blood vessels in the upper arm, then the pressure is released gradually until blood again pumps through the arteries and a pulse can be heard with a stethoscope. The sound of the pulse will disappear again when the pressure in the cuff drops below

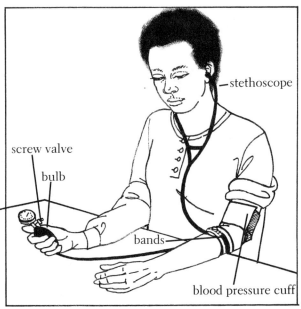

You can check your own blood pressure. Use the hand that you write with to put the cuff snuggly on the opposite arm, just above the elbow. If the cuff does not have a place to hold the stethoscope, the stethoscope should be attached with elastic to the crook of your elbow. The screw valve should be closed and the rubber bulb squeezed until the dial reads above 100. Keep pumping until you no longer hear blood pulsing with the stethoscope; pump until the dial is 20 points above the last pulse. Open the valve slowly, and listen for the sound of the pulse reappearing as the pressure drops. Note the pressure at this point, which is called the systolic pressure. Continue to watch the pressure drop, and note when you no longer hear pulsing. This represents the diastolic pressure.

the resting pressure in the vessels. The initial sound of the pulse is the *systolic reading* (first value), while the *diastolic reading* (second value) marks the point at which the pulse disappears again.

Since blood pressure varies with mood and activity, it's important that it be measured when people are relaxed and at rest. Research has shown that blood pressure values typically drop an average of 10 points between the first and second doctor visit, and 4 points from the second to the third. This pattern is attributed to anxiety. Blood pressure has also been found to drop naturally between the beginning and the end of an appointment. For this reason, unless a person's blood pressure is very high, many doctors do not make a diagnosis of hypertension until the measurements exceed 140/90 on several successive visits in which the patient has rested quietly for a half hour prior to the reading.

Some doctors even teach patients to take their own blood pressure, and have them take readings at home twice a day for a week in order to determine true resting values. To establish resting value, the blood pressure is usually measured in the morning just after arising, and another time when the person is at rest. Some doctors also advise people to take their blood pressure when they are upset to see if they react strongly to stress. Occasional high readings should not be totally ignored because they point to the fact that a person is reactive and may have hypertension or be more susceptible to it.

Doctors vary their definition of high blood pressure according to a patient's age and sex. For example, for men below 40, a reading of 140/95 is considered high; for men 40–60, high would be a reading of 150/95. A diastolic pressure of 90–95 in any age group is considered to be borderline hypertension. Some doctors will classify mild high blood pressure as 95–104, moderate high blood pressure as 105–114, and high blood pressure as anything over 115. The borderline range of 90–95 diastolic is the most controversial in terms of both diagnosis and treatment.

Once a diagnosis of hypertension is made, the doctor may attempt to determine the cause. Of all the diagnosed cases of hypertension, 90%–95% are classified as *essential* or *idiopathic* (unknown) *hypertension*; that is, hypertension that is not caused by any underlying medical condi-

tion. Essential hypertension, which is also known as *primary hypertension*, is thought to be caused by increased cardiac output, increased peripheral resistance, or increased fluid volume, all of which are of unknown origin. Often, hypertension in midadulthood is not the subject of many diagnostic tests, but is simply assumed to be essential.

The remaining 5%–10% of hypertension, which is classified as *secondary hypertension*, is caused by a variety of factors. The most common cause of secondary hypertension is oral contraceptive use: 5% of women on the pill for more than five years develop blood pressure levels above 140/90. Such hypertension is generally mild and subsides in 50% of cases when oral contraceptives are discontinued. This type of high blood pressure is most common in women over 35 who smoke, are obese, and have a family history of high blood pressure. Oral contraceptive-caused hypertension is responsible for the fact that women on the pill have five times the cardiac mortality of nonpill-users.

The other major cause of secondary hypertension is *chronic renal failure*, or decreased kidney function, which results in increased fluid volume in the bloodstream. This condition can be caused by any type of kidney disease, including infection. A very small number of people (less than 1% of all hypertensives) have secondary hypertension due to narrowing of the arteries that suppy the kidneys—a condition referred to as *renovascular hypertension*. Finally, in very rare cases, secondary hypertension is caused by adrenal hormone imbalances or renal tumors.

A doctor diagnoses the probable cause of hypertension on the basis of a complete history, physical exam, and lab tests. The history includes questions about the incidence of high blood pressure among relatives, and whether the person has had kidney disease, heart disease, or endocrine disorders. During the physical exam, the doctor will check the heartbeat and pulses, and will look carefully at the blood vessels of the eye, which show early signs of hypertension. Several lab tests will be done, including a *blood test* and *urinalysis* to check kidney function, and a *chest x-ray* and *ECG (electrocardiogram)* to make sure that high blood pressure has not affected heart function. When people with high blood pressure are under 30, have diastolic pressures of over 120, or have symptoms of kidney disease, they will be given further tests such as a *urogram (kidney x-ray)* or a *renogram (kidney scan)*.

Doctors treat primary hypertension based on the person's age, sex, history, and physical findings. Great variability exists in the way borderline hypertension (diastolic of 90–100) is treated. If people in this range have no symptoms and no serious coronary risk factors, they are often treated with nonpharmacological means, including dietary changes, stress reduction, and exercise (see section on *Self-Care*), rather than medication, and their blood pressure is monitored annually. As of 1983, The World Health Organization and the International Society of Hypertension recommended nondrug therapy for a trial of three months for patients with blood pressures below 100, and indefinitely for patients with pressures below 95. However, many doctors do treat those with values in this range with drug therapy.

If people have diastolic pressures in the range of 100–105, they are treated with drugs in order to reduce their risk of heart disease, stroke, and kidney disease. Currently, the most common drug therapy is called the *stepped care regimen*. It consists of starting the person on one drug, usually a *diuretic* (see below), and raising the dose slowly until the blood pressure drops down to 140/85. If treatment is not successful within 6–12 weeks, another drug, a *beta blocker*, which is a sympathetic nervous system depressant, is prescribed in addition. In the occasional case that an individual does not respond to the two-

drug therapy, several other kinds of drugs may be added or substituted. When people have a consistent diastolic reading of over 115, they are often started on two drugs initially, or on stronger drugs.

By far the most frequently used drugs in management of hypertension are the diuretics, of which there are a number. Due to the high incidence of hypertension, diuretics are the #1 prescription drug for people over 45, and millions of people have been treated with them during the last 20 years. Diuretics lower blood pressure because they increase the excretion of urinary sodium, which in turn lowers the body's blood volume. The most frequently chosen type of diuretics are the *thiazides (chlorothiazide, hydrochlorothiazide)*, which successfully lower diastolic pressure an average of 10–15 points. Once drug therapy is begun, it is usually continued for the rest of a person's life, except in the case of borderline hypertensives.

The thiazides generally have few short-term side effects, although people sometimes report easy fatigability, shortness of breath on exercise, tiredness, and impotence. Studies show that 15%–20% of patients actually stop treatment because of side effects. Recently, doctors have become concerned that the thiazides may have some undesirable long-term side effects as well. Studies indicate that thiazide therapy causes lowered potassium levels, high uric acid levels, and glucose intolerance. More importantly, diuretics cause an increase in blood lipid levels which is associated with an increase in heart attack rates. As a result, doctors are reconsidering whether thiazides should be the drug of choice in all cases of hypertension, especially if people have high cholesterol values or other heart attack risk factors. But until the recent studies are verified, most doctors will continue to use diuretics as the drug of choice in treating high blood pressure.

The second most commonly prescribed class

of hypertensive drugs, the beta blocking drugs, encompass several different groups. By far the most frequently used are *actenolol, propranolol,* and *timolol.* These drugs bind to beta receptors in the muscle cells of the heart and blood vessels, preventing the receptors from picking up the norepinephrine made by sympathetic nerve endings. As a result, the heart beats more slowly and less forcefully and cardiac output is lower, which lowers blood pressure. Short-term side effects of the beta blockers include fatigue, insomnia, cold in the extremities, a feeling of fuzziness, and impotence. Long-term negative side effects include raising blood *triglyceride* levels and dropping the level of protective *HDLs (high density lipoproteins),* the protective component of cholesterol. Thus some doctors question whether beta blockers, somewhat like thiazides, may increase the risk of heart attack in susceptible people. Beta blockers are contraindicated for people with asthma or heart failure. In the case of heart failure, cardiac output is already low; with asthma, beta blockers restrict widening of the airways.

If diuretics or beta blockers don't work, if there is concern about those drugs raising a person's risk of heart disease, or if the drug's side effects are particularly bothersome, there are other drugs that can be prescribed for hypertension. These drugs include *vasodilators (hydralazine hydrochloride),* and other *sympathetic nervous system blockers (Aldomet,* and *clonidine).*

A significant percentage of hypertensives fail to follow either nondrug or drug regimens. Patients often object to the side effects of their medication, or find it difficult to consistently adhere to life-style changes. Patient compliance and satisfaction are more likely if the doctor is seen regularly and if patients monitor their blood pressure at home. Hypertensive drug therapy is most effective if the doctor educates the patient regarding the risks of high blood pressure and the benefits of treatment. Drug therapy may be more effective if consistently supplemented by nondrug therapy (see section on *Self-Care*). Often this may enable the patient to alter the dosage, or type of drugs prescribed. In cases of borderline or mild hypertension, drugs can sometimes even be discontinued. Finally, doctors can generally switch a prescribed drug if people have significant problems with its side effects.

Ruling Out Other Diseases

Diagnosis of essential hypertension is a matter of accurate blood pressure readings; no other disease needs to be ruled out. Diagnosis of secondary hypertension involves establishing the underlying cause (see section on *The Doctor*).

Prevention

Dietary changes (salt and calorie reduction), stress reduction, and regular exercise can play a significant role in preventing, as well as alleviating, hypertension in a genetically susceptible person. Such life-style adjustments, including emphasis on a low-fat diet, are the most important factors in extending people's lives through the prevention of heart disease, stroke, and kidney disease.

Heart Attack, or Acute Myocardial Infarction

Symptoms

- prolonged, severe chest pain that doesn't subside with rest
- pain in mid- or left chest
- often, pain radiating down the left arm
- often, nausea
- sweating
- weakness
- dizziness
- pervading sense of something wrong
- occasionally, no pain ("silent heart attack")

Description

A heart attack is one of the most feared diseases of middle age, especially among men. Part of the mystique of a heart attack is that it often comes on without warning. Because heart attack is the leading cause of death between the ages of 40–60, the term has become almost synonymous with people facing their own mortality and coming to terms with the possibility of imminent death. This analogy is ironic because the great majority of heart attacks are not fatal.

In the United States, 1.3 million people suffer heart attacks each year. An American male has a 20% chance of having a heart attack before the age of 65. Fortunately, this figure is dropping, presumably as a result of people's willingness to lower their cholesterol intake, give up smoking, and treat high blood pressure early. Death from heart attack is also dropping significantly in the U.S. This decline is due partly to the drop in heart attacks, and partly to more prompt and effective treatment.

A *heart attack*, or *acute myocardial infarction*, refers to an episode in which some part of the heart muscle suffers permanent damage because of a sudden reduction in blood supply. "Myocardial" means heart muscle and "infarct" refers to the dead tissue. Almost all heart attacks are caused by *atherosclerosis*, a condition in which fatty deposits are laid down in the arteries (see p. 255). In the case of a heart attack, the plaques have built up in the *coronary arteries*, the arteries that supply the heart muscle itself (see illustration). As the plaques occlude more and more of the coronary arteries, it becomes harder and harder for blood to reach the heart muscle. If any area is without sufficient oxygen for a long time, cells will die and a heart attack will occur. The specific area of the heart that is damaged depends on which coronary artery is blocked. The size of the damaged area depends on the extent of the blockage, and the size of the area supplied by the occluded artery. The most common site of blockage is the *left anterior descending artery*, which causes muscle damage in the upper front portion of the *left ventricle*, the chamber that pumps oxygenated blood out from the heart to the body. The second and third most common sites, the *left circumflex* and *right*

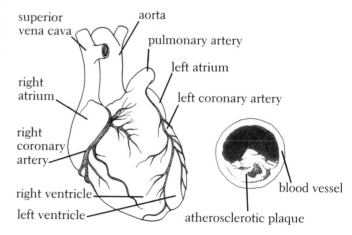

In people who experience a heart attack, plaques have built up in the coronary arteries that supply the heart muscle.

coronary arteries, also affect the left ventricle, but in different areas.

Once blood supply is cut off to a given area of the heart, the cells past the blockage begin to die. Within six to eight hours after the heart attack, the dying tissue turns pale blue and swells. Over the next seven days, the body starts to heal the damage. Within 12 hours of the heart attack, and continuing over the next 21 days, nearby functioning blood vessels send blood to the affected region. White blood cells carry off dead cells, and new connective tissue weaves across the damaged area and forms a firm scar. Almost never is a "hole" left in the heart, as is sometimes feared. Whether or not there is any residual muscle weakness depends on the magnitude of the heart attack. After a mild heart attack, there is little muscle damage and the ventricle heals well enough to function as before. After a serious heart attack, more tissue is destroyed and the function of the ventricle can be weakened.

Several incidents can trigger a heart attack. First, a prolonged increase in oxygen demand (such as exertion) can bring on a heart attack when a vessel is almost entirely blocked. Second, a *coronary thrombosis*, or blood clot, that develops at a point of significant blockage can bring on a heart attack. This situation takes place when blood platelets stick to the fatty plaque in a coronary artery. Third, if bleeding occurs in the middle of a plaque, causing the plaque to rupture or bulge, a heart attack can occur when the artery is suddenly occluded. Fourth, occasionally and for unknown reasons, an artery can suddenly spasm and constrict. Fifth, an *embolism*, a moving blood clot that lodges in a vessel can trigger a heart attack. Most heart attacks are probably the result of all these factors acting at once.

Although the exact cause of a heart attack may never be known, it is true that the great majority of heart attacks take place in people who have significant development of atheroscle-

rotic plaques. Recent studies show that a coronary artery is occluded in 70%–90% of all heart attacks. Among people who have fatal heart attacks, more than two-thirds show greater than 75% blockage of *all* three major coronary arteries.

Although heart attacks can vary greatly in severity, there is a common group of symptoms by which a heart attack can be diagnosed. With most heart attacks, the major symptom is chest pain. Generally the pain is very severe; people describe it as crushing, like a weight, tight, squeezing, viselike, or choking. Less commonly, the pain may be characterized as burning. Typically, the pain lasts for more than 30 minutes and may last for hours. The pain is generally located in the middle of the front of the chest, either directly behind the breastbone, or slightly to the left of it. Often the pain radiates down the inside of the left arm as well. Occasionally, heart attack symptoms are less typical. Sometimes they cause abdominal distress, which may be erroneously diagnosed as indigestion. In other cases, the pain affects the neck and shoulders, as well as the chest. In 10%–50% of all heart attacks, people report that they have experienced angina-like pain in the days and weeks immediately preceding the attack. Approximately 10%–20% of heart attacks are painless or *silent heart attacks*. In this case, the symptoms are shortness of breath and weakness (see below). Most remarkably, routine ECGs show that one or two heart attacks out of ten go unnoticed because they do not cause symptoms of sufficient intensity.

Other symptoms that frequently accompany a heart attack are nausea; sweating; clamminess; feelings of weakness, dizziness, or fatigue; difficulty breathing; and sudden fainting. When viewed by an observer, people who are having a heart attack often appear pale, sweaty, very uncomfortable, anxious, and restless. As opposed to a person with angina, someone suffering a heart attack is likely to pace about restlessly rather than sit, and may press a clenched fist to his or her breastbone in an attempt to counter the pain. If the person has an existing angina condition, a heart attack will be similar to angina pain, but will be more severe and will not be relieved by either rest or nitroglycerin. Interestingly, some heart attack victims also report a strong feeling of doom.

Although heart attacks do take place following exercise (13%) or extreme fatigue, they are more likely to occur during normal activity, rest, or even sleep. Heart attacks definitely occur more frequently among people who are under stress or who have recently experienced a number of life changes that bring on a period of fatigue, depression, frustration, disappointment, and/or loneliness. This cluster of feelings is sometimes referred to as the *giving-up response*. The old expressions about dying of a broken heart, or dying of loneliness, may not be completely a matter of superstition. It is known that stress causes the sympathetic nervous system to step up its activity, which increases both heart rate and *arrhythmias*, or irregularities in the heartbeat. Recent studies show that by itself stress can cause coronary spasms and arrhythmias.

Self-Care

A heart attack or a suspected heart attack should be treated by a physician (a cardiologist, internist, or family practitioner) in a coronary care unit to prevent possible life-threatening complications (see section on *The Doctor*). Anyone over 35 who experiences chest pain should call a doctor. *If there is any question of a heart attack, the sooner an individual contacts a physician and gets treatment, the better the outcome is likely to be.* A heart attack is a MEDICAL EMERGENCY. Over 50% of all deaths occur within one hour of the heart attack, 80% within four hours. Most of these deaths are caused by arrhythmias or heartbeat irregularities that will generally respond to drug therapy. The great majority of these arrhythmias occur within the first four hours after the onset of the attack. In recent years, a combination of trained CPR (cardiopulmonary resuscitation) rescue teams and mobile coronary care units that can go to the patient and begin immediate treatment has helped to significantly lower the number of deaths resulting from heart attacks.

The biggest danger to a person's life directly following a heart attack is delay. Studies show that people do not arrive at the hospital for an average of three to five hours after a heart attack. Psychiatrists think that denial and rationalization are the main factors that keep patients from seeking immediate treatment. Unfortunately, many people either believe that they will not survive a heart attack or that they will be severely handicapped by it. Neither of these beliefs is true. Between 70%–95% of people survive a heart attack, and the great majority recover completely. These survival figures would probably improve dramatically if more people knew the warning signs for a heart attack and sought treatment promptly. Often co-workers, friends, or relatives are the ones who insist on calling the doctor, whereas the heart attack victim (and sometimes his or her spouse) will tend to deny or delay. Statistics show that people who have a heart attack at work are likely to receive treatment the most quickly.

After a heart attack patient is released from the hospital, there are many beneficial self-care routines that should be followed. These routines focus on four aspects of care: 1) *reducing stress;* 2) *starting a graded exercise program;* 3) *adhering to a low-fat, low-cholesterol, low-salt diet;* and 4) *eliminating smoking.* The main concept to keep in mind is that the heart has suffered some degree of damage, and it needs adequate time to heal and rebuild strength. Except in severe heart attacks, the heart eventually regains normal function, although a scar will remain at the site where cell damage took place.

In the initial weeks after a heart attack, many patients fear that they may never lead a normal life because of the restrictions placed on their activity. It should be emphasized that the restrictions are both temporary and graded, tapering off as the damaged muscle tissue gains strength. It is also normal for patients to feel tired and depressed at this point in their convalescence. The fatigue is the result of both the damage done to the heart, and the enforced bed rest that is necessary. The depression, referred to as *homecoming depression*, is due to the patient's loss of a sense of health and intactness, as well as to fears about job loss, sexual limitations, the future, and his or her own mortality. Perhaps more than any other illness in middle age, a heart attack brings a person face-to-face with death—psychologically if not physically. Generally the depression is self-limiting and resolves within one to two months, as the person feels better and begins to resume a more normal life.

Relaxation exercises, visualization, yoga, and *meditation* are all effective means of decreasing the stress and anxiety experienced by a person after a heart attack (see p. 60). Relieving worries whenever possible and engaging in favorite hobbies or activities will also help to improve a person's outlook. In addition, any means of reducing stress and anxiety will lessen the work of the heart. The importance of stress reduction is demonstrated by the fact that it can even reduce the likelihood of a second heart attack. A study by Meyer Friedman found that if heart attack patients were able to reduce Type A behavior (see p. 265) through a counseling program that included progressive muscle relaxation, recognition of reasons for exaggerated emotional reactions, restructuring of environmental situations, and most importantly, modification of Type A habits and beliefs, these patients could

cut in half their risk of a subsequent heart attack. The Type A profile is now considered to be a complicated and controversial topic. New studies have shown that Type A people are more likely to have a second heart attack, but have a better survival rate following a second heart attack that do non-type A people. Researchers theorize that characteristics such as hostility and isolation can contribute to a heart attack, but fierce independence and a sense of being in control can help people survive once they develop an illness (see p. 51). Thus behaviorial physicians seek to reduce people's hostility, but increase their sense of control. This new view of Type A behavior is gaining credence with more and more professionals who utilize a mind-body approach to heart disease.

A second facet of a home self-care routine after release from the hospital involves a *graded exercise program*. Today, almost all doctors advise such a program. Not only does it build up people's strength safely and efficiently, it has been shown to improve their mental outlook. Through an exercise program, people regain a sense of physical well-being and develop a renewed sense of control over their own health. Typically when people are released from the hospital, they are fully ambulatory but they are generally advised to rest periodically and to refrain from lifting heavy objects. Many doctors will schedule a treadmill stress test several weeks after a person goes home. Provided the test results are favorable, the person will be encouraged to walk a certain distance on a daily, increasing basis—beginning at one block and progressing in steady increments up to a number of miles. Patients are told to keep their activity within a maximum safe-pulse rate and to stop if they experience any chest pain, shortness of breath, or undue fatigue. The amount of exercise recommended at any given point will vary depending on the severity of the heart attack, the person's performance on post-heart attack

Sex After a Heart attack

- sex or masturbation normally raises the heart rate from 80 to 90–145 beats/minute
- sex or masturbation normally raises blood pressure by 30–45 mm/hg
- for the first three to four weeks after a heart attack, foreplay is all right but not orgasm
- after three to four weeks, orgasm may be approached slowly, when the person feels ready
- many heart medicines lessen sexual interest and performance
- normal post-heart-attack depression generally lowers sexual interest for a time
- mood swings and changes in expectations affect both partners
- talking about sexual concerns is important
- exercise improves physical stamina in general
- make love when rested, one to three hours after eating, after medication is taken (if prescribed)
- *stop* if sexual stimulation causes pain in the chest, neck, jaw, or stomach, or if stimulation causes marked shortness of breath, or rapid or irregular heartbeat
- although sometimes feared, sex after a heart attack is not a frequent cause of another heart attack

stress tests, and the doctor's philosophy concerning exercise.

A third and critical factor in any post-heart attack self-care regimen involves *dietary changes* (see p. 102). A high-fat diet, such as the kind eaten previously by most heart attack patients, will only serve to further occlude already narrowed blood vessels, reducing the amount of blood reaching the heart and thereby increasing the risk of another heart attack. There is recent evidence that atherosclerotic plaques may actually shrink in the presence of low blood cholesterol levels. Thus, although such dietary changes may not be easy to maintain, they are well worth the effort.

A fourth major facet of any self-care program involves *stopping smoking*. Cigarette smoking is a known risk for coronary artery disease (see p. 263). Smoking constricts blood vessels and reduces the supply of blood to the heart. People who continue to smoke after a heart attack have a much greater risk of experiencing a second heart attack. If people have any difficulty quitting on their own, they are advised to join a group program such as Smoke-Enders.

The Doctor

The doctor (cardiologist, internist, or family practitioner) is crucial in diagnosing and treating a suspected heart attack. Diagnosis is based on a history, physical exam, and laboratory tests. In addition to a positive history of symptoms, the person often experiences skipped beats due to an arrhythmia. In a severe heart attack, there may be signs of shock due to *heart failure*, a condition in which the heart is not able to meet the body's oxygen needs. These signs include poor color, low blood pressure, cold and clammy skin, marked weakness, difficulty breathing, and a weak pulse.

Laboratory tests are very valuable in helping to diagnose a heart attack. An *ECG (electrocardiogram)*, which is done immediately, will usually show characteristic changes in the electrical patterns of the heartbeat if a person is having a heart attack. If these changes are slight, it may only be possible to make the diagnosis in relation to a previously recorded ECG. In any case, the size of the changes does not necessarily correlate with the severity of the heart attack. A *chest x-ray* may also be taken to rule out heart failure. If a person is suffering from heart failure, the heart may appear enlarged and there may be signs of fluid in the chest.

Several blood tests will be done during the next few days to determine whether or not specific enzymes are present that indicate heart muscle has been killed or irreversibly injured.

These enzymes are released by the dying cells. Unlike the ECG, the levels of these enzymes will give an indication of the severity of the heart attack. These enzymes, including *creatine phosphokynase (CPK)*, *serum glutamic oxalacetic transaminase (SGOT)*, *lactic dehydrogenase (LDH)*, and especially the myocardial-specific *CK-MB*, can be detected in the blood at characteristic times after a heart attack has taken place.

Once it has been established that someone has had a heart attack, or even if a heart attack is strongly suspected, he or she is admitted to a coronary care unit, continuously monitored with an electrocardiogram, and watched over by nurses and doctors who are specially trained to deal with the complications that occasionally take place following a heart attack. Often patients are given *oxygen*. If they are still experiencing pain, they will be given *morphine*, *nitroglycerin*, or possibly *diazepam (Valium)*.

As noted earlier, the most frequent complication following a heart attack is an arrhythmia. The increased irritability of the damaged heart makes it more susceptible to irregular heartbeats; in particular, *ventricular premature beats (VPBs)*. VPBs occur in 90% of all heart attack victims in the first four hours after admission to a coronary care unit. Normally these VPBs are not serious, but occasionally after a heart attack they can cause the heart to go into *ventricular fibrillation*, a state in which the heart flutters, but does not actually produce an effective beat. Ventricular fibrillation is the leading cause of death following a heart attack. In a coronary care unit, VPBs can be prevented or treated with stabilizing medication (e.g., *Lidocaine* or *Quinidine*).

In the last few years a new treatment has been used in treating severe, persisting heart attacks in an attempt to actually dissolve the *clot* or *thrombus* that is blocking the coronary artery. By dissolving the clot, the blocked artery can be reopened, returning blood flow to the damaged

area. Dissolving the clot both limits the damage in the affected area and keeps the clot from extending. Two different kinds of drugs are used to dissolve the clot: *streptokinase enzyme* or *tissue-type plasminogen activator (t-PA)*, which is made with recombinant DNA techniques. The drugs are simply given intravenously, or they may be given during coronary arteriography. Treatment must begin within three to six hours after the heart attack—before the damage is done. It is reserved for selected patients who can be treated within about four hours after their heart attack, who have ECG evidence of damage, and who continue to experience chest pain, indicating that the heart attack may be extending. The use of streptokinase or t-PA to dissolve the clot is a promising therapy, but it is new enough that the implications are still not understood. One study dealing with t-PA showed that the artery reopened in 66% of the patients given t-PA, as opposed to 24% in the group given a placebo. Furthermore, the t-PA group had better heart function than the control group ten days after the heart attack. The technique appears to be of great promise and is likely to be used more and more commonly. Another relatively new technique used when the heart attack appears to be extending is *coronary angioplasty*, a procedure in which a balloon catheter is inserted into the heart and expanded to widen the coronary artery at the point of damage (see p. 274).

In the case of a severe heart attack that is complicated by heart failure, powerful *diuretics* will be given to lower the fluid volume in the bloodstream, enabling the heart to pump less forcefully. Other drugs will be given to raise blood pressure and thereby increase the heart's efficiency. *Heart failure* is a condition in which the heart fails to pump enough blood to meet the body's needs. In addition to heart attacks, failure is caused commonly by prolonged high blood pressure, coronary heart disease, or heart valve disease. The symptoms of heart failure are shortness of breath during slight exercise, shortness of breath upon lying flat, weakness and fatigue, low blood pressure, and *pulmonary edema*, or fluid in the lungs.

The length of time people spend in the coronary care unit (CCU) depends on the severity of their heart attack, their subsequent progress and lack of complications, and the philosophy of their doctor. With an uncomplicated heart attack, patients move from CCU to a step-down unit within three to four days. At this point, they are encourged to spend periods of time out of bed, either walking or sitting in a chair. While they are in the hospital, they will continue to be monitored with ECGs and blood tests. They may also be given *nuclear cardiac tests*, in which a radioactive chemical is used to outline the wall of the heart, making it possible to visualize the exact damage done by the heart attack.

Following an uncomplicated heart attack, patients are released from the hospital in one to two weeks. They are advised to follow a graded exercise program, alter their diet, work to lower the stress in their life, and give up smoking (see section on *Self-Care*). In addition, many doctors now routinely put heart attack patients on *beta-adrenergic blocking drugs (see p. 272)* when they are released. Several studies have shown that these drugs lower the risk of a second heart attack in the months after the initial one. People who have severe heart attacks or complications are kept in the hospital for more than a week or two. If these people now develop heart pain after relatively little exertion, they are treated for angina (see p. 267). It is important for people to continue to see their doctor for follow-up after a heart attack. Part of the doctor's role is to help deal with the worry and depression that often occur after a heart attack.

Ruling Out Other Diseases

There are a number of causes of chest pain other than a heart attack. Strains or sprains of the chest wall muscles, ligaments, and ribs are a frequent cause of chest pain. As compared to a heart attack, this pain is generally duller, more gnawing, more localized, and more superficial. Usually such pain is made worse by moving or coughing, and can be elicited by pressing on a particular area of the chest. *Bursitis* can cause pain radiating down one arm and into the shoulder (see p. 310). *Pleurisy*, an inflammation of the lining of the lungs, causes sharp chest pain and coughing.

Anxiety, another frequent cause of chest pain, is most commonly experienced by middle-aged people who worry that they are having a heart attack. This kind of chest pain generally occurs on the left side of the chest, below the nipple. Characteristically, it involves a dull ache that persists for hours, accompanied by short stabbing pains that occur at random intervals. Such *psychogenic* or *functional chest pain* frequently occurs along with *hyperventilation*, that is, a feeling of breathlessness, and it varies with a person's activities and/or mood.

Several gastrointestinal conditions can cause pain that is confused with a heart attack, although such pain more often is brief and stabbing, or dull and burning. *Hiatus hernia* can cause midchest pain, as well as heartburn (see p. 372). *Ulcers* can cause gnawing pain in the stomach area after meals (see p. 353). A *gall bladder attack* causes pain and tenderness in the upper right abdomen and chest (see p. 372).

In general, any pain that lasts less than 30 seconds at a time is not heart pain. But any severe chest pain in a person over 35 should be evaluated by a doctor. Often the cause will not be a heart attack, but since time is such a significant factor in a heart attack, it's important that any severe or persistent chest pain be properly evaluated by a doctor.

Prevention

Much can be done in terms of long-range prevention of a heart attack. Changes in diet, exercise, and stress levels can prevent atherosclerosis and even reverse it to some extent. See the sections on *Self-Care* and *Atherosclerosis* (p. 310).

Irregular Heartbeats, Palpitations, or Arrhythmias

Symptoms

- unpleasant or nervous awareness of heartbeat
- pounding heartbeat
- feeling of heart stopping, fluttering, or skipping beats
- fast or irregular pulse
- fainting spell

Description

Under normal circumstances, the heart has a steady and predictable rhythm which results in the carefully coordinated pumping of its four chambers. The rate or speed at which the heart beats depends on an individual's activity level, emotional state, and level of fitness. Unlike the skeletal muscles, the heart muscle contracts involuntarily and without the stimulation of a nerve impulse. Each contraction or beat is initiated by a special area of cells called the *sinoatrial (SA) node*, or *pacemaker*. The pacemaker is lo-

cated near where the *superior vena cava*, the vein that returns blood from the body, joins the right chamber of the heart, the *right atrium* (see illustration).

An electrical discharge in the SA node causes the *atria*, the upper or "priming" chambers of the heart, to contract and fill the lower chambers —which in turn send blood to the lungs (via the right ventricle) and body (via the left ventricle). The electrical impulse started by the SA node travels down the heart to the lower chambers, the *ventricles*, causing them to contract momentarily after the atria. The electrical impulse reaches the juncture between the atria and the ventricles in a few hundredths of a second. Because the atria are insulated from the ventricles by a layer of fat, the impulse can only cross to the lower chambers via specialized conducting tissue called the *atrialventricular (AV) node*. The AV node delays the impulse another few hundredths of a second, which just gives the ventricles time to fill. From the AV node, the impulse spreads down the ventricles, causing them to contract. The process continues over and over again, in a rhythmic fashion, so that the atria fill and pump slightly ahead of the ventricles. If the normal sequence of events is upset, the rate or regularity of the heartbeat is disturbed, and an arrhythmia results.

The most common arrhythmias are momentary, and occur in completely healthy people. In a healthy heart, a brief interruption in the flow of blood is not significant and is quickly compensated for. Under such circumstances, arrhyth-

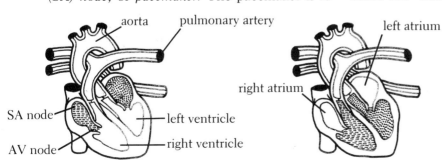

aorta   pulmonary artery   left atrium

right atrium

SA node — left ventricle

AV node — right ventricle

Each heartbeat is initiated by an area of cells called the SA *node or pacemaker. The electrical impulse causes the top chambers of the heart to contract, then crosses the* AV node *and causes the lower chambers to contract almost immediately.*

mias are rarely harmful and are not signs of heart disease. Less commonly, there are some arrhythmias that are caused by underlying heart disease and accompany a heart condition or heart attack. For people with heart disease, arrhythmias can present a serious problem because their blood flow may already be reduced.

There are several different types of arrhythmias, the most common being caused by a premature beat, either in the atria or the ventricles. These are referred to as *atrial premature beats (APBs)* or *ventricular premature beats (VPBs)*. They are caused by random discharges from outside the normal pacemaker, the SA node. If the discharge is caused by cells in the atria, an APB results; if the cells are in the ventricles, a VPB results. Both types of arrhythmias can be brought on by fatigue, emotional tension, alcohol, caffeine, or tobacco. APBs and VPBs are common in people of all ages, whether or not they have heart disease. In healthy people, premature beats have no medical significance. An APB is hard for people to notice, although they may be aware of a beat that is more forceful than usual because the ventricles have been allowed to overfill due to the long pause.

VPBs are the most common form of arrhythmia in people without heart disease. VPBs cause the ventricle to contract earlier than normal, so the pause between beats is twice as long as normal. This long pause is very obvious, and is readily perceived as a skipped beat. Both APBs and VPBs frequently disappear in people with a healthy heart as soon as they do some form of exercise. VPBs are significant in people with known heart disease (angina or heart attack), because they are associated with a higher incidence of another, more dangerous, arrhythmia called *ventricular fibrillation*. In this situation, the premature impulse doesn't cause the ventricles to contract early, it causes them to contract continuously in fine rippling motions. Fibrillation can cause death because, as long as it continues, no blood is pumped to the body.

Another common arrhythmia is *paroxysmal atrial tachycardia*, an episode of sudden rapid heartbeats that are not due to exercise or fear. It is more common among healthy young adults than people with heart disease, and it has no medical significance. Whereas a normal heart rate in healthy people is 60–100 beats per minute at rest, during an episode of tachycardia, the heartbeat ranges from 140–240—usually around 170–220. When this happens, people can feel their heart racing. These episodes usually begin suddenly, and end just as abruptly, although they can last for hours. If they persist, they can easily be treated (see section on *The Doctor*).

All the other arrhythmias are much less common and are likely to be associated with some form of heart disease. They include *atrial fibrillation*, and *bradycardia* or slowed heartbeats, and blocks in the bundle of Hiss, fibers that affect pumping in the ventricles. All these arrhythmias can be serious and should be under a doctor's treatment.

Self-Care

Skipped beats are generally not a problem in a healthy younger person and do not require treatment. However, if they are accompanied by shortness of breath or chest pain, or if they do not go away within several minutes, the doctor should be called. Because skipped beats are most often caused by stress, anxiety, tobacco, alcohol, or caffeine, they are best treated by relaxation (see p. 60). When a person is under a lot of stress and experiencing arrhythmias, it is important to deal with the cause of the stress. If a particular substance can be identified as causing the arrhythmia, it should be avoided.

Paroxysmal atrial tachycardia, or sudden rapid heartbeat, can actually be treated effectively with self-help. To stop tachycardia, people should take a deep breath, hold it, and blow out or push against a closed windpipe by contracting their abdominal muscles. Other methods are coughing, holding the breath, putting one's head between one's knees, or gagging or vomiting. All of these maneuvers break the cycle by stimulating the *vagus nerve* to the heart, which causes the heart to slow down and delays the conduction of electrical impulses from the atria to the ventricles.

The Doctor

To diagnose an arrhythmia, the doctor (a cardiologist, internist, or family practitioner) will take a medical history and perform a physical exam, paying special attention to heart sounds and pulses, and, most important, will do an electrocardiogram (ECG). An ECG (see illustration) provides a graph of the heart's electrical activity during a contraction, as the electrical potential spreads from the pacemaker down across the heart. The first part of the cycle, called the *P wave*, reflects the contraction of the atria. Next there is the *QRS complex* which represents ventricular contraction. Finally there is a *T wave*, as muscle cells in the ventricles repolarize electrically.

Aberrant patterns in the ECG sequence reveal the presence of particular arrhythmias. For example, with atrial premature beats (APBs), the P wave is earlier than normal, showing that the atria are contracting before the pacemaker. With ventricular premature beats, the QRS complex is early, showing that the ventricles have contracted earlier than normal. In paroxysmal atrial tachycardia, the heartbeat is very rapid and shows abnormal P and QRS waves.

Treatment depends on the particular arrhythmia and on the presence or absence of underlying heart disease. For those arrhythmias that require care, the most common treatment is drugs. Premature beats are only treated if a person has heart disease. In that case, APBs and VPBs are treated with *antiarrhythmic drugs* such as *quinidine, procainamide,* or *beta-adrenergic blockers* (see p. 283). Quinidine, which is made

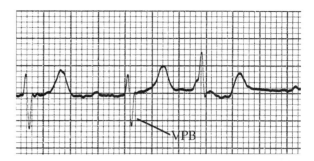

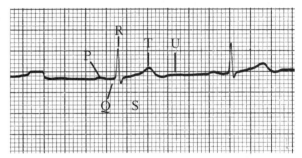

An electrocardiogram (ECG) gives a visual representation of the electrical activity that takes place in the heart during a heartbeat. Abnormalities in different parts of the ECG give an indication of various arrhythmias and heart conditions.

from the bark of the cinchona tree, depresses electrical activity in abnormal cells, but doesn't affect the cells in the pacemaker area. These characteristics make it effective against many different types of arrhythmias, including premature beats and atrial flutter or fibrillation.

PATs, or paroxysmal atrial tachycardia episodes, are initially treated with "mechanical" or nondrug measures, such as breath-holding (see section on *Self-Care*). If an episode does not respond to these treatments, the doctor can put pressure on the *carotid sinuses* in the neck, which slows the heartbeat to normal in 50% of all episodes. If the heartbeat still does not slow, one of a number of drugs can be given; the most common being *Verapamil* which slows conduction in the AV node, which carries the impulse from the atria to the ventricles.

Rarer and more complicated arrhythmias are treated with a variety of antiarrhythmic agents. In most cases, people with these arrhythmias are also being treated for other heart problems. In a few cases, when severe arrhythmias do not respond to drugs, an operation may be performed to install a *pacemaker*, an electronic device that delivers a pulse that causes the heart to beat steadily. It is used to treat various conduction difficulties, in particular, *atrialventricular block*, a condition in which the impulse from the atria to the ventricles does not conduct at the normal speed. The symptom of heart block is *bradycardia*, which is a heart rate slow enough to produce fainting or heart failure.

Ruling Out Other Diseases

It should be noted that heartbeat normally speeds up with exercise, emotion, fever, and in response to a number of drugs, including medical drugs and cocaine. Normally after exercise, resting slows the heartrate within a short period of time. *Sinus arrhythmia* is another normal variation that people occasionally confuse with an arrhythmia when they are taking their own pulse. In this case, the heart speeds up when air is inhaled, and slows down when air is exhaled. This response is due to the influence of the sympathetic nervous system (fight-or-flight response) on the vagus nerve to the heart. Acute anxiety, which can cause a *pounding heart*, is also sometimes mistaken for an arrhythmia. All of these situations can readily be distinguished by an ECG.

Prevention

Premature beats generally do not need to be prevented in a healthy person because they have no medical significance. If they are frequent and bothersome, they can be prevented by relaxing and lowering anxiety. Reducing or eliminating smoking, caffeine and alcohol will also help to eliminate palpitations or premature beats. If palpitations are a side effect of drugs such as insulin, digitalis, or diuretics, the particular dosage or drug can be altered so as to eliminate the problem.

Asthma

Symptoms

- wheezing
- shortness of breath
- coughing that may raise phlegm
- tightness in the chest
- attacks frequently take place at night

Description

Asthma, which is characterized by episodes of wheezing and difficulty in breathing, is a disease in which the *trachea*, or windpipe, and the *bronchi*, the large airways leading to the lungs, are unusually responsive to a wide variety of stimuli. As a result, a significant portion of the airway narrows—a change which is reversible, either spontaneously or with treatment. This general description of the disease has been agreed upon by asthma researchers only after much discussion, because the condition can be triggered by so many different factors and situations.

Asthma is very common: approximately 5% of the U.S. population (10 million people) have the disease. The incidence of asthma is high in childhood, drops in adolescence and early adulthood, and rises again in middle age and old age. Half the cases are diagnosed between ages 2 and 17, but a third of all asthmatics are diagnosed after the age of 30.

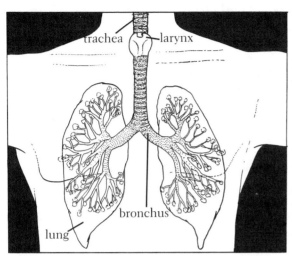

The respiratory tract includes the lungs and the bronchi (the tubes leading to the lungs). In asthma, the bronchi are unusually reactive, and narrow in response to a wide variety of stimuli.

A typical asthma attack consists of wheezing and difficulty breathing, accompanied by a cough and a tight feeling in the chest. Attacks occur more frequently at night, and can even begin during sleep. They last anywhere from a few minutes, to a few hours, to a few days. They may stop spontaneously or require medication. Between attacks people may be completely free of symptoms. People with more serious asthma may have mild symptoms even between attacks, and more severe symptoms during attacks. On the other hand, some asthmatics never have "attacks," only continuous symptoms.

For years, doctors divided asthma into two types: extrinsic and intrinsic. Currently, doctors think that most cases are a mixture of both types, but the distinction can be very helpful in understanding what triggers an attack. *Extrinsic asthma* is associated with a history of allergies to various substances. Most often, it develops in childhood, varies with the seasons, and has a distinct familial association. This type of asthma

often disappears as a child grows older. It represents about 10% of all asthma cases. *Intrinsic asthma* is not associated with allergies; it is triggered by infections or exposure to respiratory irritants. This type of asthma usually begins after the age of 30, is not seasonal, and is generally more severe than asthma that develops in childhood. Most asthmatics over the age of 35 have intrinsic asthma, although 80% of all asthmatic patients have features of both kinds.

Asthma is a complicated disease whose causes are still not well understood. With extrinsic asthma, an *allergen*, a substance that people are allergic to (e.g., dust, pollen, animal dander), stimulates special cells in the airways called *mast cells*. These cells normally protect the lungs by producing antibodies against bacterial and viral infections, but in a person with extrinsic asthma, these cells become overreactive, identifying and making antibodies against substances that aren't even germs. Once the cells recognize a particular allergen, they become covered with antibodies that pick up those allergens. When an allergen bridges two antibodies on the surface of the mast cell, the cell releases several potent chemicals, the most important of which is *histamine*. These chemicals cause the symptoms of the asthma attack. The smooth muscles surrounding the airway contract and cause the airway to narrow. Mucous cells begin producing mucus, which fills the already narrowed airway passages. Finally, the tiny capillaries nearby dilate and become permeable to fluid. This causes the area to swell, further constricting the already narrowed airway, and making it difficult to breathe.

Intrinsic asthma is not related to allergies. It is believed that this form of asthma is caused by a hyperactive parasympathetic nervous system. Among the cells lining the windpipe are special nerve endings called *irritant receptors*. When these cells pick up dirt, dust, and foreign substances, they relay a message to the brain which

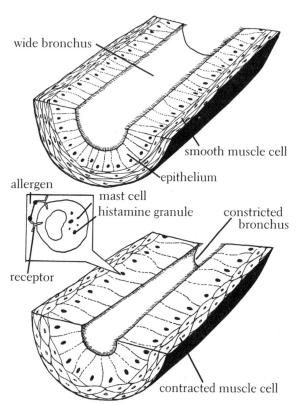

In a person with asthma, the mast cells in the lining of the bronchial tubes release histamine which causes smooth muscle cells in the bronchial walls to contract, narrowing the tubes.

causes the smooth muscle around the windpipe to contract to "protect" the lungs. Researchers think that the irritant receptors have a lower reaction threshold in a person with intrinsic asthma.

Most adults with asthma have a combination of the extrinsic and intrinsic varieties. In the mixed type of asthma, a group of foreign substances may excite the irritant receptors, and/or specific allergens may stimulate the mast cells. Once one reaction triggers an attack, the other reaction usually occurs as well.

Asthma attacks can be triggered by a wide variety of stimuli. Every asthmatic has his or her own triggers. Extrinsic asthma is triggered by whatever substances people are allergic to, including pollens, dust, fur, feathers, and foods. The most common trigger for intrinsic asthma is a cold or upper respiratory infection. Allergists theorize that a cold lowers the threshold of the irritant receptors. Airborne pollutants definitely stimulate attacks, and heavy smog increases the number of emergency room visits for adults with a mixed type of asthma. Occupational dusts and fumes can specifically trigger attacks during daytime hours, but these can occur after work hours as well. Certain occupations tend to be problematic for people with asthma, including any kind of animal work, chemical work, woodwork, or food processing jobs. In about 10% of all asthmatics, aspirin and aspirin-containing compounds can set off an attack.

Exercise can also trigger difficulty with breathing. In fact, 95% of people with asthma experience some degree of exercise-induced asthma. This type of asthma attack comes on within 5–30 minutes after the start of exercise and is thought to be caused by cold air stimulating the irritant receptors in the airway. Forms of exercise that involve the arms, such as rowing or running, are more likely to cause problems than is bike riding. Even laughing or deep breathing in cold air can set off wheezing.

Finally, asthma attacks can be triggered by emotional upsets or stress. Although asthma is no longer considered to be a psychosomatic disease associated with a particular personality type or upbringing, it is definitely affected by a person's mental state. Any strong emotion such as anger, guilt, frustration, depression, anxiety, or even joy, has been known to trigger attacks. Interestingly, placebos (medicines without active ingredients) can reduce asthma symptoms dramatically. Contrarily, the suggestion that a medication inhaler contains allergens can trigger an attack. Because mental state has such a powerful effect on asthma symptoms, relaxation, auto-suggestion, biofeedback, and hypnosis have all been used with good results by asthmatics (see p. 60).

Self-Care

Self-help is one of the mainstays of asthma treatment. When asthma sufferers understand their disease, they are better able to prevent and control attacks. Many self-help programs have been devised by asthma clinics. Basically, these programs involve educating people about the physiology of the disease, teaching them to identify the causes of attacks and their early symptoms, and helping them learn to deal with and control symptoms in the early stages. These programs teach people to avoid situations that are known to trigger attacks, and to do relaxation exercises and deep breathing exercises to help

Self-Care for Asthma

- if you smoke, stop
- avoid substances that trigger your attacks
- allergy-proof your house (see p. 251)
- avoid upper respiratory infections; treat them promptly if they occur
- drink plenty of fluids
- avoid air-polluted environments
- don't mix nonprescription with prescription medications unless recommended by the doctor
- exercise within limits; swimming is less likely to aggravate asthma than other forms of strenuous exercise
- rest if difficult breathing occurs during exercise, or use an inhaler if your doctor recommends it
- avoid exercising in cold air if that causes problems
- use inhalers properly: shake well; hold 1 inch from mouth; exhale, then press top of inhaler while steadily breathing in until lungs are full; hold breath for 10 seconds. Don't overuse inhaler, it can irritate the lungs

an attack subside. Also, an important part of any self-care program is learning to use a prescription inhaler correctly (see chart).

Asthmatics who have some degree of extrinsic or allergic asthma, as confirmed by allergy tests, are advised to "allergy-proof" their house. This involves minimizing or eliminating prolonged exposure to products that contain or harbor feathers, fur, dander, and dust (see chart, p. 251). Like people who suffer from hay fever, people with asthma are advised to humidify the air in their rooms during the winter, and possibly to use an air filter or air conditioner. It's important that the temperature not be too low, because some asthmatics are affected by the cold. Exercise is psychologically and physically helpful for asthmatics, but they must take special care when exercising and they may require medication prior to beginning exercise.

Asthmatics should not smoke, and family members who do should refrain from it in the house. Smoke not only causes bronchial irritation, it also impairs antibacterial defense mechanisms which are particularly important in the case of intrinsic asthma. As compared with asthmatics who don't smoke, those who do smoke cigarettes have more attacks, need more medicine to handle them, and even have a higher incidence of attacks requiring hospitalization. Cigarette smoke from other people has been shown to cause a reduction in flow in asthmatics' airways and an increase in their symptoms. Finally, if people are severe asthmatics or they are suffering a severe attack, they should avoid certain medications, including sedatives, tranquilizers, and sleeping pills, because they all depress the respiratory sytem. The beta-blocker *propranolol (Inderal)*, which is used to treat angina, hypertension, heart attacks, and migraines can actually trigger asthma attacks. Those asthmatics whose symptoms are stimulated by aspirin should also avoid any compounds that contain aspirin.

The Doctor

Asthma is easily diagnosed by physical exam if a person is wheezing, or by several laboratory tests, including lung function studies. Often people will recognize the cause of their wheezing, based on the experience of other family members. When listening to an asthmatic's chest, the doctor will definitely hear wheezing during an attack, and sometimes between attacks. Wheezing is most characteristic on exhalation, but may also be heard on inhalation in people with severe asthma. During very bad attacks, the chest may be so congested that the only sign is significant difficulty with breathing, but no wheezing.

Several laboratory tests are done for diagnostic purposes. A white blood cell count will be done because the cell count is frequently elevated during attacks. A microscopic inspection of the mucus or *sputum* will often show *casts*, epithelial cells that look like plugs because they have been molded in the shape of the tiny airways of the lungs. An *x-ray* of the chest may reveal more air than normal in the lungs. This hyperinflated state is due to the fact that the person is having difficulty expelling air from the lungs. Often *pulmonary function studies* will be done as well. By having people breathe into a calibrated machine, the doctor can determine exactly how much air is being moved in and out. During an asthma attack, the amount of air that people can exhale drops below normal. Pulmonary function studies not only aid in diagnosing asthma, they help the doctor determine how severe a particular attack is, and therefore how aggressively it should be treated. During or shortly after an initial attack, the doctor may order *allergy skin tests* to help determine whether a person has extrinsic (allergic) characteristics.

The doctor treats asthma attacks with *bronchodilators*, drugs that cause the bronchi to open, making breathing easier. Currently, there are a wide range of drugs available in a variety of different strengths. The drugs the doctor uses will be carefully tailored depending on the specific needs of the patient, the frequency of attacks, and the severity of the immediate attack. Treatment ranges from a maintenance regimen for a person with minimal symptoms and occasional mild attacks, to aggressive intervention for an acute episode of some severity.

The doctor treats an acute attack with *sympathomimetic drugs*, which affect the sympathetic nervous system. There are three types of receptors in the sympathetic nervous system: alpha receptors, beta 1 receptors, and beta 2 receptors. *Alpha receptors* cause constriction of smooth muscle in blood vessels, the gastrointestinal tract, and the bladder. *Beta 1 receptors* increase heartbeat, and *beta 2 receptors* cause relaxation of the smooth muscle in the wall of the bronchi, dilation of blood vessels, and tremors in the voluntary muscles.

One of the oldest sympathomimetic drugs is *epinephrine*, which stimulates all three types of sympathetic receptors. It is given as a subcutaneous injection or an inhalant (*Medihaler-Epi*). As new drugs have been developed, epinephrine use has declined because of undesirable side effects such as rapid heart rate, pallor, shakiness, headache, nausea, and vomiting. But it is still used for some sudden, severe attacks because it is such a rapid-acting, potent bronchodilator. Two other long-used sympathomimetic drugs are *isoproterenol (Medihaler-Iso)* and *isoetharine (Bronkosol)*. These inhalants affect the beta 1 and beta 2 receptors, and have side effects similar to epinephrine. More recently, a whole group of drugs has been developed that only affect beta 2 receptors. These basically dilate the bronchi without speeding up the heart. They include *metaproterenol (Alupent, Metaprel)*, *terbutaline (Brethine)*, and *albuterol (Proventil or Ventolin)*.

Almost all of the sympathomimetic drugs are available in *metered dose inhalers* that are convenient to carry and easy to administer, with proper instruction. Inhalers release the drugs in large droplets, which become increasingly smaller over distance because they lose moisture as they get farther into the airway. Since only the tiniest droplets can enter passages that are very congested, it's important to inhale the drugs slowly and deeply so that the droplets can get farther into the areas of congestion. For maximum effect, a person should hold his or her breath for 10 seconds after inhaling the medicine. Manufacturers are now making inhalers with tube spacers or reservoir systems that automatically break up the droplets.

The other class of drugs frequently used to treat asthma is the *methylxanthines*, the most common ones being the *theophyllines*, which dilate the smooth muscle in the airways by affecting the enzymes that actually cause muscle contraction. The theophyllines—including *caffeine*, which is a member of the methylxanthine family—are central nervous system stimulants. The theophyllines are usually taken in long-lasting pill form.

At the earliest sign of an attack, people should either use their inhaler, take a theophylline pill, or do both. If this treatment is not sufficient to break the attack, and the attack persists or becomes worse, the doctor should be seen. In rare cases, a severe attack can actually be life-threatening, so it's important to take severe or persistent attacks seriously. In addition to giving larger or stronger doses of sympathomimetic drugs and/or theophylline, the doctor will give oxygen, monitor the patient's breathing to adjust the dosage of medication, and if necessary give drugs and fluids intravenously. In some cases a patient may be given an automatic inhalant machine *(power nebulizer)* and/or intravenous *steroids* to aid in bronchial dilation.

Some drugs are given to prevent asthma attacks. One such drug is the inhalant *cromolyn sodium*, which acts on the mast cells to reduce their release of the chemical histamine. The drug is not effective for an acute attack. Cromolyn sodium is used for people with moderate-to-severe asthma who don't respond to bronchodilator therapy. It is also used to prevent exercise-induced asthma.

Ruling Out Other Diseases

Wheezing is generally caused by asthma, but can also be caused, more rarely, by obstructive lung disease or *emphysema*, (see p. 304) and by *heart failure* (see p. 289). Emphysema generally goes along with a history of smoking and a long-standing cough that brings up sputum; wheezing is not the main symptom and does not bring on attacks. In the case of heart failure, the person has a history of heart disease or a heart attack, significant fatigue on walking, and shortness of breath when lying down.

Prevention

Asthma itself cannot be prevented, but the attacks can be. Known triggering agents should be avoided and an allergen-free house should be maintained if a person has characteristics of extrinsic asthma. People with asthma (and household members) should not smoke and should promptly treat colds and flus. Early symptoms of an asthma attack should be treated directly to minimize the severity of the attack. Finally, stress reduction techniques can be beneficial, especially when a person's asthma is triggered by emotional factors (see p. 60).

Lung Cancer, or Bronchogenic Carcinoma

Symptoms

- coughing that generally brings up a small amount of mucus
- coughing up blood, or blood-streaked mucus
- difficulty breathing
- lack of appetite
- weight loss
- chest pain

Description

Lung cancer is the leading cause of death from cancer among men. Among women, lung cancer will soon become the leading cancer, replacing carcinoma of the breast. There has been a phenomenal and steady rise in the incidence of lung cancer over the last 50 years: in 1950, there were 18,313 deaths from lung cancer in the U.S.; in 1977, there were 90,828; and in 1986, there were over 150,000.

Approximately 85% of all lung cancer is caused by smoking. The fact that men presently get lung cancer twice as frequently as women is directly related to the number of men and women who smoke, and the length of time they've been smoking. There are several types of lung cancer. They are classified by the particular type of cell that becomes malignant, the most common being *adenocarcinoma* (35%), *squamous cell carcinoma* (35%), and *small cell* and *large cell carcinoma* (both 10%–20%). Squamous cell and small cell carcinoma are most closely associated with smoking, although the other types are also related to smoking habits.

Over the past few years, the link between lung

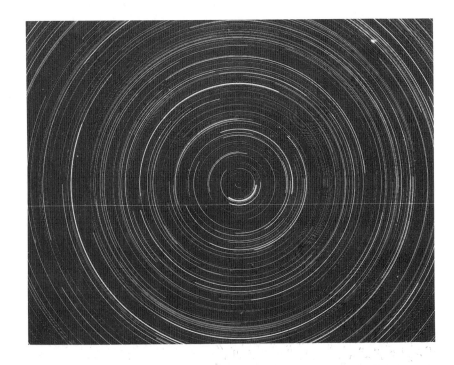

Visualizing oneself at one with the universe can help to reduce stress and improve the functioning of the immune system. Polar Star Trails. Lick Observatory.

cancer and smoking has become much clearer. Researchers no longer question whether smoking is a causal factor; more than 50 studies have demonstrated an incontrovertible connection. One of the most recent studies, the Third National Cancer Survey (TNCS), surveyed 7,500 randomly selected people and found 9.9 times the average rate of lung cancer among heavy smokers. Studies done on identical twins have ruled out a simple genetic disease. Combining data from the eight largest studies demonstrates the strength of the association between cigarettes and lung cancer: male smokers are 10 times as likely to develop lung cancer as non-smokers; heavy smokers, those who smoke more than 20 cigarettes a day, have 15–25 times the incidence of lung cancer. To put it another way, one study showed that a two-pack-a-day smoker's life expectancy was shortened by about 5½ minutes for each cigarette smoked. The strength of the association is completely *dose dependent*, that is, the rate goes up directly in proportion to the number of cigarettes smoked per day, the number of years smoking, and the depth of inhalation. It should be noted that low-tar and low-nicotine cigarettes have been found to have less of an effect than nonfiltered cigarettes. All the human data on smoking has been backed up by the results of animal experiments. Using machines that delivered smoke, dogs have been found to develop lung cancer within 2½ years. Rats who were simply kept in smoke-filled rooms have developed overgrowths of the nasal epithelial cells, and later, lung cancers. On a more positive note, studies have shown that the likelihood of lung cancer drops steadily once a person stops smoking: 15–20 years after quitting, an ex-smoker's lung cancer rate is no higher than that of a person who never smoked.

Each milliliter of smoke contains 5 billion microscopic particles. These particles are not only irritative, some of them are carcinogenic. Over 3,600 chemicals are formed in the 950-degree heat of the burning tip of a cigarette. In particular, cigarette smoke contains three different types of chemicals that affect the incidence of cancer. One group, called *initiators*, are chemicals that enter the DNA of epithelial cells in the lungs and bind directly to it, causing these cells to reproduce at an uncontrolled rate. The second group, *promoters*, consists of chemicals that do not cause cancer by themselves, but aid other chemicals that are carcinogens. The last group, the *cocarcinogens*, act directly with another chemical to cause cancer (see page 143). The most powerful carcinogenic initiator is a poly-nuclear aromatic hydrocarbon that results from the burning of the tar in tobacco. When this type of initiator is applied to the skin in mice, it causes skin cancer.

Lung cancer is diagnosed most frequently between the ages of 45 and 75, but autopsies show that the development of lung cancer is a long, slow process. It starts with the death of *cilia*, the microscopic fingerlike cells that line the airways and help to clear away mucus and foreign particles. Next, the epithelial cells lining the lungs and bronchi begin to reproduce at an accelerated rate, resulting in an overgrowth of cells. In time, the cells produced begin to appear somewhat atypical, and these unusual cells gradually replace many of the normal cells. Up to this point, the changes are reversible, and if people cease smoking, normal cells will replace the atypical ones. However, if people continue to smoke, areas of atypical cells may eventually become malignant.

The various types of lung cancer are generally slow-growing. It is estimated that most tumors have existed for five to ten years before they are discovered. For much of this time, the tumor does not cause definitive symptoms, and would not even show up on x-ray. With small, localized, or slow-growing tumors, the cure rate is quite good. If not diagnosed early, the tumor may have grown quite large, invading nearby tissue such as air passages and blood vessels. If it has metastasized, or spread to other parts of the body, the tumor can be difficult to treat, and does not have a high cure rate.

The first symptom of lung cancer is a cough that increases steadily in both frequency and severity. Often, until a person coughs up blood-tinged sputum, this symptom goes unnoticed because most smokers have chronic low-level bronchitis and have been coughing for years. A change in the character of a chronic cough is a sign that something new is happening. Another common presentation is that the smoker develops a bacterial pneumonia that does not respond promptly to antibiotics because it is in an area blocked by the tumor. When a tumor becomes large enough, a person may even experience shortness of breath and difficulty breathing due to the impairment of lung tissue. If a tumor has spread before it is diagnosed, other symptoms, such as chest or rib pain, may be present as well.

Self-Care

Several self-help regimens have been shown to improve the quality of life after lung cancer has been diagnosed. Among the most effective seem to be stress-reduction techniques such as relaxation, meditation, and guided imagery. Visualization techniques may increase the white blood cells' ability to destroy the tumor cells (see p. 67); however, the effectiveness of this technique has not been thoroughly studied. The most clearly demonstrated value of such techniques lies in their ability to minimize the negative side effects of chemotherapy and radiation. Imagery techniques have been described by Dr. Carl O. Simonton and Stephanie Simonton in *Getting Well Again;* by Dr. Bernie Siegel in *Love, Medicine, and Miracles;* by Harold Benjamin in *From Victim to Victor;* and in our book, *Seeing With the Mind's Eye.* Other alternative cancer therapies have not been studied extensively. Although none of the alternative tech-

niques have been shown to extend life in randomized studies, there is some anecdotal evidence that they both extend life and help to improve quality of life.

Currently there are a number of support groups for cancer patients and their families, such as *The Wellness Community* (213-393-1415) and *Commonweal Cancer Retreats* (415-868-0970). These groups deal with both the physical effects of cancer and cancer treatment, and the psychosocial problems faced by cancer patients. Self-help groups teach stress reduction techniques, meditation, and imagery—as well as provide support—all with the goal of enhancing the immune system. No one can predict the outcome of cancer. Remissions do occur, and therapies are constantly improving. With lung cancer, as with all types of cancer, there are a definite percentage of people who get well. A positive attitude and the existence of support networks counteract the negative effects of chemotherapy and radiation, improve quality of life, and may help to extend life.

The Doctor

Out of the 29 million annual doctor visits in which coughing is the chief complaint, the overwhelming majority are due to upper respiratory infections or bronchitis; only 1 in 300 is due to lung cancer. To diagnose or rule out lung cancer, the doctor does a careful history, a physical exam that includes listening to the chest, and several lab exams. Most often, nothing is found on the physical exam, although occasionally there may be diminished breath sounds when the doctor listens to the patient's lungs.

The most important diagnostic test is a simple *chest x-ray.* It will be compared with previous x-rays, or in questionable cases with a follow-up x-ray. Almost all cases of symptomatic lung cancer will show up on a chest x-ray. Another important test is a *cytological study* of the sputum, or phlegm; in many cases, tumor cells will actually be seen under the microscope. The final test is a *bronchoscopic examination* in which a small fiberoptic tube is passed into the bronchi to examine the questionable area seen on x-ray, and obtain a sample of the tissue. In some cases a tissue sample may be obtained through a procedure called a *percutaneous needle aspiration*, in which a needle is passed through the chest wall. If the sample is malignant, further tests will be done to see if the tumor has spread. These tests include *blood chemistries*, a *CT scan*, and possibly *lymph node biopsies*. Based on the results, a tumor is *staged* according to its size and whether it has metastasized or spread.

With most types of lung cancer, the treatment of choice is *surgical removal* of the tumor, provided it has not spread. If a tumor is not operable, *radiation* and sometimes *laser coagulation* are done to improve the symptoms. For small cell cancers, treatment involves a course of *chemotherapy* or a combination of *chemotherapy* and *radiation*.

The cure rate, or *5-year survival rate*, depends almost entirely on whether the tumor has spread. If there is no metastasis, the cure rate is approximately 70% after surgery. Overall, the cure rate is much lower, but each person's case is unique, and no one can predict the outcome.

Ruling Out Other Diseases

The vast majority of coughs are due to *colds* (see p. 208) or *bronchitis* (see p. 304), even in smokers over 40. To rule out lung cancer, an x-ray and other tests may be done.

Prevention

The people at greatest risk for lung cancer are heavy smokers 40–45 years of age or older. Some doctors advise that these people get routine sputum cytologies and/or chest x-rays in order to increase the likelihood of diagnosing lung cancer in the early stages. Although overall these tests have not been shown to cause a great increase in life expectancy, they may be important in individual cases. Also, frequent screening may make people understand the serious risk posed by continuing to smoke.

The main focus of lung cancer prevention lies in getting people to stop smoking. Thanks to massive public education, cigarette smoking has dropped from 42% of adults in 1965, to 26% in 1988. It has been found that, in addition to public education, a brief discussion of risk factors by a doctor will have a significant effect on many smokers. Studies show that 95% of the people who quit cigarettes do it by themselves. Of the remaining 5%, many are helped by group programs. The success rate of these courses ranges from 20%–50%. Once people quit, it is important to reinforce or strengthen their decision. Strategies used by various programs include support from family and friends, financial incentives from oneself or business, and relaxation techniques (see p. 60). It is also important that former smokers become aware of situations that may be precursors to relapse, including feelings of frustration, anxiety, anger, and depression, and that they take note of prosmoking social models, cues, and settings.

Bronchitis and Emphysema

Symptoms

acute bronchitis
- coughing, possibly raising of mucus
- fever
- hoarseness
- chest pain
- tiredness
- recent history of a viral upper respiratory infection

chronic bronchitis
- cough that raises mucus
- often, wheezing on exhalation

emphysema
- cough with sputum production
- wheezing
- shortness of breath and/or difficulty breathing

Description

Bronchitis is a condition in which the lining of the *bronchi*, the large airways leading to the lungs, become inflamed either due to infection or due to constant irritation. Two types of cells in the bronchial lining help to protect against damage: *goblet cells* produce mucus, and *cilia*, little fingerlike projections, move the mucus and any foreign particles out of the airway. Normally, the goblet cells produce less than a half cup of mucus per day, which people swallow without being aware of it. When the lining is inflamed or irritated, more mucus is produced and the cilia are temporarily paralyzed. As a result, mucus collects in the airways and must be cleared by reflex coughing. The type of cough associated with bronchitis comes from deep in the chest and brings up *phlegm* or *sputum*; it is accompanied by a rattling sound and sensation.

There are two types of bronchitis—acute and chronic. *Acute bronchitis* is an infection of the upper respiratory tract; it is most often caused by a viral infection, or less commonly by a bacterial infection. The infection affects the throat and bronchi. Unlike pneumonia, bronchitis does not affect the *alveoli*, the millions of tiny air sacs in the lungs. Acute bronchitis can be associated with *laryngitis* (hoarseness) or, in children, with *croup*. Typically, acute bronchitis follows a cold and is a complication of it: first people develop a runny nose and sore throat; subsequently, they develop a deep cough, which may or may not bring up phlegm. Basically, acute bronchitis heals by itself and is seldom severe in adults. If the cough persists for more than one to two weeks, and the phlegm changes from clear to yellow or green, a secondary bacterial infection may have developed which will need treatment.

Chronic bronchitis is a very different condition, with a different cause. It is defined as a cough that brings up sputum and is present for at least three months of the year during a period of two successive years, but may be present continuously. Although the exact nature of the disease is unknown, most cases are intimately associated with cigarette smoking. A much smaller number of cases are due to constant exposure to high levels of irritants such as smog or industrial air pollutants. Researchers theorize that some people with chronic bronchitis have a genetic deficiency of an enzyme that normally protects the lungs from irritants. The amount of irritants in cigarette smoke is so great that all regular smokers have some degree of chronic bronchitis, but the more the genetic deficiency is expressed, the more severe a bronchitis they would tend to have.

Symptoms of chronic bronchitis can range from *simple chronic bronchitis* as evidenced by a mild "smoker's cough" that simply causes people to cough up a small amount of clear mucus after they wake up or have their first cigarette, to *chronic obstructive bronchitis*, as evidenced by a constant cough that raises greenish mucus and is accompanied by wheezing on exhalation. Over a period of years, smoker's cough can gradually and inexorably develop into chronic obstructive bronchitis. As it progresses, people experience more and more episodes of severe bronchitis in which the cough worsens, the sputum becomes thicker, and breathing becomes more difficult.

In some smokers, simple bronchitis progresses in a somewhat different manner and develops into *emphysema*. In this case the walls between the alveoli in the lungs break down, producing enlarged air sacs that actually collapse and stick together when people exhale. In addition, the total number of air sacs decreases, so there is less surface area within the lungs for oxygen to cross over into the bloodstream. Because of these changes, people get less oxygen than normal with each breath. Initially, people only notice the difficulty they have in breathing when they exercise; but eventually, if they continue to smoke, they develop constant shortness of breath.

Few smokers have either obstructive bronchitis or emphysema alone; most have a combination of the two conditions that is referred to as *chronic obstructive pulmonary disease (COPD)*. COPD is the second or third cause of disability in older people, following heart disease and

mental illness. Most regular smokers start showing symptoms of simple bronchitis in their 40s, and symptoms of obstructive lung disease in their 50s. Approximately 25% of the population in the U.S. eventually develops either chronic bronchitis, emphysema, or a combination of the two. These individuals become progressively limited in their physical activity because of shortness of breath. On an average, they lose 50–75 ml of lung capacity per year. At some point, they begin to find active tasks difficult; eventually, they experience shortness of breath even at rest and are subject to heart failure and repeated bouts of pneumonia.

Self-Care

Acute bronchitis generally responds readily to the same self-help treatment suggested for the common cold: increasing fluids, moistening the air, and coughing up mucus (see p. 211).

The symptoms of chronic bronchitis are relieved by the self-care remedies suggested for a cold and for asthma (see p. 294). In addition, there are home measures that will help to slow sputum production and make phlegm easier to raise. Increased fluids probably help to thin the secretions and makes them easier to cough up. A *graded exercise program* will strengthen skeletal muscles for breathing and also generally makes people feel better.

The only way to stop or slow down the insidious damage being done to the lungs is to stop all forms of smoking—cigarettes, pipes, or cigars. Simply put, cigarette smoke has the greatest concentration of irritants of any substance people put into their lungs, far exceeding the pollution of the air anywhere in the environment. Long-term studies reveal that even people with chronic obstructive pulmonary disease show less loss of lung volume per year, as well as a decrease in coughing and sputum production, once cigarette smoking stops. People who have

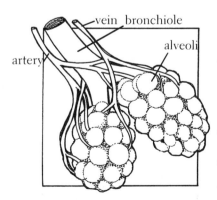

In people who have emphysema, the walls between the alveoli in the lungs break down, producing large air sacs that are less efficient than normal.

Breathing Exercises

Diaphragmatic breathing: lie on your back with your knees bent, and place one hand on your abdomen. Inhale deeply, pushing your abdomen up against your hand as you do so; let your abdomen fall as you exhale.

Pursed-lip breathing: sit or lie down in a relaxed position. Inhale normally through your nose, then purse your lips and exhale slowly against the resistance of your lips.

Staircase coughing: sitting in a comfortable position, take a slow deep breath and hold it. Then exhale in a repetitive fashion: exhale a little, then cough; exhale a little more, and cough again, etc.

---

chronic bronchitis, as opposed to more serious lung disease, can actually *restore* lung function to normal or near normal if they stop smoking. There is nothing the doctor can prescribe or do that is as important as not smoking. Many organizations (such as SmokEnders) now have programs and support groups to help people quit.

The Doctor

The doctor diagnoses acute bronchitis from a history of a cold and a deep cough, and from fluid-popping sounds, called *ronchi*, heard when the lungs are examined with a stethoscope. If there is a question of pneumonia, the doctor will order a *chest x-ray*. For acute bronchitis, the doctor will simply prescribe self-care regimens, and possibly pain medication if the person is very uncomfortable. In addition, if the sputum is yellow or green, or a sputum culture shows a bacterial infection, a course of antibiotics will be given.

Chronic bronchitis is diagnosed from a history of smoking and a persistent cough. A chest x-ray is usually done to rule out other lung diseases. *Pulmonary function studies* may be done by an internist who specializes in pulmonary

medicine and diseases of the chest, in order to assess the extent of lung function impairment. The first and most important treatment for any lung disease is to *stop smoking*. In addition, simple chronic bronchitis is treated with the same *bronchodilator agents* used for asthma (see p. 298). The bacterial infections commonly experienced by people with all types of chronic lung disease are treated with antibiotics such as *ampicillin, tetracycline,* or *trimethoprim-sulfamethoxazole.*

When simple chronic bronchitis progresses to chronic obstructive pulmonary disease (COPD), pulmonary function studies must be done on a regular basis to adjust medication and therapy. The goal of treatment is to make breathing easier and to prevent lung infections. Generally, the therapeutic regimen consists of bronchodilators and antibiotics, as needed. In severe episodes, people with COPD may be given *steroids* to make breathing easier, and *home oxygen therapy*, which is especially beneficial for sleeping. It's important to note that the sooner people with chronic bronchitis or COPD stop smoking and begin using bronchodilators, the more likely the damage to their lungs can be reversed or at least stopped.

Ruling Out Other Diseases

An x-ray helps to rule out other lung diseases such as *pneumonia* (see p. 307) or *lung cancer* (see p. 300). If wheezing is a major symptom, a person will be checked for *asthma*, in which case the wheezing can be eliminated or controlled with the proper combination of drugs. *Allergy testing* may also be done, especially if a person with chronic bronchitis does not smoke.

Prevention

Acute bronchitis can often be prevented or alleviated by promptly treating a cold with rest, fluids, and a humidifier. Such treatment is especially important for smokers and people who have a history of bronchitis.

Chronic bronchitis and COPD are among the most preventable of all severe diseases. The answer is simply to *stop smoking*. Contrary to what many people think, a smoker's cough is not a benign condition; it is an early sign of a serious progressive disease that can eventually become disabling, a disease that is associated with an increased risk of pneumonia and heart failure. Once there is evidence of chronic bronchitis, not smoking becomes imperative if people wish to avoid loss of lung function. Moreover, the earlier people are put on bronchodilators, the better their prognosis, provided they have also quit smoking.

Pneumonia

Symptoms

- fever of 103°F–105°F (39.5°C–41°C), with sweating and/or chills
- coughing that raises greenish sputum, often blood-tinged
- sometimes, coughing that produces clear sputum or no sputum
- stabbing chest pain
- sudden onset of symptoms, commonly following an upper respiratory infection

Description

Pneumonia is an infection of the *alveoli*, the tiny air sacs in the lungs, which can be caused by virus, bacteria, or *mycoplasma*, an organism that is intermediate in size between bacteria and virus. Around age 40, people most commonly experience the *viral* and *mycoplasmal* types of pneumonia. By the age of 65, *bacterial pneumonia* tends to become more common. In younger people, bacterial pneumonia is most often seen in those who are alcoholic or have a chronic illness, including AIDS.

Before the advent of antibiotics, pneumonia was one of the major killers among people who were older or who were not in good health. Now with lab tests and antibiotics, both mycoplasmal and bacterial pneumonias are readily treated, provided people do not have some underlying medical condition.

Normally, the lungs have excellent defenses against infection, as evidenced by the fact that pneumonia is uncommon, even though people are surrounded by microorganisms and routinely inhale them. Certain anatomical features make it difficult for germs to enter the lungs: the *epiglottis* closes off the top of the windpipe except during inhalation, and the frequent branching of the airways leading into the lungs acts like a filter, decreasing the chances of microorganisms reaching deep into the lungs. Whatever germs do enter the windpipe are normally carried away by the cilia, small hairlike cells that move particles out of the lungs on a bed of mucus. The cilia are aided by a natural coughing reflex. Any microorganisms that do reach the alveoli are generally destroyed by the body's own antibodies; by *macrophages*, the large white blood cells that engulf germs; or by antimicrobial agents in *surfactant*, the substance that moistens the alveoli in the lungs.

Many factors can lessen the effectiveness of these natural defense mechanisms. A serious cold or virus injures the cilia and allows mucus to build up, providing an excellent growing medium for microorganisms. Also, smoking, air pollution, and chronic bronchitis lessen the effectiveness of the cilia's functioning. If virus actually reach the alveoli, they may use up the readily available macrophages. Other factors including poor nutrition, alcoholism, and underlying conditions such as heart failure or lowered immune response also make individuals more susceptible to pneumonia. As a result, pneumonia is most common among people who are already ill or who have just had a severe cold.

A *viral pneumonia* caused by influenza and a *staphylococcal pneumonia* caused by a bacterium usually have a similar history and symptoms. Viral pneumonias can range from very mild cases hardly distinguishable from a bad cold, to severe cases similar to bacterial pneumonia. Generally viral pneumonias go away by themselves and are not severe except in people who are older or are debilitated.

Mycoplasmal or *atypical pneumonia* has a unique history and symptoms. It is caused by tiny organisms that are neither virus nor bacteria. Generally this type of pneumonia is more common among 20-year-olds than among people in midadulthood. The onset of mycoplasmal pneumonia is slow, not abrupt. Generally people have a low fever for several days, then gradually develop a severe cough that raises small amounts of white sputum and is difficult to stop. This cough also tends to persist for a longer time than with other types of pneumonia. Headache is a prominent symptom, and there is often soreness in the chest. Mycoplasmal pneumonia can produce such fatigue that people find they are unable to climb a flight of stairs.

Most often, *bacterial pneumonia* develops after a common cold or the flu. After several days, instead of getting better as they normally would, people suddenly develop severe chills, a high fever, cough, and chest pains. Their condition worsens rapidly over the next 12–24 hours. When the infection starts, the alveoli fill with fluid, and white blood cells come in to engulf the bacteria. Most people complain of pronounced lethargy, weakness, anxiety, and muscle aches. Coughing brings up greenish mucus that quite often is blood-tinged, making it appear rust-colored. There is severe, stabbing chest pain that is made worse by breathing deeply or coughing. Generally the pneumonia is in one lobe or section of the lungs, so the pain tends to be one-sided. Often breathing becomes labored, and people take frequent shallow breaths due to the pain and congestion in their lungs. In the majority of healthy people, the white blood cells eventually get the upper hand —a point that used to be referred to as "passing the crisis."

Between the ages of 40 and 65, the most common type of bacterial pneumonia is *pneumococcal*, which is caused by bacteria *streptococcus pneumoniae*. Interestingly, this microorganism is found in 10%–60% of healthy people; it only overgrows under special circumstances.

Pneumocystis carinii pneumonia (PCP) is caused by a protozoan—a simple one-celled organism. It is the most frequently diagnosed severe infection found in people with AIDS: it is seen in 64% of AIDS patients and accounts for over half of the deaths from AIDS. It is rarely seen in healthy people. PCP does respond to the antibiotics *trimethoprim-sulfamethoxazole* (Bactrim) and *pentamidine isethinoate*, but the immune systems of people with AIDS are generally not strong enough to combat the infection even with the help of antibiotics.

Self-Care

Because pneumonia can be a dangerous illness, it should be diagnosed and treated by a doctor. Mild viral pneumonias can be treated with self-care; serious viral pneumonias, and mycoplasmal or bacterial pneumonias require more treatment.

The mainstays of treatment for any type of pneumonia are bed rest and extra fluids (see p. 211). Although it may be uncomfortable, it's very important that people cough deeply and bring up mucus often. This is the only way to prevent the lungs from becoming congested.

The Doctor

Pneumonia is diagnosed by a combination of physical findings, lab tests, and x-ray, as well as a history. With a stethoscope, the doctor will hear diminished breath sounds in areas where fluid has accumulated, and crackling sounds called *rales* where fluid is popping in tiny air passages. If pneumonia is suspected, it's important to determine the type, because treatment will vary depending on whether it is viral, mycoplasmal, or bacterial. If the pneumonia is mycoplasmal or bacterial, the specific organism must be identified in order to choose the most effective antibiotic. A chest x-ray both confirms the diagnosis of pneumonia and helps to differentiate the type. X-rays show opaque areas at the site of infection: mycoplasmal or viral pneumonias commonly show patchy areas of infection; pneumococcal pneumonias generally show a dense area in one lobe. A white blood cell test will be elevated in the case of bacterial pneumonia and may be elevated slightly in the case of mycoplasmal pneumonia, but will not be elevated in the case of viral pneumonia. A *gram-stain* of the sputum will make bacteria visible; and a *culture* will identify the particular type of bacteria or mycoplasma. Mycoplasmal pneumonia will also show an elevated antibody level.

Antibiotic therapy will be started immediately in the case of a suspected mycoplasmal or bacterial pneumonia, and may be modified in one to two days when the culture results are available. For mycoplasmal pneumonia, the antibiotic of choice is *erythromycin*; for pneumococcal pneumonia, the choice is *penicillin*; for staph, it is *nafcillin*. Generally people respond rapidly to the antibiotic. In severe cases, in elderly people, or in people with serious underlying conditions, the patient is generally hospitalized, but mild cases can be treated at home. In the hospital, patients are given oxygen to assist their breathing, and intravenous fluids to prevent dehydration and to administer antibiotics.

It is important that patients see the doctor for a follow-up visit after the symptoms have resolved. The doctor will make sure the lungs are clear and check for predisposing factors that may have led to the pneumonia.

Ruling Out Other Diseases

Other than isolating the cause of the pneumonia, the doctor may want to rule out a *pulmonary infarction*, a condition in which a blood clot in the lungs causes the death of nearby tissue. This rare condition sometimes occurs when a person has been operated on, has sustained leg injuries, or has been confined to bed rest for a long time. With a pulmonary infarction there is a low fever, but no history of infection and no production of sputum.

Prevention

In general, the best prevention is prompt treatment of a cold. Vaccines for influenza and pneumococcal bacteria have been developed. They are recommended for older people and very susceptible individuals such as those with chronic heart or lung disease, or sickle cell anemia.

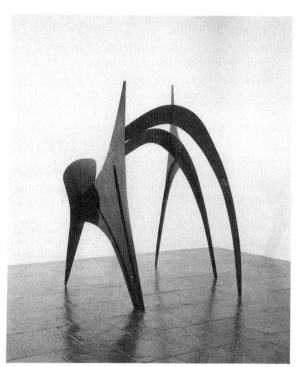

The musculoskeletal system includes the skeleton and the muscles attached to it. Together, they support and protect the body and make movement possible. Alexander Calder. The Arches. 1959. Painted steel. 106" × 107½" × 87". Collection, The Whitney Museum of American Art. Gift of Howard and Jean Lipman. 82.44.

Tendinitis and Bursitis

Symptoms

- pain and tenderness in the shoulder, elbow, wrist, thumb, hip, knee, or foot
- pain ranging from a dull ache to severe discomfort
- pain generally radiating out to the surrounding muscles
- pain on motion and/or at rest
- stiffness or limitation of movement in the affected joint
- symptoms may or may not be precipitated by strenuous activity
- symptoms may come on gradually or abruptly
- pain may be more pronounced at night

Description

Pain in the soft tissues around joints accounts for 15%–25% of the common conditions seen by a doctor. In fact, absences from work due to musculoskeletal disorders exceeded absences for heart disease, cancer, and mental illness combined. The most common causes of soft tissue pain are *tendinitis*, an inflammation of tendons, the cordlike structures that connect the muscles to bones; and *bursitis*, an inflammation of the fluid-filled sacs, called *bursae*, that cushion the joints in various areas. With each movement, a muscle-tendon complex moves the bone, and slides over the bursae. Thus tendons and bursae are subject to constant movement and friction. Tendinitis and bursitis occur most often in the shoulder, elbow, thumb, wrist, hip, knee, and foot.

The causes of tendinitis and bursitis are complex and not well understood. The two most important factors involved are probably *overuse* and *degenerative changes* that can take place with aging. Overuse is a highly variable, individual phenomenon that depends completely on the pattern and amount of exercise a person normally gets. For instance, a relatively small amount of a repetitive activity might cause an inflammation in a very sedentary person, while it might take hours of prolonged activity to cause inflammation in a person who is used to constantly moving a joint in the same way. In addition to overuse, *misuse*, that is, doing a repetitive task in an awkward manner, can sometimes provoke an inflammation.

Since tendons are not well supplied with blood vessels, both overuse and misuse can produce an oxygen deficit that causes cells to die, weakening tendon fibers and resulting in repeated microtraumas or minor injury. Moreover, even slight injuries to tendons don't heal easily because of their poor blood supply. White blood cells that come in to clear away dead and damaged tissue tend to move out of the area slowly. Both the dead tissue and white blood cells act as foreign matter, causing irritation. In response, fluid is released from surrounding cells, which puts pressure on pain nerves in the area because there is little room for swelling within a joint or tendon. Ultimately, scar tissue often forms where the injuries occur, further affecting movement. Continued use adds to the stress on the particular joint. Eventually, people may come to hold or use the joint in an awkward manner, putting unusual stress on the joint, and further slowing or preventing healing.

The problems of overuse, misuse, and slow healing can be added to significantly by degenerative changes that sometimes take place in people's joints as they grow older. By the age of 50, 25% of all healthy people show degenerative changes in their tendons. These changes include irregular borders on tendons and the splitting of collagen fibers within tendons. Such changes are seen most frequently in areas where the tendon normally rubs against bone, and they are found most commonly in people whose bones have pronounced protruberances at the ends. While such degenerative changes are known to progress with time, it is unclear whether they are due to aging alone, to years of a sedentary life-style, or to chronic overuse or misuse.

In some people there is also a tendency to build up calcium deposits in the tendons as a result of the elevated acid levels that frequently accompany the inflammatory process. Calcium salts in the fluid released by cells inside the tendons form *calcium hydroxyapatite crystals*, exacerbating any inflammation. These dry gritty crystals can eventually build up into large deposits that can be seen on x-ray. This condition is known as *calcific tendinitis*. Occasionally, pressure can force crystals out of a tendon and through the thin wall of a bursa, the fluid-filled sac that cushions certain joints. The crystals irritate the lining of the bursa, causing an acute, painful attack of bursitis.

In recent years, some doctors have come to believe in a new theory about the cause of musculoskeletal pain. It has been known for several hundred years that muscles can have painful hard spots, or *trigger points*. When these spots are pressed, they cause *referred pain* in a different location, which duplicates the pain experienced during tendinitis or a bursitis attack. Interestingly, these trigger spots are not necessarily in the tendon or muscle where the pain is —in fact, they may be some distance away and have no known anatomical connection, such as a nerve. Interestingly, these trigger points do correlate with many traditional acupuncture points. Individuals with tendinitis or bursitis will often have a tender lump at a correlating trigger point, which can readily be felt by a skilled person. Researchers theorize that the trigger points first become inflamed due to an injury or overuse. The inflammation creates a reflex muscle spasm which causes the autonomic nervous system to decrease blood flow to and stimulate the pain nerves in the *target area*. The process of injury/inflammation/muscle contraction is called the *pain-spasm-pain cycle*. Muscle tension studies show that emotional stress, including that caused by the pain itself, measurably increases the cycle of muscle contraction and pain. The concept of trigger points has led to new methods of treatment (see section on *The Doctor*).

Shoulder pain: The shoulder is the area most commonly affected by musculoskeletal conditions. Shoulder pain is second only to back pain as a reason for absence from work. Doctors believe that shoulder pain is caused, in part, by the evolutionary process of humans assuming an upright posture and developing greater mobility in their upper limbs. These profound changes were accompanied by a weakening of the attachment of the upper limbs. Unlike four-footed mammals, humans have a shallow shoulder socket which is actually held together only with muscles and tendons. Such an arrangement reduces the stability of the joint and puts additional stress on it.

The most frequent cause of shoulder pain is tendinitis of the *supraspinatus* muscle which attaches to the *scapula*, or shoulder blade. This muscle is sometimes injured by being pinched between the humerus bone of the arm and the *acromium*, the bony projection on the top of the scapula. The condition develops most frequently in people over 40 who are involved in repetitive sports or work that requires elevation and forward movement of the arm. This type of tendinitis is commonly experienced by carpenters, painters, woodcutters, gardeners, and weight lifters. Frequently people are not aware of any specific activity that precipitated an attack, although they may report a history of minor pain

and tenderness. Often the pain starts as a dull ache that involves the whole shoulder and limits forward motion. It tends to be most troublesome at night, and varies from day to day. The pain usually runs from the top of the shoulder down the outside of the arm to the elbow, even the wrist. Generally, the movement that is most impaired involves lifting the arm to the side and overhead.

When tendinitis involves calcium deposits that rupture into the bursa, the pain can come on suddenly and be so acute as to cause people to cry out at any movement of their arm. This condition is called *acute bursitis*. Although it develops abruptly, it is often preceded by a history of tendinitis. Bursitis is characterized by constant, intense pain that is not relieved by resting in any position, and is made worse by moving. Generally people with bursitis avoid moving their shoulder, and are least uncomfortable if they hold their arm against their body or immobilize it in a sling. The pain usually peaks within several days and then gradually subsides over a period of several weeks. Without proper exercise over a long period of time, stiffness and loss of movement will persist, and there can be loss of mobility in the shoulder joint (see below).

Another common site for tendinitis is the *biceps*, the muscle in the front of the upper arm. Often people who experience this type of tendinitis have recently engaged in a repetitive movement of the arm, such as tightening jar lids for canning. With this condition, pain radiates down the biceps and along the forearm. It is made worse if people try to bend their elbow while pushing up against someone's hand.

Occasionally, as a result of injury or a prolonged, untreated condition, the shoulder joint may lose a significant amount of its range of motion. This condition is referred to as a *"frozen shoulder,"* and it tends to become worse, limiting movement in the shoulder more and more. Loss of motion follows a standard sequence, which can develop insidiously when it's the result of a

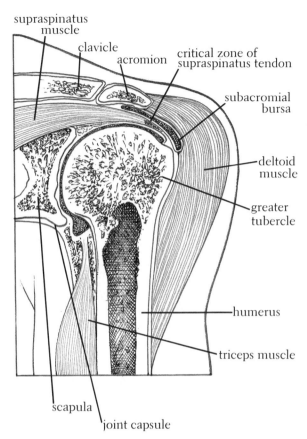

supraspinatus
muscle

clavicle

acromion

critical zone of
supraspinatus tendon

subacromial
bursa

deltoid
muscle

greater
tubercle

humerus

triceps muscle

scapula

joint capsule

*The most common cause of shoulder pain is tendinitis
of the supraspinatus muscle, which occurs when the
tendon at the end of the muscle is pinched between
the* humerus, *the bone in the upper arm, and the
acromion, a bony projection on the shoulder blade, or
scapula.*

chronic condition. First, people experience difficulty reaching behind their back to wash, put on a coat, or fasten a bra. Next, they may experience difficulty raising their arms overhead to the front or the side. This stage, which is referred to as *freezing*, is characterized by pain and increasing stiffness over a period of two to nine months. Frozen shoulder is most common in middleage, more so among women then men.

Women often first notice difficulty combing their hair, while men complain of difficulty reaching into their back pocket. Both sexes may be aware of pain at night when they roll on the affected shoulder. Finally, the joint capsule actually adheres to the top of the humerus, the upper arm bone. At this stage, called *adhesive capsulitis*, the shoulder is referred to as *frozen*. It is characterized by marked stiffness, and discomfort rather than pain. At this stage, the condition causes about a 90% loss of ability to raise the arm to the side, a 60% loss of ability to raise the arm overhead, and a 45% loss of ability to reach behind the back. *Thawing* can subsequently occur over a period of 5–24 months, during which time range of motion gradually returns; however, recovery may not be complete without physical therapy.

Elbow: The second most common site of musculoskeletal pain is the elbow. This pain is caused by a strain or tear resulting from overuse. Such minor injuries lead to swelling and can eventually cause fibrous changes in the space under the tendons that run across the elbow. By far the most common elbow condition is "tennis elbow," which causes pain around the *lateral epicondyle*, the prominence on the outside of the elbow (see illustration). Another, less common, condition is "golfer's elbow" which affects the bump on the inside of the joint.

Both elbow conditions are uncommon under the age of 40, or over 60. People cite a history of pain around the elbow while grasping an object or turning the wrist; the pain may be chronic or intermittent, and its onset may be gradual or sudden. People often complain that this condition "weakens" their grip, however, it is actually pain, not weakness, that causes them to drop objects. Picking up a heavy object or raising the wrist against resistance characteristically produces pain just below the epicondyle prominence.

These elbow conditions are caused by activities that require turning the wrist and hand back

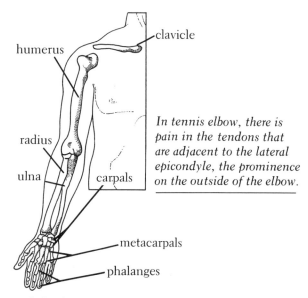

clavicle

humerus

radius

ulna

carpals

metacarpals

phalanges

In tennis elbow, there is pain in the tendons that are adjacent to the lateral epicondyle, the prominence on the outside of the elbow.

and forth repeatedly in a short period of time. The activities that are actually cited as most frequently causing the two conditions are gardening, hammering, using a screwdriver for long periods, and using a trowel in masonry work. Among tennis players, tennis elbow occurs most frequently in newer players who tend to grip the racket too tightly, especially during backhand shots.

Thumb and wrist: Repetitive activity can even cause a tendinitis of the thumb and wrist called *De Quervain's tenosynovitis.* The tendons that bend the thumb forward and back pass through a cartilage tunnel near the inside of the wrist. Activities such as pruning can sometimes cause swelling and inflammation of these tendons, producing pain on typing or grasping, especially when the thumb is bent or the wrist is turned. In fact, the characteristic diagnostic test, called *Finkelstein's sign,* involves making a fist with the thumb tucked in, and then rotating the hand inward. This motion of the hand stretches the tendons and accentuates the pain.

Hip: Among middle-aged people, the most common cause of hip pain that radiates down the thigh toward the knee is a tendinitis of the *glu-*

teal muscles, the large muscles on the side of the leg. The tendons that attach these muscles insert near the top of the *femur.* In the hip region alone, there are 18 or more *bursae* that cushion the tendons. Minor injury or overuse can cause inflammation of one or more tendons, which can spread to the bursae. Inflammation does not limit the range of motion of the hip joint, but causes a persistent dull ache down the outside of the hip and thigh, extending to the knee or below. People often are most aware of discomfort after prolonged walking or upon awakening. When the inflammation spreads to the bursae, people are troubled by pain at night, with specific tenderness at a point deep in the hip. Being overweight tends to aggravate the condition. The most frequent cause of gluteal strain is stooping over and arising with the knees kept straight, a motion which stretches these tendons to their maximum. People who have a tendency toward hip problems are advised to always bend their knees before bending their back, a habit that also relieves strain on the lower back.

Knee: The knee has a complex anatomical structure that includes at least 12 bursae that cushion the tendons crossing the joint. These tendons make possible a complicated array of movements that involve sliding, gliding, and bending. A minor injury or a cycle of disuse and overuse can produce a tendinitis in this area, most commonly among people of middle age. The main symptom is knee pain that is aggravated by movement, and is sometimes worse at night. The tendinitis may or may not cause some limitation of movement in the joint. The condition tends to be common among people whose work requires them to kneel for long periods.

Foot: Another common site of soft tissue injury is the foot. Like the tendons around the thumb, the tendons around the ankle can become inflamed due to repetitive movement, especially after prolonged, unaccustomed walking or jogging. Improper or poorly fitting footwear can press on specific tendons or put strain on the

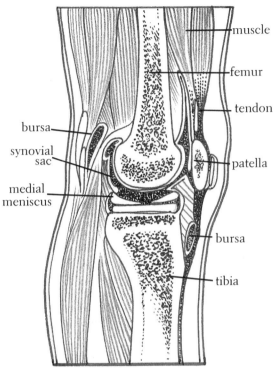

The knee is a complex joint that includes many muscles and tendons whose movement is cushioned by a number of fluid-filled sacs called bursae.

whole foot. Women who wear high-heeled shoes often have problems with the *Achilles tendon* at the back of the ankle. An inflammation of this tendon causes heel pain and may even cause "pump bumps"—little nodules on the Achilles tendon. The ends of the tendons underneath the arch of the foot can also become inflamed, causing pain and tenderness on walking. This condition frequently follows prolonged walking or standing, and is aggravated by obesity, flat feet, and poor footwear.

Self-Care

Self-help is the cornerstone of treatment for all forms of tendinitis and bursitis because these conditions tend to heal slowly. The initial treatment is *rest*: activities that put stress on the affected joint should definitely be discontinued temporarily. For example, a person with a tendinitis of the shoulder should stop repetitive activities such as pruning or painting until the acute injury begins to heal and the pain subsides. Some doctors even suggest total rest for the joint in the acute phase. For example, in the case of a shoulder bursitis they may suggest immobilizing the arm in a sling.

Physical therapy and *graduated exercises* are the most important forms of treatment. In one study comparing the various therapies for bursi-

---

Stretching Exercises to Relieve Shoulder Pain

Do these exercises two to three times a day, after taking a hot shower or applying a heat pack. Do as much of each exercise as possible; stop when it becomes painful. Start slowly; gradually increase the length of time and range of motion.

1. Leaning forward and keeping elbow straight, swing a one to two pound weight forward and back, then laterally, then in circles (see illustration). Do two to three times a day for three minutes at a time.
2. Standing sideways at arm's length from wall and holding arm straight, "walk" fingers up wall as high as possible. Repeat facing wall. Do five times in a row, two to three times a day.
3. Raise arms overhead and stretch as far as possible, keeping elbows straight. Repeat, stretching arms to side.
4. With hands locked behind neck, pull elbows backward.
5. Touch palm to lower back, then slide hand as high up the back as possible. Repeat using other hand. Alternately, pull hand up with a towel held over the opposite shoulder.
6. Hold a cane or stick at arm's length with both hands, and raise it as high as possible.
7. While standing, cross hands at wrist, then raise locked arms as high as possible, keeping elbows straight.

tis and tendinitis, it was found that there was a much improved range of motion with all forms of treatment, provided exercise was prescribed at the same time.

As soon as the pain subsides sufficiently, the joint should be taken through the appropriate range of motion exercises slowly and gently, attaining as full a range as possible. At first, range of motion exercises should be *passive*; that is, the joint should *be moved* gently with the help of the other hand, gravity, or another person (see charts). These exercises should be done two or three times a day, preferably upon arising and before going to bed. The exercises should include ones that specifically stretch the tendons (see illustrations)—especially in the case of shoulder tendinitis—in order to avoid having the shoulder become "frozen."

A number of self-help remedies can be used to control pain and prevent muscles from going into spasm, while achieving the greatest range of motion possible. When tendinitis or bursitis comes on suddenly, *ice packs* should be applied as soon as possible. An ice pack can drop the temperature of a muscle by as much as 11 degrees in an hour if applied continuously. Chilling the area tends to minimize swelling, increase function, and lessen pain by causing constriction of local blood vessels. Reduced blood flow decreases histamine release and thereby lessens the inflammatory response. Ice packs should generally be wrapped in a towel and applied for as long as necessary to control pain. It is not uncommon for people to apply ice packs intermittently for several days to minimize pain and swelling. Specifically, it is recommended that people apply ice to the affected joint shortly before going through the range of motion exercises.

Several other remedies can be used to effectively aid in pain control. Relaxation and imagery techniques (see pp. 60–67) are very useful to control pain in general, and in particular for doing stretching exercises which can be quite uncomfortable when the inflammation and swelling are at their peak. Both these techniques can radically affect a person's pain threshold,

---

Stretching Exercises for Knee Pain

Do these exercises two to three times a day, after taking a hot shower or applying a heat pack. Do as much of each exercise as possible; stop when it becomes painful. Start slowly; gradually increase the length of time and range of motion.

1. Sitting flat on floor with legs straight out, tighten the knees without moving them. Hold for several seconds, then relax; repeat 25 times.
2. Lying on back with legs straight, lift legs alternately, raising heel as high as possible. Repeat 10 times.
3. Sitting on a high bench or table, suspend a two to five pound weight (such as a handbag or small bucket) from the foot, and raise the weight by straightening the knee, 10–15 times in a row.
4. Lying on your back or sitting on a stationary bicycle, move your legs in a pedaling movement. Do for five minutes.
5. Standing on both feet and supporting yourself with a table or railing, stoop, forcing knees to bend, while keeping back straight.

Repetitive Activities That Can Produce Tendinitis or Bursitis

Shoulder	baseball and other sports
	chopping wood
	pruning
	sanding
	sawing
	weightlifting
	painting
Elbow	gardening
	masonry
	plumbing
	tennis and other racquet sports
	using a hammer or screwdriver
Thumb	cutting
	pruning

A person with bursitis or tendinitis of the shoulder should do exercises several times a day to take the joint as far as possible through its range of motion.

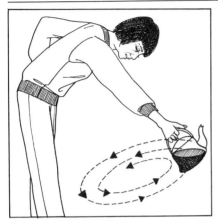

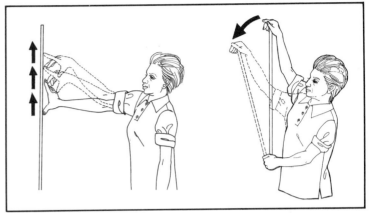

The Pendulum Exercise: *hold a weighted object straight down with your stiff arm. Swing the object in wider and wider circles; as your arm gets better, add more weight to the object.*

Wall Walking: *facing a wall, "walk" your fingers up the wall as high as you can. Go a little higher each time until you achieve full range of motion.*

The Cane Exercise: *hold a cane with your hands several feet apart. Use your good arm to push the stiff arm through its range of motion. This exercise can be done both horizontally and vertically.*

which is important because musculoskeletal pain tends to be exacerbated by emotional stress and depression. Moreover, relaxation permits muscles to stretch more readily, thereby increasing the range of motion that can be achieved.

Several over-the-counter drugs work well to lessen the pain that accompanies all forms of tendinitis. *Aspirin* is particularly effective because it is an *anti-inflammatory*. *Ibuprofen* (e.g., *Motrin*, *Advil*) is a nonsteroidal anti-inflammatory agent that is available without prescription. *Acetaminophen* (e.g., *Tylenol*) may help to control pain, but it does not reduce inflammation.

Once the acute phase of a tendinitis or bursitis is over, *heat* can be applied to the joint to promote healing. Heat increases blood flow to the area, which speeds up metabolic processes, clearing out waste products and bringing in increased amounts of oxygen. Heat also increases the ability of a muscle to stretch by as much as 2% in length and 5% in range of motion. Hot water bottles, hot baths, hot tubs, saunas, or heat lamps should be used prior to doing daily stretching exercises.

The Doctor

In the case of a simple tendinitis or bursitis, the doctor (family practitioner, internist, or orthopedist) will diagnose the condition based on a careful history and physical exam. The history includes an account of whether there was a specific injury, whether the onset was acute or gradual, a list of recent activities, and whether the individual also has any systemic illnesses such as arthritis. On physical exam, the doctor will look for swelling and tenderness, as well as pain or limitation of motion during certain movements. If the diagnosis is not obvious or if healing does not occur within the expected period, the doctor may order an *x-ray* to visualize the joint in more detail. An x-ray is not particularly useful in the case of a simple tendinitis or bursitis, but it can reveal whether calcium deposits and degenerative bone changes have taken place. *Magnetic resonance imaging (MRI)*, which provides high resolution images, and *ultrasound* may be used to aid in diagnosis.

In addition to basic self-care recommendations, doctors can prescribe a variety of treatments depending on the specific condition and the patient's preference. Several valid treatment options exist for these musculoskeletal conditions, and doctors will often give patients a choice. First, doctors can prescribe more powerful pain medications and anti-inflammatory drugs. Tendinitis, and in particular, bursitis, can be very painful and require pain medication that is more powerful than over-the-counter preparations. Doctors commonly prescribe *codeine* for this purpose. There are also a number of *non-steroidal anti-inflammatory drugs* that are very effective in reducing inflammation, thereby lessening pain and increasing the range of motion possible in the affected joint. The most common of these drugs is *indomethacin* (e.g., *Indocin*), which is very powerful, but is considered safe for short-term use (seven to ten days). Indomethacin's side effects include nausea, diarrhea, dizziness, headache, vertigo, and depression. It should be taken on a full stomach with an *antacid* to buffer it. Long-term use has been known to cause ulcers.

In addition to prescribing pain medication and an anti-inflammatory drug, the doctor may refer the patient to a physical therapist. A physical therapy program generally involves the use of cold or heat: *ice packs, ultrasound, heat lamps*, moist hot packs called *hydrocollator packs*, or *diathermy*, which uses microwaves to produce heat. After applying heat or cold, the physical therapist does *friction massage*, rubbing the affected area to increase blood flow and prevent fibrous tissue from adhering to the joint or surrounding tendons. Physical therapy also re-laxes and stretches the tendons, and helps to break up calcium deposits in the area. Finally, the physical therapist does *passive exercises*, taking the affected joint through the fullest range of motion that is possible. Gradually, the physical therapist will assign *active exercises* for the patient to do at home in order to slowly build up strength and flexibility in the affected joint. Following a severe episode of tendinitis or bursitis, individuals do better if they receive physical therapy and are assigned exercises by a professional in the proper sequence and timing.

A combination of rest, anti-inflammatory drugs, and physical therapy constitute the conservative approach to treating tendinitis and bursitis. A more aggressive approach involves local injections of a mixture of anesthetic *(procaine)* and *steroids (hydrocortisone)*. This treatment can be remarkably effective, often providing dramatic relief from pain and almost instantaneous increase in the range of motion in the affected joint, especially when there are specific points of tenderness. Injections are frequently the treatment used by sports medicine doctors for professional athletes. Many *orthopedists* consider it the treatment of choice when an individual has an acute or severe tendinitis or bursitis.

Doctors who do not use steroid injections as a first choice point out their uncommon but potentially serious side effects, including risk of infection. Steroids, by their very nature, block the body's natural healing processes, and may lessen the tensile strength of the affected tendons. Most doctors will not use steroid injections in weight-bearing joints such as the knee or ankle because of the rare possibility of rupturing the tendon. Many doctors feel that the side effects are so uncommon that the effectiveness of injections far exceeds the risks.

In any case, people who receive a steroid injection should still have physical therapy, and they cannot really use the joint actively for at least several weeks until full healing takes place. Studies of uncomplicated tendinitis show that by the end of the healing period, the results of injections and physiotherapy are no better than are the results of anti-inflammatory agents and physiotherapy. The big difference is that, with injections, the person may have less pain and more use of the joint in the first week or two.

Ruling Out Other Diseases

Systemic diseases such as *osteoarthritis, rheumatoid arthritis, and gout* (see p. 333), and a variety of neurological conditions involving pinched nerves can also cause pain around joints. Arthritis conditions can generally be distinguished by multiple involvement of joints, and by greater swelling and heat around the joint. The neurological conditions produce pain and burning along the course of a nerve, as well as numbness and weakness of the muscles controlled by the nerve. Athletic or occupational injuries involving sprains, strains, and torn ligaments (see p. 68) can also produce pain in similar sites, but a history of accident usually distinguishes an injury from an arthritis or neurological condition.

Prevention

The main principle of prevention is avoiding overuse or misuse. Individuals have customary levels of activity that their muscles are adapted to. Sudden significant increases in repetitive activities, or incorrect performance of an unfamiliar task, are the actions most likely to precipitate tendinitis or bursitis. The difficulty lies in judging what is "too much." Usually, people do not develop a problem from prolonged repetitive movement when they are under 35, although professional athletes demonstrate that with excessive activity, problems can arise even in younger people.

With increasing age and a more sedentary life-style, people have to spend increasing amounts of time warming up for certain sports or activities, and increasing amounts of time stretching out afterward (see p. 122). In addition to not overdoing, people should be careful to avoid common types of misuse with specific joints, particularly if they have demonstrated that they are prone to problems with those joints.

Often people contribute to their musculoskeletal problems without even realizing it because they develop habits that put unnecessary stress on a particular joint. For example, gardeners may raise their arms overhead to prune, rather than work from a ladder. To avoid recurrent or chronic problems, people have to modify habitual misuse patterns. In addition, it's essential that people who want to engage in certain types of repetitive activity strengthen the muscles around the joints involved through a graded exercise program. Such exercises are particularly important in the case of the shoulder, because the muscles themselves contribute significantly to the strength of the joint.

Low Back and Neck Pain

Symptoms

low back pain
- mild backache, made worse by bending or lifting, improving with rest
- acute pain in the lower back area
- muscle spasms in the lower back
- pain on bending or changing position
- pain radiating from back to thighs
- pain in the buttocks or lower extremities
- numbness and sensory loss in the legs

neck pain
- stiff neck
- pain in neck
- pain radiating to the neck and shoulders
- headache
- pain, numbness and tingling radiating down the arm

Description

Back pain, both temporary and chronic, is one of the most common complaints of Western civilization. Not surprisingly, it also consumes a significant percentage of modern medical care and is one of the chief reasons for disability. Back problems are frequently associated with occupations that require heavy lifting. During their lifetimes, almost all adults have at least one episode of back pain serious enough to limit their activities and/or keep them out of work, and 65%–80% of all adults experience some decrease in functional ability due to back pain. Approximately 3 million people have severe problems. However, most people with back problems get better, 70% within a month and 90% within 3 months.

By comparison, neck pain is almost as frequent, but far less disabling. It does not stop people from working for long; episodes usually last less than a week, and they seldom require medical treatment. Unlike back pain, neck pain is not usually occupationally related. Although neck pain is not as common as low back pain, one study found that almost 50% of all working men had at least one episode of neck pain.

Backache is not a new plague for mankind. As early as the fifth century B.C., the Chinese dealt with back problems in a book called *The Yellow Emperor's Classic of Internal Medicine*, and the Egyptians likewise referred to backache in their medical papyri. Back pain appears to be an evolutionary problem that developed when human beings began to walk upright. One expert has noted that low back pain does not afflict creatures that are swimmers, squigglers, hoppers, swingers, or flyers. When man stood upright, important changes took place in the relationship between the bones of the leg and the bones of the back, changes which caused two curves to develop in the spinal column. A *neck* or *cervical curve* develops as soon as a baby begins to hold its head up; later, a *low back* or *lumbar curve*

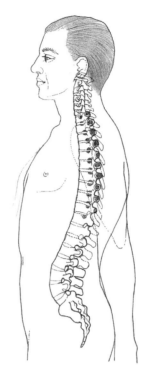

The spinal column is made up of a number of bones stacked on top of each other. Due to the upright stance that humans have assumed, the spinal column has curves in the cervical (neck) and lumbar (low back) areas which put stress on the nearby discs and joints.

develops when a baby begins to walk. This latter curve puts tremendous stress on the discs and joints of the back's vertebral column (see below). In addition to standing and walking erect, the way Westerners sit in chairs accentuates the curve of their lower back. People in Africa and Asia who squat or sit cross-legged tend to keep their backs much straighter, which is thought to account for the fact that they have little or no incidence of back problems.

In order to gain a better understanding of back problems, it is important to look at the anatomy of the back. The *spinal column* is made up of 24 individual bones called *vertebrae*, plus a fused bone at the base called the *sacrum*. Each vertebrae has two parts: a large cylindrical body in the front that bears the weight of the spine, and a posterior arch from which several bony outriggers project. The outriggers serve as attachment points for the muscles of the back,

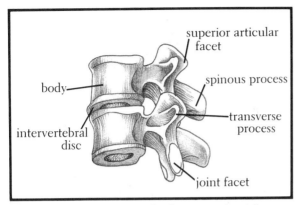

Each vertebrae in the spinal column consists of a main body and a section with outriggers. The outriggers interdigitate so as to form a gliding joint, which can become sprained if the normal motion of the joint is exceeded.

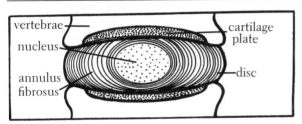

Between the main bodies of the spinal vertebrae are cartilage discs which act as shock absorbers, mediating the enormous pressures put on the spine. The discs consist of a tough outer covering called the annulus *and a soft inner core called the* nucleus.

while the arch forms a hollow canal that protects the spinal cord and nerves. The outriggers are bound to one another with ligaments, making a *gliding joint* on either side of the vertebral arch. Like all other joints, these have a definite range of motion. Although limited, the range in the gliding joints is crucial in that it allows the spine to bend and twist forward, backward, and sideways.

Between the cylindrical bodies of the vertebrae are *cartilage discs* that act as shock absorbers, cushioning the pressure put on the spinal column by sitting and walking. Such pres-

sures can be enormous; for instance, they can equal a weight of 1,500 pounds when a weightlifter raises a 100-pound weight at arm's length. Because the discs have a soft gelatinous core inside a fibrous outer casing, they readily change shape in response to pressure, much like an automobile tire. Under strong pressure the edges of the disc may actually bulge out between the vertebrae; under extreme pressure, the disc may even *herniate* or rupture, losing its gelatinous core and compressing nearby nerves and the ligaments that hold the vertebrae together.

Generally, as people grow older and become more sedentary, their back and abdominal muscles become weaker and less stretchable; as a result, more pressure is transferred to their back during lifting. Thus when older people lift objects, they are more likely to strain the gliding joints of the back or put excess pressure on a disc. Moreover, as people age, degenerative changes begin to take place in the structure of the discs themselves. Whereas 90% of all discs are normal in people between the ages of 14 and 35, above the age of 60, only 5% are. In response to biochemical changes, the discs become softer and thinner. As these changes take place, the shock-absorbing quality of the discs decreases and movement between the vertebrae becomes sloppier. Excessive mobility that stretches joints past their normal range of motion becomes increasingly likely.

Low back pain: Despite all they have learned, doctors still do not fully understand the cause of all back pain, and in some cases they have difficulty diagnosing the problem precisely. Moreover, few double-blind studies have been done to establish which treatments are most effective for specific problems. Fortunately, many cases of back pain virtually heal by themselves, and treatment is limited to self-care.

Currently, doctors believe that two problems are responsible for most back and neck pain: first, sprains and strains; and second, herniated or slipped discs. *Strains* result from stretching the ligaments that hold the vertebrae together; *sprains* result when the ligaments are partially torn. A strain or sprain causes the affected muscles of the back to go into spasm, which produces pain. The pain in turn triggers further spasms, resulting in a cycle that is difficult to stop. Sprains and strains can either be caused by a sudden injury to a relatively healthy back or they can be caused by excessive movement of the vertebral joints in a back that has some degree of disc degeneration. Injury is the reason for most acute back problems, but degeneration is also involved in the majority of chronic back problems. With chronic problems, there is often scarring and thickening around ligaments that have been torn; this scar tissue presses on nearby nerves and continues to cause pain even after the original injury has healed.

The second major cause of low back pain is a *herniated* or *slipped disc*. Until recently it was thought that herniation was the cause of most low back pain, but experts now feel that slipped discs account for less than 5% of all low back problems. Herniation can either result from a stress powerful enough to actually crush or rupture a disc, or more commonly from a series of degenerative changes. In the latter case, the cartilage that attaches each disc to the vertebrae begins to break down, increasing pressure on the disc and making it more likely to bulge out. In addition, the fibrous outer casing of the discs may eventually develop tiny tears, causing the gelatinous material in the core to deteriorate. Ultimately, a herniated disc can press on the nerve roots leading from the spinal cord to the legs (see below).

In practice, back problems are classified into two broad categories: acute and chronic. An *acute back problem* involves a sudden, dramatic impairment of function. Generally when this happens, people are executing a lifting or twisting motion. When people's backs "go out" in this manner, they are seized with sudden, profound pain, causing them to be unable to move, or to

move with great difficulty. They can stand only in a stooped position, keeping their lower back rigid, and they may even walk with their knees bent. All their movements are limited by pain and muscle spasms. Generally people with acute back pain do not have any nerve impingement, as evidenced by shooting pains and numbness in the legs. With proper self-care, this type of back problem gets better within a matter of days to weeks, and may never recur.

Some doctors believe that one type of acute back problem is due purely to muscle spasms, not to a sprain or strain of the ligaments. This condition, which has a very specific course, sometimes occurs in healthy people when they bend down and turn. The classic triggering event is an everyday action such as tying shoes, reaching for a tennis ball on the ground, or even getting out of bed in the morning; there is no history of injury or heavy lifting. Yet the people experience sudden dramatic pain that virtually immobilizes them. Doctors who are proponents of the muscle spasm theory believe the spasm is brought on by slippage in one of the lumbar joints. This type of back problem, when correctly diagnosed, can be relieved by manipulation of the spine.

Chronic back problems, involving recurrent attacks, generally signify greater disc degeneration or weaker abdominal and spinal muscles. When the discs degenerate, narrowing the space between vertebrae, and causing osteoarthritis around the posterior joints, the condition is sometimes referred to as *degenerative disc disease*. In such cases, affected individuals frequently bend or twist their back past the point of strain, and can experience discomfort whenever they stoop over, sit in soft chairs, or stand for long periods of time. Occasionally, there can be enough slippage in the lumbar joints that one vertebrae is allowed to shift slightly out of line in relationship to the vertebrae above and below it. This condition is called *spondylolisthesis*.

Chronic back problems are very common in

people who are overweight and/or have poor posture. A large abdomen or weak abdominal muscles shifts a person's center of gravity forward, accentuating the lumbar curve and keeping the spine in a hyperextended position. In this position, the spine cannot be bent forward much without strain. Occasionally during a chronic episode, people experience pain radiating to the buttocks and legs. This is referred pain from the irritated lumbar ligaments. For a small number of people, low back problems become constant and incapacitating. Doctors feel that not infrequently these people have developed a lowered pain threshold and suffer from depression, which tends to exacerbate their pain and physical limitations.

A small number of people develop *nerve root compression* due to disc herniation. Typically, these individuals have experienced gradual but progressive disc degeneration. Their histories commonly involve a number of episodes of back pain followed by recovery, possibly with back symptoms in between. Attacks generally begin with low back pain that makes it difficult to sit or stand comfortably. Less typically, people with no disc degeneration herniate a disc when they inadvertently place a severe strain on their back by lifting something unusually heavy. When this occurs, people often report a popping sound and/or a tearing feeling. Whether nerve root compression is the result of a chronic condition or an acute injury, the pain in the lower back eases, but people experience increasing pain, numbness, and tingling that radiates down one or both legs. Individuals may have difficulty standing up, raising the affected leg, or standing on the affected leg, which characteristically causes them to lean to one side. Most of the time, nerve root compression improves with medical care and does not require surgery. Swelling around the disc gradually subsides, superficial tears in the fibrous covering may even heal, and the gelatinous material that has been squeezed out of the core shrinks.

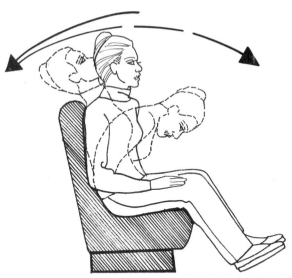

The most common cause of neck sprains is whiplash, a series of movements in which the neck moves suddenly in one direction and then recoils forcefully in the opposite direction.

Neck pain: Although *cervical* or *neck problems* are less common than ones involving the lower back, the neck area is very vulnerable to injury. The cervical vertebrae lie between the skull, a movable 8–12 pound weight, and the relatively immobile thoracic vertebrae of the chest. The muscles and ligaments around the cervical vertebrae are very likely to be strained or sprained when the head moves beyond its normal range of motion for any reason. More than half of all cervical pain is due to *whiplash* resulting from automobile collisions. When a car is hit hard in the front or back, passengers' necks are thrown forward or back, past the point of strain. As with back strain, the ligaments between vertebrae are stretched and nearby muscles experience small tears that cause bruising and swelling. If the neck is sprained, there is actually a small tear in the ligaments.

A typical story of cervical pain involves rapid bending or twisting of the neck, possibly in an unfamiliar way. At first the neck is stiff and uncomfortable to move. Next, the neck actually becomes painful and hurts distinctly on movement. If the neck and back muscles go into spasm, a headache may also result. Occasionally people may experience tingling, pain and numbness radiating down one or both arms, which may be caused either by referred pain from the injury or by nerve root compression.

Self-Care

For the vast majority of back and neck problems, self-care is the mainstay of recovery. Self-care is the treatment of choice for most sprains or strains, and even for most herniated discs. Naturally, the extent of self-care depends upon the severity of the problem. A slipped disc requires far more treatment than a mild or moderate sprain. But the outlook is favorable—more than 70% of all back and neck problems heal within a month, no matter what the treatment.

The first principle of treatment for an acute back problem is *rest*. Bed rest is advised, but it is mandatory if the problem is severe. Just as people stay off a sprained ankle, they need to "stay off" a sprained back. Individuals who can't or won't remain in bed should lie down as often as possible. In particular, they should avoid long periods of sitting because that tends to aggravate the muscle spasms. Rest and limited motion permits swelling to subside and give the ligaments and/or discs time to heal.

Bed rest allows people to get into a comfortable position, usually one that involves bending the spine. A curved position minimizes pain and possible nerve compression, thereby helping to alleviate muscle spasms. Breaking the cycle of pain and spasms is crucial to curing a backache. There are two positions that generally provide the most comfort for people with low back pain. Both involve bending the neck, hips, and knees. One position is lying on the side with knees and hips bent (perhaps with a pillow between the knees); the other is lying on the back with a pil-

low under the knees and the head. Most doctors also recommend a firm bed—either a stiff mattress or a piece of plywood between the mattress and the springs. Bed rest should be continued until the individual can walk to the bathroom without undue discomfort. This can range from one to two days for a mild sprain, to one to two weeks for a severe sprain. New studies have shown that two days of bed rest are just as effective as seven days, provided the back pain is not caused by a slipped disc. The current trend among doctors is to suggest early walking after a back episode.

The second component of self-care is the application of *heat* and *cold*. Unlike other kinds of sprains, back sprains do not produce great amounts of swelling, so heating pads are recommended more often than ice packs, but it's an individual matter. The point is to minimize the pain and stop the muscle spasms so as to permit greater stretching of the affected muscles. If a heating pad or hot water bottle doesn't work or increases the pain, the person should try ice packs wrapped in a light towel—or vice versa. Sometimes people find that alternating heat and cold provides the most comfort.

The third major aspect of self-help is *exercise*. A number of highly effective exercise regimens

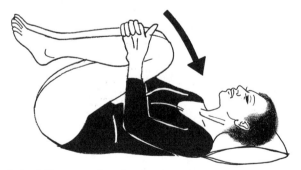

Spinal Flexion: *often low back pain can be alleviated by lying on your back or your side and gently pulling your knees up toward your chest. This position should be held for up to 5 minutes.*

have been developed by various back clinics. During the acute stage, the most important exercise is to slowly and gently flex the spine into a fetal position, which involves bending at the hips and knees and gently pulling the knees against the chest with the arms. This exercise can be done while lying on the back or the side. Generally, if done temporarily, this exercise will break a muscle spasm and sometimes can even stop an acute attack. It apparently works by releasing muscle hyperactivity. The exercise stops the muscle from continuously going into spasm by producing a smooth contraction, followed by relaxation.

A second exercise is recommended for the acute phase *only* if there is no sign of nerve root compression (e.g., there is no numbness, tingling or pain radiating to the legs). This exercise requires the help of another person. The back sufferer lies on his or her back, with knees and hips slightly bent. The therapist grasps the person's heels and lifts their legs toward their head, stopping as soon as the person becomes uncomfortable. This movement should be repeated slowly and rhythmically for two to five minutes. The rocking motion stretches the muscles of the back and tends to increase the person's ability to bend his or her back. Even with an unskilled helper, this exercise has been found to be more effective than the usual *rotation back cracking*, which involves bending the person's hips and shoulders in opposite directions (see section on *The Doctor*).

A third exercise, called *kick-ups*, basically repeats the second exercise, but is done by the back sufferer without assistance. It is generally not attempted until the acute stage is subsiding, although in mild cases it can be done almost immediately. Like the previous exercise, it should not be attempted by people with signs of root compression. To do the exercise, individuals should lie on their back with their head on a pillow and their hips and knees bent so that they form a right angle (see illustration). As

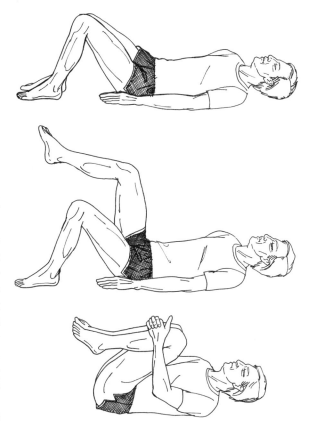

Low Back Stretch: *lie on your back with knees bent. Bring both knees to your chest, one at a time. Hug your knees until you feel a slight stretching in your lower back.*

slowly and smoothly as possible, they should raise their buttocks off the bed, letting their knees go back toward their head. Keeping their legs in the air, they should repeat a back-and-forth movement five times, and then return to the starting position, being very careful to keep their knees bent as they drop their legs down. This exercise is the major part of any *flexion-manipulation back exercise program*. To be effective, it must be done daily during the latter part of the acute stage because there is a strong tendency for the back to return to its former position of tension. Once the acute stage is over, kick-ups are often prescribed to build up the abdominal and paraspinal muscles in order to prevent further attacks (see section on *Prevention*).

There are also several exercises that are useful to relieve the pain of cervical neck strain. They basically involve gently moving the neck through its complete range of motion (see chart). In the acute stage, before the exercises are done, a warm shower should be taken or hot compresses applied to the neck.

Often, one of the underlying causes of back and neck problems is chronic muscle tension. Relaxation can be a significant factor in breaking the pain-tension cycle because tense muscles are more likely to spasm. Several different relaxation programs are commonly used in back pain clinics, including Jacobsen's *progressive muscle relaxation, autogenic relaxation, biofeedback, self-hypnosis,* and *guided imagery* (see p. 60 for instructions).

In addition to rest, heat, and exercise, over-the-counter drugs can be very useful in treating

---

Stretching Exercises to Relieve Neck Pain

These exercises are most effective if done during or after a hot shower, or after putting hot towels on the neck. Do as much of each exercise as possible; stop if the exercise becomes painful. Do the exercises two times a day.

- turn head alternately to the right and left as far as possible, relaxing in the center between turns
- slowly touch chin to chest, then lift head and look at ceiling
- bend head sideways to right and left, as if to touch ear to shoulder
- raise both shoulders as high as possible for a count of five; relax, then pull shoulders back as if to touch shoulder blades
- with hands behind back, grasp the thumb of one hand with the other hand and pull the shoulders downward toward the floor. At the same time, stand on tiptoe, and look at the ceiling. People who sit at a desk should do this exercise every two hours or so

---

the acute stages of a neck or low back episode. *Aspirin* and *ibuprofen (e.g., Motrin, Advil),* which have anti-inflammatory properties, are the most commonly suggested medications. *Acetaminophen (e.g., Tylenol)* may help to control pain, but does not reduce inflammation.

The Doctor

The doctor diagnoses the cause of neck and low back pain with a detailed history and specific physical and laboratory tests. Although there are many causes of low back problems, the most common one, a sprain, results in pain and possible muscle spasms, but little else. Back sprain can generally be diagnosed from a careful history and physical, without other tests. The physical includes feeling the back for tenderness, moving the back and legs to determine if range of motion has been impaired, and stretching the leg and knee to check for possible nerve root compression. The doctor will also do a careful neurological exam to rule out sensory loss, muscle weakness, or diminished reflexes, which can also indicate nerve root compression. Provided the history and physical do not show signs of *significant* nerve involvement or other problems, the doctor generally does no further tests.

If people do have signs of more serious nerve root compression or other underlying illnesses such as arthritis, the doctor will order various laboratory tests. A *blood test* is done to rule out nonmusculoskeletal diseases such as rheumatoid arthritis or gout. *Spinal x-rays* may be taken to establish the condition of the lumbar joints, determine the width of the spinal canal, and see if there is any sign of disc collapse. Several new tests are being used with increased frequency; a *CT (computerized tomography) scan* or *nuclear magnetic resonance (NMR) imaging* can sometimes detect anatomical problems not revealed by regular x-rays. In the past, the doctor would order a *myelogram,* a procedure which involved the injecting of dye into the spinal canal in order to visualize a possible blockage. This test is used much less frequently now, because the various new scanning techniques are noninvasive, but still provide important information.

The first step in deciding upon appropriate treatment for any low back condition is making an accurate diagnosis. Unusual or serious conditions require specific treatment, but the great majority of back and neck problems heal with time and are treated with the self-care remedies discussed above. Beyond these simple regimens, there is great diversity in the manner in which back problems are treated. Different kinds of specialists use different types of treatment. At present, back pain is treated by family practitioners, internists, physiatrists (rehabilitation specialists), physical therapists, orthopedic surgeons, neurosurgeons, neurologists, osteopaths, chiropractors, acupuncturists, body therapists, and massage specialists. Unfortunately, no double-blind studies have been done to determine the relative effectiveness of different treatments. In part, this is due to the fact that the majority of back problems heal by themselves within a short time.

Many medical schools and major medical centers now have comprehensive diagnostic and exercise programs that are run by their physical therapy or physical medicine departments. Physiatrists' programs involve graduated exercise and weaning patients off pain medications and muscle relaxants; surgery is rarely required. Exercise-based programs are considered by many doctors to be the best answer for people with chronic back problems that do not need surgery. Several different types of programs are used depending on the diagnosis and the individual physical therapy center. The three main aspects of most programs are 1) *general exercise* such as walking, swimming or jogging; 2) *flexion*, which involves strengthening the abdominal muscles through modified sit-ups or leg-lifts (see section on *Self-Care*); and 3) *extension exercises* which involve raising the back off a flat surface.

Often the exercise program is combined with education about those everyday activities that may exacerbate a person's back condition (see section on *Prevention*). Additional components of many programs include relaxation training through progressive muscle relaxation or biofeedback, guided imagery techniques, and group or individual psychotherapy sessions designed to lower the emotional stress and anxiety that people commonly transfer to the back.

Another common method of treatment is *spinal manipulation*, an adjustment maneuver in which a practitioner moves the affected joint beyond its normal range of motion, but not so far as to strain a muscle or ligament. After the back sufferer has become relaxed, the practitioner bends or turns the spine until resistance is felt, and then moves it a small distance further, so that a yielding is felt and a cracking or clicking noise is heard. One theory holds that by widening the joint space, muscle spasms are relieved. Such manuevers used to be done only by chiropractors and osteopaths, but they are now used by many orthopedists, physical therapists, and massage specialists as well. Spinal manipulation is most frequently performed in cases of

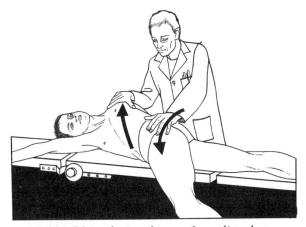

Trained health professionals can often relieve low back pain by rotating the spine slightly past its stretch point.

"acute locked back," for which it provides dramatic, immediate relief. It is also used for cases of acute or chronic back sprain, but in these cases treatment must be repeated daily or weekly to be truly effective. Spinal manipulation should not be used if there are signs of a herniated disc, such as limb pain or pain radiating below the knee, or if there is any sign of underlying disease.

Some doctors prescribe a *back brace* or *surgical corset* as part of their treatment, especially if there are signs of disc herniation or degeneration. A brace is very useful if a person must continue to do a lot of bending and lifting, because it prevents the lumbar joints from flexing or extending beyond the normal range of motion. The various corsets or braces include elastic ones; canvas supports with metal stays; metal frames; and custom ones made of fiberglass or plaster of paris. For neck sprains, *collars* are often prescribed for anywhere from ten days to eight weeks. The collar maximizes the intervertebral space and immobilizes the neck to keep the joints from going past the normal range of motion.

In addition to bed rest, some doctors prescribe *traction* or *gravity lumbar reduction* (GLR), both of which stretch the spine with weights. With conventional pelvic traction, external weights are used; with GLR therapy, people are suspended with a chest harness that makes use of the body's own weight. GLR therapy was developed at the Sister Kenny Institute as an alternative to spinal surgery for people with acute herniated discs.

Pain medication, muscle relaxants, and anti-inflammatory drugs used to be widely prescribed for back problems. In recent years, however, their use has been greatly diminished. The drugs are often not effective, and many patients actually become dependent on, or addicted to, various pain medicines and muscle relaxants. Nevertheless, certain drugs (e.g., *Valium*) may be used for *brief periods* during acute episodes or in some cases of chronic back problems.

Occasionally back problems are treated with injections of a combination of *local anesthetics* and *steroids*. This treatment is most often used if there is a specific area of tenderness, similar to a tendinitis or bursitis. The enzyme *chymopapain* is sometimes injected directly into a herniated disc in order to shrink it. Because of a 1% risk of a serious allergic reaction, chymopapain is only injected by orthopedic surgeons in an operating room. It is considered to be an alternative to surgery.

The last alternative for severe back problems is surgery. At this time, only a very small percentage of people with mechanical low back problems ever require surgery; the vast majority are cured with more conservative treatments. The only absolute indication for surgery on a herniated disc is paralysis of the legs, or the inability to control urination or defecation. Lumbar surgery is sometimes elected if conservative medical treatment fails or if people have a specific spinal deformity, such as severe disc degeneration or a narrowed spinal canal (*spinal stenosis*). Spinal surgery on the cervical area is far less common than lumbar surgery. Cervical discs do not herniate, although there may be narrowing of the spinal canal in this area. Basically there are two types of spinal surgery. One is *laminectomy*, which involves simple removal of a disc to take pressure off the spinal nerve roots. The other is *spinal fusion*, which is done in severe cases of disc degeneration: the disc is removed and a bone graft from the hip is inserted between the vertebrae to prevent movement at that point in the back.

Any spinal surgery involves a prolonged recuperation, the length of which depends upon the kind of work the patient does. Surgery is not a recommended treatment for people who are simply anxious to return to normal activity without having to follow a lengthy exercise regimen. After back surgery, the earliest people can return to sedentary work is usually 6 weeks. If their job requires much standing, walking, or bending, the recuperation time can be as long as six months. For people in the building trades or heavy industry, regular work cannot ordinarily be resumed for a year or more. In the case of spinal fusion, the graft is not fully incorporated for 9–12 months. These cautions notwithstanding, there are definitely people for whom surgery is the treatment of choice, either because of complications due to root compression, severe disc degeneration, or specific anatomical problems such as bone spurs or narrowing of the spinal canal.

Ruling Out Other Diseases

The great majority of back pain is due to sprains or muscle spasms. The second most common cause involves disc herniation (slipped disc) or degeneration. But the doctor will rule out more unusual conditions that can cause back symptoms. A detailed history and physical exam, along with other tests, can help to distinguish organic illness from pain caused by tension and anxiety, or from pain complicated by concerns about lawsuits and compensation claims. Blood tests can rule out *rheumatoid arthritis* (see p. 336), *ankylosing spondylitis*, or infection. They can also help to rule out gastrointestinal and urinary problems that can cause back pain. X-rays and/or CT scans can rule out *osteoarthritis* (see p. 334), *spinal stenosis* (narrowing of the spinal canal), *spondylolisthesis* (slipped vertebrae), compression fractures due to injury or *osteoporosis* (see p. 343), or rare bone tumors.

Prevention

There is a growing realization among professionals who deal with back problems that *prevention* is more important than *treatment*, and that factors in our modern life-style are largely responsible for the back problems we develop. Prevention involves educating people about the

---

Preventing Neck and Shoulder Strain

- keep neck straight and chin tucked down
- stand and sit up straight, with shoulders down and slightly back
- avoid looking up or reaching overhead for long periods at a time
- avoid lifting objects that are too heavy
- when driving, don't prop arm on car window or sit too low or too far back (if necessary, use a seat support to raise position)
- avoid reading or watching TV while propped on an elbow or with neck bent
- avoid sleeping on your stomach; sleep on your side or back, using a contoured neck pillow if necessary

---

causes of back problems, and showing them how to practice the basic back habits that will lower the risk of back pain and injury during daily activity (see charts). Experts believe that knowing how to use the back is the single most important factor in preventing back problems. Spine mechanics include learning the proper way to sit, stand, walk, bend over, lift, carry weights, drive, and even push or pull. It also involves advice on weight reduction, postural realignment, work habits and equipment, sleeping positions, mattresses, furniture, and other back aids.

The second part of a good spine education program involves a complete exercise program designed to strengthen abdominal and back muscles and improve posture. Good tone in these muscles is essential to a healthy back since the spine would collapse without support. These muscles are to the spine what rigging stays are to the mast of a sailboat. Exercises that are beneficial include pelvic tilts, modified sit-ups, kick-ups, leg lifts, knee bends, leg and back stretches, and relaxation exercises (see charts and illustrations). Spine education programs are very successful in dealing with back episodes and helping to avoid future ones. Such programs even help to lessen degenerative back changes, which can be accelerated by injury and excessive motion.

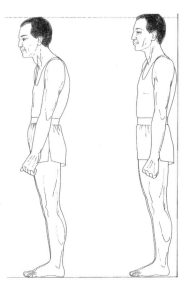

A number of basic habits help to minimize the risk of triggering low back pain during daily activities.

Good posture involves standing straight with weight distributed evenly on both feet, and the head centered over the body, in a relaxed position.

Preventing Low Back Pain

Standing:
- stand straight but relaxed, not slouched
- avoid high heels or dropped heels
- if standing for long periods, occasionally shift weight from side to side, and rest one foot on a footrest four to eight inches high

Sitting:
- sit rather than stand for long periods
- sit in straight-backed chairs that have good back support, cushions that follow body contours, and arm rests if possible
- sit with knees higher than hips—use a footstool if necessary
- avoid sitting with legs outstretched; cross ankles or use a footstool
- use a reclining chair for chronic back conditions
- slide to front of chair when getting up; slide back into chair when sitting down
- when driving, sit close to the steering wheel so as to flex knees and hips; use a back support if necessary

Bending and lifting:
- avoid lifting very heavy weights; carry several small loads if possible

- when lifting objects off the floor, keep the back straight, bend the hips and knees; never lift with knees straight
- never twist when you lift, face the object; lift straight up, using both hands; hold object close to the body
- never lift heavy objects more than 2 feet from the body or over shoulder level
- avoid straining to reach objects; reposition commonly used objects between waist and shoulder height
- avoid making beds; avoid climbing stairs
- if possible, push instead of pull; keeping back straight, push with legs and arms, not back

Sleeping:
- use a firm mattress that does not sag
- use a firm bedboard or box spring; it's as important as the mattress
- preferably, sleep on side with knees and hips slightly bent (fetal position); if sleeping on your back, put a pillow under your knees; if sleeping on your stomach, put a pillow under your hips

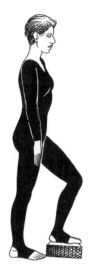
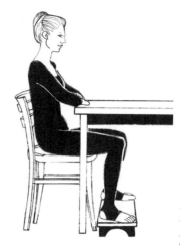

When you stand for long intervals, keep one foot forward—on a small footstool if possible; when you sit for long periods, keep both feet on a footstool, knees slightly higher than hips.

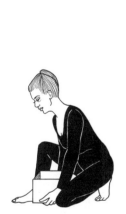
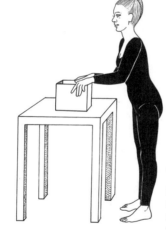

To lift an object off the ground, squat with one foot forward. To lift an object at waist height, slide the object close to you, bend your knees, and lift by straightening your knees.

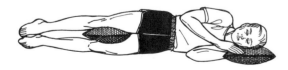
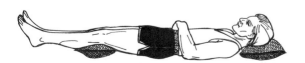

Sleep on your side with a pillow under your head and a pillow between your knees (optional). When sleeping on your back, you may find it more comfortable to put a pillow under your knees as well as under your head.

A number of exercises strengthen the muscles of the abdomen and back, and thereby help to prevent episodes of low back pain.

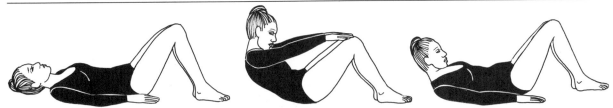

To do a modified sit-up, lie on your back with knees bent and feet on the floor. Lift your head so your chin almost touches your chest. Continue, lifting your shoulders off the floor and touch your knees with your fingertips. Do not arch your back.

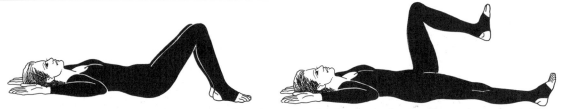

Single Knee to Chest Exercise: *lie on your back with your hands above your head and your knees bent. Move one knee toward your chest as far as is comfortable, while straightening out the other leg at the same time. Alternate legs.*

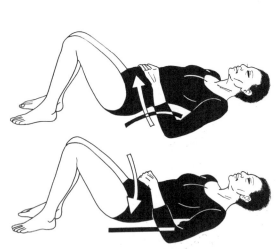

Pelvic Tilt: *lie on your back with knees bent. Tense the muscles of your lower abdomen and buttocks at the same time and hold for a count of 10. Your back should flatten along the floor.*

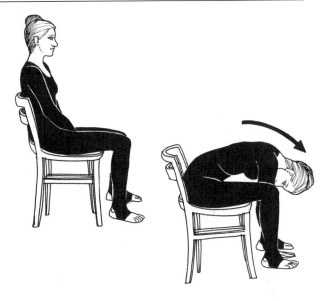

The Chair Stretch: *sit on a chair with your hands between your thighs. Bend forward until your head is between your knees.*

Arthritis: osteoarthritis and Rheumatoid Arthritis

Symptoms

osteoarthritis
- deep aching pain in the joints
- pain on movement
- increasing pain throughout the day
- joints most commonly affected are the fingers, hips, knees, feet, and spine
- pain at night
- brief morning stiffness
- joint grating or crackling upon movement

rheumatoid arthritis
- stiffness in the joints after inactivity, especially in the morning
- joint pain or tenderness
- joint swelling and warmth
- joints most commonly affected are the small joints of the hands, wrists, and feet
- swelling and tenderness are frequently symmetrical
- occasionally, a low-grade fever
- occasionally, lumps under the skin near the elbows

Description

Over 20 million people in the United States alone suffer from some form of arthritis. In terms of lost work days, arthritis is second only to heart disease. Actually, arthritis is not one, but several diseases which have different causes, different histories, and different courses. The most common of the diseases in the arthritis family is *osteoarthritis*, which affects approximately 15 million people, most of them middle-aged or older. The second most common form of arthritis is *rheumatoid arthritis*, which affects approximately 5 million people. Its incidence also rises with age. There are a number of other less common forms of arthritis, including *gout, ankylosing spondylitis*, and *systemic lupus erythematosus*.

Arthritis is one of the oldest diseases known, and has even been found in fossil remains of a swimming reptile that lived a hundred million years ago. Many modern animals are afflicted with arthritis too. In terms of human ancestors, arthritis has been found in the half-million-year-old remains of Java and Lansing man, as well as in 10,000-year-old mummies from ancient Egypt.

In common usage, *arthritis* refers to a disease of the musculoskeletal system that involves the joints. The symptoms of arthritis are decreased range of motion, pain, swelling, and tenderness in specific joints. The term *rheumatism*, which is sometimes confused with arthritis by lay people, is a general term for pain and stiffness in any part of the musculoskeletal system. It does not refer to any specific disease, but is used variously to describe the symptoms of tendinitis, bursitis, rheumatic fever, any type of arthritis, and even muscle and bone diseases.

A *joint* is the junction between two or more bones (see illustration). Most of the body's joints permit movement while also bearing weight and maintaining the body's alignment. The joints are held together by *ligaments* and the *joint capsule*: the ligaments are tough fibrous bands that stretch across the joint to connect one bone to

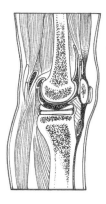

A joint is a junction between bones that permits various degrees of movement. A joint is held together by fibrous bands called ligaments and by the joint capsule itself.

another; the joint capsule is a thick fibrous envelope that encases and protects the joint. The ends of the bone are covered with *articular cartilage*, a smooth material that cushions the bones and enables them to slide over one another smoothly. The inside of the joint capsule is lined with a thin membrane called the *synovium*, which secretes the *synovial fluid* that lubricates the joint. The synovial membrane also disposes of debris that is created by friction when the bones move. In addition, the joint capsule contains many sensory nerve endings.

Osteoarthritis: Osteoarthritis, or *degenerative joint disease*, is the most common disease affecting humans and other vertebrates. In humans, degenerative joint changes are rarely seen before the second decade of life, but some degree of change is almost universal over the age of 75. By the age of 55, 80% of all individuals will show x-ray evidence of osteoarthritis. For many years it was thought that such degenerative joint changes were part of the normal process of aging, like the graying of hair, but, although the frequency of osteoarthritis does increase with age, it is no longer believed to be simply the result of wear and tear.

The causes of osteoarthritis are still not entirely clear. The disease is probably the result of a very complex interaction between physical stresses applied to the joints, the body's ability to deal with and heal those stresses, and biochemical factors that are inherited. In people who have osteoarthritis, two major changes take place within the structure of affected joints. First, the smooth, slippery *cartilage* that covers the ends of the bones and lines the joint begins to break down. This covering is extremely important because it enables the ends of the bones to slide smoothly over one another where they meet at the joint. Secondly, in people with osteoarthritis new bone formation begins at the edges of the bones that make up the joint.

Cartilage is made up of *collagen fibers*, which provide strength, and *proteoglycans*, which provide elasticity. As arthritis develops, the amount of proteoglycans decreases, causing the cartilage to lose its elasticity and making it more permeable to water, which makes it swell. Tiny areas of the cartilage soften, and then eventually develop cracks or fissures. Next, progressively bigger and bigger pieces of cartilage slough off, and this debris is broken down and removed by white blood cells. In time, large areas at the ends of bones can become bare of cartilage, making movements of the joint rough and painful. Doctors believe that this process of deterioration begins with some kind of injury to the cells that produce cartilage.

Initially, when cartilage breaks down the body attempts to heal itself. Cartilage-producing cells called *chondrocytes* proliferate and increase the synthesis of proteoglycans. Joint deterioration begins to take place only when the chondrocytes are no longer able to keep pace with the decrease in proteoglycans.

At the same time as the cartilage is undergoing degeneration, new bone growth starts at the ends of the bones, producing small bone spurs that grow out from the bone and become covered with cartilage. These spurs tend to develop in areas where there is least contact with another

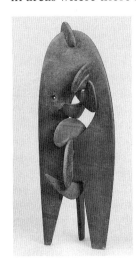

In osteoarthritis, the cartilage at the ends of bones softens and cracks off in little pieces. As a result, the bones become bare and movement becomes rough and painful. Isamu Noguchi. Humpty Dumpty. 1946. Ribbon slate. 48¾" × 20¾" × 18". Collection, The Whitney Museum of American Art. Purchase. 47.7.

surface, so joint motion does not tend to wear them down. Eventually these spurs can become large enough to affect a joint's mobility and visibly change its shape.

Pain and joint enlargement are relatively late symptoms in the development of osteoarthritis. Generally, the early stage involving the initial cartilage deterioration goes unnoticed because cartilage has no pain nerves to signal what's going on. The pain that later plagues people with osteoarthritis is due to swelling and distention of the joint capsule, as well as abrasion of the synovial lining and chafing of bone spurs on the *periosteum*, the membrane that surrounds the bone. As arthritis progresses, the joint capsule becomes inflamed due to the influx of white blood cells needed to clear away the pieces of cartilage that have broken off. Some researchers speculate that the body views these broken pieces of cartilage as foreign objects, and produces a mild allergic reaction to them.

Doctors make a distinction between *primary osteoarthritis*, which is of unknown origin, and *secondary osteoarthritis*, which develops after an insult or injury to a joint. The trauma may be a single event such as a fracture, sprain, infection, or condition like frostbite, or it may be the result of a gradual process such as poor posture, obesity, or prolonged overuse in work or sports. Currently, experts speculate that even primary arthritis may involve incorrect use of the joint to some degree. It is thought that the constant application of misdirected mechanical force may put excessive stress on the cartilage in a joint and cause it to deteriorate. Simple observation backs up this theory. People who do hard physical work are more likely than average to develop arthritis; and their arthritis tends to occur in those joints that are put under stress by the work they do. This theory is further supported by the fact that arthritis sufferers generally show more evidence of arthritis in their dominant hand, whereas osteoarthritis never develops in paralyzed limbs.

The symptoms of osteoarthritis generally appear very gradually, most commonly beginning in people over the age of 40. Deep, aching pain is the main symptom. Such pain is often difficult to localize, but occurs in the vicinity of the involved joints. At first, pain is noticed when the joint is used, but subsides when motion ceases. As the disease progresses, the ache no longer is relieved by rest. Often, pain increases throughout the day; in severe cases, the joints become continuously painful, even during sleep.

Osteoarthritis is not a systemic disease that causes generalized symptoms such as fever or tiredness, and it only occurs in specific joints. The joints most frequently affected by primary osteoarthritis are the *last* and *next-to-last* joints of the fingers, the base of the thumb, and the hips, knees, feet, and back. The knuckles, wrists, elbows, and shoulders are almost never affected by this form of arthritis. Secondary or traumatic arthritis can affect any joint that is injured, although it rarely occurs in the ankle.

Next to pain, the most common characteristic of osteoarthritis is stiffness. This stiffness only involves the affected joints, and is common upon awakening or after a period of disuse, but usually only lasts for 15–30 minutes. It subsides more quickly if a person exercises to warm up and limber up the joint. In osteoarthritis, as in all forms of arthritis, changes in weather, specific injuries, or overuse can cause pain and stiffness to worsen. Occasionally, osteoarthritis is accompanied by painful spasms in the muscles that move the affected joint.

If the disease progresses to a more severe form, joint damage can cause new symptoms that are related to anatomical changes which take place. First, narrowing of the joint space will cause the ends of the bones to rub, which often produces a crackling or crunching sound called *crepitus* when the joint moves. Second, the formation of bone spurs and the accompanying decrease in the joint space also limits the joint's normal range of motion. Third, severe arthritis eventually causes enlargement and deformity of the joint, deflecting the angles at which the bones meet.

Rheumatoid arthritis: Rheumatoid arthritis is a chronic systemic disease characterized by inflammation of the joints and surrounding tissues. Rheumatoid arthritis is difficult to diagnose because its symptoms are highly variable; the disease ranges from a single episode that is brief and mild to a chronic progressive condition that can severely limit joint movement. This particular type of arthritis occurs three times as often in women as in men, and affects over 5 million people in the United States. The incidence of rheumatoid arthritis rises with age, affecting over 10% of the population by age 65. The most common age of onset is in the 50s, although even children can develop the disease. Rheumatoid arthritis is known to occur more commonly in certain families; progress is being made in defining its genetic basis (see below). Unlike osteoarthritis, which has existed since ancient times, rheumatoid arthritis has only been described for a hundred years and may be a relatively new disease. Although the exact cause is still unknown, a tremendous amount of research has been done on rheumatoid arthritis because it affects so may people so severely.

Rheumatoid arthritis is recognized as an *autoimmune disease,* that is, a condition in which the body becomes allergic to its own tissue, in this case, cartilage. This phenomenon is thought to take place only in individuals who are genetically susceptible to the disease. Currently, most researchers believe that rheumatoid arthritis begins with a complicated series of interrelated events. Since other types of arthritis are associated with bacterial or viral infections—*rubella, hepatitis,* and *Lyme disease* being some examples—rheumatoid arthritis is thought to be triggered by an infectious agent. Unfortunately, no specific organism has yet been identified as the cause.

Doctors believe that the infectious agent invades and alters collagen cells in the joint capsule cartilage, causing a local inflammatory reaction in which one particular type of antibody, *IgG antibody,* is produced by the immune system. Subsequently, in some manner not understood, the body begins to identify this kind of antibody as a "foreign" substance or *antigen.* When this happens, the *Type A cells* in the synovial membrane that normally remove debris begin to eat up the antibodies as well. The digested products of this process cause an allergic reaction: white blood cells floating in the synovial fluid start producing large amounts of another type of antibody, *IgM antibody,* in an effort to erradicate the first kind. The second type of antibody, which is only made in this situation, is referred to as *rheumatoid factor.* They are found in the blood and synovial fluid of 80% of people with rheumatoid arthritis and are a reliable laboratory indication of the disease.

In an effort to inactivate the IgG antibodies, the IgM antibodies hook onto them and form what is called an *antigen-antibody complex.* Millions of antigen-antibody clumps become trapped in the cartilage cells and synovial fluid of the joints. In response, the body's white blood cells release a number of powerful but highly irritating chemicals (*histamine, complement, kinins,* and *lysosomal enzymes*) that cause new and expanded inflammation and tissue destruction. All these chemicals, in a protective effort gone astray, begin to destroy cartilage cells on a large scale. At the same time, cells in the synovial membrane start to multiply indiscriminately and eventually even begin to adhere to adjacent cartilage on the ends of the bones. The thickened, altered synovial membrane that results is referred to as a *pannus.* As the pannus grows, it produces more of the chemicals that dissolve cartilage. Eventually, the joint space collapses, cartilage is progressively eroded, and bone begins to dissolve under the cartilage. In advanced situations, the pannus can even invade and damage ligaments, destroying the functional ability of the joint.

Even as destruction is occurring, healing and repair of tissues are going on at the same time. During early stages of rheumatoid arthritis, before cartilage is dissolved, the process can be reversed and complete healing can still take place. Even after cartilage has been destroyed, the process can stop and some healing can take place. Doctors still do not understand what factors cause the process to stop, reverse, or continue, but they have found a linked cluster of genes, *HLA-D4*, that occurs much more frequently in people with rheumatoid arthritis. Researchers speculate that this marker represents a genetic susceptibility, either to a particular infectious agent, or to a propensity for an immune reaction to continue. A genetic predisposition would explain why rheumatoid arthritis appears to be more common in certain families.

Rheumatoid arthritis is a highly variable disease both in terms of its course and in terms of the joints that it affects. In about 80% of all cases, the disease comes on very gradually over a period of weeks and months. But occasionally the disease comes on rapidly within a matter of days. In this case there are often generalized symptoms such as fever, malaise, loss of appetite, and muscle aches. Along with, or shortly after, these initial systemic symptoms occur, joint symptoms begin.

The first localized symptom of rheumatoid arthritis may be stiffness, which is caused by the accumulation of fluid within the inflamed joint tissues. This stiffness is generally worse in the morning, after disuse, and gradually goes away as the body's lymphatic system removes the accumulated fluid. As the disease process continues, other symptoms occur, including swelling, redness, tenderness, and joint pain, all of which are symptoms of the inflammatory process. Often these symptoms are symmetrical, occurring in the same joints on both sides of the body. Sometimes people with rheumatoid arthritis also notice muscle weakness in affected joints which is out of proportion to the pain they are experiencing. This weakness is generally thought to be due to muscle atrophy resulting from disuse.

Generally, a number of joints are affected in rheumatoid arthritis, most commonly the joints of the hands, wrists, knees, and feet. Unlike osteoarthritis, the end joints of the fingers are rarely involved. If the disease progresses, it can involve the neck, elbows, shoulders, hips, ankles, jaw, or the joints where the clavicles attach to the breastbone.

In advanced stages of the disease, swelling can give joints a distinct spindle-shaped appearance. Ultimately, if severe tissue destruction takes place, the bones on either side of the joint can become oddly displaced. Such visible changes are most common in the hands. *Subcutaneous nodules* may also appear in areas subject to pressure, such as the elbow, shoulder, and back. These nodules consist of inflammatory cells walled off by a fibrous collagen capsule.

About 50% of those who are diagnosed with rheumatoid arthritis experience a few episodes and then recover completely. Some who do not spontaneously get better have mild bouts punctuated by remissions in which there are no symptoms for a month or more. In some cases remissions last for as long as 30 years. A third group of people have chronic, progressive disease with frequent inflammatory episodes, and suffer joint damage and disability. Fortunately, fewer than 3% of all those diagnosed with rheumatoid arthritis fail to respond well to treatment. A number of factors affect the frequency and severity of attacks. Exacerbations are more frequent in colder weather, and stress plays an important role in the recurrence of episodes in some people. Occasionally people can even pinpoint a specific event as triggering an episode. The event may be either psychological or physical stress, an injury, or an infection.

Self-Care

Patient education and self-care are the basis for treatment of any kind of arthritis. Arthritis is a chronic illness whose course is unpredictable and whose cause is unknown. There is no specific cure, but much can be done to alleviate discomfort and prevent progression. Unfortunately, many people believe that arthritis is invariably a crippling disease and they become depressed. Although rheumatoid arthritis is sometimes disabling, osteoarthritis rarely is. However, it's important to realize that although there is no cure for either osteoarthritis or rheumatoid arthritis, much can be done to treat it effectively. It is also important that arthritis sufferers understand what a critical role they play in their own treatment. A person's attitude about the disease, compliance with self-help regimens, and knowing when to see the doctor all strongly affect the course of the disease and a person's ability to deal with it. Realistic long-term goals vary, but generally the major goals are relative freedom from discomfort and maintenance of joint mobility. The mind has significant effects on the immune system, and studies have shown that people with a positive attitude about rheumatoid arthritis generally do better (see p. 5). Since the prognosis is better in most cases than people fear, reassurance by the doctor often plays a crucial role in treatment.

The single most important element in any self-care program lies in people educating themselves about their illness. Education is necessary in order to help patients set realistic but optimistic goals and to carry out an effective self-help program. This is especially important because, of all the common chronic diseases, arthritis is most amenable to self-management through patient education.

Through education, individuals can learn which movements, postures, and habits tend to put unnecessary strain on affected joints. This is an essential part of any good arthritis program.

In the case of osteoarthritis, avoiding strain lessens pain and increases the likelihood of cartilage resurfacing, while in rheumatoid arthritis, avoiding strain decreases the inflammatory process, and also lessens pain. Postural retraining plays a crucial role by taking excess weight off the joints during both waking hours and sleep. Proper positions for lifting and bending help to avoid damage, as do certain positions for occupational tasks and household chores. In many cases specialized instruments, such as tools with large handles, can help to relieve strain on joints.

In addition to basic education, there are a number of specific beneficial self-care measures. The first is *rest*. With osteoarthritis, the amount of rest required varies with the severity of the illness, the particular joints that are involved, and the type of work a person does. Periodic rest breaks are advised, rather than working straight through at a task. If weight-bearing joints are affected, it's worthwhile to lie down once or twice a day. Rest periods specifically aid in relieving emotional stress, which in turn helps to decrease general tiredness, muscle spasms, and pain. Often arthritis clinics suggest combining rest periods with relaxation exercises, visualization, or biofeedback (see p. 60).

In rheumatoid arthritis, rest can likewise improve symptoms and alleviate flare-ups. Complete bed rest used to be the standard treatment for episodes, but some doctors now simply advise frequent rest periods. Since rheumatoid arthritis is a systemic disease, rest tends to relieve tiredness as well as joint pain. Fatigue is such a major symptom that many rheumatoid patients nap daily.

In osteoarthritis, damaged joints cannot withstand excess stress. What is normal stress for a healthy joint can be undue stress on an arthritic joint, thereby preventing healing and hastening deterioration of cartilage. People with osteoarthritis are advised to "live within the limitations of their joints." This philosophy both relieves

---

Using Heat to Treat Arthritic Joints

- take a hot bath or shower (under 20 minutes) to decrease morning stiffness
- use hot or cold packs to reduce muscle spasms, decrease pain, and increase range of motion
- use heat pad on low or medium setting to avoid burns; never lie on heat pad or use it for more than 20 minutes at a time
- use heated pools, whirlpools, and saunas to apply heat and relax joints

---

symptoms and slows the progress of the illness. Doctors now believe that rest allows some cartilage resurfacing of the joints.

Both *heat* and *cold* are important aspects of arthritis self-care. Used appropriately, they can relieve pain and help to increase joint mobility. Heat is particularly effective in relieving the morning stiffness of rheumatoid arthritis, and even osteoarthritis. At home, heat can be applied by means of warm showers or tubs, hot packs, hot water bottles, hot compresses, electric blankets, or heating pads. During acute flare-ups, when the joints are red and hot to the touch, ice packs should be used in place of heat because cold reduces inflammation and swelling. Ice packs should be wrapped in a thin towel and applied to the affected area for as long as it is comfortable. The most convenient form to use is the refreezable ice available through camping or medical supply stores.

An important counterpart to rest is *exercise*. Obviously, for an arthritis regimen, exercise has to be carefully graded according to the severity of the disease and the amount of rest needed. Exercise is valuable for a number of reasons: it helps relieve stiffness and pain, maintains joint mobility, and strengthens surrounding muscles to maintain optimum joint function. In recent years, exercise has come to be regarded as the most instrumental factor in limiting the progression of joint disability.

As with rest, the specific exercises and amounts depend upon the severity of the illness and the joints involved. Minor arthritis requires regular exercise with some limitations; more advanced arthritis benefits greatly from a program designed and managed by a physical therapist. Normal daily activities don't necessarily qualify as an effective exercise program because people often adjust their movements to compensate for discomfort, and thus do not go through the full range of motion possible for the affected joints. Swimming is the most beneficial form of general exercise for people with arthritis. If the affected joints are in the foot, knees, hips, or back, such sports as jogging and bicycling can actually be damaging. For all but the mildest cases of arthritis, people should check with a physical therapist before engaging in any exercise program, particularly one that involves activities with repetitive or jarring motions.

Any good exercise program addresses two issues: movement and the prevention of excess strain on affected joints. Movement should be done on a daily basis after any initial stiffness has subsided, preferably after a warm bath. Generally people are advised to take affected joints through as full a range of motion as possible because this prevents ligaments and muscles from losing tone and flexibility, which leads to loss of mobility. Most recommended exercises are *isometric*; that is, they involve holding a position rather than rocking the joint back and forth. This minimizes wear-and-tear on the joint but exercises the muscles and ligaments surrounding the joint. In general, exercises should be *graded*; that is, they should never be done past the point of fatigue or pain, but they should gradually increase in number, range, and weight.

Diet is the most controversial aspect of arthritis self-care, but doctors do agree on two points: patients should eat a well-balanced diet to promote healing, and they should lose weight if they are too heavy because excess weight puts tremendous strain on all the joints. Since osteoarthritis and rheumatoid arthritis are chronic diseases without a cure, many people have been attracted to anecdotal accounts of diets that claim to provide a cure. The fact that both osteoarthritis and rheumatoid arthritis are characterized by remissions as well as flare-ups may incorrectly encourage people to believe that a particular dietary regimen may be responsible for the cause, or cure, of arthritis.

Currently no double-blind studies have demonstrated that any special diet helps people with arthritis. In fact, one study demonstrated that one of the most popular arthritis diets (no additives, preservatives, fruit, red meat, herbs, or dairy products) made no difference to a group who were on the diet, as compared to a control group. Ironically, 37% of the patients in both the diet and nondiet groups reported improvement. Researchers think these results were based on the emotional support that all the participants in the study received.

Interestingly, animal studies have shown some positive results with diet. A low-fat diet has been found to improve several forms of arthritis in rats and mice. Thus most doctors recommend a low-fat diet for arthritis patients—first because it helps to keep their weight at an optimum level, and secondly because animal studies indicate such a diet may be beneficial in itself. Another study has demonstrated improvement among animals getting a specific fatty acid that is found in some fish, but not in meat. However, patients should not focus on diet to the point of neglecting exercise and drug regimens that have been proven effective (see below).

The Doctor

An internist or rheumatologist diagnoses arthritis on the basis of a careful history, physical exam, laboratory tests, and x-rays. Osteoarthritis and rheumatoid arthritis have very different histories: rheumatoid arthritis is basically systemic and inflammatory, with symmetrical swelling; while osteoarthritis is asymmetric, and exhibits no inflammation and minimal morning stiffness. On blood tests, a diagnosis of rheumatoid arthritis is suggested by several indicators of inflammation and autoimmune dysfunction, including the presence of rheumatoid factor, a high erythrocyte sedimentation rate, a positive latex fixation, and high gamma globulin (IgG and IgM) levels. None of these indicators are elevated in osteoarthritis. In rheumatoid arthritis, x-rays show joint erosion, whereas with osteoarthritis, x-rays may reveal bone spurs, narrowing of the joint spaces, and tiny bone cysts.

The initial treatment for either osteoarthritis or rheumatoid arthritis involves the self-help regimens outlined above. If self-care is not sufficient, drug therapy may be recommended. By far the most common drug prescribed for arthritis is *aspirin*, which even though it is sold over the counter, is a fairly strong, relatively nontoxic anti-inflammatory medicine. In double-blind studies, aspirin has been found to be as effective as any of the newer, more expensive, and more toxic nonsteroidal anti-inflammatory drugs. Because aspirin's side effects are less severe, it is better for long-term use. Aspirin is thought to work by blocking synthesis of *prostaglandins*, which are a key part of the inflammatory process. To treat arthritis, aspirin is prescribed in relatively high doses. Administration is generally started at two 325 mg tablets four times a day. At these doses, some people will experience nausea and reddening or blackening of their stools due to minor gastrointestinal bleeding. This symptom should be checked to rule out other causes of bleeding. The dosage of aspirin may be increased if necessary, and should be decreased if patients experience ringing in their ears or temporary loss of hearing. To prevent stomach upset, the tablets should be taken "sandwich fashion," eating food before and after taking the tablets. Coated or buffered aspirin, or antacids may be useful for people who have trouble tolerating aspirin. It takes one to two weeks to attain levels of aspirin in the blood and synovial fluid that will achieve the desired anti-inflammatory effect. With long-term use, doctors periodically order a blood test for serum salicylate levels to adjust the dosage. In some cases *acetaminophen* (e.g. *Tylenol*), which is not anti-inflammatory, is given in addition to aspirin to increase pain control.

The second type of drug used for treating either form of arthritis is some form of *nonsteroidal anti-inflammatory*, including 1) *ibuprofen* (e.g., *Advil, Motrin*), 2) *fenoprofen* (e.g., *Nalfon*), 3) *naproxin* (e.g., *Naprosyn*), and *indomethacin* (e.g., *Indocin*). These drugs are generally given only if aspirin therapy does not provide sufficient relief. The drugs are very effective, but they have a variety of significant long-term side effects so that patients taking them must be closely monitored by the doctor. The most common side effects are stomach upset, gastrointestinal bleeding, and dizziness.

People with severe rheumatoid arthritis who do not respond to aspirin or other anti-inflammatories are sometimes given one of several drugs such as *gold preparations, antimalarial drugs*, and *penicillamines*. These drugs have been shown to prevent flare-ups, but all three types have significant side effects and must be carefully monitored. In rare unresponsive cases, patients may be given *corticosteroids* or *immunosuppressants*. Generally these drugs are only used in critical situations when other medications have not been effective.

As an adjunct to a complete exercise program, *rehabilitation doctors (physiatrists)* often prescribe various devices that are designed to reduce strain on joints, and lessen pain and deformity. These devices include *splints* for the thumb, wrist, hand and fingers; *orthotic shoe inserts* or special shoes for the feet; and leg braces, canes or walkers for the hips and knees. These aids may be used routinely or intermittently, during waking hours or during sleep. A wide variety of special large-handled tools and kitchen equipment are also available to assist people who have arthritis in their hands; they can be located through the rheumatologist or arthritis self-help groups.

In some situations, surgery may be recommended to improve joint mobility and/or relieve pain in people with advanced arthritis. A number of different surgical procedures are performed, but basically they all involve either removing the synovial membrane within the joint, fusing the joint, or replacing the joint with a metal and plastic prosthesis. Surgery is often very successful, providing relief from pain and much greater mobility.

More and more commonly for moderate-to-severe arthritis, a multidisciplinary approach is used, including a primary physician, a consulting rheumatologist, a physiatrist, a physiotherapist, an occupational therapist, and possibly a surgeon, psychologist, or social worker. In large arthritis clinics, a therapeutic plan is coordinated by an arthritis team nurse. An important goal of such a plan is to prevent joint damage and deformity. A team approach also provides psychological and emotional support, which is almost as important as physical treatment for a chronic disease like arthritis.

Ruling Out Other Diseases

There are many reasons for joint aches and pain. Perhaps the most common cause isn't even arthritis, but is *arthralgia* which is the term for joints that ache but are not swollen, red, tender, or more painful on movement. Arthralgias are typically caused by overuse, trauma, tension, or mild viruses. When the same symptoms affect muscles, it is referred to as *myalgia*. Often the distinction between arthralgia and myalgia is not clear. In this case, doctors may simply say, "It's not arthritis," or refer to the condition in general terms such as *nonarticular rheumatism*. In addition, what people perceive as joint pain is actually often pain from ligaments, tendons, or bursae (see *tendinitis* and *bursitis*, p. 310).

There are many causes of arthritic joint pain, swelling, and inflammation—osteoarthritis and rheumatoid arthritis being the most common. Other, less common forms of arthritis can be ruled out on the basis of laboratory tests and x-rays, as well as the history and physical exam that are part of the usual arthritis workup. *Gout* is an inherited metabolic disease in which uric acid crystallizes in the joints, causing attacks of acute arthritic pain in a single joint, most commonly the large joint of the big toe. A blood test will show an elevated uric acid count; also, if synovial fluid is removed from the joint, it will show the presence of crystals. *Ankylosing spondylitis* is an uncommon arthritic condition seen mostly in young men; it generally affects the spine, and in rare cases, the hands. It tests negative for rheumatoid factor and has specific x-ray findings in the sacroiliac joints of the lower back. Many *bacterial* and *viral infections* are associated with acute, temporary forms of arthritis, as well as fever, chills, and other specific symptoms. These infections include *staph* and *gonorrhea*, which are bacterial; and *hepatitis, rubella (German measles)*, and *mumps*, which are viral. *Lyme disease*, a viral disease carried by ticks, also causes arthritis, fever, and chills, as well as neurological symptoms. If untreated, the symptoms of Lyme disease can persist for weeks or months.

In rare cases, arthritic symptoms are caused by connective tissue diseases such as *systemic lupus erythematosus* or *scleroderma*. Lupus occurs primarily in young women, causing fever, skin rash, and eye symptoms, in addition to arthritis symptoms. Scleroderma symptoms include thickening of the skin and difficulty swallowing, as well as arthritis.

Prevention

Osteoarthritis accompanies aging in many people, but joint changes and damage are largely

Reducing Stress on Arthritic Joints

Wrist and hand:
• use both hands when lifting
• use outside of palm to apply pressure
• use large-handled objects or wrap handles with foam
• use glove-type pot holders
• carry shoulder purse on stronger shoulder
• avoid lifting or carrying objects, such as suitcases, by their handles

Shoulder:
• stand straight
• sleep on your back or on your good shoulder
• avoid reaching or lifting

Hip, knee, and foot:
• maintain an optimal weight
• use high chairs and raised toilet seats if getting up and down is painful
• use grab bars or rails if necessary
• use railings when climbing stairs
• take showers instead of baths if bending to sit in tub is painful

Neck:
• sleep with an orthopedic pillow
• stretch neck every 30 minutes (see p. 122)
• work at eye level
• avoid reaching, tilting head backward
• avoid cradling phone receiver with shoulder or using holder on the receiver

Back:
• sleep comfortably (see p. 331)
• roll to side and slide out of bed, rather than sitting up first
• avoid sitting in soft furniture for long periods of time

preventable. The main principle of prevention is a graded exercise program and joint protection which involves avoiding overuse, trauma, or positions that cause wear on affected joints (see charts and section on *Self-Care*). Weight reduction and good posture are important adjuncts to any plan for joint protection.

There are no specific prevention guidelines for rheumatoid arthritis since its cause is unknown. However, like osteoarthritis, the joint damage caused by rheumatoid arthritis can largely be prevented (see above) if people adhere to a well-designed self-care program.

Osteoporosis

Symptoms

- no initial symptoms
- upper or lower back pain that is acute or chronic
- loss of height and postural changes
- fractures of the vertebrae, hips, or wrists

Description

Osteoporosis is a condition in which there is "too little bone"; that is, the density of the bones decreases to the point that they can no longer support the body. Eventually the bones can become so thin and brittle that a fracture results from a fall or straining effort that normally would be harmless. These fractures are regarded as "pathological" because the force involved is so much less than what is usually required to cause a break. Not only do the bones break more easily if people have osteoporosis, they heal more slowly, and are more likely to break again. If the disease is severe, people may never regain full mobility.

Recent studies have shown that osteoporosis is a problem of enormous proportions world-

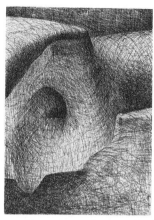

A *high-calcium diet and regular exercise help to protect against osteoporosis. Henry Moore.* Rocks, Arch, and Tunnel. *Plate XVI from* Elephant Skull. *1970. Etching, printed in black, 13⁹⁄₁₆″ × 9³⁄₄″. Collection, The Museum of Modern Art, New York. Gift of the artist and Gallerie Gerald Cramer, Geneva.*

wide. It is estimated to affect 15 million people in the U.S. alone, causing 1.3 million fractures annually. Osteoporosis generally begins in midadulthood and increases with age. Up to the age of 65, osteoporosis is six times more common in women than in men; above age 75, it is only twice as common in women. Many doctors now believe that there are two types of osteoporosis: *postmenopausal osteoporosis*, which affects people 50–65 years of age (predominantly women), and *senile osteoporosis*, which affects a large number of women and men over the age of 75.

In the early stages of bone loss, osteoporosis produces no symptoms. When bone loss becomes significant, fractures begin to occur, often in the spine. The spinal vertebrae contain two different types of bone: *cortical* or dense bone, and *trabecular* or sparse bone (see illustration). Loss of trabecular bone produces problems more quickly than does loss of cortical bone. Vertebrae begin to collapse when trabecular bone loss reaches 11%. This point is reached by 20% of Caucasian women by the age

trabeculae
growth plate
spongy bone
bone marrow
compact bone

Bones have dense areas called cortical bone *and less dense areas called* trabecular bone. *Vertebral fractures caused by osteoporosis involve the loss of trabecular bone.*

of 60. The only symptom of such vertebral collapse is loss of height. On the average, adult females lose .15 cm per year. Vertebral *crush fractures* actually begin to occur when trabecular loss reaches 14%. A woman with a crush fracture typically is one at high risk, about 20 years postmenopause, who simply lifts or turns with moderate force, then experiences mild to severe back pain for days or weeks. Generally the pain is initially episodic, but eventually becomes chronic. On the average, women with advanced osteoporosis experience one vertebral fracture per year. Without successful treatment, multiple fractures can produce a loss in height of 4–8 inches, and a spinal distortion referred to as *dowager's hump* or a *dorsal kyphosis*.

In later stages, there is significant loss of cortical, or dense, bone which can result in fractures of the hip or thigh. Such fractures have been called a "dreadful complication" of osteoporosis because they can actually be life-threatening. In the U.S. alone, there are 200,000 hip fractures per year, mostly among people above 65. The death rate for these people in the ensuing year is 10%–20% due to complications of surgery and lack of mobility.

There are a number of factors that increase the risk of developing osteoporosis. By compiling a list of risk factors, a profile emerges of the women who are most at risk. Small-boned women tend to be more susceptible than large-

boned women because they have less bone mass to begin with. Blacks have a significantly larger frame size on the average than do whites; as a result, they are much less likely to develop osteoporosis. Our genetics cannot be changed, but many of the other risk factors can be adjusted to decrease the likelihood of losing bone mass.

Although the definition of osteoporosis is simple, the causes are complex and probably involve multiple factors, all of which contribute to the development of bone loss. Contrary to popular misconception, bones are living tissue. Up into adulthood, the bones keep increasing in mass. Then bone mass levels off, and a regular cycle of loss and replacement evolves. Special areas of bone contain cells called *osteoclasts*, whose job is to dissolve bone, constructing little tunnels. Simultaneously, other cells called *osteoblasts* construct new bone and fill in the tunnels. When the processes of resorption and formation are equal, bone mass is stable. In people with osteoporosis, there is either too much resorption or too little formation; as a result, bone mass decreases.

Starting around midadulthood, everyone begins to experience a steady decrease in bone mass. This loss has been demonstrated through a new technique called *photon beam absorptiometry*, which allows extremely accurate measurement of the thickness of a bone. Interestingly, men lose about .17% per year, while women lose about .19% until menopause begins, at which point women begin to lose 1.01% per year—a fivefold increase. At those rates, the average woman will lose over 30% of her bone mass by the age of 80, the average man about 8%. With a longer life expectancy, more and more people can expect to undergo significant bone loss and the fractures that result from it.

In the first seven years after menopause, women experience an 8% greater loss of bone than before menopause. A number of studies link this acceleration to the decrease in *estrogen* that occurs with menopause. It has been found that women who have both ovaries surgically removed before the normal age for menopause are also subject to a rapid loss of bone. Lack of estrogen causes bone to be more sensitive to the body's *parathyroid hormone*, which causes calcium to be dissolved out of bone tissue. If women are given supplemental estrogen, calcium is better absorbed into bone. Indeed, studies have shown that women on supplemental estrogen have only one-fifth the bone loss of women who were not given estrogen. Women taking supplemental estrogen lost an average of .05% per year, while women not taking supplements lost 1.04%. When supplementation was started within three years after menopause, there was actually some *increase* in bone mass. Not only did the women given estrogen have less bone loss, they had fewer fractures. However, supplemental estrogen therapy remains controversial because of possible side effects (see section on *The Doctor*). After menopause, the major source of estrogen women have is body fat that is converted to estrogen. Thus heavy women have been found to suffer less bone loss than very thin women. Above 180 pounds, almost no women have been found to develop osteoporosis; below 140 pounds, more women have osteoporosis than don't. Approximately 75% of the women with osteoporosis weigh between 100–140 pounds.

Another factor affecting bone loss is the availability of calcium in the diet. Bones contain 99% of the calcium in the entire body. Premenopausal women require 1000 mg of calcium per day for their normal dietary needs. This amount is higher than some minerals because a certain amount of calcium is normally lost in urine and feces. Postmenopausal women need 1400 mg of calcium daily because after menopause women absorb calcium from digested food in the bowel much less efficiently. However, studies have shown that the average middle-aged woman only gets 550 mg of calcium per day after menopause. Women who are on a low-calorie diet generally get even less. To meet the calcium requirements for nerve transmission and other needs, the body withdraws calcium from the bones if the diet does not provide enough.

The recommended daily allowance (RDA) for calcium is 800 mg, which is 25% less than a premenopausal woman needs, and 75% less than a postmenopausal woman needs. Not surprisingly, some studies have found that bone loss is less in women who take extra calcium. Women given supplemental calcium lost an average of only .22% bone mass per year, as opposed to an average loss of 1.18% in women not taking supplemental calcium. The women who were getting more calcium also had fewer fractures. In countries like Finland, where high levels of calcium are consumed, the fracture rates among women are the lowest in the world. Interestingly, small amounts of Vitamin D are necessary for absorption of calcium from the intestine, but paradoxically, high doses of Vitamin D begin to cause bone resorption. Vitamin D is produced by the skin when it is exposed to sunlight, and it is added to milk in moderate amounts.

Exercise is also thought to be a factor that affects osteoporosis; it has long been known that lack of mechanical stress results in bone loss. Prolonged bed rest may cause a drop in bone mass of as much as 4%. Similarly, a broken bone in a cast will lose bone mass even as it is healing. Weightlessness in space has been found to cause 5% bone loss within the duration of one Skylab mission. Researchers believe that bone cells grow in response to mechanical strain or stimulation. This theory is supported by the fact that many athletes have been found to have a higher than average bone mass, specifically in those bones that are put under weight-bearing stress by their particular sport. On the other hand, swimmers, who are essentially exercising in a situation of diminished gravity, do not show increased bone mass. Studies of moderate exercisers versus nonexercisers have found that the exercisers had 27% more bone mass in the thigh bone than did nonexercisers. Last, and most impressive, it has been found that among 80-year-old women in a nursing home, those who did light-to-moderate exercise for 30 minutes three times a week showed a 4.2% increase in bone mass compared to a matched group who did not exercise.

Several other life-style and dietary factors affect bone loss. Of these, smoking is the most significant risk factor. The negative effects of smoking are threefold: smokers do not absorb calcium efficiently from their food; they tend to be thinner; and smoking is associated with earlier-than-normal menopause. By itself, early menopause increases a woman's risk of osteoporosis because it means more years of lowered calcium absorption. Interestingly, breastfeeding, and perhaps pregnancy itself, is associated with greater bone mass. This effect may be due to increased calcium in the women's diet or calcium supplementation during this period. On the other hand, breastfeeding and multiple pregnancies may both increase the risk of osteoporosis if women have poor nutrition during pregnancy or lactation. High caffeine intake is another risk factor because caffeine increases the excretion of calcium in the urine, but it has not been found to be a major factor. Alcohol is also associated with bone loss. Heavy alcohol consumption not only specifically decreases calcium absorption, it is associated with poor nutrition in general. Finally, a high protein diet, especially one that is high in meat, is associated with a loss of calcium because protein is converted to ketoacids in the normal digestive process, and these compounds carry calcium out in the urine.

Self-Care

Although symptoms are not evident in mid-adulthood, bone loss is beginning to occur in the majority of women, and even in men. Thus self-help measures should be instituted well before

---

Preventing Osteoporosis

- increase dietary calcium (see p. 105) by eating more calcium-rich foods and taking dietary supplements if necessary
- three to five times a week, engage in weight-bearing exercise such as walking, jogging, or racquet sports
- stop smoking
- avoid excessive alcohol consumption
- consider hormone replacement therapy if you have developed osteoporosis or are at high risk for it; risk factors include a small slender frame, early menopause, loss of both ovaries

---

the age at which symptoms begin, especially in those people who are at high risk. Risk factors include being female, slender, postmenopausal, and Caucasian; experiencing an early menopause; smoking, drinking alcohol, eating a low-calcium diet, and a sedentary life-style. The more of these factors that apply, the more at risk a person is.

The first part of self-help treatment is a *high-calcium diet* and adequate *Vitamin D.* Many physicians believe that 1500 mg of calcium per day by itself is enough to prevent or reverse osteoporosis. This calcium can be acquired either through diet or through supplementation. The best sources of calcium are dairy products: an 8 oz. glass of milk contains 300 mg of calcium, almost one-third of the daily premenopausal requirement. (Low-fat or nonfat dairy products are recommended because they contain less fat, a risk factor for a number of other diseases.) Leafy green vegetables contain calcium, but it is unclear how much of it is absorbed. Supplementation is an inexpensive, safe source of calcium. Calcium is available in tablet form (200 or 500 mg), and is found in calcium carbonate antacids, such as *Tums* (220 mg). Although most people get enough Vitamin D, those who eat only small amounts of meat or dairy products and do not get much sun may need supplemental Vitamin D. Vitamin D should only be taken in low doses, in conjunction with calcium, because it is toxic in high quantities.

Another important self-help measure is getting adequate *exercise*. In terms of preventing osteoporosis, people should engage in a weight-bearing exercise at least three times a week. Exercise needn't be excessive to be effective; even regular brisk walking will suffice. In addition to maintaining or increasing bone mass, exercise helps to build up the muscles that support the skeleton. Moreover, exercise enhances balance, flexibility, and gait, all of which enhance a person's mobility and decrease the likelihood of falls.

Finally, stopping smoking, keeping alcohol consumption moderate, and keeping caffeine intake low will all serve to maximize calcium absorption. It should be noted that these measures are basic guidelines for good health in terms of preventing a number of other illnesses.

The Doctor

Doctors currently recommend treating osteoporosis to prevent the fractures and complications that occur when bone loss reaches a certain point, but they vary in their efforts at diagnosis and treatment. Some doctors recommend *photon beam absorptiometry* to check for bone loss in middle-aged women who are at high risk. Because the procedure is expensive and its long-range value for routine use has not been established, it is not advised for all women. However, many doctors advise that all adult women follow the self-help measures outlined above.

For years, the major treatment to prevent osteoporosis in women has been *estrogen replacement therapy*. Optimally, treatment is begun soon after menopause takes place, and continues for life. Although this therapy is effective in preventing bone loss and subsequent fractures, it remains the subject of serious medical contro-

versy. Past use of supplemental estrogen by itself has definitely been associated with an increased incidence of cancer of the uterus. Some studies have shown that among women on supplemental estrogen there are seven times as many uterine cancers as among women in a control group. In general, the higher the dosage and the longer replacement is continued, the greater the risk of malignancy. Unlike other chemically induced cancers, the latency period for estrogen-induced cancer is only three to six years.

New evidence has shown that by combining the hormone *progestin* with estrogen therapy, the increase in the uterine cancer rate can be eliminated. As a result, many doctors now routinely prescribe estrogen and progestin together. Current therapy varies, but basically it involves three weeks of low doses of estrogen tablets, usually in combination with progestin during the last 10 days of the cycle. After one week off, the cycle is repeated. It is common for women to remain on supplemental estrogen for 15–20 years. Provided women take progestin as well as estrogen, their risk of uterine cancer has not been shown to be increased (see p. 429). If doctors prescribe estrogen therapy, many of them require their patients to undergo a pelvic exam and Pap smear every six months to check for cancerous or precancerous changes in the uterus and cervix.

Past problems with estrogen replacement have led to a wide difference in attitude and therapeutic practice among doctors. Some doctors will not prescribe estrogen replacement at all; others will prescribe it only for women who are at high risk for osteoporosis, such as slender smokers who experience early menopause. The 1984 National Institutes of Health (NIH) Consensus Conference on Estrogen Replacement Therapy recommended estrogen therapy for osteoporosis prevention in Caucasian women who had both ovaries removed before age 50, and said it should be considered for Caucasian women who are at increased risk of osteoporosis because of natural early onset of menopause, extreme thinness, or smoking. The NIH conference generally indicated that decisions to treat women outside of these categories should be made on a case-by-case basis after a discussion between physician and patient of the risks and benefits of treatment. Likewise a panel of the National Cancer Institute felt that estrogen replacement therapy should be used only for women who are at high or moderately high risk for developing osteoporosis.

In addition to causing uterine cancer, estrogen replacement has other side effects which include inducing monthly menstrual bleeding, breakthrough bleeding, fluid retention, breast tenderness, headache, leg cramps, and less commonly, gallstones and blood clots in the leg veins. For years there has also been a question as to whether estrogen replacement is associated with a higher incidence of breast cancer. Most research has not found an association, but some newer studies have found an elevated risk after long-term administration of estrogen (9–15 years). Another drawback is that if estrogen therapy is discontinued, bone loss begins again and, in fact, is *accelerated* to an average of 2.5% per year, which is more than double the normal postmenopausal rate. One study found that if women discontinued estrogen therapy after four years, their bone loss equalled that of women who had no therapy by the end of eight years.

Currently there is also debate about the effect of estrogen therapy on the incidence of heart attacks in postmenopausal women. One major study found that estrogen lowered the risk of heart attack, while another study indicated that it substantially increased the risk of heart attack and stroke, especially among women who smoked. The addition of progestin to estrogen therapy also appears to raise the risk of heart attack, but the significance of this is debatable.

On the other hand, estrogen does help eliminate some of the undesirable symptoms of menopause, including hot flashes, vaginal dryness, and vaginal shrinkage. However, many doctors feel that for the majority of women these symptoms can be treated without estrogen (see p. 428).

Several experimental drugs are being used to treat osteoporosis after fractures occur. *Sodium fluoride* has been shown to stimulate osteoblast cells within the bones, and has been shown to significantly increase the formation of bone and decrease the incidence of bone fractures. Although it seems to work best in large doses, studies show it may even be beneficial in the doses found in fluoridated drinking water. The other experimental drugs in use are the hormones *calcitonin* and *calcitriol*, which inhibit bone resorption.

Ruling Out Other Diseases

Until recently, osteoporosis was generally first diagnosed when people suffered fractures. Now, increasingly, it is diagnosed at earlier stages in high-risk women with the use of *photon beam absorptiometry* or *CAT scans*. Other bone diseases that cause bone loss are rare and can be ruled out on the basis of blood tests.

Prevention

Osteoporosis is a disease that can be prevented. In general, the necessary measures are not excessive. Moreover, many are the same as those recommended for a generally healthy lifestyle (see section on *Self-Care*). The emphasis on calcium is unique to osteoporosis, but calcium is a basic mineral that is associated with no harmful side effects.

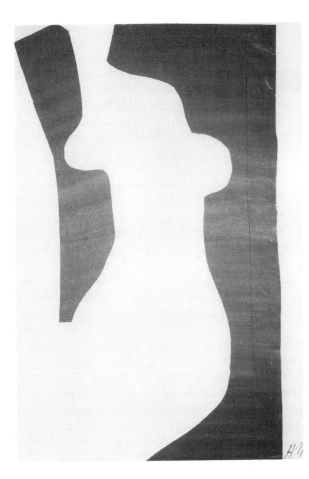

The gastrointestinal system, which breaks down and absorbs food, is significantly influenced by diet and stress. Henri Matisse. Venus. 1952. National Gallery of Art, Washington. Ailsa Mellon Bruce Fund, 1973.

349

Acute Gastroenteritis: Stomach Flu, Food Poisoning, and Traveler's Diarrhea

Symptoms

- nausea
- abdominal cramping
- vomiting
- diarrhea
- often, headache and muscle aches
- often, fever
- possible history of exposure to tainted food

Description

There are many causes of acute disturbances of the digestive tract that result in vomiting and/or diarrhea. Generally, these upsets are caused by infectious agents such as viruses, bacteria, or parasites, or by a *toxin*—a poisonous chemical produced by viruses or bacteria. The toxin or infectious agent may be contained in food, or spread from person to person. Both vomiting and diarrhea are the body's mechanisms for quickly ridding itself of the infectious agent or toxin. Commonly, *food poisoning* refers to disturbances associated with food intake, in particular ones that affect groups of people and are not accompanied by a fever. *Infectious gastroenteritis* refers to disturbances that are more often accompanied by a fever and spread from person to person. There is much overlap between the two types of disturbances because they are both ultimately caused by an infectious agent. The

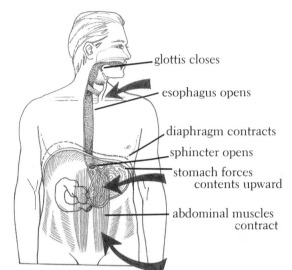

glottis closes

esophagus opens

diaphragm contracts

sphincter opens

stomach forces contents upward

abdominal muscles contract

Vomiting is a natural mechanism for ridding the stomach of noxious substances. First, the abdominal muscles contract, then the esophageal sphincter opens and the diaphragm contracts sharply.

symptoms are much the same no matter what the cause, but the incubation period, severity, and mode of transmission vary.

With toxins, the *incubation period*, or time before symptoms occur, is generally very short because the toxin has already been produced by the infectious agent in food. The most common toxin is produced by *Staphylococcus aureus.* Other frequent offenders in this group are *Clostridium perfringens* and sometimes toxic strains of *Escherichia coli (E. coli)*. With a toxin, the *incubation period* is only one to two hours after eating. The particular agent causing food poisoning often remains unidentified unless if affects a number of people, for instance, at a picnic, dinner, or restaurant. Food poisoning is not accompanied by a fever; there is no inflammatory process, since no bacteria or virus is growing and reproducing in the digestive tract. The toxin simply binds to cells in the lining of the *jejunum*, the lowest part of the small intestine, causing the cells to release large amounts

of fluid. Characteristically, this type of gastroenteritis begins suddenly and causes a number of urgent bowel movements consisting of large volumes of very watery diarrhea. The process is self-limiting, peaks in approximately 10 hours, and subsides within a day.

A different type of gastroenteritis results when a virus, bacterium, or parasite actually invades cells of the small and large intestine and begins to reproduce there in large numbers. The body sends in white blood cells to fight the infection, which causes local inflammation and a fever. The incubation period for this type of gastroenteritis is longer because it takes some time for the agent to reproduce in numbers sufficient to cause symptoms. Common bacterial infections are caused by *Shigella, Salmonella, nontoxic Escherichia coli,* and *campylobacter jejune.* They can spread through food, contaminated water, or hand-to-hand contact. With bacterial infections, symptoms begin 12–24 hours after exposure. Often there is much cramping and pain due to the inflammation, but the diarrhea is relatively small in volume.

A viral gastroenteritis generally takes longer to cause gastrointestinal symptoms; the incubation period is 18–48 hours. Viral strains, most commonly the *Norwalk virus* and the *Snowmountain virus,* are only spread from person to person, not by means of food. Specific symptoms of a viral infection include an abrupt onset of vomiting and/or diarrhea, along with flu-like symptoms such as headache, muscle aches, and fever. A viral gastroenteritis usually lasts 48–72 hours and goes away by itself.

Traveler's diarrhea is very common and typically occurs about three days after arrival in a new location. It is thought to be due to infectious agents, most often an unfamiliar strain of *E. coli* bacteria, or an unfamiliar virus. However, unfamiliar food and drink, as well as anxiety are also thought to play a role. After people become adapted to a particular bacterium or virus, they no longer develop symptoms.

Self-Care

The various types of gastroenteritis are not usually serious, and they all tend to be self-limiting. Symptomatic self-care is usually all that's needed. Treatment consists of drinking plenty of fluids and giving the digestive tract a rest from solid foods. It's important to drink as much fluid as is lost, especially if the diarrhea and/or vomiting is profuse and prolonged. Clear fluids such as water, weak tea, soda, and electrolyte-replacement solutions like *Gatorade* are all that should be taken until the diarrhea subsides. Over-the-counter preparations such as *Pepto-Bismol* slow down the diarrhea and may be very helpful, but are generally not necessary. In fact, it's often better to let the diarrhea run its course because it helps to clear the body of the infectious agent. If there is vomiting, liquids will be tolerated best if they are drunk in very small amounts at frequent intervals.

Once the vomiting and diarrhea subside, people can begin to eat a bland diet of rice, toast, cereal, and plain pasta. Fruits, roughage, spicy foods, coffee, and alcohol should be avoided until cramping stops and bowel movements attain a normal consistency. Milk and fatty foods should also be avoided or eaten in small amounts because the abraded intestinal lining temporarily has difficulty digesting fats, milk, and sugar. The more severe the gastroenteritis, the longer a person should remain on clear liquids initially, and then on bland foods.

The Doctor

Generally, gastroenteritis is a self-limiting disease that does not require treatment by a doctor, but the doctor should be called if a person has severe abdominal pain, has bloody stools or vomit, or shows signs of dehydration such as the skin remaining wrinkled after it is pinched. Food poisoning can occasionally cause bloody stools and cramping that is severe enough to warrant

---

Diet for Stomach Flu

For vomiting:
- until vomiting stops, drink clear fluids such as water, soda (flat, without bubbles), apple juice, or bouillon; drink little but often
- when vomiting stops, begin eating small amounts of bland foods, such as rice, bananas, applesauce, crackers, toast, dry cereal without sugar

For diarrhea:
- drink clear fluids (see above) in small amounts; avoid milk which is hard to digest; continue clear fluids only for up to two days
- avoid solid foods, especially fruits that make stools loose (apricots, prunes, melons); as diarrhea slows, begin eating small amounts of bland foods (see above)

---

pain medication. Dehydration occurs when a person's fluid intake does not keep up with fluid loss. Often dehydrated people will complain that they are thirsty or that their mouth feels dry. They will also urinate infrequently, and their urine may be a dark yellow or orange color.

The doctor will do a *white blood cell count* to test for infection and a *stool culture* to determine if the gastroenteritis is caused by bacteria. If the culture is positive for the bacteria *Shigella (bacillary dysentery)*, a course of antibiotics is often given. One of two broad-spectrum antibiotics—*trimethoprim-sulfamethoxazole* (e.g., *TMP-SMX, Septra*) or *ampicillin*—are generally prescribed.

The doctor will treat any significant dehydration with intravenous fluids, either in the doctor's office or in the hospital. If a person is having difficulty keeping fluid down because of vomiting, he or she may also be given an anti-nausea medication.

There is some controversy about what is the best treatment for traveler's diarrhea. Generally the condition goes away by itself; however, it can be especially annoying and difficult to cope with when people are traveling. The nonprescription preparation *bismuthsubsalicylate (Pepto-Bismol)* is a favorite of many experienced travelers. It has been shown to reduce the volume of diarrhea by half, and to speed up the normal recovery time by about one day.

Some doctors prescribe *diphenoxylate with atropine* (e.g., *Lomotil*) for diarrhea, but others are reluctant to because it often prevents the body from ridding itself of the infection and causes constipation afterward. *Iodochlorhydroxyquin (Entero-vioform)*, which was once widely used abroad, is no longer used because it is not very effective and it can cause damage to the nervous system. Some doctors prescribe the antibiotic *TMP-SMX* to treat or even to *prevent* traveler's diarrhea. When traveling to areas known to cause diarrhea, TMP-SMX can be taken preventively starting about a week before an individual leaves.

Ruling Out Other Diseases

For a severe or prolonged gastroenteritis, the doctor may do a stool culture to determine if the cause is viral, bacterial, or possibly parasitic. The most common parasite in the U.S. and Europe is *Giardia lamblia*, a one-celled flagellate. Giardia is suspected if a person has acute diarrhea with bulky, greasy stool, and is very tired. Another parasite is *Entamoeba histolytica*, a single-celled animal common in tropical areas. *Amebic diarrhea* is suspected if a person has recently traveled to an endemic area. Repeated bouts of diarrhea, especially if they are bloody, can be caused by intestinal inflammation, including *regional enteritis* or *ulcerative colitis*, which is distinguished from bacterial or amebic diarrhea by the absence of an infectious organism in a stool culture. Persistent mild diarrhea that is not bloody is called *functional diarrhea* (see p. 358); it can be due to emotional causes.

Changes in bowel habits—including blood in the stool—can also be caused by *cancer of the colon* (see p. 362), but the symptoms do not usually appear suddenly or disappear by themselves.

A history of vomiting without diarrhea can be caused by pregnancy, diabetes, a recent head injury, or a new medication. Despite the many conditions that can cause diarrhea and vomiting, the diagnosis of gastroenteritis is usually readily made from the patient's history.

Prevention

Food poisoning is prevented by proper refrigeration of food and by cooking at high enough temperatures for a long enough time. The most common culprits in food poisoning are picnic foods containing meat, fish, or egg products which are left unrefrigerated for too long. Common examples are potato salad, egg salad, chicken, turkey, ham, pork, and fish. Commercial mayonnaise is generally not a problem because it is more acidic than is homemade. Another common source is food that is defrosted very slowly and then cooked incompletely.

Travelers' diarrhea is most common in tropical countries that lack good sanitation and refrigeration, but it also affects foreign travelers to the U.S. The main prevention is the famous maxim of avoiding all unchlorinated water, including ice cubes and tap water for tooth brushing. In addition, travelers should avoid uncooked vegetables or fruits that can't be peeled. High-quality, portable charcoal water filters are now available.

Prevention of bacterial and viral gastroenteritis is largely a matter of careful hygiene. As with viral and bacterial colds, the germs are spread by fecal-oral transmission. Thus, careful hand washing, especially before food preparation, is important. People who have gastroenteritis should wash their hands thoroughly after going to the bathroom. Use of disinfectants such as bleach or Lysol on surfaces may also minimize the spread of germs when a member of the household is ill.

Peptic Ulcer

Symptoms

- pain in the upper middle abdomen
- often, nausea and vomiting
- often, a poor appetite

Description

A *peptic ulcer* is an eroded area in the *mucosa*, the top layer in the lining of the stomach and the *duodenum*, which is the upper part of the small intestine. Ulcers in the stomach are referred to as *gastric*, those in the intestine as *duodenal*. Although the cause of ulcers is not precisely known, most of them are related to overproduction of *hydrochloric acid* and *pepsin*, a digestive enzyme.

Ulcers are relatively common. In the U.S., they affect up to 25% of men and 16% of women; however, only 5%–10% of people have symptoms of sufficient intensity to cause them to seek treatment. Duodenal ulcers are over five times as common as gastric ulcers. Duodenal ulcers are most common in the age range 25–50, while gastric ulcers are most common between the ages of 40 and 70. It is interesting to note that the disease apparently did not exist or was uncommon before 1900. Equally mystifying, for unknown reasons the incidence of ulcers has been dropping steadily at about 8% per year over the last decade.

The main symptom of ulcers is frequent *dyspepsia*, or indigestion. However, only a small percentage of people with dyspepsia ultimately turn out to have a peptic ulcer as diagnosed by lab tests. Most people with a history of indiges-

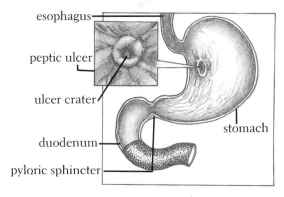

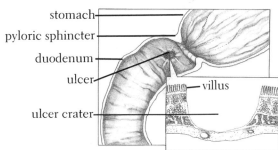

An ulcer is an eroded area in the lining of the stomach or the duodenum, the upper part of the small intestine.

tion have what is referred to as *functional dyspepsia* or *functional bowel disease* (see p. 358), which is thought to be due to psychological stress, anxiety, or dietary intolerances. Functional dyspepsia is simply indigestion of unknown origin, unrelated to erosion of the lining of the gastrointestinal tract.

Doctors have long recognized that the digestive tract, which is under the control of the *autonomic*, or automatic part, of the nervous system, is exquisitely sensitive to emotional states. The autonomic nervous system causes bowel motility to slow in times of fear or stress, and increase during periods of relaxation. Also, when people become angry or upset, the secretion of hydrochloric acid and the digestive enzyme pepsin increases markedly and stomach motility becomes hyperactive.

The classic story of an ulcer is pain or discomfort in the mid-to-upper abdomen, near the bottom of the *sternum*, or breastbone. It used to be said that the pain generally was of a burning or gnawing quality, began one to three hours after eating, was relieved by food or antacids, and often awakened people at night. It is now recognized that ulcer pain is more typically episodic, with stabbing pain for a short time, interspersed with longer periods that are free of symptoms. By comparison, functional dyspepsia is more likely to cause persistent pain, but does not awaken people.

The physiology of how an ulcer develops is still not well understood. Under normal conditions, the lining of the digestive tract produces a mucus gel that forms a protective coating to prevent digestive juices from eroding the lining. In addition, the lining produces *bicarbonate*, an alkaline chemical that neutralizes acid. The amount of acid produced by the digestive tract is increased in response to several biochemical factors. First, whenever people think about food, the specially adapted endings of the autonomic nerves leading to the stomach release the neurotransmitter *acetylcholine*, which stimulates acid secretion. Second, whenever there is food in the stomach, the digestive hormone *gastrin* is released. Third, whenever *mast cells* in the lining of the stomach release *histamine*, more acid is produced.

About 50% of people with duodenal ulcers have acid secretion rates that are well above normal. This excess is thought to be the main cause of duodenal ulcers. Doctors also think that some people secrete less stomach mucus, or the mucus they produce has less of a neutralizing effect. Doctors speculate that there may be a genetic predisposition to one or both of these factors, since ulcers do seem to be more common in some families.

There are several life-style factors that also seem to be linked to ulcers. Emotional stress is associated with increased acid production and an increased incidence of ulcers. Studies have demonstrated that some people develop increased acid secretions and ulcers during stressful periods, but that when the stress is relieved, acid production decreases and the ulcers heal.

There is also a significant link between smoking and ulcers. A greater percentage of ulcer patients smoke than do people without ulcers. The more people smoke, the greater the likelihood of their having ulcers, the more severe their ulcers will be, and the more ulcer complications they will experience. Finally, smokers with ulcers are less likely to heal than ulcer patients who do not smoke. Research has shown that the nicotine in cigarettes actually decreases the amount of bicarbonate secreted into the duodenum by the pancreas, indirectly raising the acid level of the intestine. Interestingly, many smokers notice that they get indigestion when they smoke a number of cigarettes in a short time.

Certain foods and beverages are also known to increase the secretion of acid in the stomach. These substances, which are called *secretagogues*, include alcoholic beverages, beverages containing caffeine, decaffeinated coffee, milk, and cream. Alcohol, in addition to being a se-

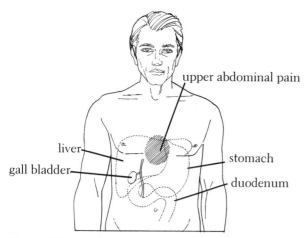

liver
gall bladder
upper abdominal pain
stomach
duodenum

Upper abdominal pain can be caused by conditions of the esophagus, stomach, duodenum, or gallbladder.

cretagogue, is a direct irritant. Several studies indicate that dietary fiber may play a protective role against ulcers. One study has found that people in Northern India who basically eat a soft diet have higher ulcer rates than people in Southern India who eat a diet that is higher in fiber.

A number of prescription and nonprescription drugs are also known to cause or exacerbate ulcers. *Aspirin* and aspirin-containing compounds can actually erode the lining of the stomach. People on high doses of aspirin are more likely to have ulcers. *Nonsteroidal anti-inflammatory drugs* that are often taken for joint pain can directly damage the mucosa and reduce bicarbonate and mucus production. This makes them particularly ulcerogenic, especially when taken regularly over a long period of time. Nonsteroidal anti-inflammatory drugs include *ibuprofen* (e.g., *Motrin, Advil*), which is available over the counter, and *indomethacin* (e.g., *Indocin*), which is a stronger drug, available only by prescription. Steroids may also increase the likelihood of ulcers, especially *prednisone* when given in large doses for long periods.

Although ulcers generally respond well to the present treatment regimens, they can lead to serious complications. If an ulcer erodes into a blood vessel, it can cause significant loss of blood. If the blood is vomited up, it can be bright red, black, or the color and texture of coffee grounds. When blood passes through the intestine, it can either be bright red if the bleeding is rapid, or have a black, tar-like look if the blood moves more slowly through the intestine and is "digested." Such bleeding is always a MEDICAL EMERGENCY, and should be seen by a doctor immediately. Another ulcer complication that requires emergency treatment is *perforation*, a situation in which the ulcer erodes through the wall of the stomach or duodenum. The major symptom of perforation is severe unrelenting upper abdominal pain. A third serious complication of ulcers occurs when the duodenum becomes obstructed as a result of severe swelling of the tissues around the ulcer. In this case the symptoms are nausea and vomiting.

Self-Care

Self-care plays a very important role in both treating peptic ulcers and preventing their recurrence. Self-care, like drug therapy, is based on the principle of "No acid, no ulcer." There is much that can be done to lower acid production. First, ulcer patients are advised to deal with stress and reduce the level of tension in their life, rest, get adequate sleep, modify their diet, and use visualization/relaxation techniques (see p. 67).

In the 1960s and 1970s, diet was the principle means of treating ulcers. Ironically, the regimen then recommended, called the *ulcer sippy diet*, advised eating frequent, bland meals and drinking cream at hourly intervals initially, then decreasing to every few hours. In the last 10 years, this diet has been totally rejected based on new research findings. First, it was found that milk products did not neutralize stomach acid, but in fact increased the secretion of acid. Next, controlled studies showed that a bland diet actually didn't affect stomach acid levels and didn't speed ulcer healing. Finally, it was found that frequent small meals also increased the production of acid.

The current medical advice is simply to eat regular, nutritious meals that are high in fiber and to avoid food and beverages that increase ulcer symptoms. In addition to these general guidelines, people are told to avoid alcohol, caffeine drinks, decaffinated coffee, and chocolate. All ulcer patients should give up smoking completely because it retards healing, even if medication is taken.

Nonprescription *antacids* (e.g., *Mylanta, Maalox, Gelusil, Alternagel,* and *Amphagel*) have long been used as an effective means of neutralizing stomach acid. They not only relieve symptoms, they help to heal ulcers. Because they need to be taken in large quantities, antacids should be taken according to a doctor's directions (see below). Ulcer patients should not use antacids that contain *calcium carbonate* because after temporarily neutralizing acid secretions, they can cause an acid rebound. Ulcer patients are also warned to avoid aspirin-containing compounds, steroids, and nonsteroidal anti-inflammatory agents because they can damage the mucosa.

The Doctor

The doctor may suspect an ulcer based on the patient's history, but confirms the diagnosis with either an *upper gastrointestinal (GI) x-ray* or with *endoscopy*, a procedure in which a slender fiberoptic instrument is passed down the gastrointestinal tract in order to examine the lining of the stomach. An upper GI x-ray is generally done first because it is easier and less expensive, but x-rays miss 20%–30% of all ulcers. If a person has a negative x-ray, but is very symptomatic, the doctor may recommend endoscopy. If an x-ray reveals a suspicious-looking gastric (stomach) ulcer or the ulcer does not heal, endoscopy will be done in order to rule out the possibility of a malignancy. About 3% of all stomach ulcers that appear benign on x-ray prove to be malignant. Most stomach cancer occurs in people who are over 60.

Drugs developed during the last 10 years have radically affected the treatment of peptic ulcers. The drugs are not necessarily more effective than the old regimens that involved frequent, large doses of antacids, but they are much more convenient. Instead of drinking large amounts of liquid antacids seven times a day, patients now simply take pills once or twice a day. The most commonly prescribed drugs are *H2-receptor antagonists* that block histamine from binding to the cells that produce acid in the digestive tract. The first of these antagonists, called *cime-*

tidine (Tagamet), is taken once or twice a day. The drug can cause breast enlargement and impotence in men. A newer drug, *ranitidine (Zantac)*, is stronger and has fewer side effects. It is also taken once or twice a day. Both of these new drugs reduce acid secretion by 75%–95%, and have been shown in studies to heal ulcers within four to six weeks in 70%–80% of all patients. The newest drug, called *famotidine (Pepcid)*, is more potent than the others and is taken only once a day. Interestingly, in the same ulcer study, *placebos*, medicines containing no active ingredients, healed the ulcers in about 50% of the people in the control group. A significant percentage of people, up to 70%, experience recurrences of ulcers. Cimetidine and ranitidine have been shown to prevent recurrences, and are prescribed for up to a year in severe cases.

The second type of ulcer treatment is *antacid therapy*, which has been used for a number of years. Studies have shown that antacids will only lower acid levels enough to promote healing when taken in quite large doses (2 T., or 30 ml) seven times a day, one and three hours after meals and at bedtime. Smaller or less frequent doses will relieve pain, but may not heal the ulcer. Tablets do not work as well as liquid antacids because they do not coat the stomach. All the magnesium- and aluminum-based antacids work equally well and are nonprescription, so the choice is quite literally a matter of taste. Another factor to take into account is that the magnesium antacids sometimes produce loose stools, whereas the aluminum ones can be constipating.

A third treatment regimen for peptic ulcer uses a medicine that enhances the natural protective mechanisms of the digestive tract rather than reducing the amount of acid produced. This medication is an aluminum hydroxide salt called *sucralfate (Carafate)*, which coats the stomach, but is not absorbed. It comes in pill form and is taken four times a day.

Currently all three types of medical regimens

are considered effective; the choice is made by the patient in conjunction with the doctor. Generally, doctors initially suggest the H2 blockers because of their convenience.

Both bleeding and perforation are serious complications that constitute a MEDICAL EMERGENCY. They affect approximately 25% of all ulcer patients, of whom 15%–20% experience bleeding, 6%–10% perforate, and 5% develop an obstruction in the duodenum. For each of these conditions, the ulcer patient is hospitalized and treatment is begun immediately. About 85% of the time, the bleeding stops by itself. When it does not, either endoscopy and cauterization (heat sealing), or surgery must be performed. Perforation may be treated medically or surgically, although surgery is usually necessary. Obstruction in the duodenum is initially treated medically with nasogastric suction, but sometimes requires surgery in addition.

Ruling Out Other Diseases

In most cases, frequent or long-lasting indigestion or dyspepsia is not caused by ulcers; most cases are considered to be indigestion of unknown origin *(functional dyspepsia)*, which is ruled out by an upper GI series or endoscopy. The same symptoms can also be caused by *chronic gastritis* or *duodenitis*, a long-term in-

flammation of the digestive tract that can be caused by a variety of factors, including drugs, stress, and alcohol. Short-term gastritis can be caused by viruses, bacteria, or alcohol (see p. 349). Long-term symptoms of indigestion can also be caused by *hiatus hernia*, a condition in which the contents of the stomach regularly backs up into the esophagus. This condition usually has heartburn as its major symptom (see p. 377).

Prevention

Since ulcers are very strongly affected by lifestyle factors, there is much people can do to avoid their occurrence and recurrence. Prevention is particularly important when there is a family history of ulcers or a personal history of long-standing, mild, upper abdominal discomfort. The main principle of prevention is to lower digestive acid production (see section on *Self-Care*). Since there is strong data linking stress to stomach motility, acid production, and ulcers, stress reduction should be the key factor in prevention (see p. 58). This approach should be backed up by eliminating tobacco and alcohol, increasing fiber, and avoiding foods that cause stomach upsets. A focus on prevention is imperative because ulcers tend to be a chronic disease that recurs in 70%–80% of all patients.

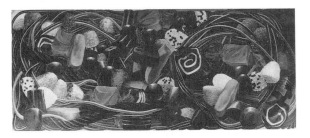

Ulcers are not the cause of most indigestion. Kay Kurt. Ever Eat Anything That Made You Feel Like Saturday Night on Tuesday Afternoon. 1968. Oil on canvas. 60″ × 144″. Collection, The Whitney Museum of American Art. Gift of Margery and Harry Kahn. 73.64.

Irritable Bowel Syndrome, Nervous Indigestion, Spastic Colon, Irritable Colon, or Functional Dyspepsia

Symptoms

- abdominal pain or distress
- constipation
- diarrhea
- excess gas or belching

Description

Irritable bowel syndrome, or *IBS*, is a broad term referring to several types of altered bowel function that are not caused by any specific disease. IBS is by far the most common gastrointestinal disease, and is the major reason people see gastroenterologists, doctors who specialize in diseases of the digestive tract. In fact, irritable colon or nervous indigestion ranks equally with the common cold as a reason for missing work. Some authorities estimate that as many as 30% of the population in the U.S. have IBS at any one time.

The major symptoms of IBS are abdominal pain or discomfort, constipation, diarrhea, and gas. The pain associated with this condition is highly variable in terms of severity, location, and duration. Discomfort often occurs after meals, and is relieved by passing gas or having a bowel movement; it rarely wakes a person at night. Pain is most common in the left lower quadrant, although it can sometimes occur under the left rib cage. Sensations of fullness, lack of appetite, and nausea are common. Often these feelings will be accompanied by burping and gas, a combination for which Ogden Nash coined the term "burbulence." Symptoms range from mild indi-

gestion to severe abdominal pain requiring hospitalization.

Another symptom that may be associated with IBS is severe episodic rectal pain just above the anus, which lasts for a few minutes, then disappears by itself. This pain, called *proctalgia fugax*, is caused by a spasm in the *pubococcygeus muscle*. The spasm is not caused by any organic disease and does not require treatment. Although it can occur in people who do not have IBS, it is more common in people with IBS. It is relieved by upward pressure on the anus or a hot bath.

Most doctors divide IBS into two types: one which is associated with constipation, the other with diarrhea. By far the most common is *spastic colon*, the type that produces constipation. Bowel movements are infrequent and are passed with difficulty. Characteristically, this condition produces a bowel movement that consists of small, hard "rabbit pellets." The other, less common, form of IBS is referred to as *painless diarrhea*. In this condition, the stools are usually semiloose but not watery, often come on urgently, and may be associated with abdominal cramping. With this type of IBS, bowel movements are most frequent in the morning, and may contain mucus. Occasionally, people will have a combination of both types of IBS, their stools alternating between small hard pellets and diarrhea.

Although doctors are not certain of what causes IBS, they have long recognized that both types of IBS are associated with emotional factors. Studies have found that both initial onset and recurrences are linked with periods of high emotional stress. It has also been found that people with IBS have higher emotional stress in their lives than do people in control groups who do not have the disease. Situations of severe stress, such as exams or military service, can definitely bring on *transitory disorders of bowel function*. The connection between emotions and bowel function is not surprising, since digestion and bowel motility are regulated by the *autonomic nervous system*, which controls the fight-or-flight response and the relaxation response. The *sympathetic branch* slows down gastrointestinal motility, or movement; while the *parasympathetic branch* increases bowel movement. They both work in response to thoughts and emotions.

Recently, researchers have done studies attempting to measure colon motility during stressful interviews. Normally, the colon has slow contractile movements that move fecal matter along the intestine. If the movements become either too fast or too slow, normal stool production is disrupted. Studies on stress interviews show that when people became hostile or defensive, their bowel motility increased a great deal, causing a squeezing motion that slowed the stool's transit and allowed more water to be absorbed from it. On the other hand, when people reacted to the stress interview in a passive or depressed manner, their bowel motility decreased. Such a decrease is associated with rapid transit of the stool, which means little water is absorbed by the colon.

Other studies have demonstrated special characteristics of the bowel that are associated with IBS symptoms. It has been found that IBS patients are more sensitive to pressure in the rectum, and are more likely to feel rectal pain. As a group, people with IBS have slower bowel contractions and are more reactive to digestive hormones. Doctors have also observed that IBS patients are more reactive than normal to rapid ingestion of cold liquids, highly seasoned foods, coffee, and meals that are high in carbohydrates.

Dr. T. P. Almy, one of the main researchers investigating bowel motility, concludes that disturbances of colonic function are "normal bodily manifestations of emotional tension," similar to other autonomic nervous system activities such as sweating or blushing. Almy feels that IBS patients simply represent the most reactive part of the normal spectrum of bowel motility. In addition, he believes they may be more easily aroused by stressful situations or events. Almy believes that colic in babies and stomachaches in young children that are relieved by a bowel movement are early manifestations of IBS.

A number of studies have found that there is a familial link associated with IBS; that is, people who have a parent with IBS symptoms are more likely to have the condition themselves. Some researchers speculate this is due to a genetic tendency of the bowel to be more reactive, or a tendency of the person to be more reactive to stress in general. Other researchers speculate that the familial link may be based on learned behaviors. Bowel habits are routines that people learn, and children can unconsciously acquire maladaptive patterns. Investigators have linked IBS to clusters of personality characteristics. As compared with patients who did not have IBS, those who did were found to be more likely to be anxious.

Self-Care

Once the diagnosis of IBS has been made by a doctor, one important aspect of treatment is self-care. The first self-care routines are dietary. People with IBS should eat a wide range of foods, but avoid those that have repeatedly upset them. For one person this might be cold liquids; for another, spicy foods. Many doctors advise IBS patients to gradually increase the amount of fiber in their diet, since studies have shown that fiber tends to normalize transit time through the intestine. Most people are aware that increased fiber is a treatment for constipation but may be surprised to learn that fiber not only speeds up lengthy transit times, it also tends to slow down rapid transit times by adding bulk to the stool. Additional bulk also drops the pressure in the colon, which decreases uncomfortable sensations. Although studies have shown that a high-fiber diet makes a great percentage of IBS pa-

Self-Care for Constipation

- respond promptly to urges to have a bowel movement, but realize that a daily bowel movement is not necessary for health
- when possible, make a point of having a bowel movement at the same time each day, and do not be hurried
- avoid medications that cause constipation, such as magnesium antacids
- avoid laxatives and cathartics, because the body can become dependent on them
- increase foods with fiber (see p. 95)
- avoid refined grains such as white rice, white flour, cream of wheat
- drink plenty of fluid—at least six glasses per day
- get daily exercise
- use psyllium seed stool-bulking agents (e.g., Metamucil) on a regular basis

tients feel much better, some carefully controlled studies raise questions as to whether patients are reacting to the fiber, or to the placebo-effect of changing their diet. However, given the many health benefits of increased fiber, everyone should be on a high-fiber diet anyway, especially those IBS patients who are troubled by constipation. In addition to a high-fiber diet, IBS patients are advised to use high-fiber *psillium hydrophilic mucilloid* (e.g., *Metamucil* and *Konsyl*) on a regular basis, starting at one T. per day. If symptoms persist, the dosage can be increased slightly. For the psyllium to be most effective, a person also has to drink four to eight glasses of water per day.

The other major self-care measures for IBS are reducing stress and dealing with anxiety. Relaxation and meditation exercises can be immediately helpful and should be used on a continuing basis (see p. 60). Likewise, activities that are particularly enjoyable, such as sports or outdoor exercise, help to reduce stress and increase general feelings of pleasure and well-being. From a long-term perspective, it's important for IBS patients to identify anxiety-producing situations and gain insight into the personality characteristics that tend to make them anxious. Although individuals can do much of this on their own, counseling can often be invaluable.

The Doctor

Diarrhea, constipation, and abdominal pain are general symptoms that are associated with a number of conditions. No one test positively identifies IBS; rather, its diagnosis is established by ruling out other diseases that have the same symptoms. Because IBS is the most frequent reason for these symptoms, such workups most often come out negative.

The doctor begins with a careful history to assess the significance and severity of the symptoms. An individual's history, combined with his or her age, determines what laboratory tests the doctor decides to do. In a young person with mild symptoms, the doctor may order no lab tests; but with an older person who has a change in bowel habits, a work-up will be done to rule out other diseases (see below). A blood test will be done to check for anemia, which would indicate internal bleeding. If diarrhea is a symptom, stool cultures will be done to check for the presence of bacteria or parasites (see p. 349). Depending upon the person's age and specific history, *sigmoidoscopy* and/or a *barium enema* will be done. Sigmoidoscopy is a procedure in

Self-Care for Functional Indigestion

- avoid overeating
- eat slowly and chew food thoroughly
- avoid fried or fatty foods
- avoid gas-producing foods if they don't agree with you (e.g., beans, cabbage, onions)
- avoid alcohol and cigarettes
- don't eat when you're upset
- learn to identify and deal with stress (see p. 58)
- exercise daily

which the doctor uses a special instrument to examine the lower colon; a barium enema provides a diagnostic x-ray of the intestine. A presumptive diagnosis of IBS will be made if all these tests are negative.

The symptoms of IBS often decrease dramatically when people are told they do not have any organic disease. A negative work-up lays to rest many fears and eliminates one area of stress in their lives. The doctor will recommend dietary adjustments, and may have the patient avoid milk to see if he or she is one of the small number of IBS patients who have a lactose intolerance. Psillium hydrophillic muscilloid (e.g., *Metamucil*) will be recommended. In addition the doctor will discuss the kinds of stress and anxiety the person is under, and recommend relaxation, meditation techniques, or biofeedback training. For patients with severe and disabling symptoms, the doctor may recommend a support group or psychotherapy.

If severe symptoms do not respond to these therapies, there are several drugs that can be prescribed, but they do not cure the disease, and they do have side effects. For constipation, *anticholinergic drugs* (e.g., *Propantheline* or *Trydihexethyl*) may be given to slow excess bowel motility. For severe diarrhea, *diphenoxylate with atropine* (e.g., *Lomotil*) may be given for a short time. In some cases, doctors may also prescribe pain medication (e.g., *Demerol*), tranquil-izers, or antidepressants for short-term use. Antidepressants apparently affect the central nervous system pain nerves from the bowel. All these drugs can help to give temporary relief of symptoms, but support or counseling is usually necessary to get at the cause of the problem.

Ruling Out Other Diseases

A complete work-up for IBS enables the doctor to rule out other causes of the symptoms such as *gastroenteritis* (see p. 349) or *diverticulitis* (see p. 369), both of which can produce pain and fever. The work-up will also rule out *regional enteritis (Crohn's disease)*, a chronic inflammatory bowel disease; *ulcerative colitis*, a chronic inflammatory disease of the colon; and *cancer of the colon* (see p. 362). Both ulcerative colitis and cancer of the colon can produce blood in the stool.

Prevention

People who have a familial or personal history of nervous indigestion or a reactive bowel may be able to prevent IBS symptoms. A high-fiber diet and stress reduction measures (see section on *Self-Care*) can help to normalize bowel motility. It is particularly important that "susceptible" people become aware of, and learn to deal with, those situations and factors that tend to upset their digestive tract.

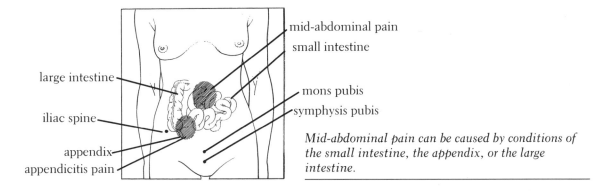

Mid-abdominal pain can be caused by conditions of the small intestine, the appendix, or the large intestine.

Colon Cancer, or Adenocarcinoma of the Colon

Symptoms

- rectal bleeding
- abdominal pain
- changes in bowel habits, including constipation, diarrhea, or narrowing of the stools
- unexplained weight loss
- unexplained anemia

Description

Colon cancer is the most common malignancy in the U.S., surpassing even lung cancer and breast cancer. The U.S. rate of 49.1 cases per 100,000 people is one of the highest in the world. The generalization that the more developed the area, the higher the rate of colorectal cancer holds true not only worldwide, but even within individual countries. Thus the incidence of colon cancer is high in North America, Europe, and New Zealand, and low in South America, Africa, and Asia. Likewise, rates of colon cancer are higher in the northern U.S. than in the South, and higher in urban areas than in rural areas. Studies show that when people migrate from a country or area of low incidence to one of high incidence, in a relatively short time they attain rates similar to those of their new locale. Even more interesting, statistics show that rich people in developing countries such as Colombia have a high colon cancer rate, while poor people have a low rate.

Based on a careful study of statistics like these, cancer experts theorize that colon cancer, like many other forms of cancer, is influenced by environmental factors. Researchers believe that diet plays a key role, particularly a diet that is high in fat and animal protein. In a large study of 28 countries, it was found that colorectal cancer occurred in direct proportion to the amount of meat ingested, specifically beef. In Australia, colon cancer rates dropped 20% between 1955 and 1965, when there was a corresponding drop in the amount of beef eaten. In New Zealand, where beef intake did not decline, rates of colon cancer remained the same.

Experts have developed a complex theoretical model for the way in which diet causes colorectal cancer. Research has shown that the foods people eat determine which bacteria grow in their intestine. People who eat a diet that is rich in meat have a greater population of anaerobic *clostridia* bacteria, and fewer aerobic *lactobacillus* bacteria. The anaerobic clostridia are very active bacteria that break down amino acids, cholesterol, and, most important, bile acids from the gall bladder. Many of the resulting compounds are *carcinogenic*, that is, cancer-causing; or *cocarcinogenic*, that is, they help another chemical cause cancer. Both people and animals with high anaerobic bacterial counts have higher rates of colon cancer.

On the positive side, a number of dietary factors have been shown to help prevent colon cancer. Foods such as broccoli, cauliflower, brussels sprouts, turnips, and cabbage increase the amount of two intestinal enzymes—one that breaks down carcinogens and cocarcinogens formed by anaerobic bacteria, and another enzyme that acts as a barrier to carcinogens. As a group, these vegetables are referred to as the *cruciferous* family. Studies have shown that people who frequently eat these vegetables have lower rates of colon cancer.

Another protective factor against colon cancer is *fiber*. It has long been recognized that Africans who eat a diet high in fiber and roughage have a low incidence of colorectal cancer. Fiber causes food to pass more rapidly through the digestive tract, which means that carcinogens have less contact with the mucosal cells lining the intestine. In addition, components in fiber called *lignin* and *pectin* bind directly to bile salts and their breakdown products, and carry them out of the bowel so that they cannot be absorbed by the body.

A number of other substances have a protective effect against colon cancer as well. *Antioxidants* such as *selenium*, *Vitamin C*, and *Vitamin E* prevent the breakdown of bile salts. These compounds have been shown to be effective in preventing cancer in several animal studies. Other animals studies have shown that *lactobacillus bacteria*, which are present in some yogurts, are associated with inhibition of tumors. Finally, soybeans are known to contain a *protease inhibitor*, which prevents the breakdown of protein and has been associated with lower rates of colon cancer. Experts speculate that this substance may be a factor in the relatively low rate of colon cancer in Japan.

Although diet is the major factor determining rates of colon cancer, there are other factors that influence an individual's susceptibility as well. Worldwide, the rates of colon cancer are very low below the age of 40, rise sharply after the age of 50, and reach a peak around the age of 75. This pattern can probably be attributed to the fact that cancer is a disease that normally takes many years to develop. Genetic factors play a definite role: people with more than one relative who has had colon cancer have a threefold greater risk and are more likely to develop the disease at a younger age. People with only one relative who has had colon cancer are not shown to be at significant risk.

A number of medical conditions increase the likelihood of colon cancer. One is *benign adenoma polyps*, which are overgrowths of epithelial tissue that develop into a tumor that is flat or hangs on a stalk. Unless such polyps are very large, they have no symptoms other than occasional bleeding. Although only 1% of small adenoma polyps are malignant, they are all removed because it's believed that they are precursors of carcinomas. Some types of adenoma polyps are more likely to become malignant than others. *Ulcerative colitis*, a condition in which the colon is chronically inflamed, also carries a higher risk of colon cancer, as does a history of female genital cancer. Several rare genetic conditions put people at much greater than average risk, including *familial polyposis*, a condition in which the intestine has thousands of tiny *polyps* or growths, and *Gardener's syndrome*, which is another familial polyp condition.

Symptoms of colon cancer vary according to the location of the malignancy. Rectal bleeding is a very important symptom that often appears even before a change in bowel habits. Studies show that 60%–90% of people with cancer of the colon experience bleeding. Generally a bowel movement is accompanied by a small amount of bright red blood, and possibly mucus, although the blood can be so slight and so mixed in that it is not visible.

About 50% of all colon cancer occurs in the left colon (see illustration). Cancer in the *left colon*, which includes the rectum, tends to

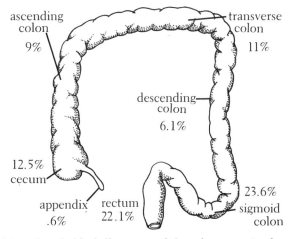

More than half of all cancers of the colon occur in the first 25 cm. (approximately 10 inches) of the colon. The other half are found in the descending, transverse, and ascending colon.

cause "obstructive symptoms." People experience a gradually progressive constipation, and/or a reduction in the diameter of the stool because the malignancy tends to narrow the diameter of the colon and make it more difficult for stool to pass. Occasionally, this gradual constipation may be interrupted by periods of diarrhea. Symptoms of cancer in the *right colon* are somewhat different because at this point in the intestine, fecal matter is still liquid. Moreover, a small amount of blood mixing with the stool in the right colon generally goes unnoticed. Often the first sign of cancer of the right colon is vague abdominal discomfort or pain. Other signs of cancer at this site are anemia due to blood loss, and/or weight loss. Cancer of both the left and right colon can be signaled by abdominal pain ranging from dull to sharp. In later stages, cancer of the left colon, as well as the right, is typified by weight loss and anemia.

One of the difficulties in diagnosing cancer of the colon is that the symptoms are so nonspecific. Subtle changes in bowel habits and/or vague abdominal pain are common to many people in our culture. They are rarely caused by cancer of the colon in people in their 20s and 30s who are not in one of the high-risk groups. Bleeding, which is a more specific and disturbing symptom, is rarely caused by cancer of the colon in the under-40 age group. As people grow older, the likelihood of cancer increases, but cancer of the colon is still not the most common cause of bleeding or a change in bowel habits. The characteristics of bleeding can also vary: a small amount of blood on the toilet paper is much more likely to be from *hemorrhoids* or *anal fissures* (see p. 366). Nevertheless, it is very important to rule out cancer in the case of a change in bowel habits, abdominal pain, and/or bloody stools, especially in people over 50.

Self-Care

Cancer of the colon must be diagnosed and treated by a doctor. The most important thing that people can do to take care of themselves is to see a doctor at the first sign of a problem. When cancer of the colon is treated early, the cure rate is 80%–90%. Unlike some cancers, colorectal cancer is very curable. Presently there are a number of support groups whose purpose is to work with people who have cancer. The groups offer support to help improve a person's attitude and teach stress reduction, meditation, and imagery techniques to enhance functioning of the immune system (see p. 302).

The Doctor

Based on a person's medical history, the doctor will evaluate the symptoms and assess whether or not there is a history of polyps, colorectal cancer, or ulcerative colitis. First, the doctor will do a *digital rectal exam*, and a *vaginal exam* in women. A rectal exam may reveal the presence of hemorrhoids or fissures that might cause bleeding. It will also reveal approximately 15% of tumors of the colon. If an individual is over 40 and has changes in bowel habits or bleeding, the doctor will usually order a *sigmoidoscopy*. There are two types of sigmoidoscopes, a rigid one and a flexible one. Generally the flexible ones are preferred because they are less uncomfortable for the patient, and they enable the

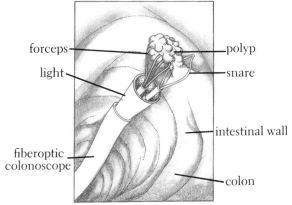

Colonoscopes allow doctors to locate and remove colon polyps without abdominal surgery.

doctor to see more. Depending on the suspected likelihood of colon cancer, the doctor may also order *a lower GI x-ray*, called a *double contrast barium enema*. Together, sigmoidoscopy and a barium enema can detect the great majority of colon cancers. If a polyp is seen on the x-rays, or if the first tests are negative but suspicion remains high, the doctor will order *colonoscopy*, a procedure in which a long fiber-optic instrument is used to examine the entire colon and remove any polyps in order to determine if they are malignant.

If cancer is diagnosed, surgery is performed to remove the tumor and an area around it. In many cases only a portion of the colon and nearby lymph nodes are removed, and the ends of the intestine are simply rejoined. If the tumor is located close to the anus, or if the cancer is advanced, it may be necessary to do a *colostomy*, a procedure in which the intestine is attached to a new opening on the abdomen. If a *CT scan* reveals the cancer has metastasized, or spread beyond the colon, surgery may be supplemented with *chemotherapy* or *radiation*.

When colon cancer is diagnosed early, it is highly treatable. With surgery, the *cure rate* for tumors that have not spread is 80%–90%. The cure rate for all tumors, including those that have metastasized, is over 50%. In the majority of cases, surgery does not necessitate a colostomy.

Prevention

Although the rate of colon cancer is very high in this country, there is a great deal that can be done to prevent this form of cancer. There is no absolute proof that a low-fat and/or high-fiber diet reduces the risk of colon cancer, but studies strongly indicate that this is the case. *Primary prevention* involves eliminating the agents that contribute to colon cancer (see section on *Description*). *Secondary prevention* involves early detection and removal of premalignant tumors. Unlike other types of cancer, it is now believed that screening for colorectal cancer is justified for people over 40 who are at average risk, as well as for those who are at higher risk because of their medical history. Large studies are in progress to determine what type of screening is the most accurate, most cost-effective, and most acceptable to patients.

As of 1980, the American Cancer Society made a series of recommendations for the screening of people who had no symptoms and were of average risk: 1) People should have an annual *rectal exam* beginning at age 40. 2) Beginning at age 50, people should have an annual *fecal occult blood test*, specifically a *Hemoccult test*, which involves checking the stool for hidden blood three days in a row. 3) *Sigmoidoscopy* is recommended, at ages 50 and 51, and every three to five years thereafter if the two initial exams reveal no polyps. 4) If polyps are found on the initial sigmoidoscopies, they should be removed, and colonoscopy should be done annually to detect any new polyps. Some doctors feel the number of colon cancers detected by routine sigmoidoscopy is not sufficient to justify this procedure, but other doctors feel that some schedule of routine sigmoidoscopy is reasonable in light of the fact that cancer of the colon is the most common malignancy in the U.S.

Hemorrhoids and Anal Fissures

Symptoms

hemorrhoids
- rectal bleeding
- anal protrusions or skin tags
- vague discomfort or pain in the anal area
- mucous discharge
- itching sensation around the anus

anal fissures
- severe pain on defecation
- gnawing pain between bowel movements
- rectal bleeding

Description

Hemorrhoids are simply veins in the anal area that have become enlarged. They are among the most common of human diseases, occurring in 50% of people by the age of 50. There are two types of hemorrhoids, internal and external. *In-ternal hemorrhoids* are widenings in the veins which are in the upper part of the rectum and are covered by the mucosa that lines the rectum. *External hemorrhoids* are widened veins, covered by skin, that lie outside the anus. They can be seen and felt as small bulges or skin tags around the anal opening. Because both types of veins are part of the same network, most people have a combination of internal and external hemorrhoids. Hemorrhoids vary greatly in size, and both the internal and external types sometimes protrude from the anus during a bowel movement. Very mild internal hemorrhoids or external hemorrhoids do not protrude, so they cannot be felt.

There are several theories as to what causes hemorrhoids. One theory maintains that elevated pressure in the veins causes them to bulge. According to this theory, human beings became more susceptible to this condition when they assumed an upright stance. Pregnancy and straining to have a bowel movement further elevate the pressure in the veins and are thought to promote the development of hemorrhoids. Interestingly, hemorrhoids are rare in areas of the world where people tend to have soft stools due to a large amount of fiber in their diet. Another theory holds that hemorrhoids are not actually varicose or enlarged veins at all, because they contain bright red oxygenated blood, whereas veins normally carry dark red, oxygen-depleted blood. According to this theory, hemorrhoids are thought to be connections between arteries and veins that bleed and swell when they are rubbed or strained.

People often are unaware of hemorrhoids until they bleed. Bleeding is usually noticed as a bright red streak on the toilet paper, or as a spot of blood on the stool. Eventually the bleeding can become sufficient to cause blood to spurt or drip with a bowel movement. Alternately, hemorrhoids may be noticed only when they progress to the point that they prolapse, or protrude from the anus. Initially they will slide back in at

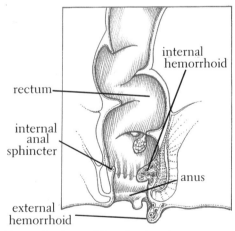

Hemorrhoids are dilated veins that can occur either around the anus or inside the wall of the rectum. Rectal polyps are outgrowths of the mucous membrane that lines the rectum.

the end of the bowel movement by themselves, but eventually, they may have to be pushed back in manually with lubrication. Usually the last symptom to be noticed is pain, which can vary from mild to significant. Hemorroids can also cause itching and slight incontinence.

Occasionally, a hemorrhoid develops a blood clot which blocks off one particular blood vessel. When this occurs, a lump may suddenly appear in the anal area, and produce an intense pain that may continue for several days. This condition is referred to as a *thrombosed hemorrhoid*. The problem is not harmful and usually disappears spontaneously within a week.

An *anal fissure* is a tear in the skin around the anal opening that is accompanied by swelling which causes pain in the sensitive nerve endings nearby. Often fissures are caused by straining to pass hard, dry stools. Unlike hemorrhoids, fissures cause intense pain during defecation, as well as gnawing pain between bowel movements. Fissures are so tender that sometimes merely touching the area causes tremendous pain. As a result, when people have a fissure, they often avoid having a bowel movement, which can lead to additional problems with constipation. Fissures do sometimes bleed, but usually less profusely than hemorrhoids.

Self-Care

Small hemorrhoids require no treatment, but to avoid making them worse, straining to defecate should definitely be avoided. A *high-fiber diet* (see p. 95) and/or *psyllium-seed bulk laxatives* (e.g., *Metamucil*), plus four to eight glasses of water a day, will make the stools generally softer. *Sitz baths* or warm baths will help to relieve pain. For a thrombosed hemorrhoid, one to two days of bed rest may help to relieve pressure, and warm baths and/or cold compresses may help to alleviate pain. Many over-the-counter hemorrhoid preparations are sold, but they are generally not recommended by doctors

Self-Care for Hemorrhoids
• avoid constipation (see p. 360) • sit in a hot bath for 10–15 minutes two to three times a day • instead of toilet paper, use witch hazel compresses or a soapy washcloth to clean perineal area after a bowel movement • avoid sitting or standing for long periods of time

because they aren't very effective and people can become allergic to the topical anesthetic they contain.

The treatment for anal fissures is the same as for hemorrhoids: sitz baths, a high-fiber diet, and stool softeners. The pain can also be relieved by nonprescription *anusol suppositories*, which contain a mild anesthetic. In general, an anal fissure heals by itself within several weeks.

The Doctor

The doctor diagnoses hemorrhoids by inspecting the anal area and doing a digital rectal exam. Internal hemorrhoids that do not protrude can be more difficult to diagnose. If there is significant bleeding in a person over 40, the doctor will also do *sigmoidoscopy* and/or a *barium enema* to rule out the rarer possibility of cancer of the colon.

If hemorrhoidal symptoms are severe, or the hemorrhoids become inflamed or thrombosed, the doctor will remove them by one of several methods that can be done in the office. An internal hemorrhoid may be treated with *rubberband ligation*, a minor procedure in which the hemorrhoid is tied off. After about a week, the hemorrhoid will slough off for lack of blood supply. Alternately, internal hemorrhoids can be injected with *sclerosing solutions*, chemicals that gradually cause them to block off; or they can be removed either by laser or through a freezing technique called *cryosurgery*. If a thrombosed external hemorrhoid is large enough, it may be removed under local anesthetic. Finally, if hemorrhoids become severe enough, they may need to be removed surgically in the hospital in a procedure called a *hemorrhoidectomy*. This is recommended especially when there is a large amount of tissue that tends to remain protruded after bowel movements.

An anal fissure can often be diagnosed from a simple visual inspection of the anal area. A digital rectal examination will be done if it is not too painful. The doctor will recommend stool softeners, and may prescribe *anesthetic lubricants* to relieve pain. In the unlikely event that a fissure does not heal naturally, it can be repaired surgically in the hospital.

Ruling Out Other Diseases

Cancer of the colon (see p. 362) and *diverticulitis* (see p. 369) will be ruled out by sigmoidoscopy, a barium enema, or colonoscopy, if bleeding has been a significant symptom, especially if the patient is over 40.

Prevention

The most important preventive measure for hemorrhoids and anal fissures, as for other conditions of the colon, is a high-fiber diet. This type of diet adds bulk to the stool, making it softer and easier to pass, and lessening the likelihood of straining on defecation. Drinking sufficient fluids and establishing regular bowel habits can also help to avoid constipation. It's important that people promptly heed their body's signals and go to the bathroom when they feel the need. However, people do not need to have a bowel movement every day, and it is not advisable to sit on the toilet and strain when they feel no urge.

Diverticular Disease: Diverticulosis and Diverticulitis

Symptoms

mild, or *simple*
- intermittent cramping pain over the lower left abdominal area
- tenderness in the lower left abdomen
- often, no symptoms

severe
- significant lower left abdominal pain
- altered bowel habits: constipation, occasionally diarrhea
- often, fever
- rarely, rectal bleeding

Description

Diverticula are little outpouchings, or hernias, in the lining of the colon which protrude through the muscular wall of the colon. *Diverticular disease* is the term used to describe the symptoms produced by these outpouchings, in particular when they become infected and/or perforated. These outpouchings have been found to be extremely common in Western cultures, and their incidence increases directly with age. Diverticula are rare in people under 30, but by the age of 60, 20%–50% of people in the U.S. have developed them.

The majority of people with diverticula have no symptoms, a condition that is referred to as *diverticulosis.* In the past, the assumption was that the diverticula did not cause symptoms because they weren't inflamed, but doctors now believe that many of these people actually have chronic or intermittent lower abdominal pain that is often overlooked or ascribed to other causes such as *irritable bowel syndrome* (see p.

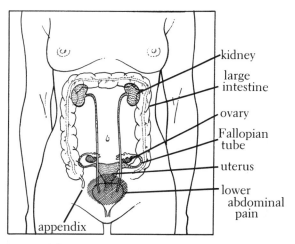

Lower abdominal pain can be caused by conditions of the colon, bladder, or uterus.

358). Frequently these people also have chronic constipation, alternating with episodes of diarrhea. As long as the symptoms are mild, people often do not even seek treatment. The only way doctors and patients become aware that diverticula are the cause of these symptoms is if the outpouchings are observed on a sigmoidoscopic or x-ray exam.

The degree to which people are symptomatic is thought to relate to the size and number of diverticula, and, more importantly, the degree to which they are inflamed. When an outpouching becomes seriously inflamed, it can develop a microscopic perforation, or hole, that allows tiny amounts of fecal material to fester in the wall of the colon. When the resulting inflammation or infection is very severe, the wall of the colon can swell and become partially blocked. The infected state is referred to as *diverticulitis,* or inflammation of the diverticula. The symptoms of diverticulitis are pain and often fever. The infection can vary from mild to serious enough to require hospitalization. Occasionally, diverticula bleed; this can be a cause of significant rectal bleeding, but only 10%–30% of people with diverticulosis ever experience rectal bleeding, and usually it is not even noticed. In recent years, doctors have come to realize that diverticulosis and diverticulitis are not actually two separate conditions, but are part of a continuum which is now referred to as *diverticular disease of the colon.*

Researchers have developed a theory of how diverticula develop. Normally the colon squeezes in a regular rhythm which moves fecal material through the intestines at a slow but steady rate. These movements cause the colon to form ridges made up of thick and thin muscular bands, giving the colon a corrugated appearance. The bands that protrude inward become thickened, while the bands that protrude outward become thinner. Pressure normally rises in the colon when the bands squeeze. If the pressure is chronically high, outpouchings tend to develop in the weakest areas of the thin bands. The areas most naturally susceptible to herniation are the points where tiny blood vessels go through the muscular layer of the colonic wall to reach the lining. When fecal material

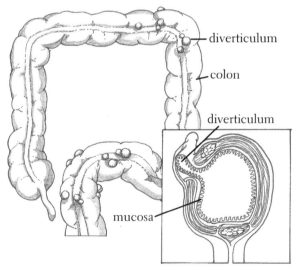

Diverticuli are tiny outpouchings that develop in the wall of the colon as a result of chronic high pressure. These outpouchings can become infected when bacteria and fecal material become lodged in them.

become lodged in the outpouchings, they can become inflamed and infected.

Doctors speculate that a number of different factors can cause pressure to be unnaturally high in the colon. In Western countries, the main factor is thought to be a lack of fiber in the diet. The human colon is adapted to work most efficiently when the stool has a high bulk content, such as was found in the diet of early humans. This early diet was high in uncooked fruits and vegetables, and unprocessed grains. On the other hand, the highly refined diets of today's Westerners produce a digested material that is largely absorbed in the small intestine, leaving a small, highly processed residue to pass into the large intestine, or colon. Researchers postulate that to handle this small amount of low-bulk fecal matter, the colon squeezes into more and more bands in order to slow down the transit time. Otherwise, the fecal matter is not kept in the colon long enough to absorb the necessary water content, and the stool tends to be very loose or watery. Thus a low-fiber diet not only produces a small amount of bulk, it causes higher pressures in the colon. The bulkier the stool, the wider the colon is stretched as the fecal matter passes. Somewhat paradoxically, the wider the colon, the lower the pressure against the walls, and the less likely diverticula are to develop.

These new theories about diverticula are backed up by cross-cultural epidemiological studies. Remarkably, diverticular disease was unknown 100 years ago. It has only been with the invention of roller-milling, which takes the fiber out of flour, that the disease has become common. It is still uncommon in Africa, India, and the Middle East, all of which generally have a high-fiber diet. However, people in those countries who eat a Western diet or who move to Western countries often develop the disease.

Another factor thought to be associated with diverticular disease is stress. The reason for this may not seem as readily apparent, but stress directly affects the autonomic nervous system which regulates the motility, or movement, of the colon. If people become anxious or are under stress, the movements of the colon decrease in frequency, thereby slowing the transit of fecal material, and causing it to become drier and harder. Again, stress is thought to be more common in industrialized countries with their hectic, competitive life-styles (see p. 40). One researcher has postulated that a major cause of diverticular disease has to do with the inaccessibility of the commode in Western life and our social constraints on passing gas in public. Both of these factors also tend to increase pressure in the colon.

Self-Care

In the past, asymptomatic diverticular disease was left untreated, although the symptom of mild constipation might be treated with laxatives. Ironically, people with symptomatic diverticular disease were told by doctors to eat a low-fiber diet to avoid "irritating and obstructing the diverticula." Current recommendations advise a high-fiber diet (see p. 95) for everyone with diverticular disease, except during acute attacks. In addition, many doctors suggest that people take *natural or synthetic bulking agents*, such as *psyllium hydrophilic mucilloid* (e.g., *Metamucil* or *Konsyl*) and make sure they drink four to eight glasses of water daily. Finally, patients are advised to avoid unnecessary stress in their life and learn to deal with unavoidable tensions (see p. 58).

Self-Care for Diverticulosis

- eat a high-fiber diet (except during attacks)
- exercise daily
- don't smoke
- avoid alcohol
- learn to identify and deal with stress (see p. 58)
- try to adopt a positive attitude about life

The Doctor

Diverticular disease is diagnosed from a history, a physical exam, and lab tests. The diverticula can be visualized either by a *sigmoidoscopic exam* or a *barium enema*. Mild diverticula are treated entirely with self-care (see above). If people have a fever and significant pain, they will be treated with a course of a *broad-spectrum antibiotic* (e.g., *ampicillin*, *cephalothin*). Generally, most attacks aren't severe, and they respond readily to antibiotics. During an attack, doctors temporarily advise a low-fiber diet to avoid irritating the colon until the infection subsides.

If an attack causes severe enough nausea and vomiting or uncontrollable pain, the patient will be hospitalized and given antibiotics and intravenous fluids to prevent dehydration. If patients do not improve, develop complications, or have recurrent infections, surgery may be considered to remove the diseased section of colon. Only 4%–10% of patients hospitalized for diverticulitis require surgery.

Ruling Out Other Diseases

A barium enema differentiates diverticular disease from *irritable bowel syndrome* (see p. 358) or *cancer of the colon* (see p. 362).

Prevention

Research indicates that a high-fiber diet is the major factor in the prevention of diverticular disease, and also lessens the likelihood of hemorrhoids, irritable bowel syndrome, cancer of the colon, and even diabetes. For many people, adopting a high-fiber diet requires a real commitment to seriously altering their normal diet by refraining from eating processed foods and making an on-going effort to eat more foods that are high in fiber. Often, one of the easiest ways to increase fiber is to take a bulking agent (e.g.,

Metamucil or *Konsyl*) every day. Increasing fiber is a lifelong process, and the earlier people switch to a high-fiber diet, the healthier they are likely to be—especially if they are over 40, have any of the symptoms of diverticular disease, or have had diverticula diagnosed on a sigmoidoscopic exam. In addition, people should drink plenty of fluids, attempt to establish regular bowel habits, and work to lower the stress in their lives (see p. 58).

Gallbladder Disease: Gallstones and Gallbladder Attacks

Symptoms

gallstones
- often, no symptoms
- pain in upper middle or upper right abdomen, possibly radiating to the right shoulder or upper back *(biliary pain)*
- pain that starts slowly, builds to a steady peak, then goes away after several hours
- occasionally, nausea and vomiting

acute cholecystitis
- pain begins as above, then localizes to upper right abdomen, and does not go away
- lack of appetite, nausea, and often vomiting
- yellow skin color (jaundice)
- low fever

Description

Gallstones, or *cholelithiasis*, is one of the most common conditions of the digestive tract. Most people who have gallstones aren't aware of

them, and never have any symptoms at all, but in 10%–20% of these people, the stones block the gallbladder, causing it to contract painfully. In about 20%–50% of people who experience one or more attacks, the gallbladder becomes inflamed or blocked, requiring hospitalization and treatment.

The *gallbladder* is a muscular, pear-shaped organ about three to four inches long, whose function is to store and concentrate *bile*, a digestive juice made by the liver. Bile is an emulsifying agent that lowers the surface tension on fat molecules, making it possible for them to be broken down by *pancreatic juices*. The liver makes about a quart of bile per day. From the liver, bile passes down the *hepatic duct*, which becomes the *common bile duct* after it is joined by the *cystic duct* coming from the gallbladder (see illustration). Near the site where the common bile duct empties into the *duodenum*, or small intestine, the common duct is also joined by the *pancreatic duct*. Passage of these digestive juices from the common bile duct into the duodenum is controlled by the *sphincter of Oddi*. If the duo-

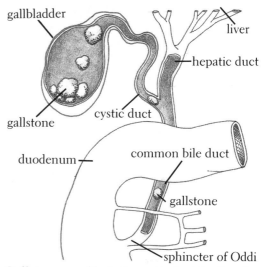

Gallstones can block the cystic duct leading from the gallbladder, or they can become lodged in the common bile duct which leads to the small intestine.

denum is empty of food, the sphincter of Oddi remains closed, and bile accumulates in the common duct, eventually backing up into the gallbladder, where it becomes concentrated as water and various salts are absorbed. When food containing fat enters the duodenum, the sphincter opens and the gallbladder contracts, forcing bile into the small intestine.

Bile is made up of *bile salts, bile pigments, lecithin,* and *cholesterol.* Cholesterol is an insoluble substance that becomes soluble only when it is joined to bile salts and lecithin. When there is too much cholesterol as compared to bile salts, the cholesterol precipitates out, forming *cholesterol gallstones,* which account for 75% of all stones found. The bile in people with this type of gallstone has a higher percentage of cholesterol than does normal bile. A second type of gallstones, called *pigmented gallstones,* are composed of dark, yellow-colored *bilirubin* (digested red blood cells) and *calcium salts.* Less is known about why this type of stone forms, although it occurs with certain forms of *anemia* in which red blood cells are broken down more frequently than usual.

In the U.S., approximately 10% of men and 20% of women develop cholesterol gallstones in midadulthood. A number of factors increase the likelihood of developing gallstones. The incidence of gallstones increases with *age,* peaking between ages 55 and 65. Due to a link with the female hormone *estrogen,* women are two to four times as likely to develop gallstones as men. From puberty until menopause, women's bile has 15% more cholesterol than men's. Since increased amounts of estrogen are produced during pregnancy, the likelihood of gallstones increases with the number of times a woman has been pregnant. Likewise, women who have been on *estrogen replacement therapy* (see p. 429), or even *birth control pills,* are more likely to eventually develop cholesterol gallstones.

A number of risk factors for cholesterol gallstones have to do with nutrition. *Obesity* itself is

a predisposing factor: people who are 20% overweight have two times the risk of gallstones, and very obese people have almost six times the risk (see p. 445). In addition, the bile of people who are overweight, regardless of whether they have gallstones, is higher in cholesterol than the average person's. Ironically, *dieting* can also increase a person's risk. When people diet, the percentage of salts in their bile drops; as a result, less cholesterol can be dissolved and more is precipitated out in the gallbladder. Once people lose weight, however, their risk of gallstones decreases. Ideally, people who are overweight should lose weight once and keep it off.

Several other nutritional factors also play a role in the formation of gallstones. High levels of *cholesterol* and *triglycerides* in food are associated with higher levels of cholesterol in bile, and thus with higher numbers of gallstones. Studies have shown a dramatic rise in the incidence of cholesterol gallstones in Japan since the Japanese have adopted a diet higher in fat. Although there is increasing evidence linking a high cholesterol diet to this type of gallstones, studies large enough to merit national recommendation have yet to come out. A *low-fiber diet* also seems to correlate with an increased risk of cholesterol gallstones. One animal study has demonstrated that a low-fiber diet results in higher cholesterol levels in bile. Other studies have shown that if people supplement their diet with bran, the level of cholesterol in their bile drops below the level necessary to form stones.

The risk factors for the less common, pigmented gallstones are somewhat different. The incidence of these stones also increases with age, but other risk factors include alcoholism or cirrhosis of the liver, hemolytic anemias, and gallbladder infection caused by cholesterol stones.

The symptoms of gallstones vary depending upon whether or not the stones block one of the ducts. The majority of stones cause no symptoms because they lie in the gallbladder and do not affect its functioning. Among people who have gallstones that are diagnosed inadvertently, it has been found that 70%–90% have no symptoms for as long as 10–25 years. Those who develop symptoms usually do so within five years.

The most common symptom caused by gallstones is *biliary pain*, not infection or blockage. Biliary pain, or what is frequently referred to as a *gallbladder attack*, results when a stone temporarily blocks either the cystic duct leading from the gallbladder, or the common duct leading to the duodenum. Doctors speculate that this pain is the result of the gallbladder contracting spasmodically, or the result of pressure building up in the gallbladder. If the stone moves back from the mouth of the gallbladder, or, more commonly, passes into the duodenum, the attack subsides by itself. General, ill-defined gastrointestinal symptoms such as bloating, indigestion, and discomfort are not believed to be due to gallstones because they occur as often in people who do not have gallstones as in those who do.

Characteristically, biliary pain comes on gradually in either the upper middle, or upper right, side of the abdomen. Over a period of 15–30 minutes, the pain builds to a peak of intensity, then gradually disappears over the next several hours. The pain is normally steady, not intermittent; and it may radiate to the back or the upper right shoulder. Typically, the pain is not made worse by movement. The pain may also be accompanied by nausea and vomiting. Many people believe that attacks are precipitated by a fatty meal, and that may be the case, but studies have yet to prove it.

The timing of attacks is unpredictable and varies greatly in frequency: some people have episodes within weeks of each other, some months or years apart. Of people who have had one episode of biliary pain, only 30%–60% will have subsequent attacks. Within five years, 10% of those who've had an attack will develop a gallbladder inflammation; within 20 years, 20%–50% will develop an inflammation (see below).

The most common complication of gallstones is an acute inflammation of the gallbladder wall, which is called *acute cholecystitis*. It is due to a stone blocking the cystic duct, which causes excess fluid to accumulate in the gallbladder. As a result, the lining of the gallbladder becomes inflamed, and may even become infected. Acute cholecystitis starts like a biliary attack, but because one of the ducts remains blocked, the attack does not subside. Instead of going away after several hours, the pain localizes to the upper right abdomen and does not disappear without medical care. In addition to nausea and vomiting, a fever develops, as well as tenderness in the immediate area of the gallbladder. Approximately 20% of the time, colored pigment salts trapped in the gallbladder are reabsorbed into the bloodstream in sufficient quantity to give people a slightly yellow or jaundiced color.

Another serious complication of gallstones is *choledocholithiasis*, a condition in which a stone blocks the common duct leading to the duodenum. In this situation, no bile can pass into the intestine from the liver or the gallbladder, and the bile ducts and bile often become infected. With choledocholithiasis, there is a variable clinical course ranging from no symptoms if the duct is only partially obstructed, to significant symptoms. People commonly have a fever, chills, and biliary pain. There is usually significant enough jaundice that the whites of the eyes, as well as the skin, become yellow. Eventually, the urine may turn dark due to colored bile pigments that are filtered out of the blood by the kidneys. In severe cases of choledocholithiasis, the liver can even become infected.

Self-Care

Symptomatic gallbladder disease requires treatment by a doctor. However, a low-cholesterol, high-fiber diet may play a role in treating cholesterol gallstones in the future. There have been no definitive studies in humans showing that such a diet actually dissolves gallstones, but some animal studies suggest that this may be possible.

The Doctor

The doctor diagnoses gallstones on the basis of a physical exam, laboratory tests, and several diagnostic procedures. The typical findings vary depending upon whether or not a stone is blocking a duct, and which duct is blocked. Asymptomatic gallstones do not show up on a physical exam or blood tests, but they may be diagnosed accidentally from an abdominal x-ray, abdominal ultrasound, or abdominal surgery that is being done for other reasons.

The treatment for asymptomatic or "silent" gallstones has been a matter of controversy for years. Until recently, many doctors recommended *cholecystecomy*, a surgical procedure in which the gallbladder is removed. Their decision was based on the assumption that most stones would eventually cause complications, and that postponing surgery would carry a greater risk for an older patient, especially one whose gallbladder was infected. Thus doctors reasoned that since the gallbladder is not necessary for the digestion of food, it was better to remove the gallbladder when a person was young and healthy. Currently, most doctors do not recommend cholecystectomy for asymptomatic gallstones because reliable studies have shown that most gallstones do not cause problems. Moreover, medical and surgical improvements have made it safer to operate on older people even when the gallbladder is infected. However, gallbladder removal may be recommended for diabetics because they can experience severe complications from gallstones.

When a person complains of simple biliary pain, usually nothing is found on physical exam or lab tests. Gallstones are diagnosed on the basis of *ultrasound* and/or a gallbladder x-ray called an *oral cholecystogram*, which involves having a person swallow tablets of *iopanoic acid* or *tyropanoic acid*, a substance that is picked up by the gallbladder. Occasionally these tests fail to show stones that are present.

Some doctors recommend surgery after a first attack because such a high percentage of people having one attack have subsequent episodes, and may experience complications. Other doctors do not recommend surgery unless a person has recurrent attacks. Still other doctors recommend medical therapy with drugs containing *chenodeoxycholic acid* (e.g., *Chenix*), which dissolves cholesterol gallstones. These drugs, which contain natural bile acids, are effective in only 13%–50% of all cases, and must be taken for 6–24 months. The medicine has several side effects, including elevated blood cholesterol levels and diarrhea. The drug is only effective for small cholesterol stones in a functional gallbladder. A new, nonsurgical technique, *lithotripsy*, which uses ultrasound to fragment gallstones, is being studied and used experimentally in the treatment of uncomplicated gallstones. Currently, drugs that dissolve cholesterol gallstones must be taken after the procedure. If it proves effective, it may be used increasingly, as ultrasound fragmentation is now used to break up kidney stones.

Generally people with suspected *acute cholecystitis*, an inflammation of the gallbladder caused by a stone blocking the cystic duct, are admitted to the hospital for diagnostic tests and treatment. The physical exam shows upper right abdominal tenderness, and often, the gallbladder can be felt. The white blood cell count is high due to the inflammation, and if the person is jaundiced, the *bilirubin level* is also high. Several other blood values, *alkaline phosphatase* and *serum transaminase*, will also be elevated. *Abdominal ultrasonography* is used to visualize the size and location of stones. The diagnosis is confirmed by a new test called *hepatobiliary scintigraphy (HIDA scan)*, which involves injecting a low-level radioactive tracer into the bloodstream. Within 15–30 minutes the radioactive material appears in the ducts; a blockage is indicated if none of the material can be seen in the gallbladder.

If acute cholecystitis is confirmed, a person is treated with supportive measures until surgery can be performed. To stop the gallbladder from going into spasm, the person is taken off oral food and given intravenous antibiotics and pain medication, if necessary. A nasogastric tube is inserted through the nose and down the esophagus into the stomach to draw off excess fluid and gas. Within two to three days, the gallbladder is removed surgically. In the past, surgery was often delayed for six to eight weeks until the infection had been treated with a course of antibiotics, but recent studies have shown that early removal of the gallbladder actually reduces both complications and the length of hospital stay.

People with suspected *choledocholithiasis*, a stone in the common duct, are also hospitalized for diagnosis and treatment. These people generally have upper right abdominal tenderness, a high white cell count, a very high bilirubin if they're jaundiced, and high alkaline phosphatase, serum amylase and liver function tests. The combination of significant jaundice and elevated lab values tends to indicate that a stone is blocking the common duct. The diagnosis can be verified, and other conditions ruled out, by *endoscopic retrograde cholangiopancreatography (ERCP)*, a procedure in which a thin fiberoptic tube is passed down the esophagus, through the stomach, along the duodenum, and into the common duct. Dye is injected through the tube in order to visualize the blockage on x-ray. If a stone is found in the duct, the person will be stabilized and given intravenous fluids, antibiotics, and pain medicine if necessary. Within a day or two, the gallbladder and the stone will be surgically removed.

Ruling Out Other Diseases

A gallbladder attack can be confused with other conditions that affect the upper abdomen, such as *ulcers* (see p. 353), *irritable bowel syndrome* (see p. 358), an *infection of the pancreas*, *angina* (see p. 267), *acute hepatitis*, and less commonly, with *abdominal cancers* (see p. 362). With ulcers, the pain is generally more burning, and it tends to occur shortly after meals. With angina, the pain is brought on by exercise; also, it is more likely to be located under the breastbone, and has a sensation more like tightness or gas cramps.

Prevention

At present, there are no definitive studies on prevention of gallstones, but research points to the fact that a low-cholesterol, high-fiber diet may help to prevent and possibly dissolve cholesterol gallstones. Animal studies support the theory that a high-cholesterol diet leads to the formation of this type of gallstones, and that reduction of cholesterol intake actually causes the stones to disappear. In any event, a low-cholesterol, high-fiber diet has no negative side effects, and in fact, has beneficial effects in terms of a number of other diseases, including heart disease, diabetes, diverticulitis, and cancer of the colon.

Hiatus Hernia and Reflux Esophagitis, or Gastroesophageal Reflux Disease

Symptoms

- burning or pain under the breastbone (heartburn)
- sour regurgitation, especially at night
- in some people, slight difficulty swallowing

Description

Reflux esophagitis is a condition in which the contents of the stomach or duodenum come back up into the esophagus. X-ray studies have shown that small amounts of material come back up into the lower esophagus all the time, but generally the problem is so mild that no treatment is sought. If a significant amount of material comes up often, symptoms become more pronounced. The most common symptom of reflux is *heartburn*, which can vary from a mild burning sensation after meals, to constant pain under the *sternum*, or breastbone. Heartburn may be accompanied by regurgitation of stomach contents into the mouth.

Generally, when people eat they are sitting in an upright position, so gravity aids muscular contractions in moving the food from the esophagus to the stomach (see illustration). When food reaches the stomach, the lower esophageal sphincter opens reflexively, but while digestion is taking place, the sphincter is normally closed, which keeps the contents of the stomach from refluxing. During digestion, the stomach churns and churns, and finally squeezes the partially digested food through the *pyloric valve* into the *duodenum*, the upper part of the intestine.

Doctors currently think that heartburn is largely due to an abnormality of esophageal per-

istalsis, or improper functioning of the esophageal sphincter. Studies have shown that in people with reflux esophagitis, the sphincter has less muscle tone than normal, and exerts less pressure to remain closed. If the pressure in the stomach during digestion is greater than the pressure exerted by the lower esophageal sphincter, partially digested food will reflux into the lower part of the esophagus. Strong pressure in the stomach can even cause sour regurgitation into the mouth. The burning sensation characteristic of heartburn is due to the fact that stomach acids in the refluxed material irritate the lining of the esophagus.

Doctors used to think that heartburn was caused by a *hiatus hernia*, an anatomical condition in which a small part of the stomach protruded out of the abdominal cavity into the chest cavity, through a widening in the opening of the diaphragm that the esophagus passed through. New research has shown that 30%–75% of the people in a study had hiatus hernias, yet only 5% complained of significant heartburn. Moreover, some people who are bothered by reflux esophagitis definitely do not have a hiatus hernia. Therefore, the role of a hiatus hernia in heartburn is now considered less important, although it may occasionally add to a person's symptoms.

Hiatus hernia is a condition in which the junction between the stomach and the esophagus slides above the diaphragm.

Self-Care

Esophageal reflux or heartburn is a condition that responds well to self-care. Approximately 85%–90% of people who have esophageal reflux are helped by a combination of self-help measures. The first measure recommended is to raise the head of the bed 6″–8″, either by putting blocks under the head of the bed, or by putting a plywood wedge under the mattress. This change in angle puts gravity to work, and greatly reduces the number and length of heartburn episodes at night.

A number of factors related to eating habits tend to either relieve or exacerbate reflux symptoms. Studies have shown that antacids and foods containing protein increase the tone of the sphincter; while fatty foods, chocolate, coffee (decaf or regular), caffeine, peppermint, and alcohol decrease the tone. Although no studies have been done thus far, it appears that certain foods give some individuals more gastric distress than others. Foods that are often cited as bothersome are onions and spicy foods. Small meals definitely seem to be tolerated better than large ones; people should also avoid lying down or going to bed within two or three hours after eating a meal.

Studies show that cigarette smoking makes heartburn worse. Also, anything that raises the general pressure in the abdomen should be avoided, including being overweight, wearing tight belts or girdles, and bending over for long periods of time. Anatomical and hormonal changes during pregnancy cause a temporary increase in abdominal pressure, as well as decreased tone in smooth muscles, including the sphincters. As a result, heartburn tends to be more common during pregnancy.

If self-help measures do not prove effective, heartburn may be relieved by over-the-counter antacids containing either *magnesium* or *aluminum hydroxide* (e.g., *Maalox, Digel*). These medications may be taken after meals and/or before bed, as directed on the label.

The Doctor

The doctor diagnoses esophageal reflux based on a history of the characteristic symptoms. Unless the symptoms are severe, the doctor will initially just recommend self-help measures. The doctor may also order a procedure called a *barium swallow* to visualize the esophagus and help to eliminate other conditions. Occasionally the test may enable the doctor to actually observe the reflux.

If self-care measures do not prove sufficient, the doctor may prescribe medications, such as *metochlopramide (Reglan)*, which increases sphincter pressure and causes the stomach to empty more quickly. Other drugs that are sometimes used include *cimetidine (Tagamet), ranitidine (Zantac),* or *famotidine (Pepcid)* that block the secretion of gastric acids, and therefore lessen the likelihood of acid reflux. These are the same drugs that are used to treat ulcers (see p. 531). In very severe cases, further diagnostic tests may be ordered, and surgery may be considered to reinforce the lower esophageal sphincter.

Ruling Out Other Diseases

If esophageal reflux causes sharp pain under the breastbone, it must be differentiated from *angina* (see p. 353) or a *heart attack* (see p. 386). An electrocardiogram (ECG) will be done if a heart attack or angina is suspected.

Prevention

Avoiding smoking and certain foods (see above), as well as moderating alcohol consumption, will help to maintain the tone of the esophageal sphincter. In addition, for people who are very heavy, weight loss will also help to lower abdominal pressure and may prevent esophageal refluxing.

ENDOCRINE

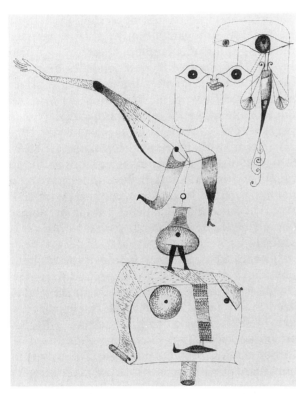

The hormones produced by the endocrine glands control metabolism and keep the body in delicate balance. Paul Klee. A Balance-Capriccio. 1923. Pen and ink, sheet: 9" × 12⅛". Collection, The Museum of Modern Art, New York. A. Conger Goodyear Fund.

Diabetes Mellitus

Symptoms

- often, no symptoms, but a high blood glucose level
- frequent urination
- increased thirst
- increased hunger
- weight loss
- weakness and fatigue
- dizziness, headaches, and blurry vision
- frequent skin infections and vaginal yeast infections

Description

Diabetes mellitus is a disease caused by several factors, each of which causes the pancreatic hormone *insulin* to be produced in low amounts or to be less effective than normal. As a result, glucose, a sugar, cannot be used or stored properly in the body and builds up in the bloodstream at higher than normal levels, producing a number of symptoms. Diabetes is extremely common; it is estimated that the disease affects 10 million people in the U.S., or 5% of the population. Currently, the incidence of diabetes is increasing at 5% a year, and the number of people with diabetes is expected to double in 15 years. Diabetes is the third major killer in the U.S., a fact many people do not realize. Diabetes predisposes people to small blood vessel abnormalities of the retina, kidney, and nerves, and it doubles their chances of heart attack and stroke.

379

Historically, diabetes is a condition that has been recognized since Egyptian times. It has been described in records from early Egypt, Greece, and India. In China, it was noted for characteristically making the urine sweet and sticky. The term diabetes comes from the Greek word for "siphon" or "pass through," which refers to the frequent urination that is a classic symptom of uncontrolled diabetes. "Mellitus," the Latin word for honey, was added to the name in the 1600s.

Any attempt to define diabetes becomes complicated because the disease is extremely complex in both its causes and its effects. In 1978, the National Diabetes Data Group reclassified diabetes into two separate syndromes. *Type I*, or *insulin-dependent diabetes mellitus (IDDM)* is a condition in which people secrete very little or no insulin. These people develop very high levels of blood sugar and toxic levels of *ketoacids* from the rapid breakdown of fat, which can put these people into a *diabetic coma*. Without outside insulin, Type I diabetics cannot survive. Type I diabetes usually develops before the age of 45, most often in childhood between the ages of 11 and 13. This class of diabetes used to be referred to as *juvenile onset, ketosis-prone,* or *brittle diabetes*. Although the onset of the disease is sudden, it is thought that the condition may actually develop over a period of weeks to months. New research links Type I diabetes to genetic factors and an as-yet unidentified virus. It is thought that after exposure to certain viruses, genetically susceptible people develop antibodies against the cells in their pancreas that produce insulin. Although it is known that viruses, genetics, and the autoimmune system are all involved, the exact mechanisms behind Type I diabetes have not yet been worked out. The hope is that a test can be devised to identify the presymptomatic stage, and in the meantime, that some kind of immune intervention can be developed to prevent the destruction of all the insulin-producing cells in susceptible people.

The drug *cyclosporin* is currently being tested for that purpose.

The second class of diabetes, *Type II* or *non-insulin-dependent diabetes mellitus (NIDDM)*, is a condition in which people remain able to produce a significant amount of their own insulin. Generally, these diabetics do not go into diabetic coma and are not dependent on outside insulin for survival, although they may need outside insulin to maintain proper blood-sugar levels. The onset of Type II diabetes most frequently takes place after the age of 45. Former names for Type II diabetes are *maturity* or *adult-onset diabetes*, or *stable diabetes*. Ninety percent to 95% of all cases of diabetes are Type II. The great majority of these diabetics, 80%–90%, are obese. Type II diabetes tends to run in families. Some doctors believe there may be a combination of types, or a continuum of subtypes, because many diabetics' symptoms do not completely match either the Type I or Type II profiles.

To gain a basic understanding of the complex physiology of diabetes, it is important to understand something about the way sugar is metabolized in the body, and the role insulin plays in that metabolic cycle. In the intestine, all foods are broken down into three basic constituents—carbohydrates, proteins, and fats. These constituents are then processed into even simpler forms: carbohydrates are broken down into a simple sugar called *glucose*; proteins are broken down into *amino acids*; and fat is broken down into *fatty acids*. When glucose reaches the bloodstream, it is taken up by cells throughout the body; in muscle cells it is used for energy, in brain cells it is used for essential brain functions, and in liver cells it is transformed and stored in the form of *glycogen*. The hormone *insulin* regulates the storage and mobilization of glucose. Insulin enables glucose to pass into all the different types of cells. Normally when food has been digested after a meal, the level of glucose in the blood does not rise suddenly. Anticipation of food causes a signal to be sent to the *beta cells of the pancreas*; insulin is actually released before the meal and causes digested sugar to be taken up steadily by cells as it enters the bloodstream.

Like other hormones, insulin is a protein made up of amino acids. Once insulin is produced in response to a rise in blood glucose, it enters the bloodstream from the pancreas and circulates for a mere four to eight minutes. By the time, all the molecules of insulin have become bound to receptors on the surface of individual cells throughout the entire body. Once an insulin molecule has been picked up, the cell can transport glucose across the cell membrane. Unused glucose is stored in the liver as *glycogen*, and can be converted back to glucose by a hormone called *glucagon*. Glycogen is reconverted whenever a low blood sugar level shows that the body needs more energy, such as occurs during exercise.

People with noninsulin-dependent diabetes mellitus (NIDDM) experience several problems with their insulin. First, they are often relatively *insulin deficient*; that is, they do not produce a normal amount of insulin in response to a given amount of blood sugar produced by a meal. In essence, they produce too little insulin, too late. Between meals, some of these people may produce enough insulin, but their bodies cannot adjust to heavy loads. Researchers postulate that these people's pancreatic cells may not recognize glucose as readily as do normal pancreatic cells. Second, most patients with NIDDM are also *insulin resistant*; that is, their bodies have trouble efficiently using the insulin they produce. Insulin resistance has two causes: 1) there are too few insulin receptors on cells throughout the body, and 2) the enzymes and glucose transport proteins in the cells do not work appropriately to bring glucose into the cells. Finally, people with NIDDM have a problem with the way their liver cells reconvert glycogen to glucose. Normally, when insulin is taken up by the liver cells, the cells respond by not breaking

down any more glycogen. However, in people with NIDDM the cells keep on breaking down glycogen, thereby increasing the amount of glucose in the bloodstream. Thus when people with NIDDM eat a meal, three factors may cause their blood sugar levels to be above normal. First, their insulin secretion may not increase normally in response to the food. Second, their insulin may not work properly in any of their cells, including the liver. Third, their liver may break down more glycogen than they need.

High levels of blood sugar cause two sets of problems—one immediate and one long-range. The immediate symptoms are those by which diabetes is often recognized: increased urination, greater than normal thirst, increased appetite, tiredness, blurred vision, and frequent infections. The increase in urination results from the fact that the kidney, which cannot handle too much glucose, stops reabsorbing glucose in the normal way, and lets it pass into the urine. As part of this process, extra water is carried out with the glucose. This unusual loss of water causes people to become slightly dehydrated and therefore thirstier than normal. People also become unusually hungry because their body does not make efficient use of their food—excreting sugar rather than metabolizing it. As a result, people feel tired because their cells are not getting sufficient energy. Blurred vision is caused by excess fluid that collects in the lens of the eye as a result of the body trying to dilute excess sugar that accumulates there. It is believed that people with NIDDM get frequent skin and other infections because their white blood cell reproduction is impaired. Vaginal yeast infections are more common also, probably due to high glucose levels and the acidity of the vagina. All these symptoms are common to both types of diabetes.

People with Type I diabetes, who make little or no insulin, may also build up ketones in their blood if they do not get the extra insulin they need. Ketones are a product of the breakdown of fatty acids, which are metabolized when carbohydrates are not available. At a sufficiently high level, ketones cause nausea and vomiting, and eventually a coma. This condition, called *diabetic ketoacidosis*, is a MEDICAL EMERGENCY.

In addition to the immediate effects of high blood sugar levels, which can be controlled through diet and exercise, insulin, or other medications, there are a number of long-term complications that are ultimately more dangerous. These complications are much more common with insulin-dependent diabetes, but they can also occur with Type II. Basically, the long-term effects involve the deterioration of large and small blood vessels. The main question in diabetic research today is whether or not strict control of glucose levels can avoid these long-term problems. At present, research seems to indicate that strict glucose control is associated with fewer severe complications of the tiny blood vessels, although some diabetics whose glucose has been poorly controlled for years suffer few complications. A definitive study has yet to be done. Evidence for the benefits of *tight control* comes from several diverse sources. Studies of animals on a high-glucose diet, especially those with diabetes that has been induced, show that these animals eventually develop damage in the small blood vessels of the eye and kidney. When blood sugar levels are controlled, the damage doesn't develop, doesn't progress, or even improves to some extent. In humans, large-scale retrospective studies have shown that blood vessel damage was most likely to occur in people who had uncontrolled glucose levels. Small-scale prospective studies that have followed diabetics for several years have found that people who maintain good control show fewer retinal problems. Such studies indicate that strict glucose control will probably lessen, and may even prevent or improve, damage to the tiny blood vessels of the eye, kidney, and nerves.

On the basis of biochemical evidence, doctors have developed theories as to how and why high glucose levels cause damage to the small blood vessels. In the body, glucose becomes attached to hemoglobin (Hgb), a protein that is found in the red blood cells and carries oxygen to the cells. The combination of the two is called *glycosylated hemoglobin*. Since red blood cells live for approximately 120 days, glycosylated hemoglobin tends to build up over several months. In diabetics, glycosylated hemoglobin levels tend to be high when they are not in good control. This measurement is the basis for an important new test, called the *glycohemoglobin test*, which can indicate the average blood sugar over the previous two months, reflecting the effectiveness of long-range glucose control. This discovery of the binding between glucose and hemoglobin has caused speculation that glucose can bind to many proteins in body tissues. And indeed it has been found that another sugar, *sorbitol*, binds to proteins in blood vessel walls and nerve cells. Once bound, the sugars alter the water-balance in cells, causing them to take in more water to maintain a normal level of dilution, which in turn, causes cells to swell. This swelling may be responsible for the damage to blood vessels that is the basis of long-term diabetic complications.

The most common complication of diabetes is the effects on the small blood vessels, a condition referred to as *microangiopathy*. Very frequently, the changes in small blood vessels are associated with changes in the nerves which are referred to as *neuropathy*. Neuropathy is of unknown cause, although doctors speculate it may be due to poor blood flow or altered metabolism in the nerve cells themselves. Neuropathy can cause tingling, numbness, burning, and pain in the lower limbs, feet, or hands. Numbness and lack of feeling may make people less conscious of foot injuries, and more likely to put unusual pressures on the feet, which often results in sores and ulcers. Foot care is of major importance because uncontrolled diabetics generally do not heal well due to poor circulation. In addition, neuropathy can affect the autonomic nervous system, which controls the body's automatic functions. As a result, diabetics sometimes suffer from indigestion, diarrhea, constipation, an overly full bladder, urinary tract infections, fainting, and/or impotence.

Damage to the small blood vessels of the eyes causes the veins in the back of the eye to develop tiny leaks, a condition called *retinopathy*. There are two types of retinopathy: proliferative and nonproliferative. *Nonproliferative, or background retinopathy*, is by far the most common type, affecting approximately 30% of all people who have had diabetes for five years. In this case, minor blood vessel changes are seen but the eyesight is not usually affected, although the condition can be a precursor to real damage. Capillary leakage can cause swelling of the *macula*, the sharp-focus area of the retina, which can impair vision. *Proliferative retinopathy*, which is fairly uncommon, especially among Type II diabetics, is a condition in which the tiny blood vessels in the eye overgrow. Eventually this can lead to large breaks in the blood vessels or even detachment of the retina. Both of these conditions are serious and require treatment. Another eye condition that is more common in diabetics is *premature cataracts*, which are opacities of the lens. They are similar to cataracts developed by old people, but they occur at a younger age, are related to the length of time people have had diabetes, and are more likely if diabetics do not maintain good control of glucose levels.

Microangiopathy can also cause *nephropathy*, a thickening of the *glomeruli*, the tiny filtering units of the kidney. Nephropathy is a gradually developing condition, first signalled by the appearance of protein in the urine. If it continues to progress, it can cause severe kidney damage and even kidney failure. Nephropathy, neuropathy, and retinopathy all tend to occur together; they are all the result of the progression of small blood vessel disease.

Macroangiopathy, which affects the large blood vessels, is the major long-term threat to diabetics. This condition is actually an accelerated form of *atherosclerotic disease* (see p. 255), in which fatty deposits build up in the walls of the arteries. It is the cause of heart attacks, strokes, and reduced blood flow to the lower legs, which sometimes leads to leg ulcers and even gangrene in diabetics. Atherosclerosis is more frequent than average in diabetics, comes on earlier, and is more severe. Because diabetics are unable to break down fats efficiently, they tend to have high blood levels of all types of fats, especially LDLs, or low density lipoproteins, which are associated with an increased heart attack rate (see p. 260). Diabetics also have low levels of protective HDLs, or high density lipoproteins. It has also been found that their lipoproteins become bound to glucose, and behave abnormally. The atherosclerotic process is probably exacerbated by the fact that microangiopathy causes swelling and blood vessel damage, creating an ideal site for blood platelets to stick and subsequently, for fatty plaques to develop.

Researchers have long acknowledged that *obesity* is a contributing factor in the development of Type II diabetes. Over 80% of people with this disease are overweight. Studies have shown that obese people generally have a higher-than-normal level of insulin in their blood at all times, but they have a low number of insulin receptors on the fat cells in their tissues. Researchers hypothesize that constant overeating, which is responsible for most obesity, causes the production of high levels of insulin in order to get digested food (glucose and fat) out of the bloodstream and into the tissues. The problem is that with fewer insulin receptors, the cells don't take up glucose efficiently, so blood sugar levels begin to rise higher and higher. However, studies have shown that when people go on a reduced-calorie diet, blood levels of insulin decrease, the number of insulin receptors in their cells increases, and blood sugar levels drop. A low-calorie diet can often effectively control Type II diabetes by bringing insulin production back into balance with blood sugar levels. Insulin balance occurs even before people lose weight.

Self-Care

Self-care is crucial in the treatment of both types of diabetes. In the case of Type II diabetes, self-care can often eliminate the need for medication; in the case of Type I diabetes, self-care is essential in maintaining good blood sugar control and avoiding the complications of insulin therapy.

The most essential concept in diabetes self-care is *dietary control*. The first step is weight loss, if it is necessary. A dietitian determines a person's ideal weight based on his or her height and activity level, and then figures the *daily caloric intake* required to maintain this weight. For most Type II patients, simply not exceeding this level will immediately lower glucose levels and eventually bring about weight loss if people are above their ideal weight. Once diabetics reach their ideal weight, they are likely to achieve lower blood glucose levels, lower blood lipid levels, higher insulin levels, and less insulin resistance (more insulin receptors). In addition to determining the recommended daily caloric intake, the dietitian will divide this figure among protein, carbohydrate, and fat, and apportion it throughout the day, avoiding a large concentration of calories at any one meal. Currently, dietitians advise lower protein levels (15% of total calories), higher carbohydrate levels (50%–55%), and lower fat levels (30%–35%) for diabetics. In addition, diabetics are cautioned about drinking, because alcohol is so high in calories that it makes it difficult to maintain a balanced diet.

It used to be thought that all diabetics should totally avoid sucrose, or regular sugar. Many diabetics found this total sugar restriction very dif-ficult to comply with. Doctors now believe that a small amount of sucrose is acceptable (5% of the carbohydrate load) if it is eaten in a mixed-meal context and spaced throughout the day. In recent years, *fructose*, a natural sugar similar to glucose but 30% sweeter, has been recommended as a substitute for sucrose. Studies show that fructose is absorbed more slowly from the gastrointestinal tract and is metabolized differently by the liver, so that there is less of a rise in glucose and insulin levels after a meal. Not all diabetic clinics agree with the value of substituting fructose for sucrose, because eventually insulin is needed to break down any sugar. *Sorbitol*, or *sugar alcohol*, and *xylitol*, which are found naturally in certain fruits and seaweed and used in many "dietetic" foods, have also been recommended for diabetics because they eventually metabolize to fructose. Like fructose, these sugars are absorbed more slowly from the gut than sucrose, and they do contain calories. The latest research seems to indicate that pure sucrose may not elevate blood sugar levels any more than do complex carbohydrates, such as potatoes, provided sucrose is taken as part of a meal. If further research bears this out, there may be less limiting of sugars in diabetic diets. However, diabetics would still have to watch their sugar intake because sugar adds empty calories to the diet, which affects both insulin balance and obesity, the major problems for most diabetics.

The American Diabetic Association has developed *exchange lists*, citing foods that are equivalent in proteins, carbohydrates, or fats, so as to make it easy for people to substitute within a wide variety of foods and still stay within their dietary guidelines. These exchanges can be very helpful in maintaining a balanced diet while adhering to a set number of calories. They are particularly important for people with Type I diabetes, who must carefully balance caloric intake with insulin dosage and exercise levels.

For many years diabetics have been told to

use artificial sweeteners such as *saccharin* and more recently, *aspartame (Nutrasweet)*. This was suggested so that diabetics would have the taste of sweetness without ingesting sugar or adding to their calories. Not only were these products available in bulk, they were also used in many prepared foods that were marketed for diabetics. Serious question has been raised as to whether the artificial sweeteners are healthy. Studies have shown saccharin to be a weak carcinogen that is linked to the development of bladder cancer in animals. In any case, these foods are not necessary for maintenance of a proper diabetic diet, although they have certainly assuaged the sweet tooth of many diabetics (and nondiabetics as well).

Fiber has long been recognized as an important component of the diabetic diet. In fact, in preinsulin days, leafy green vegetables were a mainstay of the diabetic's diet, providing a sense of fullness without adding many calories. Recent research has again accentuated the importance of fiber. Large amounts of fiber (10–15 gms per meal) have been found to decrease the rise in blood glucose levels after meals, thereby decreasing the amount of insulin needed by both Type I and Type II diabetics. It is thought that fiber accomplishes this by slowing down carbohydrate digestion and delaying the emptying of the stomach. Researchers have found that a high-fiber diet has occasionally enabled diabetes to go off oral medication or even insulin. Some doctors question whether it is an increase in fiber that brings about these dramatic results, or whether it may be other factors in the diet, such as a high proportion of carbohydrates as opposed to protein or fat.

In recent years doctors treating diabetics have come to place more and more importance on diet, as opposed to medication. At this point, there are many therapists and clinics that believe that a very large percentage of Type II diabetics theoretically could be maintained on diet therapy alone, without medication. The problem is, too few diabetics are both disciplined and serious about their diet. In part, this may be due to the fact that many doctors treating diabetes do not spend much time educating their patients about diet. Nutritionists and dietitians seem to have more success in convincing diabetics to adhere to a prescribed diet.

It has long been known that *exercise* affects blood sugar levels and the production of insulin. At many diabetic clinics, exercise is a major focus of diabetic therapy, along with diet and insulin, particularly for Type II diabetics. In addition to helping with weight loss, a long-term exercise program has a preventive effect against heart disease, for which diabetics are at increased risk. Exercise drops blood sugar levels, thereby decreasing the need for insulin, and it makes muscle cells more sensitive (i.e., less resistant) to insulin, so that more sugar is brought into the cells by a given amount of insulin. Among Type II diabetics, those who exercise *regularly* utilize their glucose more efficiently even when they are not exercising. One study found that after eight weeks of exercise, Type II diabetics had to produce only half as much insulin after meals as they needed prior to their exercise program. It should be cautioned that a Type II diabetic who is overweight and sedentary should not abruptly begin a rigorous exercise program if they are over 40 and/or have high blood sugar levels. First, they should be evaluated by their doctor for heart and foot problems, and then they should begin a graded exercise program that starts out slowly (see p. 116).

Stress reduction also plays an important role in diabetes therapy. It is known that the hormones produced under stressful conditions, *epinephrine, norepinephrine, glucagon,* and *cortisol,* directly raise blood glucose levels and counteract insulin. Not surprisingly, stress and anxiety often cause diabetics to go out of insulin balance. Thus many doctors advise diabetics to practice relaxation exercises and attempt to lower life stress (see p. 60).

Diabetics need to pay special attention to *good hygiene* (see chart). Decreased foot sensation and blood flow that may result from damage to the nerves and blood vessels make injuries common and harder to heal. For that reason, diabetics are advised to keep their feet clean and inspect them daily. Likewise, it is very important to wear shoes that fit properly and cause no friction, and to check socks for small foreign objects. Minor injuries should be treated promptly; washing and covering injuries with sterile gauze will lessen the chance of infection. The doctor should be contacted if there is any sign of infection, such as redness, swelling, or pain. Diabetics also need to pay special attention to flossing and brushing their teeth; dental problems are three times more common than normal in diabetics. Diabetics are also more susceptible than normal to skin infections, and should keep their skin clean and dry. Women diabetics are particularly susceptible to vaginal yeast infections (see p. 398).

Diabetics are routinely advised to *stop smoking*. Smoking constricts the tiny blood vessels in the feet, increasing the likelihood of foot problems. Even more important, smoking increases diabetics' chances of heart attack and stroke, which are already higher than average.

Self-monitoring is the key to making sure that all these self-care measures are keeping glucose levels in strict control. All diabetics, especially those on medication, should check their urine and their blood glucose levels regularly, and adjust their medication and life-style accordingly.

The Doctor

Diabetes is diagnosed by testing the amount of glucose in the blood. First a *fasting glucose test* is done after a person has not eaten for 8–12 hours. The normal range is 65–110 mg of glucose/deciliter. If the glucose finding is over 140 on more than one occasion, a person is diagnosed as diabetic. When the fasting glucose results are borderline, a *glucose tolerance test* is done. In this test a glucose mixture is drunk after an overnight fast, and then blood and urinary glucose levels are determined at one-, two-, and three-hour intervals. Generally a diagnosis of diabetes is made if the blood level is over 180–200 mg at two hours, and at one or more of the other readings.

Currently, there is tremendous emphasis on patient education and self-care in the treatment of diabetes. Given the chronic nature of the illness, and the fact that insulin production is part of a feedback loop, it becomes crucial that diabetics understand the nature of the disease and participate actively in treating themselves with life-style changes as well as medications. Currently, there is a trend toward a combined health-team approach to diabetic care. Often a patient is seen by a doctor, a nurse, a health educator, a dietitian, and a social worker. The object is to tailor an individual program for each patient, based on the type of diabetes they have and the treatment it requires. Patients and their families have to understand the disease itself, what the dietary requirements are, how urine and blood are tested for glucose levels, how medication should be taken if it is prescribed (either oral medications or injected insulin), how to deal with acute complications (coma) and other illnesses, and how to maintain good foot care (see section on *Self-Care*).

The treatment for diabetes varies depending on the type and the severity. *Type II diabetes* is initially managed with diet and exercise in most cases. Treatment is monitored by testing the amount of sugar in the urine or blood. When blood sugar exceeds a threshold, usually about 180 mg/deciliter, sugar begins to spill over in the urine. If blood sugar levels do not drop in response to an aggressive dietary regimen, an oral medication or insulin injections will be prescribed in addition.

The oral diabetic medications, which were developed in the 1950s, only work for some Type II diabetes. Their exact mode of action is not well understood, and it is unclear why they work for some diabetics and not for others. These compounds initially stimulate insulin production to some extent, but the effect declines after several months. In the long run, these medications lower blood sugar levels by decreasing the cells' resistance to insulin. The greatest advantage of the medications is that they do not require injection. Currently, there are a number of oral medications, including the most common, *chlorpropamide* (e.g., *Diabinase*) and *tolbutamide* (e.g., *Orinase*), as well as *tolazamide* (e.g., *Tolinase*), *acetohexamide* (*Dymelor*), *glipizide* (*Glucotrol*), and *glyburide* (e.g., *Micronase, Diabeta*). Some are taken once a day, some up to three times a day.

In 1960, the University Group Diabetes Program (UGDP) did a study that raised the question of whether oral diabetic medications increased the likelihood of death from heart attacks or strokes. The methodology of the study has been called into question, and 20 years after there was still no consensus among physicians,

and no good study had been done to resolve the controversy. The FDA concluded in 1983 that the UGDP study, while not conclusive, did provide sufficient evidence to support a warning of a possible risk of increased cardiovascular mortality. The FDA added that the primary form of treatment for Type II diabetes should be diet, exercise, and weight reduction, but that where such a program had clearly failed, physicians should advise their patients of the advantages and risks of oral medications, and jointly make a decision about their use. Most doctors believe that the oral medications are safe, but some do not prescribe them. Oral medications are most often prescribed for nonobese people with mild Type II diabetes or temporarily for more severe, obese, Type II diabetics until their diet, exercise, and weight reduction program drops their need for medication. Oral medications are also prescribed for patients with severely elevated fasting blood sugars (greater than 230 mg/deciliter) who do not respond to, or will not comply with, dietary therapy. This last group may also be managed on injectable insulin.

Insulin was discovered in 1922 when a young Canadian doctor and his lab assistant found that an extract made from the pancreas of healthy dogs could save dogs who were dying of diabetes. Before this, Type I and severe Type II diabetes were fatal. Insulin is available in a number of forms, concentrations, and release times. For years, insulin was made by refining a pancreatic extract from either beef or pork. In more recent years, recombinant DNA techniques have enabled drug companies to produce in the laboratory insulin that exactly matches the type produced by the human body. All kinds of insulin are effective, but some people have allergies to a particular type. Insulin is available in either 40- or 100-unit strengths. It must be injected since it is broken down in the digestive tract before reaching the bloodstream.

Insulin is available in three different release speeds: *regular* or *semilente* (rapid release), *lente* or *NPH* (slow release), and *ultralente* or *PZI* (very slow release). The body's own insulin, as well as the regular form of medication, reacts within minutes and clears from the body within five to seven hours. While this works very effectively when insulin is made as needed within the body, the short-acting form of medication means that most people would have to inject themselves several times a day. For that reason, it was very helpful when researchers determined a way to slow the breakdown of injectable insulin. The slow release and very slow release forms are either made into large, slow-dissolving crystals with zinc, or are bound to a protein that slows the absorption of insulin by the cells.

A typical Type II diabetic on insulin therapy takes one insulin shot of lente or NPH insulin daily before breakfast. They also test their urine or blood to verify that they're getting the correct dosage. For more severe Type II diabetics or Type I diabetics, there is a wide variety in treatment plans; most take more than one shot and/or mix the types of insulin. In certain severe cases of Type I, diabetics can have a *continuous subcutaneous insulin infusion pump* (CSII) attached to an abdominal vein. In combination with a home blood testing regimen, the pump provides greater flexibility and control over insulin release.

The most common problem associated with oral or injectable medication is *hypoglycemia* or *low blood sugar*, which results when the medication in effect "works too well" and drops the blood sugar below the level necessary to function alertly. The two most common causes of hypoglycemia are eating too little or too late, or exercising more than usual. The symptoms of hypoglycemia are usually anxiety and nervousness, sweating, shakiness and dizziness. The treatment is to eat something with sugar, such as orange juice or special glucose tablets. If ignored, hypoglycemia can eventually cause drowsiness, fainting, or unconsciousness. Although hypoglycemia can occur with oral medi-

cation use, it is most frequently experienced by people who inject insulin.

Good diabetic control involves managing blood sugar levels carefully. Neither insulin nor oral medications obviate the importance of dietary control and exercise. Good control is important for preventing and treating complications that affect the eye and kidney. Diabetics should see their doctor at regular intervals, usually every three to four months, to determine whether they are staying in balance. Generally, a blood test for glucose, a urine glucose, and a urinary protein test will be done. Another very useful test is the glycosylated hemoglobin test, which measures how well blood sugar levels have been controlled over the past several months. If necessary, adjustments will be made in diet or medication (when prescribed). At routine intervals, the doctor will monitor blood pressure and cholesterol to make sure these values are not elevated, thus increasing the risk of heart disease. In addition, the doctor will examine a diabetic's eyes for retinal changes and feet for a decrease in sensation and pulses. Often an internist or endocrinologist will refer patients to an ophthamologist for annual eye checkups. If retinal changes are seen, the ophthamologist will follow the patient closely. *Retinal hemorrhaging* is treated by *photocoagulation*, a technique in which a laser is used to cause clotting in the leaky capillary.

Ruling Out Other Diseases

The typical diabetic response to a fasting glucose test rules out other diseases.

Prevention

Type I diabetes cannot be prevented, but the hope is that an immune therapy will soon be able to prevent damage to pancreatic cells following infection. Type II diabetes is a different story. Many investigators feel that Type II incidence could be cut in half by preventing obesity and getting people to follow good dietary habits. Effective weight control; a low-sugar, low-fat, and low-calorie diet; regular exercise; and not smoking are especially important for people who have a family history of diabetes or women who have a history of *gestational diabetes* during pregnancy.

Complications of both Type I and Type II diabetes are thought to be largely preventable through careful control of blood sugar levels. Heart disease, which is the major cause of death among diabetics, is also thought to be largely preventable through lowered fat and cholesterol intake. Complications in pregnancy can also be avoided with careful control.

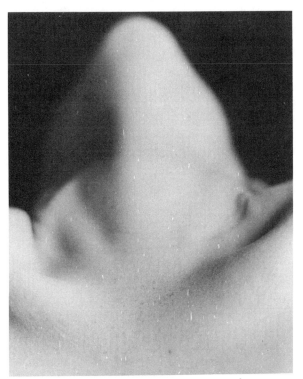

The thyroid is an endocrine gland, located in the neck, which controls the body's metabolic rate. Flight. Photo by Michael Samuels.

Thyroid Disease: Hyperthyroidism and Hypothyroidism

Symptoms

hyperthyroidism (thyroid excess)
- nervousness, anxiousness, and emotional lability
- hand tremor
- fatigue
- weight loss combined with increased appetite
- rapid heartbeat, or palpitations
- poor tolerance of heat
- increase in frequency of bowel movements
- often, swelling of the neck around the Adam's apple and bulging eyes

hypothyroidism (thyroid deficiency)
- tiredness, lethargy, weakness
- intolerance of cold
- decreased sweating
- slow heartbeat
- weight gain combined with lack of appetite
- swelling of hands, face, limbs
- dry, puffy skin
- constipation

Description

The *thyroid* is an endocrine gland located in the neck that manufactures and secretes *thyroxine*, the hormone that controls the body's basic metabolic rate. Thyroxine affects the functioning of 13 or more enzymes that work within the cells to break down carbohydrates and proteins. The effect of thyroxine on overall metabolism is striking: a lack of it can halve the metabolic rate, while an excess can double the rate. In addition, thyroxine directly affects the heart, the nervous system, and the gastrointestinal tract. By caus-

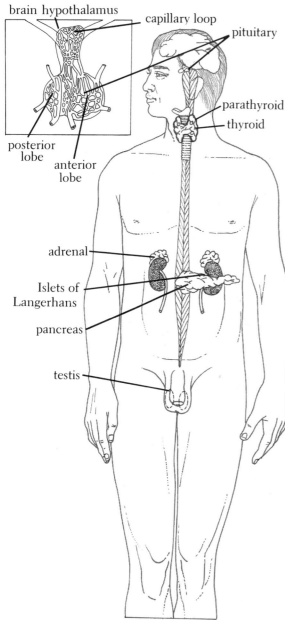

The thyroid, which is located in the neck, is one of the glands in the endocrine system. The thyroid produces the hormone thyroxine which controls the body's metabolic rate. The thyroid is controlled by a feedback system from the brain's hypothalamus and the nearby pituitary gland.

ing the heart to pump harder and blood vessels to widen, thyroxine gets food to the cells more quickly and speeds up the body's breakdown of nutrients. Thyroxine also speeds up nervous system activity and reflexes, and increases gastrointestinal motility. Finally, thyroxine helps to raise body temperature by increasing the amount of energy utilized within each cell.

The thyroid gland is controlled by a feedback system in the brain. When thyroxine in the bloodstream drops below a certain level, a part of the brain called the *hypothalamus* releases a hormone called *thyrotropin-releasing hormone (TRH)*. This hormone, in turn, causes the *anterior pituitary gland* in the brain to produce *thyroid-stimulating hormone (TSH)*. The thyroid produces thyroxine in direct proportion to the amount of TSH released. Using iodine and a protein as raw materials, the thyroid produces thyroxine and stores it, releasing it only when TSH in the bloodstream enters the thyroid. In addition to making thyroxine or *T4*, the thyroid makes tiny amounts of an extra-strength thyroxine, *T3*. Most T4 and T3 is bound to a protein when it is released into the bloodstream, to insure that it circulates throughout the body.

The thyroid is the only endocrine gland that can either release too little or too much hormone, in both cases causing illness. Thyroid disease is fairly common: hyperthyroidism affects 2%–3% of women and .3% of men in the U.S.; hypothyroidism affects 1½% of women and .15% of men. Although both diseases can affect people at any age, the greatest number are diagnosed between the ages of 30 and 50. Both hyperthyroidism (excess hormone) and hypothyroidism (too little hormone) tend to progress if left untreated.

Currently, researchers speculate that in most cases hyperthyroidism and hypothyroidism are the result of an *autoimmune reaction* in which the body becomes allergic to its own thyroid tissue. In people with hyperthyroidism, it has been found that the body is producing an antibody called *thyroid-stimulating immunoglobulin (TSI)*, which works like thyroid-stimulating hormone but is much more powerful. Interestingly, receptor sites in the thyroid pick up the antibody TSI in preference to the hormone TSH. Unlike the hormone, the antibody in not produced in response to low blood levels of thyroxine, but seems to be produced constantly by the white blood cells. In the case of autoimmune hypothyroidism, which is also known as *Hashimoto's thyroiditis*, the white blood cells produce antibodies to the thyroid tissue itself, eventually destroying the gland.

Hyperthyroidism: This condition is a dramatic illness, because increasing the body's metabolism has wide-ranging consequences. The typical hyperthyroid person appears agitated, speaks rapidly, moves quickly, complains of feeling anxious, and may even have a tremor of the hands. As a result of the disease, people may find themselves losing weight effortlessly or being able to eat large amounts without gaining any weight. Women often experience shortened menstrual periods with less bleeding than normal. Heart palpitations may result from the increase in metabolic rate, and hyperactivity may sometimes cause insomnia and/or extreme fatigue. People with hyperthyroidism often complain of intolerance to heat, and experience increased sweating and discomfort in high temperatures. Often their skin will feel hot and moist, and they may wear light clothing even in cold months. Hyperthyroidism is usually accompanied by a high metabolic rate, bulging eyes, and diffuse enlargement of the thyroid gland, which is called a *goiter*. This triad of symptoms is referred to as *Grave's disease*. For unknown reasons, people who develop protruding eyes may complain of unusual tearing, irritation of the eyes, and sensitivity to light. The onset of the disease can take place relatively suddenly in a matter of weeks, or more gradually over a period of months.

Historically, it has been noted that the onset of hyperthyroidism often follows some sort of severe emotional stress or psychic trauma. Although not all doctors agree, some doctors postulate that stress by itself can alter the functioning of the immune system, causing it to produce antibodies to the thyroid. Hyperthyroidism also has a definite familial pattern, with the condition being more common in people whose parents had it. Researchers have found a group of inherited immune changes on chromosome 6 that are more frequent in people with this disease than normal.

Hypothyroidism: Whereas people with hyperthyroidism basically have all their body processes speeded up, people with *hypothyroidism* (too little hormone) are basically slowed down. The symptoms of hypothyroidism are less dramatic than the opposite disease, and the illness generally comes on very gradually—so gradually that people may not associate the changes with an illness. People with hypothyroidism are often tired, lethargic, and weak. They are troubled by cold temperatures, wear layers of clothes, and like to turn the heat up. Their skin tends to be dry and cool. Often their skin also tends to be rough and yellowish from the buildup of *carotene*, a protein found in hair and nails. Puffiness of the hands, face, and feet is typical; this symptom, which is referred to as *myxedema*, is due to sugar building up under the skin. Women with hypothyroidism often have menstrual periods that are longer and heavier than normal. People with hypothyroidism tend to have little appetite but gain weight, and are likely to be troubled by constipation as a result of a decrease in bowel motility.

Self-Care

Both diseases are treated by a doctor. There is no specific self-help regimen for hypothyroidism, but for hyperthyroidism there are measures that are an adjunct to medication and improve the way patients feel. Paradoxically, people with hyperthyroidism should schedule times for rest and relaxation, and avoid strenuous activities until they are stabilized on medication. In many cases, bed rest is initially necessary because so much energy is being used just to maintain body functions. Stress reduction is useful because people with hyperthyroidism tend to be anxious, emotionally labile, and overly reactive to stress, even though they are not making higher than normal levels of stress hormones. Large amounts of thyroxine tend to mimic the stress hormones in their effects. In some cases reducing stess and removing psychic trauma may bring about a dramatic improvement, and possibly even cause the disease to remit. Because people with hyperthyroidism burn so much energy, they feel better if they eat a high-calorie, high-protein diet that is high in vitamins, especially B-complex. If their nutrition is poor, people with hyperthyroidism can go into negative nitrogen and calcium balance, which may intensify their feelings of exhaustion.

The Doctor

Both of these thyroid conditions are diagnosed on the basis of a history, physical exam, and lab tests. The history includes questions related to the specific symptoms; the physical exam includes careful palpation of the thyroid and observation of the thyroid when the person swallows. If there is any question of a thyroid problem, the doctor will order a *T4* or a *free T4 test* to determine the amount of the hormone in the bloodstream. This simple blood test will reveal whether a person is hyper- or hypothyroid. If the test is borderline or doesn't agree with the patient's symptoms, other tests can be done. These include a *T3 test*, a *radioactive iodine uptake*, a *thyroid scan*, a *T3 uptake*, or one of a number of other tests. In hypothyroid cases, the doctor will also order a test for the pituitary hormone *thyrotropin* or *TSH*. Older tests, such as the *protein-bound iodine* or the *basal metabolism* are no longer used because the newer tests are more accurate.

Hyperthyroidism (excess hormone) is treated in two stages. Initially, patients are given drugs to suppress their thyroid's production of thyroxine. Both *propylthiouracil (PTU)* and *methimazole (Tapazole)* prevent iodine from being bound to a protein in the thyroid. It takes several weeks before the full effects of this treatment are noticed. After two to four weeks, another round of thyroxine tests will be done to measure the drop in thyroxine level, and the dosage will be readjusted. In 10%–50% of cases, this period of thyroxine suppression will relieve the symptoms, and no further medication will be necessary. Doctors think that the medicine does not actually cure the disease, but temporarily lowers thyroxine while the body returns to normal production by itself.

In most cases, however, people will need further treatment for their hyperthyroidism. Three options are available: continued medical treatment with an antithyroid drug, treatment with radioactive iodine, or surgery. The decision is based on how severe the symptoms are and how well the person reacts to the first phase of treatment. None of the treatments is ideal; each has its own advantages and drawbacks. The first option is a lower dose of the antithyroid medication for 6–24 months, with follow-up tests at routine intervals. If lab tests show less and less need for medication, people may eventually be taken off the drug, or they may be put on a long-term maintenance dosage. The disadvantage of this treatment is that there is a rare chance of a toxic reaction to the drug, and patients must continue to be monitored. Antithyroid drugs are generally the treatment of choice for people under the age of 18.

The surgical solution, which has been used for many years, involves removal of most of the thyroid gland. Surgery is recommended for people who do not respond to antithyroid medication, or for those who have a greatly enlarged thyroid. After patients have received a complete course of antithyroid medication, they are given *iodine* for one to three weeks prior to surgery in order to reduce the number of blood vessels in the thyroid. In expert hands, this treatment is totally curative 90%–98% of the time. The disadvantages to surgery are the general risks of anesthesia and surgery, the discomfort that follows surgery, and a 50%–60% risk of eventually becoming hypothyroid.

The third option for hyperthyroidism is treatment with one to two doses of *radioactive iodine* (^{131} I). The iodine is taken up by thyroid cells and destroys them. This treatment has several possible disadvantages. First is the concern over the long-term effects of radioactive therapy—possible cancer, leukemia, and/or birth defects. Follow-up studies since the 1940s do not substantiate these concerns, but radioactive treatment often does make patients hypothyroid. Some doctors elect not to use radioactive therapy in people under an arbitrary age, which may be 20, 30, or 40 years, and some do not recommend it for women of childbearing age. But currently it is thought to be the first choice of remedies for people above the chosen age cutoff.

The treatment of hypothyroidism (too little hormone) is much more straightforward and has fewer complications. Patients are simply given the appropriate amount of either natural or synthetic thyroxine. Follow-up thyroid tests are used to establish the correct dosage. Many older people have been on thyroxine replacement therapy for years. Often they were diagnosed before the advent of sophisticated thyroid testing and follow-up. In such cases, many doctors will periodically discontinue medication for three weeks and retest to determine if these people actually still need medication. It should be emphasized that thyroxine is not a "pep pill" to be taken if a person simply has low energy. In fact, taking thyroxine will cause the thyroid gland to produce less of the hormone in order to keep the metabolism in balance.

Ruling Out Other Diseases

Thyroxine testing will determine whether thyroid problems are the cause of nervous anxiety, fatigue, menstrual disorders, and/or metabolic imbalances, all of which can be due to a number of other causes. Both *benign nodules* and *cancer of the thyroid*, which is uncommon, cause a characteristic lump or painless swelling in the thyroid area. These conditions have none of the symptoms of hyperthyroidism and generally do not result in elevated lab values.

Prevention

There is currently a question as to whether stress or psychic trauma may sometimes play a role in triggering hyperthyroidism in susceptible people (see section on *Description*). Certainly there is nothing harmful about minimizing the amount of stress normally encountered since it has been established that a number of other conditions are caused by stress (see p. 277).

G E N I T O U R I N A R Y

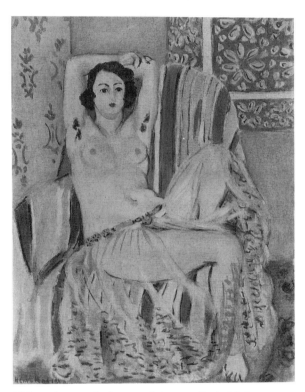

Although sexual pleasure does not diminish in midadulthood, and often is even enhanced, the reproductive and urinary systems are subject to conditions that affect both sexual function and people's perception of their own sexuality. Henri Matisse. Odalisque with Raised Arms. 1923. National Gallery of Art, Washington. Chester Dale Collection.

Urinary Tract Infections

Symptoms

lower urinary tract infection (bladder or urethra)
- frequent urination
- burning pain on urination
- cloudy, dark, or bloody urine
- foul-smelling urine
- pain or ache just above the pubic bone
- upper abdominal pain
- fever and/or chills

upper urinary tract infection (kidney)
- all of the above symptoms
- back pain and tenderness just below the ribs (flank pain)
- sudden onset of fever
- occasionally, vomiting and headache

Description

An infection can affect any part of the urinary tract, including the *urethra*, the *bladder*, or the *kidneys* (see illustration). Symptoms vary somewhat according to which area is involved. Most often, urinary tract infections are caused by bacteria, although they can be caused by yeast or viruses. Normally, the urinary tract and urine are sterile; that is, they are free of bacteria or other microorganisms, except at the entrance to the urethra where there are often microorganisms, most commonly *staphylococcus* bacteria.

The urinary tract has natural homeostatic means of preventing infection. Urine is normally acidic and contains high concentrations of urea; both these factors tend to prevent microorganisms from growing in it. Also, the process of constant excretion flushes the system out on a regular basis. Finally, the membrane that lines the urinary tract (and vagina) has a number of mechanisms for fighting infection, including surface antibodies and an acidic pH.

Urinary tract infections (UTIs) develop when microorganisms manage to overcome all these natural defenses. It is thought that generally the source of the bacteria is fecal matter from the intestinal tract. Feces normally contains high quantities of *E. coli* bacteria, the type that causes 80% of all UTIs. Interestingly, UTIs are much more common in women than in men. The reason is believed to be anatomical: in women, the urethral opening is very close to the anus, and the bladder is less than an inch from the urethral opening (as opposed to several inches in a man). This proximity probably makes it much easier for *E. coli* to enter the urinary tract in women.

The incidence of urinary tract infections rises steadily by age in women so that by their 60s, about 9% of all women experience an infection. The reason for this general rise is unknown, but there are several specific factors that are associated with an increased frequency of UTIs in women. First, women are more likely to develop an infection when they experience a sudden increase in the frequency of intercourse—a phenomenon sometimes referred to as "honeymoon cystitis." Doctors believe that the infection is encouraged by irritation of the urethral opening. Secondly, women are more prone to urinary tract infections during pregnancy. This is thought to be due to several factors, the most important being increased pressure on the bladder from the enlarging uterus.

Urinary tract infections among men are actually rare, occurring in only 0.03% to 0.05% of men. Often, infections are caused by a urethral obstruction that slows the flow of urine. Because of the frequency of obstructions, men with urinary tract infections are generally seen by a urologist, a doctor who specializes in diseases of the urinary tract, to rule out this possibility. Urinary tract infections in men become increasingly common after the age of 40 due to enlargement of the prostate gland, which acts like an obstruction (see p. 403).

Urinary tract infections are associated with a specific set of symptoms. Some of the symptoms are due to the infection itself, others to irritation of the very sensitive lining of the urethra and bladder. Symptoms of irritation include the need to urinate more frequently than usual, and burning or pain in the urethra during urination. If the bladder itself is irritated, there may be pain or discomfort in the area just above the pubic bone. With an infection, there may also be fever and the urine may be cloudy and foul-smelling. All of the symptoms can range from mild to quite severe. Doctors estimate that half the time, women have such mild symptoms they do not even seek treatment, and allow the infection to go away by itself in a matter of days. More pronounced symptoms will cause women to seek treatment and will be readily recognized should they recur. These symptoms are present with *cystitis* (infection of the bladder), kidney infections, and *urethritis* or *acute urethral syndrome* (inflammation of the urethra). The incidence of these three conditions is about equal.

Often, UTI symptoms simply reflect *irritation* of the extremely sensitive lining of the urinary tract, as opposed to *infection* of the tract. About half the time that symptoms occur, there are not many microorganisms present. This condition is called *acute urethral syndrome*. It is most frequently caused by low numbers of chlamydia bacteria (see p. 398), which are sexually transmitted, but it can be caused by mechanical irritation (intercourse, tight clothing) or chemical irritants.

A kidney infection is likely to be accompanied by several symptoms in addition to increased fre-

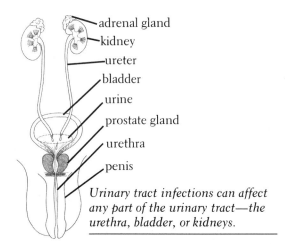

— adrenal gland
— kidney
— ureter
— bladder
— urine
— prostate gland
— urethra
— penis

Urinary tract infections can affect any part of the urinary tract—the urethra, bladder, or kidneys.

quency of urination, burning on urination, and bladder pain. These other symptoms include shaking chills, sudden onset of a fever, and back pain just below the ribs (flank pain). Finally, both kidney and bladder infections are often accompanied by cloudy, dark, or bloody urine. If untreated, serious kidney infections can impair the kidneys' ability to remove metabolic wastes from the blood. Chronic infections sometimes cause permanent scarring of the kidney tubules that produce urine. Prompt effective treatment prevents the possibility of such damage.

Self-Care

A diagnosed UTI should be treated with antibiotics, but self-care measures can help to relieve symptoms of irritation such as bladder pain and burning on urination. The sooner self-care measures are instituted, the more effective they will be. The first self-help measure is to drink large amounts of fluids, up to 8 oz. of liquid per hour. This is actually a major part of treatment, in addition to helping to relieve symptoms. Copious amounts of liquid flush out the urinary tract, removing bacteria and decreasing the rate at which they can multiply. Liquids also help to make the urine less concentrated, which makes it burn less.

Alcohol, tea, coffee, and citrus juices should be avoided because they can irritate the lining of the urinary tract and make burning sensations worse. Many doctors recommend cranberry juice in an effort to acidify the urine and lessen burning, but others question the efficacy of this treatment. To relieve discomfort some doctors now recommend making the urine alkaline with 1 teaspoon of baking soda in a glass of water every three to four hours. This remedy should not be used by people with high blood pressure who are on a salt-restricted diet.

Finally, sitting in a warm bath often helps to relieve urethral irritation. To relieve bladder pain, *acetaminophen* (e.g., *Tylenol*) may be taken. Aspirin and Vitamin C should be avoided because they tend to acidify the urine.

The Doctor

The doctor does a history, physical exam, and lab tests to diagnose a urinary tract infection. The history includes questions about the symptoms, their onset, and recent sexual activity. The doctor will also want to know if the person has had previous UTIs or is pregnant. During the physical exam, the doctor will tap on the person's back to determine if there is kidney pain. The doctor will also order a *urinalysis,* a microscopic examination of the urine to check for bacteria, and a *urine culture* to specifically identify the type of bacteria and determine which antibiotic the bacteria are most sensitive to.

Since there are normally bacteria around the tip of the urethra, a *clean-catch urine sample* must be obtained for testing. The area around the urethral opening should be washed with water, and urine should not be collected as the person first begins to void. A small sample should be taken mid-stream. For women, it is important to spread the labia so that the stream does not pick up any bacteria from the perineum. Even with these measures, a urine sample will normally contain up to 10,000 bacteria per milliliter of urine. When there is a urinary tract infection, the bacteria will number 100,000 per milliliter or more, and there are often red or white blood cells present in the urine as well. If the infection involves the kidneys, the urine sample may contain clumps of white blood cells called *casts*.

Both simple bladder infections and kidney infections are treated with broad-spectrum antibiotics several times a day for 7–10 days. Several *antibiotics* are commonly used, including *sulfisoxazole, ampicillin, amoxicillin,* and *trimethoprim plus sulfamethoxazole*. In addition to the antibiotic, the doctor will recommend self-help measures. Generally a UTI responds rapidly to treatment: bacteria in the urine disappear within a day; symptoms disappear within two to three days. If symptoms persist longer, or return within several weeks, another urinalysis will be done, as well as a repeat urine culture to determine what antibiotic the bacteria will be sensitive to. The new antibiotic will be prescribed for 10 days to a month.

In the case of repeated UTIs, the person will be referred to a urologist for an *intravenous pyelogram (IVP)*, or *urogram*, which is an x-ray that determines if there is any obstruction in the urinary tract. If there is no obstruction and the infection persists, the doctor may prescribe a three to six month course of a *urinary antibacterial agent*, such as *methenamine mendelate*, in conjunction with an acidifying agent like Vitamin C which enhances the effect of the antibacterial agent. The doctor will also advise drinking large amounts of liquids at frequent intervals.

Ruling Out Other Diseases

Simple symptoms of irritation—burning on urination, increased frequency of urination, and lower abdominal pain—can be due to *urethritis*, an inflammation of the urethra. Causes of urethritis are irritation, infection of the urethra with low numbers of organisms, such as *chlamydia*, or a vaginal infection (*yeast* or *candida, trichomonas, gonorrhea,* or *G. vaginalis*, see p. 298). All of these infections are diagnosed by laboratory smears and cultures. A urethritis is suspected when there is irritation but no urinary tract infection. Urethritis accounts for painful urination about 50% of the time, while UTIs account for the other 50%. Urethritis is five times as common as UTIs in sexually active women.

Generalized abdominal pain can be due to various gastrointestinal conditions including *gastroenteritis* (see p. 349) and *gallbladder attack* (see p. 372). *Back pain* can be caused by musculoskeletal strain (see p. 319).

Prevention

Studies have shown that a high fluid intake can help to prevent bladder infections. Often doctors advise women to wipe themselves from front to back after urination and defecation in order to keep fecal bacteria away from the urethral opening. This practice is especially important for women who have a history of urinary tract infections. Doctors also recommend that women urinate after intercourse and perhaps drink a glass of water to help flush out bacteria that may have entered the urethra. For women who have a history of UTIs related to sudden increases in sexual activity, doctors may prescribe one or two antibiotic pills after frequent intercourse as a means of prevention.

Preventing Bladder Infections

- drink large amounts of liquid—eight glasses of water a day will flush bacteria out of the bladder
- urinate as soon as you have the urge; urinate often
- wipe perineal area from front to back to avoid bringing fecal bacteria in contact with the urethra
- avoid feminine sprays and bubble baths that may be irritating to the urethra
- wear loose cotton underpants and pants
- urinate after intercourse
- use lubrication for intercourse in order to avoid urethral irritation

Infectious Diseases of the Reproductive Organs, Including Vaginitis, Urethritis, and Sexually Transmitted Diseases

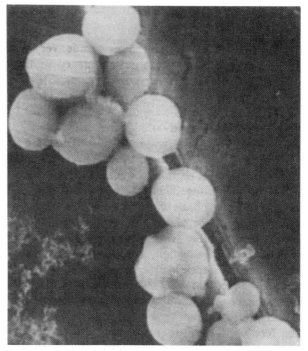

Yeast infections are a common cause of vaginitis in women. Electron micrograph: Candida albicans. Magnification: 5,000 X.

Symptoms

yeast, candidiasis, or *Candida albicans*
- intense vaginal itching
- burning on urination
- occasionally, redness and swelling of the labia
- curd-like, white vaginal discharge with yeasty odor

trichomonas vaginalis
- occasionally, slight penile discharge
- profuse, frothy, greenish vaginal discharge
- discharge often heaviest in women just after the menstrual period
- labia can be swollen or tender
- possible burning on urination in men and women

nonspecific vaginitis, Gardnerella vaginalis, or *G. vaginalis*
- increased grayish white vaginal discharge
- fishy, ammonia-like odor to the discharge
- no associated itching or pain

Chlamydia trachomatis
- burning on urination
- increased frequency of urination
- occasionally, discharge from the penis or vagina
- possibly, no symptoms
- occasionally, signs of tubal infection, salpingitis, or pelvic inflammatory disease (P.I.D.) in women
  - lower abdominal pain and tenderness
  - fever
  - often occur around the time of a menstrual period

gonorrhea
- often, no symptoms
- discharge from the penis or vagina
- burning on urination in both men and women
- occasionally, signs of pelvic inflammatory disease (see above)

toxic shock syndrome
- sudden onset of fever over 102°F.
- vomiting and diarrhea
- sunburn-like rash
- dizziness due to a drop in blood pressure
- usually develops within 5 days of onset of menstrual period, and is associated with tampon use

Description

There are a number of infectious diseases that commonly affect the genital organs in both men and women. These conditions are caused by a diverse group of organisms, ranging from the virus-like bacteria, *Chlamydia trachomatis*, to microscopic plants such as yeast. Some of these organisms are normal inhabitants of the reproductive tract that overgrow; others are invaders that are most often transmitted through sexual contact.

This wide group of diseases is often addressed together because they cause many of the same basic symptoms. In men, these conditions frequently cause a *urethritis*, an inflammation of the tube leading from the penis to the bladder. The symptoms of urethritis are burning on urination, increased frequency of urination, and often a discharge of some sort from the penis. The most common conditions that men develop are gonococcal urethritis, caused by the bacteria *Neisseria gonorrhoeae*, and nongonococcal urethritis, 40% of which is caused by *Chlamydia trachomatis*. Most cases of urethritis in men are derived from sexual contact, although there are cases of urethritis in men that are either irritative or nonsexually transmitted. The exact cause of a urethritis can only be established by laboratory tests.

Infectious diseases of the reproductive system cause a wider and generally more pronounced group of symptoms in women. The symptoms include burning on urination, a vaginal discharge, and pain or itching around the vulva and entrance to the vagina. There is also a larger number of organisms that commonly cause these symptoms in women. Although each organism has a somewhat specific pattern of symptoms (see p. 398), the final diagnosis can only be made through laboratory tests. In women, the most common syndrome is *vaginitis*, an inflammation of the vagina and/or labia (as opposed to the urethritis that men develop). The three most common causes of vaginitis are a yeast infection

(candida), a nonspecific vaginitis (most likely due to *Gardnerella vaginalis*), and a trichomonas infection. Occasionally several organisms may be present at the same time. Gardnerella and trichomonas are usually transmitted by sexual contact, but yeast is a normal inhabitant of the vagina that may overgrow, especially before the menstrual period. Yeast infections occur more often in women who are pregnant, have diabetes, eat a high sugar diet, or who are taking birth control pills, supplemental estrogen, antibiotics, or steroids.

Gonorrhea is another frequent cause of burning on urination and vaginal discharge. There are currently 1–2 million cases of gonorrhea in the U.S. each year. It is estimated that 50%–85% of women and 10% of men do not exhibit symptoms when they develop gonorrhea. Not only does this allow the infection to spread more widely, it is potentially serious because gonorrhea is a major cause of infertility in women. Gonorrhea is virtually always spread by sexual contact: a woman has about a 75% chance of catching gonorrhea from an infected man, whereas a man has only about a 25% chance of catching it from an infected woman. This difference is due to the fact that women receive a large dose of the bacteria in a man's semen.

The most significant complication of bacterial infections is *salpingitis*, an infection of the Fallopian tubes in women that can result in infertility or ectopic pregnancies, in which the egg implants outside the uterus. This condition is also referred to as *pelvic inflammatory disease*, or *PID*. Almost 15% of women who have gonorrhea develop PID. The symptoms are abdominal pain and tenderness, vaginal discharge, and fever; but these signs may be so mild as to go unnoticed. Gonorrhea accounts for about half of all cases of PID, while other organisms, especially chlamydia, account for the rest. PID can also be caused by a strain of streptococcal bacteria. PID was three to five times more common among women who used an intrauterine device

(IUD) for birth control, because the IUD acted as a foreign body that inflamed the uterus and made it more susceptible to infection. Today, IUDs are not used in the U.S. Tubal infection can cause scarring of the Fallopian tubes which prevents eggs from passing into the uterus, thereby making a woman infertile. Approximately 15% of women become infertile after one PID infection, and as many as 75% become infertile after three or more infections.

If urethritis is not due to gonorrhea, the most likely cause is *Chlamydia trachomatis.* In recent years, chlamydia has become the most common sexually transmitted disease in the U.S. Chlamydia is also the cause of *urethral syndrome,* a condition in which women have all the symptoms of a urinary tract infection—burning on urination, frequency, and bladder discomfort—but do not show enough bacteria to meet the diagnostic criteria for a urinary tract infection. A chlamydial urethritis tends to be a milder disease than gonorrhea, particularly in men.

The risk of getting sexually transmitted diseases depends greatly on the number of sexual contacts a person has. The more different partners an individual has, the more likely he or she is to contract urethritis or vaginitis, and the more likely it is to be caused by a sexually transmitted organism such as gonorrhea or chlamydia. The more monogamous two partners are, the less likely they are to contract urethritis or vaginitis, and the more likely such an infection is to be caused by yeast or one of the less common bacteria. Statistically, the highest rates of sexually transmitted diseases are found in unmarried, sexually active people between the ages of 15 and 35, and in homosexual males.

Toxic shock syndrome (TSS) is a systemic illness caused by a toxin produced by the bacteria *Staphylococcus aureus.* Over 90% of the cases occur in menstruating women who are using tampons. The staph bacteria are thought to multiply in tampons, especially in high-absorbency synthetic tampons, as opposed to cotton or rayon tampons. Researchers think that the toxin produced by the staph enters the bloodstream through small ulcers or abrasions in the vaginal wall. Toxic shock syndrome is a rare (6 cases per 100,000 menstruating women per year), but potentially serious disease that most often occurs in women under 30. Presumably these women have not been exposed to the bacteria previously and therefore have not developed antibodies to it. Any menstruating woman who experiences TSS symptoms should remove a tampon if she is wearing one and seek medical attention promptly. TSS was first reported in 1978. At that time it had a fatality rate of 15%. Although it is serious, improved treatment has greatly reduced the possibility of mortality. TSS has a high rate of recurrence (about 33%), so women who have had it are advised to discontinue all tampon use.

Self-Care

Any person with symptoms of urethritis should see a doctor because the symptoms may be caused by an infection of the urinary tract (see p. 394) or by a sexually transmitted disease, both of which are responsive to treatment. As an adjunct to medication, people with UTIs or urethral syndrome should drink large quantities of liquids and avoid irritating foods (see p. 397).

Any woman with more than one sexual partner and symptoms of vaginitis should see a doctor to rule out the possibility of gonorrhea or chlamydia, conditions which should be treated. There are many self-help regimens that can be used for vaginal infections caused by yeast, trichomonas, or *G. vaginalis.* Often mild infections caused by these organisms will go away by themselves, but if the symptoms are bothersome, women will be helped by douching daily with *white vinegar* and water (4 T. vinegar to 1 qt. of water). For G. vaginalis, some doctors recommend douching with 2 T. of the antiseptic *betadine* to 1 qt. of water, or with a mixture of plain *yogurt* and water which reintroduces lactobacillus, a beneficial bacteria, into the vagina. In addition to douching, women with infections should wear all-cotton underpants and avoid panty hose or tight-fitting clothes. Women with a vaginal infection should also dry the genital area thoroughly after bathing and avoid scratching or rubbing it. They should minimize intercourse temporarily because it tends to be irritating; if they do have intercourse, they should use lubrication and have their partner use a condom to avoid passing the infection to him. Also, men are often asymptomatic carriers of trichomonas, and occasionally are carriers of yeast, in which case they may repeatedly infect their partners.

The Doctor

The doctor does a history and physical to diagnose a urethritis, vaginitis, or sexually transmitted disease. Based on the person's specific symptoms and recent sexual activity, the doctor will suspect one condition or another, and do laboratory tests. If a woman complains of symptoms of vaginitis, a pelvic exam will be done and a sample of the discharge will be taken. A *saline suspension* is done to test for trichomonas or G. *vaginalis*, a *potassium hydroxide smear* to test for yeast, and a *gram-stain smear* to test for gonorrhea. *Cultures* may also be done for gonorrhea and chlamydia. In a man with urethritis, the doctor will do a gram-stain for gonorrhea. For a urethritis without vaginitis in a woman, a doctor will do a urinalysis and cultures for gonorrhea and chlamydia if applicable.

For a woman with a mild yeast infection, the doctor may simply recommend cleaning the genital area with soap and water or douching as recommended under *Self-Care*. Generally, however, the doctor will prescribe vaginal suppositories or creams containing either *nystatin* or newer drugs called *clotrimazole (Mycelex)* or *mi-*

conazole nitrate (Monistat) for one to three days. Occasionally women complain that miconazole burns, but it seems to be more effective than nystatin. In recurrent cases, the doctor will repeat the creams or eventually prescribe oral nystatin. Occasionally, the doctor will treat the woman's partner if he is suspected of being a carrier.

Trichomonas is generally treated with *metronidazole* (e.g., *Flagyl, Prostat*), an oral medication. Metronidazole is effective but can have significant side effects, including gastrointestinal cramps, lack of appetite, nausea, vomiting, and diarrhea. Nausea is more likely if the drug is taken with alcohol. Finally, the drug has been shown to cause mutations in bacteria and cancer in mice. Although there is no evidence thus far that it has caused cancer in humans, metronidazole is not recommended during the first 16 weeks of pregnancy. Many doctors routinely use metronidazole because they see few problems with it, but some doctors avoid prescribing it. Most doctors now recommend that a woman's partner be treated at the same time to prevent reinfection. They also suggest that asymptomatic male partners use condoms until treatment is finished.

G. *vaginalis*, or nonspecific vaginitis, is generally treated with either *ampicillin* tablets or with *metronidazole* (e.g., *Flagyl, Prostat*), the drug discussed above. Not all doctors advise metronidazole in this case, since an effective alternative exists and the condition is even less troublesome than trichomonas. In cases of G. vaginalis, both sexual partners are generally treated.

Gonorrhea is treated with one of several recommended antibiotics, each equally effective. *Tetracycline* can be taken orally for a week; *amoxicillin* or *ampicillin* can be taken in a single dose accompanied by one dose of oral *probenecid*; or two injections of *penicillin* G can be given, along with one dose of *probenecide*. Tetracycline has the advantage of also being effective against chlamydia, which is now known to coexist with gonorrhea 45% of the time. Chlamydia by itself is treated with oral *tetracycline*. Due to the fact that these diseases are transmitted sexually, it is important that a person's sexual partners be treated at the same time to prevent reinfection and stop the spread.

A follow-up culture should be done a week after treatment for gonorrhea and/or chlamydia is completed. During this time people should refrain from intercourse. If the person has been treated for gonorrhea with penicillin and has had no sexual contact, but the repeat culture is positive, it is assumed that the particular strain of gonorrhea is penicillin-resistant. The person is then treated with a single injection of *spectenomycin* or oral *tetracycline*. However, if a person has been reinfected through sexual contact, he or she will simply repeat the initial treatment. If a woman is diagnosed as having PID, she will be given higher doses of one of the three drugs.

Ruling Out Other Diseases

Laboratory tests are used to differentiate one cause of urethritis or vaginitis from another. Postmenopausal women sometimes develop an *irritative vaginitis* from dryness caused by a drop in their estrogen levels (see p. 426). Burning on urination can also be due to a *urinary tract infection* (see p. 394). Pelvic inflammatory disease has to be differentiated from other causes of lower abdominal pain, including *appendicitis* and *ectopic pregnancy*.

Prevention

The likelihood of developing a yeast infection, which causes a nonsexually transmitted vaginitis, can be reduced by keeping the genital area dry and avoiding irritation. Tight-fitting pants and materials that do not breathe, such as synthetics and leather, should be avoided. This is particularly important for susceptible women. Yeast infections seem to be more common in women who are overweight, take birth control pills, have just taken a course of antibiotics, are pregnant, or have diabetes. Women who eat a lot of sweets and are troubled by yeast infections may find it helpful to lower the amount of sugar in their diet.

Sexually transmitted diseases can largely be prevented by changes in life-style or use of condoms. Monogamous relationships, checking new partners' sexual histories, and/or lowering the number of sexual contacts will all help to reduce the likelihood of contracting any of the various sexually transmitted diseases. Used properly and carefully, condoms are an effective means of reducing the spread of sexual diseases, although they do not eliminate the risk entirely, since they can slip off or tear, and infectious organisms could be present on, or spread to, genital areas not covered by the condom. The advantages of condoms are that they are a convenient safety factor that lacks side effects and can enhance sexual pleasure by delaying male orgasm. Their disadvantages are that they reduce sensation and interrupt lovemaking so people do not always use them reliably.

Prostate Disease: Prostatitis, Enlarged Prostate, and Prostate Cancer

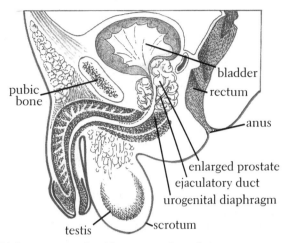

If the prostate gland becomes enlarged, it can put pressure on a man's urethra and cause problems with urination.

Symptoms

prostatitis (inflammation of the prostate)
- pain in the perineum (area between the anus and the penis), lower back, or penis
- burning on urination
- increased frequency of urination
- discharge from the penis
- fever

enlarged prostate
- narrow, weak urinary stream
- difficulty starting and stopping urination, dribbling
- increased urination at night, causing men to wake from sleep
- inability to urinate

cancer of the prostate
- often, no symptoms
- symptoms of enlarged prostate (see above)
- pain in the lower back

Description

The *prostate* is a small, walnut-sized gland in men that lies below the bladder (see illustration). The *urethra*, the narrow tube that leads from the bladder to the tip of the penis, passes through the prostate. The prostate produces a milky fluid which is mixed with seminal fluid during ejaculation, and gives semen its characteristic cloudy appearance. Sperm from the *testes* mixes with seminal fluid from the *seminal vessicles* and subsequently joins with prostatic fluid to make *semen*. The function of prostatic fluid is unknown, but it has an alkaline pH which is thought to neutralize the acid pH of the vagina, thereby making the sperm more motile.

The prostate is very tiny up until puberty when it begins to enlarge in response to increased amounts of male hormones. During puberty the prostate grows from 4 g. to 20 g. After puberty, the gland stops enlarging until about the age of 45. At this point, one of two things happens: either the prostate gradually decreases somewhat in size, or it begins to grow again at a substantial rate.

The pattern of middle-age prostate enlargement is referred to as *benign prostatic hyperplasia (BPH)*. It is the most common form of nonmalignant growth in adult men. A study in Sweden found the incidence of BPH to be about 60% at 45–60 years of age, about 75% at 60–70 years of age, and 95% above age 70. The incidence of BPH is high in Europe, low-to-average in the United States, and low in Asia. It is not known why some cultures have much higher rates of BPH than others. What is known is that prostate enlargement is definitely related to two factors: male hormones and age. BPH has not been found in men under 40, nor in men who underwent castration prior to puberty. Animal studies have shown that the administration of male hormones can produce BPH in dogs, which are the only animal other than man who spontaneously develops the condition.

Prostatic enlargement is not a problem in itself; the difficulty lies in the fact that the enlarging prostate often compresses the urethra which passes through it. At first, the *detrusor muscles* which initiate urination are able to contract more forcefully and overcome resistance caused by the narrowing of the urethral tube, but if the diameter of the urethra eventually becomes sufficiently reduced, a man will start to have difficulty urinating. As the urethra becomes increasingly compressed, men develop a group of symptoms referred to as *prostatism*. These symptoms include narrowing of the urinary stream and weakening of its force, hesitancy or difficulty beginning to urinate, difficulty stopping the flow of urine and a tendency to drip or dribble, a need to urinate more frequently at night, and a feeling that the bladder is not being completely emptied following urination. In fact, the amount of urine present in the bladder after urination, *the residual urine*, is greater. As BPH progresses, the amount of urine generally left in the bladder continues to increase. As a result, men have to urinate more and more often during the day and at night. Men with these symptoms are more likely to experience bladder infections, and ultimately the urethra may even become blocked, so that a man is unable to urinate. Benign enlargement of the prostate has a highly variable course. The great majority of men experience mild symptoms with no change for many years, but 10% experience worsening symptoms and need surgery to relieve very bothersome symptoms and/or to avoid complete blockage.

The second most common disease of the prostate is *prostatitis*, an inflammation of the prostate. Although it can occur at any age, it is most common in men between the ages of 20 and 50. Usually the cause is unknown, although a certain percentage is caused by bacteria. The sign of a bacterial infection is an ascending inflammation of the urethra which is called *urethritis* (see p. 399). Most bacterial infections are caused by *E. coli*, although they can be caused by the sexually transmitted bacteria, N. *gonococcus* and *chlamydia* (see p. 398).

There are two types of prostatitis, acute and chronic. *Acute prostatitis* has a sudden onset of genital pain, most commonly in the perineal area between the anus and penis, but occasionally in the scrotum, penis, or lower back. Along with pain, there are fever, chills, burning on urination, increased frequency, and a urethral discharge. Acute prostatitis is caused by bacteria. *Chronic prostatitis*, which is a milder condition, is much more common. It is associated with slight burning on urination, increased frequency, a scanty discharge, and pain in various parts of the genital area. The most common form of chronic prostatitis is nonbacterial in origin. The condition is baffling to doctors; for patients, it is an annoying problem that does not respond readily to treatment.

Up to the age of 60, *cancer of the prostate* is a rare cause of prostate problems; above the age of 60, it becomes increasingly common, until by age 80, 5% of men will have developed it. It is included here because it can cause some of the same symptoms as benign prostate hyperplasia. Since a malignancy causes a growth in the prostate, it can also cause blockage of the urethra and lead to hesitancy, straining to start urinating, reduction in the force and width of the stream, dribbling at the end of urination, a feeling of incomplete emptying of the bladder, and increased frequency.

The cause of cancer of the prostate is unknown. Studies have not correlated its incidence with environmental factors such as smoking, fat intake, alcohol use, or chemicals. Like BPH, the growth of a prostate cancer is influenced by the presence of male hormones, but BPH does not predispose a man to prostate cancer. In fact, the tissue that is affected is entirely different: BPH involves the gland cells that produce prostatic fluid; a malignancy affects cells in the lining that surrounds the gland. Unlike BPH, prostate cancer does not cause a soft, diffuse enlargement of the gland; rather, it creates a small, hard lump. If a malignant lump is removed before it metastasizes, the cure rate for this type of cancer is very high.

Self-Care

Benign prostatic hyperplasia is basically treated with self-care unless the symptoms become severe enough to make surgery necessary (see section on *The Doctor*). Most often, however, surgery is not a clear-cut decision. Although BPH is known to progress, its pattern of growth is unpredictable. Generally it takes 15–20 years for symptoms to become significant. At that point, the symptoms may stabilize or even regress for months or years at a time. One study found that at any one time, half the patients with BPH were improving or remained unchanged. Men also react very differently to the inconvenience of their symptoms. For example, some men react strongly to having to urinate several times a night; others are unconcerned.

Several life-style habits can help to relieve BPH symptoms and help to prevent *urinary retention*; that is, the inability to urinate. Men with BPH should avoid drinking large amounts of fluid within a relatively short time. To prevent their bladder from becoming distended, they should urinate whenever they feel the urge. Distension can cause the thickened muscle of the bladder wall to lose its tone, making it even more difficult to urinate. It is important to note that alcohol has a diuretic effect; that is, it increases urine production. The combination of alcohol and drinking large amounts of liquid can exacerbate symptoms even in men who generally have only minor symptoms. Both antihistamines and the combination of alcohol and fluids are

common causes of acute urinary blockage in men who do not even have BPH.

Some doctors believe that the prostate gland can become "congested," making BPH symptoms worse. Adherents of this theory believe that the best means of alleviating this congestion is regular intercourse or masturbation.

There are several self-help measures that help to minimize the discomfort of a prostate infection. It's important to continue taking in fluids to keep up urination, but not to drink fluids in large quantities. Measures that will ease prostate discomfort include sitting in warm bath (sitz bath) and avoiding acidic foods. Sodium bicarbonate (1 tsp. baking soda to a glass of water) helps to make the urine less acid, thereby reducing bladder irritability. This measure is not recommended for long-term use or for people with hypertension because sodium bicarbonate is high in salt. If necessary, *acetaminophen* (e.g., *Tylenol*) may be taken for pain.

The Doctor

The doctor diagnoses benign prostatic hyperplasia from a history and physical exam. On *rectal exam*, the doctor will feel a diffusely enlarged gland that may be either firm or soft. The degree of enlargement that is felt does not necessarily correlate with the severity of the symptoms. The doctor may also have the patient urinate to establish the degree to which there is straining, narrowing of the stream, etc. A *urinalysis* will be done to rule out infection, and a *blood test* will be done to check kidney function. If the symptoms are severe, the doctor may order a *urogram*, an x-ray of the bladder and the urethra. The doctor may also pass a *cystoscope* up the urethra in order to visualize the neck of the bladder and see how the enlargement of the prostate has affected the urethra. Although most patients find the exam uncomfortable, it does reveal important information.

There is no drug therapy for benign prostatic

hyperplasia, and surgery is advised only under certain circumstances. Impairment of kidney function is a definite indication for surgery. Urinary blockage (retention) or recurrent urinary tract infections are also frequently cited as reasons for surgery. Finally, surgery may be the joint decision of the patient and the doctor when the patient finds the symptoms of BPH unacceptable. The choice to operate is often individual and subjective.

Currently, there are three different surgical procedures used to correct BPH. Over 90% of the time, prostate tissue is scraped out through the urethra, a procedure called *transurethral resection of the prostate (TURP)*. It is done in the hospital, generally with spinal or epidural anesthesia, sometimes with general anesthesia or a local. A special instrument with a light and an electrical loop is inserted into the urethra. The loop is used to scrape out the prostate in small pieces, which are flushed out of the bladder at the end of the operation. A special urinary catheter is left in the urethra so that the bladder can be irrigated for one to two days after the surgery. It is not unusual for men to have bleeding for a few more days, and increased frequency and urgency of urination for a period of time after the operation. Because men are more susceptible to urinary tract infections shortly after the surgery, they are routinely put on antibiotics. The operation does not cause impotence, but often causes men to have "dry orgasms" because the ejaculate goes up into the bladder, which is not a problem. About 5% of the time patients develop a postsurgical narrowing of the urethra which must be opened with a cystoscope. As many as 10% of patients ultimately require a repeat operation because not all the prostatic tissue was removed initially. The other two types of prostate removal are done with an incision through the lower abdomen just above the pubic bone. They are not often used for BPH, except for cases in which the prostate is very enlarged.

Bacterial prostatitis is diagnosed by laboratory exams, a *urinalysis*, a *blood count*, and a microscopic exam and culture of the prostate secretions. When a bacterial infection is suspected due to a fever, chills, and a discharge, antibiotic therapy is started at once. The most common choice is *trimethoprim-sulfamethoxazole*, which is taken two times a day for 30 days. Nonbacterial infections are often treated with the *antibiotics tetracycline* or *erythromycin*, which seem to be effective. For nonbacterial prostatitis, some doctors advise prostate massage.

Cancer of the prostate, which is rare in men under 60 years of age, can often be diagnosed by physical exam, but must be confirmed by biopsy. On a rectal exam, the doctor will find a hard lump in the prostate that feels unlike the rest of the tissue. Treatment depends upon whether or not the cancer has spread. If it has not, the prostate is surgically removed through an incision between the scrotum and the anus. The prognosis is excellent if the cancer has not spread, and good even if it has metastasized. If spread has occurred, surgery may or may not be done, and radiation, chemotherapy, and estrogen therapy may be used.

Ruling Out Other Diseases

In some cases, symptoms from enlargement of the prostate must be differentiated from prostate infection. Burning and urgency tend to indicate a *urinary tract infection (UTI)* (see p. 344). To differentiate a prostate infection from a UTI, several lab tests must be done, including a urinalysis and a microscopic examination and culture of the prostatic fluid. In general, BPH is easily diagnosed, but occasionally a cytoscopic exam is necessary to rule out other uncommon causes of prostate symptoms.

Prevention

At present, there is no known prevention for BPH or cancer of the prostate, although with early detection, prostate cancer is often curable. Since prostatitis is sometimes caused by an ascending infection of the urethra, minimizing the spread of sexually transmitted diseases may help to lower the incidence of prostate infection (see p. 402).

AIDS, or Acquired Immunodeficiency Syndrome

Symptoms

- unusual weight loss and loss of appetite
- persistent diarrhea
- persistent fever and/or night sweats
- swollen lymph nodes
- profound fatigue
- sudden appearance of painless, colored (pink to purple) patches, lumps, or nodules on the skin or mucous membranes (Kaposi's sarcoma)
- skin or mucous membrane ulcers (herpes simplex)
- nonproductive cough and shortness of breath (*Pneumocystis carinii* pneumonia)
- whitish coating on tongue and throat, mouth pain, and difficulty swallowing (oral candida)

Description

Acquired immunodeficiency syndrome (AIDS) is a condition caused by a virus, in which the body's immune system becomes damaged and thus is less able to fight infection. AIDS was first recognized in 1981 when the Centers for Disease Control (CDC) in Atlanta began recording cases of a number of young homosexual or bisexual men who developed *Pneumocystis carinii pneumonia* or *Kaposi's sarcoma*, a malignant skin tumor—diseases which had previously been rare in young people. Based on a small number of cases, the CDC recognized a new disease, and defined AIDS as the presence of a "reliably diagnosed disease," such as Kaposi's sarcoma or *P. carinii* pneumonia, that indicates an immune defect not due to a recognized cause. Because AIDS is a new disease, and there is a great deal of ongoing research into its epidemiology and treatment, information about AIDS is being constantly changed and updated at a rate so fast that it is difficult to deal with it within the confines of any book.

In the U.S., the disease has predominantly stricken homosexual men and intravenous drug users of both sexes. It has also been found in a small number of hemophiliacs and recipients of blood transfusions, as well as in Haitians living in the U.S. Also at high risk are the sexual partners of anyone in the above groups, and babies born to mothers with AIDS.

The spread of the disease has been dramatic and alarming. By 1988, over 46,000 cases had been identified in the U.S. alone, and the disease had also been identified in Europe, Africa, and Canada. AIDS has a very high incidence in central Africa, mostly in Zambia, Zaire, and Rwanda, where it affects women as often and in as great numbers as it does men, and is primarily spread heterosexually. Based on the existing epidemiological studies, scientists speculate that the virus originated in remote areas of Africa, possibly even as a disease of nonhuman primates. The disease is currently thought to have spread from Africa via several routes.

Although the disease has spread rapidly around the world, it has not been found to be transmitted by casual contact. Thousands of health-care providers and family members have been in close contact with AIDS patients without contracting the disease. Virtually every case of AIDS has been linked to intimate sexual contact or direct exposure to contaminated blood or blood products. No case of AIDS has been proven to be spread by hugging, touching, contact with clothing, sneezing, coughing, or eating food prepared by someone who has AIDS. Even though there is a very small amount of the virus present in the saliva and tears of people with AIDS, no cases have been spread by these means. Likewise, no cases have been proven to be spread by insects. However, a number of practices are associated with a high risk of transmission of the virus: use of contaminated blood or blood products; use of contaminated needles, syringes, bulbs, or cookers; unprotected intercourse, either anal or vaginal, with an infected partner, and ingestion of an infected partner's seminal fluid.

In 1984 it was established by researchers in France and the U.S. that AIDS is transmitted by the *human immunodeficiency virus (HIV)*, which at one time was called "LAV" by its French discoverers and "HTLV-III" by its American discoverers. HIV is a special type of virus called a *retrovirus* because, unlike regular viruses, it has a special way of reproducing. Usually a virus simply reproduces itself, killing the cell it has entered in the process. Retroviruses don't kill the cells they enter—instead they merge with them. Retroviruses carry their genetic information on a single strand of RNA rather than on a double strand of DNA. The retrovirus contains an enzyme that converts its viral RNA into double-stranded viral DNA. This enzyme is called *reverse transcriptase* because this highly unusual method of making DNA is the opposite of normal protein synthesis. The new viral DNA moves from the *cytoplasm* into the *nucleus* of the cell, where it merges with the DNA of the host cell. From then on, whenever that cell or any of its offspring reproduce, they produce an altered cell that has viral genes built into the chromosomes in its nucleus.

Only three retroviruses have been identified. One is HIV. Another is a feline leukemia virus that produces immunosuppression in cats. The third is HTLV-I which produces leukemia or

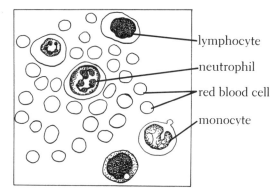

Lymphocytes are an important part of the body's immune system: they produce antibodies and regulate the immune process.

lymphomas in humans; it is most commonly found in Japan. All of the retroviruses specifically attack a type of immune cell called the *helper T-lymphocyte.* Lymphocytes are special cells in the blood and lymph systems that help to fight off infection. There are two types of lymphocytes: *B-lymphocytes*, which make antibodies when stimulated, and *T-lymphocytes*, which regulate the whole immune process. Among the T-lymphocytes are helper T-lymphocytes which help the B-lymphocytes produce antibodies, and suppressor T-cells which slow down the immune response. The helper T-lymphocytes play a key role in the immune response: they help B-cells recognize foreign invaders, and they produce a substance that makes the B-cells multiply. The HIV virus specifically attacks the helper T-cells. Lack of sufficient T-cells means people's defenses are lowered and they are much more susceptible to infections that the immune system of a healthy young person normally fights off easily.

Unless all of the aberrant cells are somehow destroyed, a person will remain infected. People who have been exposed to the virus usually develop detectable levels of antibodies against the virus within 6–12 weeks. The antibodies demonstrate that the body is attempting to fight the virus, but generally the immune system is unable to fend off the virus because it has become weakened.

Researchers now have some idea of the course or natural history of what happens after a person becomes infected with the HIV virus. Not everyone who is exposed to the virus becomes infected with it. The likelihood of infection appears to be related to the number of times a person is exposed, and the number of virus organisms transmitted in each exposure. Thus there is a high risk of developing AIDS from blood transfusions from infected donors, a significant but smaller chance of developing AIDS from sharing needles and drug paraphernalia with an infected addict, and a very small chance for a medical worker to develop AIDS from a single accidental needle stick. Likewise, with sexual contact, the chances of becoming infected rise with increased numbers of encounters with an infected person or people.

In some people who are exposed, the virus grows throughout their system and they become infected. These people produce antibodies to the virus; greater than 99% of these people will have a positive HIV-antibody test. Currently, two tests are used to identify infection with the HIV virus. The *enzyme immunoassay (EIA)* is the first test to be done. Because there are occasional false-positive results with the EIA, if the test is positive, it is repeated and followed by another test, usually the *Western blot*, which is more sensitive.

The course of an AIDS infection is still unknown, in that it is not certain what percentage of people who are HIV-positive will develop AIDS or in what period of time. People who are persistently infected but don't develop symptoms carry the virus and are capable of passing it on to others. It is these carriers, rather than people with diagnosed AIDS, who constitute the major reservoir of the infection and are basically responsible for the spread of the disease. Carriers carry the virus in their blood, specifically in the white blood cells that are attempting to fight the virus. These white blood cells spread the disease to the white blood cells of another person when they come in direct contact with the blood or mucous membranes of that person.

For months to years, the virus can multiply in the cells of an infected person, but not necessarily produce symptoms of disease. Eventually, a large number of people who have been infected develop some symptoms of infection. Researchers currently estimate that roughly 25%–50% of infected people go on to develop AIDS. The time between being infected with the virus and actually developing some symptoms is referred to as the *incubation period*. In terms of AIDS, the range of the incubation period has been particularly difficult to establish because AIDS is such a new condition and because the exact time of exposure is often hard to determine precisely. By studying earlier frozen blood samples of current AIDS patients, researchers have been able to calculate the time that lapsed between the first appearance of HIV antibodies in the blood and the first appearance of AIDS-related symptoms. Studies have shown that the incubation period varies from three to ten years, with a mean of seven years. It is also known that the number of people, both homosexual and heterosexual, who have been infected by the virus worldwide is truly enormous. Because of the long incubation period, a substantial number of people were infected before the disease was even discovered. As of 1988, scientists estimate that between 1,000,000 to 1,500,000 Americans have been infected with the virus. In 1985, studies showed that 10%–70% of homosexuals and 50%–65% of IV drug users in high-risk areas such as New York City and San Francisco were antibody-positive, and that 10%–60% of steady heterosexual partners of drug users and bisexuals were antibody-positive. As of 1988, 0.04% of people who were screened for blood donations were found to be antibody-positive, which is a better overall reflection of the percentage of people who have been infected.

When AIDS was initially discovered in homosexual men in 1981, scientists also identified a corollary syndrome that they called *AIDS-related complex*, or *ARC*. When the HIV virus was discovered in 1983, it became clear that ARC was an early form of AIDS, and was caused by the same virus. This condition is not recognized by the CDC for reporting purposes, but its present definition by the National Institutes of Health (NIH) is the presence of two unexplained symptoms of AIDS and two abnormal laboratory values. Another AIDS-related disease is called *lymphadenopathy syndrome (LAS)*, which is defined as lymph nodes larger than 1 cm in diameter in three sites for three months, in the absence of any other underlying medical cause. Approximately 33% of patients with LAS have no symptoms other than swollen lymph nodes. Another group of men with LAS have one or more fungal or bacterial skin infections, including herpes or yeast. Currently, doctors are unable to predict which people with LAS will eventually develop AIDS, although it is estimated to be 10%–30%.

As of 1988, the CDC has redefined AIDS as an illness characterized by one or more "indicator" diseases such as Kaposi's sarcoma or *Pneumocystis carinii* pneumonia. There are now two long lists of indicator diseases, the list being much more extensive if the person also tests positive for HIV antibodies. Because there are no symptoms of a damaged immune system, by itself, the symptoms of AIDS are the symptoms of whatever disease or opportunistic infection the person gets as a result of a lowered immune response. For example, if people with AIDS have pneumonia, their symptoms are the symptoms of pneumonia. Because AIDS patients are susceptible to a broad spectrum of illnesses, they can have a wide variety of symptoms, ranging from skin rashes to coughs to diarrhea to mental disorientation.

The first AIDS patients commonly had *Kaposi's sarcoma* (KS). Its symptoms are the sudden appearance of pink to purple patches, nodules, or painless bruiselike areas on the skin or on the mucous membranes of the mouth, nose, or anus. Kaposi's sarcoma is an unusual cancer not generally seen in people under 60 or in residents of North America. As of 1985, only 6% of AIDS patients had had KS. As of 1987, 65% of all AIDS patients developed *Pneumocystis carinii* pneumonia. Its symptoms are a fever and chills; a dry, hacking, nonproductive, persistent cough; shortness of breath; and chest pain. The cough lasts longer than a flu and is not associated with smoking. In addition, AIDS patients often get a variety of other illnesses. They develop chronic, progressive ulcers of the skin and mouth from *herpes simplex*; a white coating and pain in the mouth, and difficulty swallowing from oral *candida* infections; chronic diarrhea due to one of many organisms; and meningitis, encephalitis, and neurological damage from a number of organisms. Most of these infections are rare in people with healthy immune systems. In people with a compromised immune system, these diseases are very difficult to treat, and most often one of them eventually proves fatal for people who have AIDS.

AIDS has now become the leading cause of death for men aged 25–44 who have never married, many of whom are homosexual. The scope of the social and medical problem that AIDS represents is still not well understood. Because of the magnitude of the problem, research is going on at a rapid rate, with the promise of new knowledge of the disease and the hope that a vaccine can soon be developed that will be effective. New material can be expected to update the information given here, as well as changes in the definition and classification of the disease.

People who have AIDS, and even people who are infected with HIV (test positive) but do not show symptoms, should take precautions that they do not spread the virus to others. Most counselors advise that people with AIDS inform their sexual partners, past and future, and that they use safe sex practices. Moreover, they should not share any items that could be contaminated by blood or semen, and they should notify any medical personnel who care for them, including their dentists. Women of childbearing age who test positive should get counseling from a gynecologist. These women have a significant chance of transferring the infection to their baby, either *in utero*, during childbirth, or during nursing. Moreover, pregnancy will make these women more vulnerable to opportunistic infections because pregnancy normally lowers the effectiveness of the immune system.

Self-Care

In general, the medical aspects of AIDS are so serious as to require treatment by a doctor. However, self-care has a role to play at several levels. People with AIDS or ARC need tremendous emotional support; the psychosocial problems created by these illnesses are enormous. They include both the physical, economic, and emotional problems of a young person faced with a life-threatening illness, and the special problems of a person with a disease that excites public fear and social stigma. The extent of these problems make support and self-help education crucial. Such care is best given by the multispecialty clinics and AIDS support groups that have evolved to meet the crisis. In many cities, the gay community has become well organized and effective in its support of people with AIDS.

A number of hospitals in cities with a high incidence of AIDS have developed model programs for taking care of AIDS patients. Generally, they utilize medical care from a number of specialities, as well as the services of psychiatrists, social workers, and representatives from community organizations. Social workers and community representatives help AIDS patients deal with medical crises and arrange for home care between hospitalizations. The Shanti Project of San Francisco not only maintains ongoing support groups for patients and their family and friends, but counsels patients about caring for themselves, and even provides low-cost housing. The San Francisco AIDS Foundation has a telephone hotline and referral lists of people who can provide financial and social assistance. A group called AIDS Alliance has educational and recreational programs, and organized retreats. Although cities with large numbers of AIDS patients tend to have the most services, specialized multidisciplinary care is now being found in many smaller cities and hospitals as well. Further information can be obtained through the AIDS Hotline (800-342-AIDS or 202-245-6867) or the National Gay Task Force (800-221-7044).

Medical workers who work with AIDS believe

Prevention for People with AIDS

- avoid exposure to infection through others' coughing, sneezing, bodily wastes, open cuts, or sores
- avoid using other people's toothbrush, razor, or unclean food utensils
- be certain your doctors and medical workers know you are immunodeficient before you accept any immunization
- clean and cover wounds promptly; avoid cuts if you have a low blood platelet count
- avoid travel to areas where sanitation is poor
- avoid toxoplasmosis and other animal-borne diseases; wear rubber gloves when handling pet wastes
- take antibiotics only when prescribed, in order to avoid developing fungal infections such as yeast
- avoid mood-altering drugs because they can weaken the immune system
- eat a well-balanced diet, avoid stress and fatigue, and use relaxation and imagery to help build up the immune system (see p. 68)

Source: Adapted from L. Mass, "Medical Answers About AIDS."

that there is much that people with AIDS can do to minimize or prevent opportunistic infections and strengthen their weakened immune system. Careful hygiene will help avoid exposure to germs (see chart), while a balanced diet (see p. 102) and stress reduction (see p. 58) can help to build up the immune system. There is a growing body of evidence in psychoneuroimmunology that relaxation and imagery techniques, as well as attitude (see p. 51), can have significant effects on immune functioning, including the production of helper T-cells. While studies have not dealt specifically with AIDS patients, they do deal with the immune system and may well be applicable to AIDS patients. At the least, these kinds of self-care measures have been found to improve quality of life in people with other types of life-threatening illnesses.

The Doctor

AIDS is confirmed by the presence of a reliably diagnosed disease indicative of an immune system defect, that has no underlying medical cause. Repeated enzyme immunoassay HIV antibody tests that are positive and a positive Western blot test confirm that a person has been infected, but do not mean a person has developed AIDS unless he or she also has an indicator disease. A blood test measuring the ratio of helper T-lymphocytes to suppressor T-lymphocytes is used to demonstrate an immune deficiency.

As of 1988, there is still no definitive treatment that can cure AIDS. Currently, a two-part approach to treatment is being used. First, the indicator disease is treated with specific therapies. AIDS patients are treated for Kaposi's sarcoma or whatever opportunistic infection they have. Kaposi's sarcoma is treated, often successfully, with radiation and/or chemotherapy. Infections are treated with appropriate antibiotics. For example, *P. carinii* pneumonia is treated with *sulfamethoxazole-trimethoprim* or *pentam-*

Precautions for AIDS Care Givers

- wear gloves when handling syringes or body fluids
- wear a gown if any body fluid will come in contact with your clothes; wear a mask if body fluid might become airborne
- use only disposable needles and dispose of them properly in designated containers
- clean up spills of body fluids with a solution of 10% household bleach and water
- wash hands thoroughly after close contact with body fluids of people who have AIDS

Note: Household members who are not *sexual* partners of AIDS patients are at minimal or no risk. No cases of AIDS have been known to spread merely through casual contact.

Source: Adapted from L. Mass, "Medical Answers About AIDS."

---

idine isothionate. Candida (yeast) infections are treated with *nystatin* or *clotrimazole* (see p. 401). Herpes simplex infections are treated with *acyclovir.*

Secondly, new drugs are being used that have the promise of either enhancing the immune system or killing the virus. As of 1988, a drug called *azidothymidine* (e.g., AZT, *zidiovudine, Retrovir*) has shown significant promise in keeping AIDS patients alive, and in preventing people with AIDS from developing opportunistic infections. It is the first drug to be recognized for decreasing mortality and preventing infections. The drug stops the progression of the disease by breaking the viral DNA before it slips into the nucleus of healthy cells. After administration of the drug, the level of helper T-lymphocytes often rises significantly. Other drugs in the research stage are also designed to attack the manner in which the virus replicates. AZT is being tried on people with ARC as well as AIDS to see if early administration can prevent AIDS infections from occurring. The initial results have been encouraging.

Ruling Out Other Diseases

Severe opportunistic infections and/or Kaposi's sarcoma rarely occur in young people without AIDS. On the other hand, LAS is more difficult to diagnose since there are many causes of swollen lymph nodes and viral-type symptoms in young people. Lymph nodes normally become enlarged when the body is fighting off any infection, whether it is caused by a virus or a bacteria. Thus people at low risk for AIDS should not become frightened if they do experience swollen lymph nodes. Uncommonly, swollen lymph nodes can also be caused by cancer, either *lymphoma* or *Hodgkin's disease*. If there are other symptoms of malignancy in addition to the swollen lymph node, a biopsy will be done. However, this is not common. There are many causes of the more general symptoms such as cough, weight loss, diarrhea, fatigue, and night sweats. However, people who have these symptoms and are also at high risk should definitely see a doctor.

Prevention

Because no vaccine has yet been developed for AIDS, education about transmission and informed life-style changes provide the best protection against getting AIDS. There are four known routes for transmission of AIDS or HIV infection: sexual contact, intravenous drug use, contact with contaminated blood products, and congenital transmission from an infected mother to a newborn.

Sexual transmission, the major means of infection, depends on the number of sexual encounters a person has and the likelihood that one or more partners are infected with the virus. Multiple sexual partners and/or sexual contact with someone at high risk greatly increases a person's chances of becoming infected. In the gay community, the chance of infection from an occasional sexual encounter is very high. The risk

is lowest for two people involved in a strictly monogamous relationship that have not had any other contacts for a number of years.

Statistically, in the general heterosexual population, the risk of sexual contact is still far below 1%. But in any group where the prevalence of infection is high, it is imperative that safe sex practices be used to prevent contact with blood, semen, or vaginal secretions. This means abstaining from intercourse, avoiding intercourse without the use of condoms, or knowing the sexual history of one's partners (and *their* partners). It has been said that from the point of view of AIDS, when people have sex with someone, they have sex with all the partners that per-

---

AIDS Prevention

- be knowledgeable about the sexual history, preferences, and risk status of sexual partners
- safe sex includes anything that does not involve exchange of any body fluid, including rubbing, massaging, kissing skin, and mutual masturbation
- do not engage in unprotected vaginal or anal intercourse with a partner who is at risk or whose sexual and drug history is unknown; males should put on a condom before they have contact with any body fluids; condoms should be used with a gel, foam, or cream that contains the spermicide 5% nonoxyol-9
- theoretically, oral-genital contact of any kind, and even deep mouth-to-mouth kissing, carries some risk
- avoid mood-altering drugs, including alcohol, during sex because they can impair judgment
- do not share any object that comes in contact with blood, such as IV drug paraphernalia, and even toothbrushes and razors; such objects can be sterilized by boiling in water for 15–30 minutes, or by soaking them in 40% alcohol (10 minutes) or 1 c. of household bleach to 10 c. of water and then rinsing them
- take sensible precautions around people with AIDS to avoid exposure to body fluids (see additional chart)

son has had for the last five to ten years. Whenever people have intercourse with someone at risk or with someone whose history they do not know, they should use condoms (see p. 402). Diaphragms and spermicides do not provide adequate protection in this regard. To be effective, condoms must be put on *before* a man enters his partner because control of ejaculation is not precise, and there can be semen leakage before ejaculation.

AIDS prevention among intravenous drug users is even more difficult. The virus is readily transmitted by needles, so it's essential that people do not share or even reuse drug paraphernalia. This is not currently a problem in hospitals or medical facilities because in the U.S. sterile disposable needles are routinely used.

Use of contaminated blood or blood products has been responsible for the transmission of a low number of AIDS cases—543 cases among 15 million people up through 1987. Since the development of the antibody test, combined with a screened volunteer donor system, the risk of infection by transfusions of blood and blood products has been reduced to between 1 in 100,000 and 1 in a million. Factor VIII concentrates for hemophiliacs are now heat-treated to eradicate the virus. Despite the low risk, people sometimes choose to donate blood for themselves or family members prior to elective surgery.

Abnormal Uterine Bleeding: Hormonal Changes, Fibroids, Cervical Cancer, and Uterine Cancer

Symptoms

- unusually heavy or light vaginal bleeding
- usually long or short periods
- irregular spacing between periods
- spotting between periods
- pain or discomfort during periods
- in some cases, no symptoms

Description

During much of their reproductive years, most women experience great regularity in their menstrual cycles. Typically, women tend to be so regular once menstruation becomes established that they are quick to notice variations from their normal pattern. Yet at some point almost every woman experiences some sort of bleeding change that she considers abnormal or atypical. The great majority of these variations are caused by conditions that are not serious, and they result from a wide variety of situations. But occasionally abnormal uterine bleeding is caused by a condition that may require treatment, such as uterine fibroids or a tumor. Since these conditions increase in frequency in women over 35 years of age, it's always important for women in this age range to check out abnormalities in their menstrual cycles.

A menstrual period is the result of a complex interplay of anatomical and endocrine factors, which are discussed at length elsewhere in this book (see p. 424). In brief, on a monthly basis the timing program in the brain's hypothalamus signals the pituitary gland to release two hormones: *follicle-stimulating hormone (FSH),* which causes an egg to mature in one of the ovaries, and *luteinizing hormone (LH)*, which causes a mature egg to be released into the Fallopian tube. The *corpus luteum*, the case that surrounds the egg, produces two other hormones: *estrogen*, which causes a thickening of the lining of the uterus, and *progesterone*, which causes the growth of tiny glands in the uterine wall. If conception and implantation do not take place, the corpus luteum shrinks and stops producing estrogen and progesterone. As a result, the uterine lining stops growing and the surface sloughs off and is expelled as a *menstrual period*, a discharge consisting of blood, uterine cells, and hormones.

The normal menstrual cycle varies from 24–34 days, while the normal duration of a menstrual period is 1–8 days, the average being 3–5 days. The amount of menstrual blood expelled with a period varies from mere spotting to 80 ml, or approximately one-half cup. Interestingly, studies have shown that only half the women who complain of heavy bleeding are actually losing more than 80 ml. Although there is a wide range in quantity of flow, each woman generally has periods of similar amount and length. This is not surprising since both factors are determined by hormonal levels, and those levels tend to be the same from one month to the next.

Many factors can cause changes in women's normal menstrual patterns. By far the most common reasons for abnormal periods in women of reproductive age are *pregnancy* and *miscarriage*. In addition to normal conceptions, it is estimated that many fertilized eggs fail to develop properly and are sloughed off in a period that is delayed and is generally heavier than normal.

Another common cause of abnormal uterine bleeding is the use of *estrogen*. This category includes premenopausal women taking birth control pills and postmenopausal women on estrogen replacement therapy (see p. 429). If one or more birth control pills are missed, women often experience *breakthrough bleeding* or spot-ting between periods. With low-dose birth control pills, women sometimes miss a period altogether. By definition, the periods experienced by postmenopausal women on estrogen are "abnormal." Generally, women on supplemental estrogen experience regular bleeding, either during the interval between pills or even during the pill cycle.

Women also experience menstrual irregularities due to *variations in hormonal levels* that result from stress, illness, diet, exercise, and unknown causes. These are considered to be normal variations, as opposed to those caused by specific medical conditions. There is no question that emotional stress, such as conflicts at home, problems at work, or worries over children, can affect the hypothalamus and cause changes in menstrual cycles.

In recent years doctors have come to realize that the tremendous increase in strenuous exercise among many women is a frequent cause of menstrual irregularities and even *amenorrhea*, which is the lack of a period for three or more cycles. Such problems are common among women who run long distances, dance seriously, or are involved in competitive sports. Researchers believe that regular menstrual periods are dependent upon maintaining a certain critical percentage of body fat: weight loss of 10%–15% or more below what is normal for one's height, or a drop in body fat to less than 22%, seems to cause amenorrhea. Occasionally women who exercise very strenuously disrupt their hormonal patterns even if they maintain the necessary percentage of body fat. Researchers think this is due to the high levels of natural opiates, called *endorphins*, that are produced by heavy exercise. Likewise, women who drop more than 10%–15% below ideal body weight—for instance, those with *anorexia nervosa*—often experience amenorrhea even though they do not exercise strenuously.

Another cause of menstrual change is lack of ovulation or ovulating at the wrong time, which causes *dysfunctional uterine bleeding*. Failing to ovulate is much more common than is ovulating at an unusual time. Such anovulatory cycles cause periods that are irregular as to timing and flow. This type of menstrual period occurs most frequently at *menarche*, when girls are just starting to menstruate, and in the years prior to *menopause* (see p. 424). An anovulatory cycle results when the corpus luteum produces estrogen in the first half of the cycle, but not progesterone; the result is an unopposed thickening of the uterine lining. In the presence of variable estrogen levels and low amounts of progesterone, the lining can vary widely in thickness and menstruation can occur at unpredictable times. Typically, the menstrual period is delayed and heavy.

Abnormal uterine bleeding can also result from a number of conditions of the uterus, cervix, or ovaries, including but not limited to malignancies. These conditions are much less common than the causes listed above, but their incidence goes up with age. For women in mid-adulthood, it's important to rule out gynecological conditions as the cause of abnormal bleeding, especially when a postmenopausal woman who is not on estrogen therapy experiences bleeding. In that case, none of the hormonal causes of abnormal bleeding apply. A number of gynecological conditions can cause abnormal bleeding at different ages, including *cervical* or *uterine polyps*, which are endometrial growths that grow on a stalk; *cervicitis* or *vaginitis*, that is, an inflammation of the cervix or vagina (see p. 398); *atrophic vaginitis*, a functional lack of lubrication that develops in pre- or postmenopausal women (see p. 426); *uterine fibroids*, which are benign uterine growths; *endometriosis*, which involves abnormal growth of uterine tissue outside the uterus; *tubal infections*; *ectopic pregnancy*, that is, a fertilized egg that implants outside the uterus; as well as *cancer of the uterus* and *cancer of the cervix*.

Among the most common of these conditions

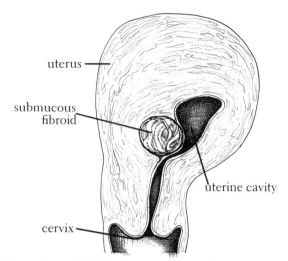

Approximately 20% of women over 35 develop uterine fibroids—growths consisting of smooth muscle and connective tissue. Fibroids can be asymptomatic, or they can cause heavy or irregular bleeding.

is *uterine fibroid tumors*, or *myoma of the uterus*. Fibroid tumors are by far the most common growths of the female reproductive system. More than 20% of all women over 35 have fibroids, growths that consist of smooth muscle and connective tissue. Fibroids generally grow in groups, and they range in size from microscopic to very large. They can be completely asymptomatic, or they can cause heavy or irregular uterine bleeding. Most often, such bleeding takes the form of heavy or prolonged menstrual periods, but it can also cause bleeding between menstrual periods. Depending on their size and location, fibroids sometimes cause urinary frequency and abdominal discomfort. Often fibroids shrink with menopause, sometimes dramatically.

Far less common, but much more serious, are malignancies of the reproductive tract, which are potentially life-threatening. The most common of these is *endometrial carcinoma*, or *cancer of the uterus*. With early diagnosis and treatment, this cancer has an excellent cure rate. In the U.S. in 1985, there were 37,000 cases of uterine cancer diagnosed, but only 2,900 deaths. The incidence of uterine cancer is low before the age of 45, rises sharply between ages 45 and 55, and peaks in the 60s. Like many other cancers, endometrial carcinoma is more common in affluent Western cultures; the incidence is low in Japan and in underdeveloped countries. Some researchers speculate that this difference is due to dietary habits.

Between 1970 and 1975, there was a dramatic rise in the number of uterine cancers in the U.S., especially among women aged 45–65. This rise is thought to be associated with the relatively new use of estrogen replacement therapy for menopausal women. In controlled studies it has been shown that women on estrogen replacement are at much greater risk for endometrial cancer than are women who do not take estrogen. The risk increases with the dosage of estrogen and the length of time the hormone is taken. More recent studies have indicated that with the addition of a progestin, estrogen replacement therapy apparently does not cause higher rates of uterine cancer (for a more detailed discussion, see p. 430).

In addition to estrogen, there are several other factors that put women at higher than average risk of developing cancer of the uterus. These include late menopause, hypertension, diabetes and, most importantly, obesity. Women who are 20 lbs. overweight are three times as likely to develop this cancer; women who are 50 lbs. overweight are nine times as likely. Researchers think this is also an effect of estrogen. In postmenopausal women, estrogen is no longer made in the ovaries; it is synthesized largely in fat cells from adrenal hormones. Thus women who are overweight have much higher postmenopausal estrogen levels than women who are thin.

The major symptom of uterine cancer is abnormal uterine bleeding. Thus uterine cancer has to be ruled out in any postmenopausal women who have uterine bleeding or in premenopausal women over 35 who have heavy, prolonged bleeding. It should be noted, however, that less than 10% of postmenopausal bleeding is due to cancer of the uterus. Most is caused by three other conditions: *uterine polyps: hyperplasia*, which is stimulation of the uterine lining by some form of estrogen, either external or internal; or *fibroids*. Of diagnosed cases of uterine cancer, 75% are postmenopausal, 15% occur around the time of menopause, and only 10% are premenopausal. Uterine cancer tends to have a high cure rate because it usually exhibits symptoms—that is, abnormal bleeding—at a relatively early stage in its development. Moreover, in the majority of women, the cancer will not have metastasized outside the uterus when it is diagnosed. The cure rate for uterine cancer that has not spread is over 90%.

Cancer of the cervix is a much less common, but more invasive cancer. For this reason, it is very important to diagnose it in the early stages. The *cervix*, the bottom of the uterus, protrudes into the vagina (see illustration); the opening in the cervix is referred to as the *cervical os*. The tip of the cervix, where the vaginal lining meets the uterus, is made up of *squamous epithelial cells*, a rapidly-dividing type of cell that con-

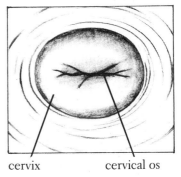

cervix   cervical os

The bottom of the uterus, which projects into the vagina, is called the cervix; *the opening is called the* cervical os.

stantly renews itself. The inside of the cervix is lined with *columnar epithelial cells*, a slower-growing type of cell which secretes mucus. Between the two types of cells is a border called the *transformation zone*. For reasons not well understood, the cells in this area are particularly susceptible to the slow development of abnormalities that are precursors to cancer.

Studies have found that several sexual factors are linked with abnormal cells in the transformation zone of the cervix. For decades it has been known that cervical cancer is rare among nuns and other sexually inactive women. More recently, studies have found that the incidence of cervical cancer is higher than average among women who first had intercourse at an early age, and among women who have had a large number of sexual partners. A study has also found that the rate of cervical cancer is higher among women whose husbands were previously married to a woman who developed cancer of the cervix. All of these factors point to some sort of sexual transmission of the disease, although the exact means of transmission has not yet been established.

Recently, two viruses have specifically been linked to cervical cancer: *herpes simplex virus (HSV)* and *human papillomavirus (HPV)*. Studies show that women who have had genital herpes have an increased incidence of cervical cell changes. Also, one study found that 90% of women who have cervical cancer have antigens to HSV, as compared with only 10% of women in a control group who had not had cervical cancer. Papillomavirus, or HPV, is a group of viruses that cause warts, including genital warts. Two of the viruses in the group, HPV-16 and HPV-18, have been found in cancerous cervical cells. Internal genital warts are often seen near cervical cancers, but no study has been done on the association between genital warts and cervical cancer. Nevertheless, researchers do not doubt that cervical cancer is linked to some subclass of the papillomavirus. External genital

warts, ones that occur on the vulva in women, are caused by HPV-6; they have not been shown to be related to cervical cancer. Interestingly, other studies have shown that smokers have four times the incidence of cervical cancer as nonsmokers. Researchers think that nicotine acts as a cocarcinogen or promoter, helping the virus cause changes in cervical cells.

Currently, there is significant debate among researchers as to whether the use of oral contraceptives may actually increase the chances of cervical cancer. Several studies suggest a relationship between cervical dysplasia and cancer, and the use of birth control pills for over three years.

It is believed that all these environmental factors cause slow changes in the cells at the junction between the inside and outside of the cervix, a condition which is referred to as *cervical dysplasia*. Between 1.2% and 3.8% of women show these early cervical changes; the incidence is highest between the ages of 25–35. As dysplasia involves more and more of the epithelial tissue, the cells take on a more and more cancerous appearance. When all of the cell layers have undergone change, the condition is referred to as *carcinoma of the cervix in situ (CIS)*. Recently the whole process has been given the name *cervical intraepithelial neoplasia (CIN)*. CIN changes are divided into 3 grades: CIN 1, mild dysplasia; CIN 2, moderate dysplasia, and CIN 3, severe dysplasia. Doctors estimate that between one-third and two-thirds of all cervical dysplasias (CIN 1) progress to cancer. About one-third go away by themselves, for unknown reasons. However, the percentage that become cancerous is so great that they should all be treated by a doctor.

In 1943, Dr. Papanicolaou developed a technique for scraping and grading cells from the cervical transformation zone. This test, which has become an important screening procedure, is called the *Pap smear* or *cervical smear*. Because it is easy to do, relatively inexpensive, and highly effective in diagnosing cervical cancer in the early stages, the Pap smear has become widely accepted by both patients and doctors. Since the inception of the Pap smear, there has been a 50% drop in the mortality rate of cancer of the cervix. Women who are screened regularly have only one-sixth the invasive cancer rate of women who are not screened.

For years, the American Cancer Society recommended annual Pap smears for women once they became sexually active. As of 1988, the society recommended that women initially have a Pap smear annually for three successive years, and thereafter as recommended by their doctor. Frequent screening is recommended for women who are at higher than average risk. Although the high-risk category has not been defined clearly, many experts would include the following criteria: first having intercourse within one to two years following onset of menstruation, use of birth control pills, a history of herpes infections or internal venereal warts, and/or smoking. For these women, yearly Pap smears are recommended until the age of 60. The American Cancer Society stopped recommending an annual Pap smear for all women because cervical dysplasia precedes cancer of the cervix *in situ* by an average of seven years. However, many gynecologists still do the test every year because they believe that it provides the maximum safety.

The average age at which women develop cancer of the cervix is 51. In the early stages, there are no observable symptoms, although both dysplasia or cancer can be identified on a Pap smear. In later stages, the major symptoms of this form of cancer are abnormal bleeding (usually between menstrual periods in a premenopausal woman), and a cervical discharge. Frequently, the bleeding is noticed after intercourse or straining; however, such bleeding is most often due to other, noncancerous cervical conditions. If detected early, before any spread has occurred, cervical cancer has a 99% cure rate.

The overall cure rate is lower because not all women have regular Pap smears. If cancer of the cervix is not diagnosed in the early stages by a Pap smear, it is much more likely to spread to the lymph system.

Self-Care

There are important self-help techniques that apply to certain causes of abnormal uterine bleeding; however, severe, persistent, or recurrent changes in premenopausal bleeding, as well as any postmenopausal bleeding, should be brought to the attention of a doctor to rule out any condition that requires treatment. It is reassuring to know that most of them are not a cause for worry.

When menstrual changes are caused by diet, exercise, or stress patterns, much can be done by women themselves. In terms of nutrition, it's important that women eat a well-balanced, low-fat diet that allows them to maintain their weight at, or near to, the ideal amount for their size. Smoking, alcohol, and caffeine should be avoided entirely, or their use limited. Exercise should be kept within reasonable bounds, especially if women experience amenorrhea. Stress

---

Self-Care for Menstrual Cramps

- do moderate exercise of any kind
- stay warm—take a hot bath or apply a heating pad or hot water bottle to back or abdomen
- gently but firmly massage the abdomen and/or lower back
- assume an all-fours position with head down to help alleviate severe cramps
- traditional remedies are drinking herbal teas or alcohol in moderation
- some women find foods high in calcium or vitamin B_6 may be helpful
- many nonprescription pain relievers may help, including aspirin, acetaminophen, and ibuprofen (which specifically lessens uterine pressure)

should be minimized by relaxation techniques (see p. 60), life-style changes, meditation, and/or counseling.

Several self-help techniques have been shown to improve the quality of life after cancer has been diagnosed (see p. 302).

The Doctor

A woman should consult her gynecologist about certain types of abnormal bleeding, including all postmenopausal bleeding, menstrual periods that last more than 10 days, periods that are unusually heavy or light, recurrent heavy periods, periods that occur less than 21 days or more than 35 days apart, or uterine bleeding that occurs at any time between menstrual periods. *Ovulation bleeding*, that is, a single episode of spotting that occurs between menstrual periods about the time of ovulation, is quite common and is not considered a problem. One very heavy period, occurring at the normal time, is also not generally considered to be a problem. However, if a woman ever feels anxious or concerned about menstrual changes, she should talk with her doctor.

The treatment of abnormal uterine bleeding depends completely on a woman's age and the cause of the problem. A diagnosis is made on the basis of a history and a physical that includes a pelvic exam and lab tests. The doctor will want to know if a woman is taking any type of estrogen, and will inquire about stress, diet, and exercise, as well as past menstrual history. In particular, the doctor will ask detailed questions about the timing and quantity of abnormal bleeding, including the number of pads or tampons used.

On the basis of the history and pelvic exam, the doctor will often be able to establish the cause of irregular bleeding in a younger woman. For example, the doctor will be able to feel fi-

broids, or see a polyp or evidence of vaginitis or cervicitis. The doctor will also do a *Pap smear* to check for cervical dysplasia, a blood test to see if heavy bleeding has caused anemia, and a pregnancy test if there is any possibility of pregnancy. If the pregnancy test is positive, the doctor may do an ultrasound test to help rule out an ectopic, or tubal pregnancy. If it appears that a woman is experiencing dysfunctional uterine bleeding due to lack of ovulation, especially in a woman under 35, the doctor will generally prescribe estrogen and/or progesterone to normalize the lining of the uterus. There are many different hormone regimens, including straight progesterone, straight estrogen (which produces a heavy period referred to as a *medical D&C*), or birth control pills, which are a combination of the two hormones.

If doctors believe that a woman over 40 has dysfunctional bleeding as a result of ovulatory irregularities, they will often perform a *D&C (dilatation & curettage)*, in which the cervix is dilated and the lining of the uterus is scraped out. D&Cs are the most common type of gynecological surgery. Gynecologists often do the procedure in the office or on an outpatient basis at the hospital. The woman is given a sedative and a local anesthetic called a *paracervical block*. If a polyp is seen, it will be removed, but small asymptomatic fibroids are simply observed and left.

If a D&C reveals the presence of large fibroids that are causing pain or anemia, they may be removed at a later time under general anesthesia. In that case, if a woman wishes to have future pregnancies, only the fibroid will be removed. This procedure is called a *myomectomy*. If a woman is premenopausal and does not wish any further children, the doctor may do a *simple hysterectomy*, removing the uterus but leaving the ovaries. Often a simple hysterectomy can be done vaginally without an abdominal incision.

A D&C is the usual treatment any time a woman experiences postmenopausal bleeding, unless she is on estrogen/progesterone therapy. In that case, she will normally have a light period. However, if she has unusually heavy bleeding or bleeding between periods, the doctor will discontinue hormone therapy and do a D&C. If the lab report shows that the uterine cells are normal, further treatment will depend on the cause of the abnormal bleeding. If the pathology report reveals uterine cancer, a *hysterectomy* will be done through an abdominal incision. In addition to the uterus, the Fallopian tubes and the ovaries will be removed since they are involved in 8% of all cases. If the tumor has spread, other therapies such as radiation may be used.

If a woman has an abnormal Pap smear, further tests are performed, including *colposcopy*. In this procedure, the cervix is painted with a stain such as iodine in order to locate questionable cells, and a tissue sample is removed for biopsy with the aid of a special microscope. Further treatment varies depending on the depth and spread of abnormal cells. For noninvasive, small lesions that can be seen with colposcopy, the area is treated with *cryosurgery*, a freezing technique, or with *carbon dioxide laser surgery*. Neither technique requires anesthesia. For severe dysplasia or cancer *in situ*, *conization* is done, a procedure in which a cone-shaped section is removed from the cervix. If cervical cancer *without* spread is found in a young woman who still wishes to have children, the doctor will do nothing further, but will follow the woman closely. When a biopsy or conization reveals cervical cancer in an older woman, a hysterectomy will be done. If there is no evidence of spread, the doctor may do a *vaginal hysterectomy* in which only the uterus is removed. If there is evidence of spread, *a radical abdominal hysterectomy* may be done in which the ovaries, Fallopian tubes and lymph nodes are removed in addition to the uterus. Often, *radiation* treatments will also be used to eliminate any remaining cancerous cells.

Ruling Out Other Diseases

The preceding discussion has dealt with the most common causes of abnormal uterine bleeding, both pre- and postmenopausal. Broadly speaking, the causes are either hormonal changes (including pregnancy), which are more common in younger women, or organic diseases of the reproductive system, which are more common in older women. The causes are differentiated by a history, physical exam, lab tests, and, in some cases, the results of a D&C. Less frequently, abnormal uterine bleeding is caused by systemic disease, including *clotting disorders* or *thyroid conditions* (see p. 379), or by an *ovarian condition*. Occasionally, women confuse uterine bleeding with bleeding from a *urinary tract infection* (see p. 394), *hemorrhoids* (see p. 366), or a *vaginal irritation* (see p. 398).

Prevention

Menstrual irregularities due to stress, poor nutrition, or overexercising can be avoided by making positive life-style changes. Preventive measures are especially important for women who notice that their cycles are susceptible to upsets (see section on *Self-Care*).

There are no methods for preventing polyps or fibroids. Neither is considered a serious illness, and little research has been done on the causes or factors associated with their development. Abnormal bleeding due to birth control pills or postmenopausal estrogen therapy can be avoided by adjusting dosages or discontinuing therapy.

Interestingly, much is known about both primary and secondary prevention of cervical and uterine cancer. Primary prevention addresses the causal factors and prevents the illness from occurring; secondary prevention deals with early diagnosis and effective treatment of these conditions. A number of factors affect the primary prevention of cervical cancer. It is thought that young women should delay intercourse until their cervix attains maturity, or use barrier forms of contraception (condoms or diaphragms). The adolescent cervix seems particularly susceptible to cellular change. Good hygiene and prompt treatment of any venereal disease, especially genital warts and herpes, should also help to lower the incidence of cervical cancer. Women of all ages can lower their risk of this type of cervical cancer by keeping the number of their sexual contacts low, by not using birth control pills for long timespans, and by using barrier forms of contraception which help to prevent the spread of the papilloma viruses. Finally, giving up smoking will markedly decrease a woman's chances of developing cervical cancer. In terms of secondary prevention of cervical cancer, Pap smears taken at regular intervals continue to be very effective, and are especially important for women at high risk (see p. 419).

Primary prevention for uterine cancer involves both life-style factors and medical treatment. Weight control starting early in life and a low-fat diet (see p. 102) reduce the risk of developing uterine cancer in later life. In addition, most cancer experts question the routine prescription of postmenopausal estrogen replacement therapy, which has been linked with a higher incidence of uterine cancer. However, estrogen/progesterone combinations are thought to be a safer option for women who choose to use estrogen replacement therapy (see p. 429).

In terms of secondary prevention, that is, early diagnosis and treatment, women should see their gynecologist for any uterine bleeding after menopause, and women at higher-than-average risk for uterine cancer should have pelvic exams every 6–12 months, including regular Pap smears, which can occasionally suggest some types of uterine abnormalities. Women at higher risk include those with a history of obesity, diabetes, hypertension, postmenopausal use of estrogen, anovulatory periods, or no history of full-term pregnancy.

Menopausal Syndrome

Symptoms

- irregular menstrual cycles, followed by cessation of menstruation at an average age of 51
- light or heavy bleeding
- longer menstrual cycles
- hot flashes or flushes
- night sweats
- vaginal dryness and/or soreness
- occasional pain on intercourse
- headaches
- dizziness
- anxiety or depression

Description

From a medical standpoint, *menopause* simply refers to a woman's final menstrual period, or the cessation of menstruation. The medical term *climacteric* refers to the span of time during which a woman passes from the reproductive to the nonreproductive part of her life. The climacteric includes a pre- and postmenopausal time in addition to menopause itself, and thus it can only be identified retrospectively. In popular usage, the word "menopause" is used like the term "climacteric," to refer to the transitional time that generally spans several years in a woman's late 40s and early 50s. For this discussion, we will use menopause in the lay sense.

Like the onset of menstruation, menopause is a normal part of the female reproductive cycle. Basically, menopause occurs when a woman's estrogen and progesterone production undergo a radical drop, which causes a number of physiological changes in addition to the end of menstruation. Some of the ensuing changes are viewed positively by most women—for instance, few are unhappy that they no longer get menstrual periods. Other changes, such as hot flashes and vaginal dryness, may present problems for a number of women. Because women complain about the problematic changes, many doctors tend to regard menopausal symptoms as a condition requiring treatment.

Not all cultures consider menopause and its associated physical changes as a problem. In part, this may be due to sociological factors. In many cultures women enjoy increased status and greater freedom after menopause. For example, among the Rajput caste of India, women must remain veiled and housebound before menopause; after menopause, they are allowed to go about widely in society. Interestingly, these women are not reported to experience negative symptoms in conjunction with menopause. On the other hand, a sociological study in Israel showed that the women in transition, with the least support from their culture in terms of traditional roles or modern freedoms, had the most problematic physical symptoms associated with menopause.

In many cultures, the positive aspect of not bearing more children is emphasized, and physical symptoms of menopause are simply given little notice. It may be that physiological freedom from childbearing has less positive status in our culture due to greater knowledge of, and use of, birth control. Moreover, since our culture has come to put such extreme emphasis on youth and beauty over the last few decades, menopause has become linked to a loss of status due to the negative aspects of "aging." Thus women in this society may tend to concentrate on the problematic aspects of menopause.

Given our cultural background and the lack of emphasis on the positive aspects of menopause, the climacteric has come to be looked upon by many women as basically negative. Misconceptions and fears have arisen linking menopause with instant aging and the end of sexuality. Such attitudes can often make physical symptoms seem worse than they actually are. In addition, even in our ostensibly more open times, many women feel the same embarrassment over menopausal symptoms that they felt about symptoms at the onset of menstruation. Once again, women tend to allude to problems and physical necessities in veiled terms, rather than discussing them frankly and matter-of-factly. Perhaps women are also disturbed by their inability to reliably predict or direct the responses of their body in relation to menopause.

Our culture seems to have a philosophical preference for controlling nature rather than living in harmony with it; thus we ultimately look for ways to "cure" the symptoms of menopause, rather than deal with them. During the 1960s, a book called *Feminine Forever* popularized medical treatment with supplemental estrogen, known as "estrogen replacement therapy," as a means of remaining young, staying sexually attractive, and avoiding the "horrible" symptoms of menopause. Although there had been no long-range studies on the consequences of this treatment, doctors prescribed estrogens to a significant number of women. It has been estimated that as many as 50% of postmenopausal, middle-class American women took estrogen in the mid-1970s. When studies showed a link between estrogen therapy and uterine cancer, doctors and women alike were forced to reconsider the routine use of supplemental estrogen. The emergence of the self-help and holistic medical movements, as well as the feminist movement, spurred people to reconsider the classification and treatment of menopause as a "disease." The use of supplemental estrogen, and the attitudes that underlie it, are being reevaluated and, often, replaced with self-help measures and a more positive view of menopause as a natural process that is a landmark in a woman's sexual life, but not the end of it.

Menopause is the result of a complex interaction between hormones, eggs, and the body. A woman starts to make eggs in the third week of embryonic life. At 20 weeks, a female fetus achieves her maximum number of eggs—about

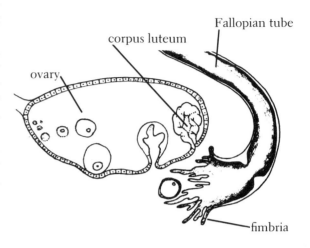

During a menstrual cycle, an egg emerges from one of the ovaries, enters the Fallopian tube and moves down into the uterus. Estrogen and progesterone are produced by the follicle, *the egg case that is left behind when the egg emerges from the ovary.*

7 million. No new eggs are formed after seven months of gestation. For unknown reasons, the number drops down to 2 million by birth, and 300,000 by puberty. At menopause, there are few eggs left, and those eggs that are left no longer ripen and leave the ovary in response to hormonal stimulation. A total of only 400 or 500 eggs are actually ovulated between *menarche*, which is the beginning of menstruation, and menopause. The other hundreds of thousands of eggs undergo *atresia*, a process in which the egg case initially enlarges in response to hormonal stimulation, but then simply dissolves.

At puberty, the *pituitary gland* in women begins producing two important hormones—*follicle-stimulating hormone (FSH)*, which stimulates the growth of cells in the egg case or *follicle*, and *luteinizing hormone (LH)*, which basically causes the egg case to rupture and the egg or *ovum* to move out of the ovary into the *Fallopian tube* that leads to the uterus (see illustration). In response to FSH and LH, the *folli-*

cle, or egg case, surrounding a few of the eggs temporarily becomes an active endocrine organ that produces several different hormones at varying times in the menstrual cycle. The cells surrounding the ovum start to produce *estrogen* at the beginning of the menstrual cycle, reaching a peak just before ovulation takes place. During the first part of the menstrual cycle, estrogen causes the wall of the uterus to thicken and the glands in the wall to deepen. Estrogen causes the appearance of secondary female sexual characterisitics such as development of breasts, pubic hair, and wider hips; and it continues to affect the female sexual organs throughout life. In addition to estrogen, the developing follicles also produce small amounts of *androgen*, the male sex hormone.

About the middle of the menstrual cycle, a brief surge of luteinizing hormone causes ovulation to take place. Although several follicles have grown and produced estrogen since the beginning of the cycle, generally only one egg case enlarges significantly. This egg pops out of the ovary in response to the rise in LH; the other eggs simply undergo atresia and dissolve.

Meanwhile, the cells in the follicle surrounding the ovulated egg enlarge and form a structure called the *corpus luteum*, or "yellow body." The corpus luteum itself rapidly begins to produce significant amounts of estrogen, as well as large amounts of *progesterone*, a hormone whose role is to help maintain pregnancy. During the second part of the menstrual cycle, following ovulation, progesterone causes a further thickening of the uterine wall and an increase in its blood vessels. Progesterone also signals the uterine glands to start accumulating nutrients in preparation for implantation of the egg. If implantation does not take place, the corpus luteum dies, and the production of estrogen and progesterone drops precipitously to very low levels. This sudden drop causes the blood vessels in the lining of the uterus to contract, and the lining is sloughed of as a menstrual period.

Menopause comes about when a woman's eggs are all used or they no longer respond to follicle-stimulating hormone. When this happens, two results ensue: follicles no longer produce estrogen or progesterone, and therefore the uterine wall no longer thickens and sloughs off on a monthly basis. Nevertheless, the pituitary continues to produce FSH and LH—in fact, it produces them in larger quantities.

As a woman approaches menopause, the developing follicles produce lower and lower amounts of estrogen, causing the preovulation part of the menstrual cycle to be shorter and shorter, and causing ovulation to take place earlier in the cycle. The post-ovulation part of the cycle does not change in length. Thus, the average length of a woman's menstrual cycle that was, for example, 35 days at age 15, 30 days at age 25, and 28 days at age 35, becomes as short as 23 days after age 45. As menopause actually nears, marked menstrual irregularities become common. It is not unusual for premenopausal women to experience both long and short cycles, although the length generally starts to increase once again. As menopause approaches, periods also vary between light and heavy, although it is more common for them to be light. Women who enter menopause before the average age of 51 generally have a shorter time of such irregularities, while women who enter menopause after age 51 often have a longer time of irregularities.

The irregularities in menstrual cycles are caused by the fact that the follicles of the last eggs vary in the amount of estrogen and progesterone they produce. Some follicles produce lower amounts of estrogen and progesterone, while others produce a burst of estrogen and normal amounts of progesterone. Sometimes a follicle grows, but ovulation does not even take place, which results in very light flow. Such anovulatory cycles become more and more common as menopause nears. Ultimately, the majority of women experience longer and longer cycles, with lighter and lighter bleeding, finally tapering off to spotting. It is less common for women to continue to produce large amounts of estrogen shortly before menopause, and therefore experience heavy periods.

Once a middle-aged woman has not experienced a menstrual period in 6–12 months, a retrospective diagnosis of menopause can be made. With the cessation of menstrual cycles, signs of a decrease in estrogen begin to occur, although estrogen production does not stop entirely. As stated earlier, women normally produce the male hormone androgen; this androgen is metabolized into estrogen in fat cells of the body, primarily, and in liver and muscle cells. The more fat cells a postmenopausal woman has, the more estrogen she tends to produce. This estrogen can be present in amounts equal to the lowest levels of a normal menstrual cycle, but it is less potent. A woman's adrenal glands also produce low amounts of progesterone and *testosterone*, a male hormone that stimulates the growth of facial hair.

Since estrogen tends to enhance cell growth (e.g., in the lining of the uterus), the drop in estrogen that comes with menopause causes a number of atrophic changes in the female genital system. The ovaries, Fallopian tubes, and uterus itself shrink in size. For women with fibroids or endometriosis, this decrease in size is beneficial. Lower estrogen also causes the folds in the vaginal wall to flatten and the vagina to become smaller, especially in women who have not born children vaginally. At the same time, the mucous membrane lining in the vagina thins, and the cervix decreases in size and produces less mucus. The combination of dryness and thinness makes the vagina more susceptible to abrasion; sometimes during intercourse or douching, a woman may even experience slight vaginal bleeding. The labia majora shrink in size too, and there may be some loss and coarsening of pubic hair. Like the cervix, the *Bartholin's glands* at the entrance to the vagina also produce less mucus. The lining of the bladder and urethra also shrink and become thinner, which can lead to more frequent urination, and in some cases to more frequent bladder infections. Finally, there is a reduction in the fat content and glandular tissue of the breast. Since the skin does not shrink, the breasts generally develop a more flattened appearance.

All these changes notwithstanding, there is no evidence that a woman experiences any physically-based lessening of sexual desire. In fact, the postmenopausal rise in the male sex hormone *androgen* experienced by women often increases their interest in sex by sensitizing the clitoris and affecting the hypothalamic area of the brain that controls sex drive. The "apparent" rise in androgen is due to the fact that estrogen no longer opposes the effects of the male hormone. Sociological and psychological changes in women's lives after menopause may also heighten their interest in sex. Women no longer have to be concerned with the possibility of unwanted pregnancy, their children are often grown and fairly independent, and their husbands have frequently reached a stable point in their careers. Thus many women and their mates find themselves with more time, less distractions, and a continued interest in sex.

The most frequently reported problem associated with menopause is *hot flashes*—feelings of heat or burning that are followed by sweating. These sensations last anywhere from a few seconds to 10 minutes, often occurring in waves. Generally a flush begins in the head and face, and spreads down to the neck and breasts, and may or may not continue to spread over the rest of the body. The sweating that follows affects the whole body, but is most prominent in the upper body. The amount of perspiration actually produced varies greatly. When flashes occur at night, a woman will suddenly awake feeling hot and sweaty. Hot flashes are often preceded by a brief feeling of pressure in the head, and some women experience heart palpitations. About 75% of all menopausal women experience hot flashes. The symptoms are most common in the first year or two after menopause, and tend to drop thereafter, but 25%–50% of all women are still having them five years after menopause. About half the women who experience hot flashes do not report them as a problem and characterize them as mild.

Although the cause of hot flashes is still unknown, much has been learned about them. At one time hot flashes were considered to be psychosomatic, but it is now recognized that they represent a real instability in the blood vessels of the skin. Studies have shown that skin temperature rises by as much as 14°F during a hot flash, and peaks within 10 minutes. This elevation and subsequent drop in skin temperature is followed by a .5°F drop in core body temperature. The temperature of the skin does not fully return to normal for 40 minutes.

Flushes are related to *estrogen withdrawal*, rather than lack of estrogen. They are actually not experienced by women who have never produced estrogen due to a congenital lack of ovaries, but they are uniformly experienced by women who have both ovaries removed surgically. Similarly, flashes are immediately experienced by women who stop estrogen replacement therapy.

Researchers speculate that bursts of luteinizing hormone released by the pituitary reset the body's thermostat in the hypothalamus. Normally, the hypothalamus regulates body temperature through sweating and blood vessel dilation. Sweating cools the body by evaporation; widening of the vessels under the skin radiates heat away from body. Although hot flashes are not an average response shared by everyone in a room, they are a reaction to changes in temperature. Postmenopausal women recognize that flashes are often precipitated by environmental cues such as hot weather, hot rooms, a warm bed, hot beverages, spicy foods, alcohol, caffeine, and emotional upset. Apparently the hypothalamus adjusts to

hormonal changes within several years after the onset of menopause.

Emotional disequilibrium, anxiety, irritability, and depression are feelings commonly experienced by women of menopausal age. It is unclear whether these feelings are related to the physical changes of menopause or are indirectly due to the pressures and life changes experienced by women of this age. Research has not proven one side of the argument or the other, but currently points to the fact that emotional symptoms are largely the result of social/emotional factors such as a perceived loss of youth, children leaving home, marital problems, financial problems, and career changes. On the other hand, it is known that emotional lability is often associated with the hormonal changes experienced by women. Other examples of this are the mood swings experienced during pregnancy and the postpartum period, both of which are psychologically stressful as well. Interestingly, some double-blind studies have found that women on estrogen replacement therapy showed no less emotional disequilibrium than did those taking a placebo. Other studies have supported the idea that estrogen improves mood and outlook.

Menopause affects women's health in ways other than menopausal symptoms. Two potentially serious medical conditions, *heart attack* and *osteoporosis*, increase significantly after menopause (see p. 284 and p. 343). In the case of heart attack, postmenopausal women's rates gradually increase and become equal to those of men of the same age. This increase is thought to be due to the fact that menopause is associated with a rise in cholesterol levels, averaging 16 points. However, estrogen/progestin replacement therapy does not prevent this rise; in fact, it may even increase the cholesterol level. In regard to osteoporosis, it is postmenopausal women who are at the greatest risk. Dietary changes—in particular those that lower cholesterol intake and raise calcium levels—are useful in decreasing the incidence of these diseases. Estrogen replacement therapy does slow bone loss as long as the therapy continues; however, this protective effect drops off fairly quickly when estrogen is discontinued.

Self-Care

Generally, self-care measures are sufficient for dealing with most cases of menopausal symptoms. Hot flashes are an outward sign of a normal hormonal process. Gynecologist Dr. Sadja

---

Self-Care for Menopausal Symptoms

General:
- get aerobic exercise three to five times a week
- eat a varied, healthy diet
- avoid crash dieting or being too thin (the fat cells in the body produce estrogen)
- stop smoking—cigarettes interfere with ovarian function
- decrease alcohol, which causes a decline in ovulation
- decrease caffeine, which increases irritability
- learn to identify and deal with stress (see p. 58)

Hot flashes:
- wear layers of loose, cool, cotton clothing that can be removed
- keep the house cool, especially the bedroom
- drink cool beverages frequently

Vaginal dryness:
- avoid vaginal irritation due to excess soap
- wear loose cotton underpants and pants
- use vaginal lubricants: creams, vegetable oils, or water-soluble jellies
- during intercourse, spend more time in foreplay because sexual response is slower
- have sex or masturbate frequently (sexual arousal seems to stimulate vaginal lubrication)
- do Kegel exercises to strengthen vaginal muscles
- discuss the use of estrogen creams with your doctor if these methods are not adequate

---

Greenwood, author of *Menopause Naturally*, suggests that hot flashes need to be accepted with humor, much like adolescent acne. Since hot flashes resolve naturally as the body reaches a new equilibrium, the goal is to live with them as comfortably as possible. For women who've always been troubled with feeling cold, flashes may not represent such an onerous problem. In many cases, hot flashes can be prevented by avoiding situations known to trigger them. During this stage, women can keep cool by dressing in lighter clothes or in layers that can easily be removed. It will also help to keep the house thermostat down and sleep with less covers. Menopausal women should definitely keep up their exercise, but need to wear lighter clothes and spend more time cooling down after exercise. In addition, it is advisable to avoid caffeine, alcohol, and hot drinks if these substances tend to trigger flashes. Smoking should definitely be discontinued because it is known to interfere with ovarian function and to decrease estrogen levels.

Vaginal dryness and soreness usually respond to self-help measures. It is important to treat these symptoms because they can be disturbing and diminish sexual pleasure. It should be noted again that these symptoms have nothing to do with sexual sensitivity, drive, or attractiveness. A number of nonprescription lubricants are available, including creams, oils, and non-water-soluble and water-soluble jellies (e.g., *K-Y jelly* and *Lubifax*). These lubricants can be used anytime, but are an especially important aid during foreplay. By menopause, the natural lubrication of the vagina takes longer to achieve. Doctors also notice that postmenopausal women who are sexually active or who masturbate show fewer signs of vaginal shrinkage and dryness. It is thought that sexual activity increases the amount of androgen produced in the ovaries, and that it, like estrogen, affects the vaginal mucosa. If the vagina is sore or tender, women may be more comfortable during intercourse if they assume the position on top be-

Kegel Exercises

- Kegel exercises increase strength in the muscles of the pelvic floor, i.e., the muscles around the vagina and urethra
- to identify the muscular sensations, intentionally start and stop the flow of urine several times when going to the bathroom; to avoid muscle strain, do not try this when your bladder is very full or you are tired
- practice the exercise when *not* urinating; contract the muscles for 3–5 seconds, then relax completely; do the exercise 5–10 times in a row
- practice at any time, whether standing, sitting, or lying down; the exercise can also be practiced during intercourse
- Kegels improve a woman's bladder control and enhance sexual satisfaction

cause it allows them greater control over their partner's penetration.

During the years preceding menopause, several life-style changes may help to control the irregularity of menstrual periods and/or heavy bleeding. The goal of all self-help measures is to keep estrogen levels as regular as possible, since the eggs tend to produce varying amounts of estrogen during the climacteric. Both smoking and alcohol are known to decrease estrogen production and by themselves can cause short, erratic periods. In addition, some women find that high caffeine intake also causes irregular periods. Very heavy exercise on a regular basis, as well as crash dieting and excessive weight loss, are also known to suppress ovulation, and therefore affect estrogen production.

Stress reduction can be very helpful for women in both the immediate pre- and post-menopausal years (see p. 58). Relaxation can help to relieve many of the emotional upsets associated with menopause and with premenstrual syndrome. Many women find that in learning to cope more effectively with marital, job, and financial problems, they have fewer problems with irregularities in menstrual periods before

menopause, and with postmenopausal symptoms such as headaches, dizziness, anxiety, and depression. The more interests women have, and the greater their sense of fulfillment, the more accepting and flexible women can be about the changes that take place during this period of their lives (see p. 70).

The Doctor

Since the years before menopause are characterized by irregularity in menstrual periods, a diagnosis of menopause cannot be made until a woman in her late 40s or early 50s has gone for six months without a period. If a woman experiences very heavy periods or frequent spotting between periods, she may be advised to have a D&C *(dilatation and curettage)*, a procedure in which the lining of the uterus is scraped out. Most often a woman's heavy periods are caused by hormonal imbalances that commonly precede menopause, but a D&C will rule out any problems, and may help to make periods more normal. D&Cs are usually done on an outpatient basis under local anesthesia, either in a doctor's office or in the hospital.

A great deal of controversy still surrounds the treatment of menopausal symptoms with *estrogen replacement therapy*. Currently, over one-third of all American women above the age of 50 are put on estrogen replacement. As long as it is continued, replacement therapy does relieve hot flashes and vaginal dryness, and will reduce the bone loss of osteoporosis. But there is little evidence that it will eliminate the emotional symptoms sometimes linked with menopause, or that it will prevent aging. Moreover, since flashes and vaginal dryness are caused by the withdrawal of estrogen, these conditions do develop whenever estrogen therapy is discontinued.

Currently, there are compelling medical reasons against *routine* use of estrogen replacement therapy. There is a definite increase in the risk of uterine cancer, a risk that goes up the longer estrogen is taken. It has been found that adding a progesterone-like hormone called *progestin* eliminates this risk, but it may increase the risk of heart attack and stroke. By itself, estrogen use doubles the risk of gallstones (see p. 372), and there is some question as to whether estrogen may increase the risk of breast cancer (see p. 431). Estrogen replacement therapy is generally contraindicated for women with fibroids, gallstones, liver disease, thrombophlebitis, diabetes, and for women who have had cancer of the breast, uterus, or ovary.

At the present time, estrogen is most frequently given as *conjugated equine estrogen* (e.g., *Premarin*). For days 1–25 of each calendar month, estrogen is given; in addition, unless a woman has had a hysterectomy, *progestin* is given on days 16–25. No medication is given from day 26 until the end of the calendar month, at which time a woman will generally have a light, painless period.

Women who have a great deal of vaginal soreness and dryness that do not respond to nonprescription lubricants are often treated with *estrogen creams* (e.g., *Premarin cream*). These low-dose estrogen creams are applied nightly with an applicator to the sore area for 5–10 days in a row, and thereafter every 3–4 days or twice a week. The use of Premarin cream thickens the vaginal wall and helps to relieve soreness, but does not increase vaginal lubrication to premenopausal levels, so lubrication is still recommended before intercourse. Although women do not achieve as high a blood level with estrogen cream as they do with estrogen tablets, there is concern that even this topical estrogen may increase the incidence of uterine cancer. Thus some doctors recommend that women who use estrogen cream regularly take 10 days of progestin tablets every six months.

Currently, some doctors prescribe estrogen on a routine basis, some prescribe it on a case-by-case basis, others rarely prescribe it. Women should take estrogen replacement therapy for menopausal symptoms only after evaluating with their gynecologist their own health history and risk factors, the general risks and benefits of replacement therapy, and the degree of discomfort they are experiencing due to their symptoms. In discussing estrogen therapy with her doctor, a woman should ascertain the doctor's own philosophy about it, and if she does not agree, switch to a physician who has a similar attitude about the drug. Estrogen replacement therapy should not be undertaken lightly or simply as a beauty aid.

Ruling Out Other Diseases

Under the age of 40, cessation of menstrual periods may be due to a variety of causes, including pregnancy, stress, weight loss, regular strenuous exercise, birth control pills, or hormonal imbalances. Blood tests for FSH and LH levels will establish if the cause is premature menopause.

Hot flashes with no other symptoms can be caused by various medical conditions, including *hyperthyroidism* (see p. 389), *diabetes* (see p. 379), and general infections. Such flashes tend to be of longer duration than those caused by menopause and do not localize in the area of the head.

Postmenopausal vaginal soreness may be due to a *vaginal infection* such as *yeast* or *trichomoniasis* (see p. 398), in addition to lack of lubrication. Infections are often accompanied by itching or a vaginal discharge. They can be ruled out by a pelvic exam and lab tests.

Heavy menstrual flow or spotting before menopause may be due to a variety of uterine or hormonal causes, including *fibroids*, or more rarely, *cancer of the uterus* (see p. 414). These can be ruled out on the basis of a D&C and an examination of the tissue.

Prevention

It is important to reiterate that menopause is a natural part of a woman's life cycle and not an "illness." Most of the undesirable symptoms associated with menopause respond to simple self-care measures. Stopping smoking and reducing alcohol consumption can help to prevent both the premenopausal symptoms of irregular periods and the postmenopausal symptoms of hot flashes. Continued sexual activity and supplemental lubrication with nonestrogen creams or gels can help to minimize vaginal soreness.

Breast Lumps or Tumors, Including Fibroadenomas, Fibrocystic Disease, and Breast Cancer

Symptoms

fibroadenomas
- typically, a small, round, firm lump in the breast
- lump is separate from surrounding tissue, has clear borders and is somewhat movable
- lump is not tender
- lump doesn't grow or change with menstrual periods
- most commonly occurs in younger women

fibrocystic disease
- breast pain and tenderness
- discrete, soft, rubbery lump(s)
- lump(s) separate from surrounding tissue and have clear borders
- lump(s) often appear and disappear rapidly
- lump(s) often fluctuate in size and tenderness during a menstrual cycle
- multiple lumps are common; both breasts may be involved
- most commonly occurs in middle-aged women; rare after menopause

breast cancer
- typically, a firm-to-hard breast lump of varying size
- often, edges are not clear and lump is fixed to underlying tissue
- lump is not tender
- lump steadily increases in size
- most common in women over 50

Description

Breast lumps are a common reason for women to see a doctor. Because of concern about breast cancer, most women are alarmed when they discover a lump in their breast. Yet despite the fact that carcinoma of the breast is a relatively common cancer in our culture, most women with a breast lump do not have breast cancer. In women under 30, the great majority of lumps are either fibroadenomas or fibrocystic breast disease. In women between the ages of 30 and 50, fibrocystic disease remains by far the most common cause of breast lumps. In postmenopausal women aged 50 and over, breast cancer is still relatively uncommon, but a greater percentage of lumps that develop at this age are malignant.

Fibroadenomas: Fibroadenomas are benign tumors that are small, firm, round or oval lumps that are not tender to the touch. Most often, they occur within 20 years of puberty, and they are rare after menopause. Generally, fibroadenomas feel separate from the breast tissue around them, they tend to be movable, and their borders or edges are distinct. They range in size from pea-sized to 2″ in diameter, but they are generally small and do not fluctuate in size from month to month. About 10% of the time, there is more than one lump, either in one or both breasts. Occasionally, a fibroadenoma that has gone unnoticed for years will be found in a middle-aged woman whose breasts have shrunk somewhat after menopause.

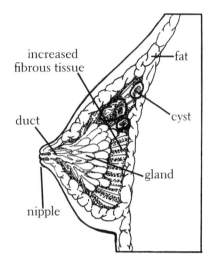

increased
fibrous tissue

fat

duct

cyst

gland

nipple

In fibrocystic breast disease, fluid-filled sacs, or cysts, develop in one or both breasts, and the amount of fibrous tissue in the breast(s) increases. One out of five women develop cysts at some point.

Fibrocystic disease, or mammary dysplasia: Fibrocystic disease is by far the most common breast disease. The main symptom of this disease is pain and tenderness in one or both breasts, often increasing noticeably between the time of ovulation (approximately 14 days after the first day of the last menstrual period) and the menstrual period. This pain and tenderness is often accompanied by a discrete lump or lumps in one or both breasts. These cysts tend to be soft, rubbery masses with fairly distinct edges. They can appear and disappear rapidly, and they generally fluctuate in size during menstrual cycles, being largest and most painful right before the onset of the period, and smallest and least uncomfortable right after a period.

About 16% of all women seek medical attention for breast pain at some time during their life. Fibrocystic disease encompasses a wide variety of conditions, ranging from tender, lumpy breasts to discrete cysts with specific microscopic characteristics. Tender, lumpy breasts are generally considered a variant of normal breast tissue, but are still classified as fibrocystic disease by doctors. The condition is most common in women between the ages of 30 and 50. When the breasts shrink after menopause, multiple residual cysts can often be felt.

Since fibrocystic disease fluctuates with the menstrual cycle, researchers speculate that estrogen levels play a role in the disease. This theory is supported by two facts: the condition generally disappears with menopause (when estrogen levels drop), and women who are on estrogen replacement therapy continue to experience problems. It is not known whether the symptoms are due to estrogen-caused fluid retention or to the effects of other hormones. Fibrocystic disease has also been linked to *methylxanthines*, a molecule found in caffeine, chocolate, and colas. Studies have shown, and many women corroborate from experience, that eliminating methylxanthines from the diet lessens breast pain and reduces the size of cysts. But definitive results remain to be established.

Fibrocysts are always of concern, not only because of the pain they can produce, but because they are common among women in the age group when breast cancer first occurs in substantial numbers. Moreover, one variety of fibrocysts is associated with an increased risk of breast cancer. Women who exhibit this type should be examined carefully at frequent intervals (see below).

Breast cancer: *Breast cancer* first appears as a small, firm-to-hard lump with indistinct borders. The lump is not tender to the touch, does not fluctuate with menstrual cycles, and most often is fixed to underlying tissue, either muscle or skin. If untreated, breast cancers grow progressively larger. Eventually other symptoms become apparent. Because the lump is attached, the breast develops a dimpled look over the lump as the skin retracts. The skin may become reddened, and the affected breast may appear asymmetrical or larger than the other one.

Most breast cancers—over 90%—are discovered by women themselves, not by physical exam or mammogram. Although different types of breast carcinomas vary in the speed at which they develop, they are basically not fast-growing.

The average tumor enlarges at a slow, steady rate, doubling in size in 100 days. This means they do not reach 1 cm, the size that can be felt, for eight years. Breast cancer tends to metastasize, and if not detected, it often spreads to lymph nodes in the armpit.

Although the cause of breast cancer is still unknown, much has been learned about the *risk factors* associated with it. Studies have shown that the most likely causes are a genetic tendency combined with specific hormonal factors. It has long been known that women are more likely to develop breast cancer if there is a history of breast cancer among their first-degree relatives, that is, in a mother or sister. If the relative developed cancer after menopause, the risk is only 1.2 times greater than normal, but the risk is 3 times as great if the relative developed cancer *before* menopause, 5 times as great if cancer developed in both breasts after menopause, and 9 times as great if the cancer was premenopausal and affected both breasts. Although a number of women have a family history of postmenopausal breast cancer, only a fairly small number of women have a family history of premenopausal cancer in both breasts.

Certain hormonal factors associated with a woman's menstrual history may also put her at higher than average risk. Early onset of menstruation (under 12), late menopause, lack of children or only one child, and having one's first child after 35 are all associated with an increased risk of breast cancer. Interestingly, breast cancer virtually never develops in women who lose both ovaries at a young age.

The incidence of breast cancer varies from country to country. Overall, the incidence is highest in the developed nations (with the exception of Japan), and the lowest in the undeveloped nations. These differences are generally accredited to *fat in the diet*: Western countries tend to eat a high-fat diet as compared to undeveloped countries. Interestingly, studies have shown that breast cancer in Japan is higher in

areas where diets are richer in fat; similarly, rates are higher among Japanese women who move to the United States. In addition to such epidemiological studies, animal research has also linked fat consumption to breast cancer. In several studies, the more fat that experimental animals were fed, the more breast tumors they developed. Apparently fat does not *cause* the tumors, but does enhance their growth. A high-fat diet has been shown to affect levels of the natural hormones estrogen and prolactin. On the other hand, animals fed fish oils that are high in *omega-3 fatty acids* actually had tumor rates that were lower than average.

Many recent studies provide convincing evidence that alcohol consumption is another factor associated with a higher risk of breast cancer. The rates are 40%–60% higher in women who are moderate drinkers (three drinks or less per week), and almost double in women who consume more than three drinks per week. The association between alcohol and breast cancer is more significant among premenopausal women and women who are thin. Experts now recommend that women at high risk definitely curtail their alcohol consumption, and further they suggest that lowering alcohol consumption will lessen the chances of breast cancer for any woman.

The last important risk factor for breast cancer is simply *age*. The incidence of breast cancer increases directly with age, rising dramatically after menopause. In North America, the annual rate is 53 cases per 100,000 for women aged 35–40; 156 cases per 100,000 for women aged 45–50; and 228 cases per 100,000 women aged 65–69. Currently, breast cancer is the most common cancer among women in the U.S.: 1 out of every 11 women will develop breast cancer at some point in her life. This risk is sufficiently high that women should do all they can to lower their risk of developing breast cancer, and to increase the chances of detecting it early.

Doctors assess women in terms of all the risk

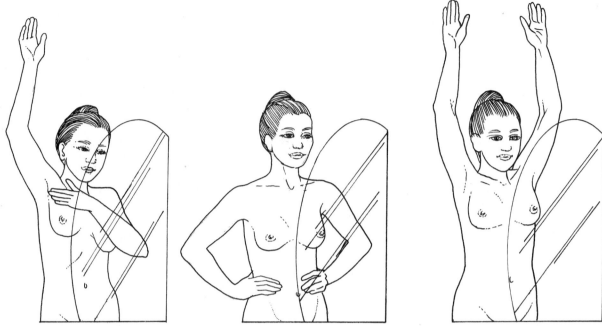

Monthly Breast Self-Exam begins with a visual inspection in front of a mirror. Women should look for changes in size, shape, and dimpling of both breasts and nipples.

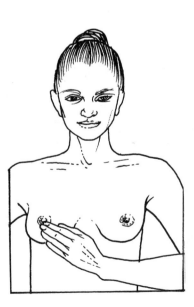

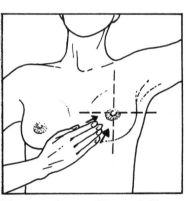

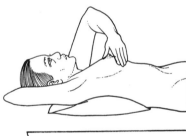

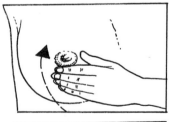

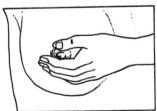

The second part of Breast Self-Exam involves feeling all four quadrants of the breast with the fingertips of the opposite hand. The fingertips should be pressed into the breast tissue gently, but firmly, with small, circular motions. Finally, each nipple should be squeezed to see if there is any discharge.

factors in order to identify those women who are at greater than average risk. Individuals with several factors are at greater than average risk. These women are followed more closely than is the average woman. Nevertheless, most women who develop breast cancer are simply at risk for dietary and age reasons, not because of family, menstrual, or pregnancy history.

Early detection of breast cancer: Over the last 20 years, great progress has been made in diagnosing breast cancer in the early stages before it has spread. Although early detection methods have definitely reduced the death rate from breast cancer, researchers feel that the survival rate could be increased even more dramatically if screening were more widely promoted and used. Early detection programs include breast self-examination, breast exam by a doctor, and mammography. It has been shown that a program utilizing these techniques can significantly lower the death rate in women over the age of 50. Currently, it is estimated that only 25% of women examine their breasts regularly, and only 11% of doctors prescribe mammography at routine intervals.

One of the most effective means of detecting breast cancer is known as *Breast Self-Exam (BSE)*, a technique in which a woman examines her own breast both visually and by touch. The American Cancer Society (ACS) recommends that all women over the age of 20 examine their breasts on a monthly basis. Premenopausal women should do the exam seven to eight days after the start of each period; at this point the breasts are least likely to be lumpy from hormonal changes. A woman should check for breast symmetry and skin dimpling by examining her breasts in a mirror while her arms are held at her sides, then overhead, and on her hips. Next, a woman should lie down and feel each breast and armpit area for lumps, using the fingertips of the opposite hand. A new technique called *MammaCare*, which is believed to be even

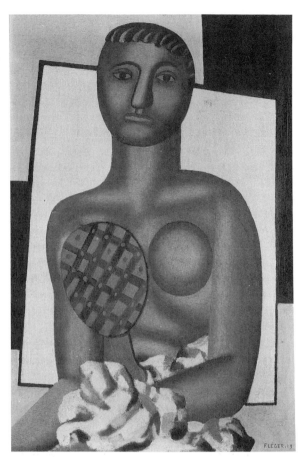

It is reassuring to know that most breast lumps are not malignant, but it is very important that women check their breasts on a regular basis and see their doctor if they discover a lump. Ferdinand Leger. Woman with Mirror. 1929. National Gallery of Art, Washington. Chester Dale Collection.

more effective than the traditional self-exam method, teaches a woman to detect lumps in a simulated breast model that matches the nodularity of her own breasts. The American Cancer Society also provides training classes and most doctors give women verbal instruction and a pamphlet on examining the breasts. The importance of self-examination is attested to by the fact that 90% of all tumors are discovered by women themselves.

Another method of early detection is *mammograms*, which are soft-tissue x-rays that are taken with special equipment. Approximately 40% of the tumors picked up by this type of x-ray are too small to be felt by hand. Tumors as small as 1 mm (.039 inches) can be visualized, and detection may occur as much as two years earlier than it would by manual exam. The value of mammography has been shown by several large-scale studies. The Health Insurance Plan of New York found that mammography was only of benefit between 50 and 60 years of age, but that within this age range, those receiving mammography had only 60% as many deaths as did a control group that did not get mammography. A 1982 American Cancer Society study showed that 80% of tumors identified by mammography had not yet spread to the axillary lymph nodes under the arm, whereas only 45% of tumors picked up by manual exam had not spread. This is very significant because survival rates from breast cancer are much higher if the tumor has not spread.

For years physicians were slow to make use of mammography due to concern over cost, radiation exposure, and the high rate of false positives. Mammograms vary from low-cost screening programs (e.g., *MammoVans*) to higher fees for private radiologists. Many health plans now cover routine mammograms. In terms of both money and doctor hours, it would be impossible to examine all 50–60-year-old women annually. Radiation exposure has also been a concern because radiation has been shown to cause certain types of cancer. However, the new low-dose machines only emit .1–.4 rads per 2-view exam. As a result, the benefits of mammography far outweigh the average risk of radiation for women in their 40s and 50s.

The American Cancer Society and American College of Radiology have issued a joint set of guidelines for use of mammography as a screening tool for asymptomatic women. They suggest that a woman have a *baseline mammogram* sometime between the ages of 35 and 40. This mammogram should be used as a basis for comparison with later mammograms. They recommend that women between the ages of 40 and 50 get a mammogram every one to two years. Above the age of 50, women are advised to get a yearly mammogram. Women who have a higher than average risk for any reason should have an annual mammogram above the age of 40.

Mammography does not replace manual examination because many tumors are *not* picked up by mammography. Between 11% and 40% of tumors that can be felt by hand escape detection on x-ray. Small tumors in very dense tissue, especially in young women, may be difficult to see on x-ray. The American Cancer Society recommends that women have their breasts examined by a doctor every three years between the ages of 20 and 40, and annually thereafter. Women at higher than average risk should have a yearly exam starting before the age of 40.

Foods and Drugs That May Aggravate Fibrocystic Breast Disease*

Foods
coffee
caffeinated tea
cola sodas
chocolate

Commonly prescribed drugs
Cafergot
Darvon
Empirin with codeine
Percodan
Theophylline medications

Nonprescription drugs

Anacin	Empirin compounds
Bromo Seltzer	Excedrin
Cope	Midol
Dexatrim	NoDoz
Dristan	Sinarest
Empirin	Vanquish

---

* *These substances contain* methylxanthines.

Self-Care

Self-examination of the breasts is an important means of detecting breast lumps. Breast cancer should be ruled out in the case of any lump, and this can only be done by a physician. Several self-help techniques have been shown to improve the quality of life after breast cancer has been diagnosed (see p. 302).

Self-care measures may be very helpful if a woman is diagnosed as having fibrocystic breast disease. A caffeine-free diet is recommended by many doctors since it helps to relieve symptoms in some women. Because pain is very subjective, and because most women are upset by the thought of breast cancer, women who have premenstrual breast swelling and tenderness may find that their symptoms are greatly relieved just by going to the doctor and being assured that they do not have breast cancer. Some women who experience discomfort because of fibrocystic breast disease are helped by wearing a well-fitting support bra. A bra can even be worn to sleep when tenderness is significant. Small, unverified studies seem to indicate that breast discomfort may be decreased by supplements of *Vitamins B1, E,* and *pyridoxine.* Pyridoxine should be taken as directed because high doses can cause neurological problems. *Evening primrose oil,* which contains *essential fatty acids (EFAs),* is also under evaluation as a dietary supplement therapy.

The Doctor

The doctor diagnoses the type of breast lump on the basis of a physical exam, a mammogram, and if necessary, lab tests. Often the physical exam will give an indication of what the lump is, based on its consistency, location, and movability. The doctor will also evaluate a woman's medical history and ask questions that will help to assess her risk status. Most women coming to a doctor with a breast lump do not have cancer, especially if they are under 50 and have no risk factors. But any lump should be carefully evaluated.

The work-up for a breast lump varies with the characteristics of the lump, the risk status of the woman, and the doctor's approach. In a woman under 30, a lump that feels like a fibroadenoma will be removed and biopsied to rule out cancer. Most often, this will be done on an outpatient basis, under local anesthesia. If doctors suspect fibrocysts in women 30–50, they will insert a needle into the lump. If fluid is withdrawn and the lump disappears thereafter, a diagnosis of fibrocystic disease is confirmed, and the woman is followed for this condition. Women who persistently have significant breast pain and lumpiness that does not respond to self-care therapies are occasionally given hormonal medication to reduce breast pain and nodularity. Although studies have shown some of these drugs to be effective, they do have side effects and their long-term effects are unknown.

When the diagnosis of a lump in a middle-aged woman is questionable, the doctor is likely to order a mammogram. In 90% of all cases, the doctor can correctly diagnose the lump from the mammogram, but because the mammogram is not definitive, a biopsy is done to make the final determination. Several types of biopsy can be done, and the doctor has a variety of options at this point. Two types of *needle biopsy* are available: *fine needle aspiration* simply removes a few cells for microscopic analysis, whereas *core needle biopsy* uses a special needle to remove a small core of tissue for examination. Both types of needle biopsy are done on an outpatient basis.

If the needle biopsy is negative, but the physical findings or the mammogram are suspicious, further tests will be done. Currently, the National Cancer Institute recommends a two-step approach in which an *open biopsy* is done first and the lump is surgically removed, often as an outpatient procedure using a local anesthetic. If the results of this biopsy are negative, nothing further will be done. If the lump is malignant, further surgery will be done within a week or two. This two-stage plan represents a change from the previous medical approach to a suspicious lump. In the past, a woman was admitted to the hospital for a biopsy, and definitive surgery was performed at the time of the biopsy if the results of an immediate *frozen sample* showed a malignancy. The two-stage approach gives a woman a chance to adjust to her diagnosis psychologically and, if she desires, to seek a second opinion about her diagnosis and the treatment recommended. When the lump is malignant, other tests may be done to ascertain whether or not the tumor has spread. The tests generally done are a *mammogram* of the opposite breast, a *chest x-ray*, and a *blood panel*. A *bone scan* may be done if there are specific indications for it. Tissue from the original biopsy will also be tested to see if it has *estrogen* or *progesterone receptor sites* that would make the tumor responsive to hormonal therapy, if that becomes necessary at a later date. Tumor cells often have receptors for these hormones, which means that chemotherapy can be specifically targeted at the tumor cells.

The surgical procedures or options recommended for breast cancer depend on the size and spread of the tumor, the type of malignant cell, and the medical philosophy of the doctor. Currently, within the medical community there continues to be a major controversy as to what type of surgery is most effective. Until the mid 1970s, the standard treatment was a *radical mastectomy* in which the entire breast, the underlying pectoral muscle, and the lymph nodes in the armpit were removed. The procedure was traumatic for women not only because of the diagnosis, but because the physical effects were so extreme. Moreover, since early detection methods were not as widely used then, many breast tumors had already spread by the time they were discovered.

In subsequent years, the radical mastectomy was replaced by a *modified radical*, in which the breast and lymph nodes were removed, but the pectoral muscle was not. The results of this operation were much more satisfactory both cosmetically and functionally.

More recently, several other types of operation have been used as an alternative to the modified radical. *Simple* or *total mastectomy* involves removal of the entire breast, but not the pectoral muscle or the axillary lymph nodes. Increasingly, doctors also recommend *breast reconstruction* in which a lifelike implant is inserted to replace missing breast tissue and a nipple is constructed, if necessary, out of genital tissue. Such reconstruction is done at a later date.

Segmental mastectomy or *lumpectomy* involves the removal of the tumor and a small area around it. This procedure is usually accompanied by *axillary dissection*, in which the lymph nodes in the armpit are removed. In almost all cases, segmental mastectomy is combined with later *radiation therapy*, which is not necessary if the breast is removed. Although it continues to cause controversy, the lumpectomy is being used as an alternative to the modified radical mastectomy more and more often on the basis of several recent studies. Recent research shows that *chemotherapy* should be done in conjunction with a lumpectomy.

One major clinical trial recently sponsored by the National Cancer Institute studied 2,100 women with breast cancer: one group received a modified radical mastectomy; a second group received a lumpectomy with lymph node removal; and a third group received a lumpectomy, node removal, and subsequent radiation. The five-year survival rate was approximately the same for all three groups. Because the women who received radiation had a lower rate of recurrence in the opposite breast, a number of doctors now recommend lumpectomy and radiation for many of their patients. Several other studies have also found no difference in survival rates between women who received the various forms of treatment. However, the practice of doing radical mastectomies remains the standard for many physicians, who feel that the long-range effectiveness of lumpectomy will not be fully proven for some years. The controversy over treatment of breast cancer remains so great that several states, including California and Massachusetts, have passed laws requiring doctors to advise women of the various treatment alternatives that exist.

Even among doctors who endorse lumpectomy, there is still some question as to which women should have this procedure as opposed to more extensive surgery. Some doctors recommend lumpectomy only for tumors under 2 cm in diameter, while others consider it an option even if the tumor is 4–5 cm in diameter. For tumors bigger than 5 cm, a modified radical is recommended by almost all doctors. A radical mastectomy, which includes removal of the axillary nodes and the pectoral muscle, is not often recommended anymore.

Based on more recent studies, researchers now think that breast cancer is somewhat systemic, in that it has a tendency to metastasize in some women. Thus, whereas doctors used to routinely do a radical mastectomy in the hope of preventing the spread of the tumor, they now feel that removing more surrounding tissue may not generally be that useful. What seems to be more effective is doing *adjuvant*, or additional, *therapy* if necessary. The consensus of recent conferences is that women who have evidence of malignancy in the axillary nodes should receive either chemotherapy or hormonal therapy in addition to surgery. Most women who have cancerous nodes are over 50 and have tumors that are positive for estrogen receptors. These women are generally given a new drug called *tamoxifen*, which is an antiestrogen agent.

Because the initial treatment does not always prevent breast cancer from spreading, doctors check women frequently following breast cancer surgery. For the first three years, women are generally examined every three to four months, then every six months for five years, and thereafter every six to twelve months. Following treatment, these women are also advised to examine themselves monthly and to have an annual mammogram.

The earlier breast cancer is diagnosed, the better a woman's prognosis. At this time, a tumor that has not spread to the lymph nodes has a 70%–95% cure rate. The cure rate for a localized tumor that is estrogen-positive is 90%. Even when the tumor has spread to the lymph nodes, the 5-year survival rate is still good. Breast cancer cure rates are improving steadily due to earlier detection and the effectiveness of newer, more refined chemotherapy and hormonal therapy techniques.

A number of factors seem to help women cope more effectively with the physical and psychological effects of breast cancer. The two-stage procedure and the alternative of more cosmetically acceptable surgeries, combined with strong support groups and greater general knowledge about breast cancer, have helped to alter the way women view this disease. The hope is that a more positive outlook will encourage women to check their breasts regularly and get mammograms at recommended intervals.

Ruling Out Other Diseases

A breast lump can be due to one of several conditions. Most breast lumps are not cancerous, but since breast cancer can be life-threatening, it is very important that any lump be seen promptly by a doctor in order to establish its cause.

Prevention

Most doctors now believe that the risk of breast cancer is lower among women who eat a low-fat diet and drink a minimum of alcohol. The National Cancer Institute is currently sponsoring large-scale studies to ascertain the value of a low-fat diet. Since this type of diet has no harmful effects and is also thought to decrease the risk of many other diseases, women of all ages would be well-advised to reduce their fat consumption (see p. 102). Recent research tends to support the theory that certain vitamins and minerals, such as selenium, may play a role in the prevention of breast cancer. Such long-range prevention factors are especially important to women who are at greater than average risk for breast cancer.

OBESITY

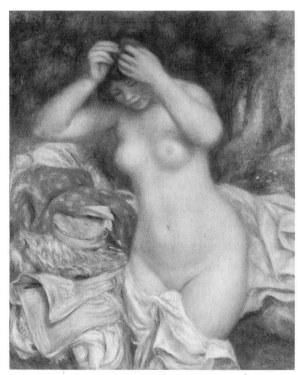

Obesity is one of the most common reasons for doctor visits, and dieting is the most common form of self-treatment. Auguste Renoir. Bather Arranging Her Hair. *1868. National Gallery of Art, Washington. Chester Dale Collection, 1962.*

Obesity and Dieting

Symptoms
- weight approximately 20% or more above normal (see charts)

Description

Obesity is an extremely common problem in industrialized nations. Although most people think of obesity primarily in terms of its esthetic and social effects, its physical and psychological effects are even more serious. There is increasing evidence that obesity leads to, or aggravates, a wide variety of serious illnesses, including heart disease, adult-onset diabetes, gallstones, osteoarthritis, and complications of pregnancy. It has long been known on the basis of actuarial tables that obesity significantly lowers life expectancy. In the past, it was thought that this effect was only demonstrated when obesity was greater than 30%, but more recent studies have shown that life expectancy is actually longest at 10%–20% *below* the average weight as shown in most tables.

Obesity is not the simple disease it was once thought to be. At this point, doctors debate whether obesity is a disease in itself, or a symptom of many diseases that have a variety of causes. The definition of obesity has varied throughout medical history, but basically it refers to a situation in which an individual has a greater than normal amount of fat or *adipose tissue*, the result of which is a significant impairment of health.

441

Desirable Weights for Men and Women According to Height and Frame, Ages 25 and Over

HEIGHT (IN SHOES)*	WEIGHT IN POUNDS (IN INDOOR CLOTHING)		
	Small Frame	Medium Frame	Large Frame
Men			
5′ 2″	112–120	118–129	126–141
3″	115–123	121–133	129–144
4″	118–126	124–136	132–148
5″	121–129	127–139	135–152
6″	124–133	130–143	138–156
7″	128–137	134–147	142–161
8″	132–141	138–152	147–166
9″	136–145	142–156	151–170
10″	140–150	146–160	155–174
11″	144–154	150–165	159–179
6′ 0″	148–158	154–170	164–184
1″	152–162	158–175	168–189
2″	156–167	162–180	173–194
3″	160–171	167–185	178–199
4″	164–175	172–190	182–204
Women			
4′10″	92– 98	96–107	104–119
11″	94–101	98–110	106–122
5′ 0″	96–104	101–113	109–125
1″	99–107	104–116	112–128
2″	102–110	107–119	115–131
3″	105–113	110–122	118–134
4″	108–116	113–126	121–138
5″	111–119	116–130	125–142
6″	114–123	120–135	129–146
7″	118–127	124–139	133–150
8″	122–131	128–143	137–154
9″	126–135	132–147	141–158
10″	130–140	136–151	145–163
11″	134–144	140–155	149–168
6′ 0″	138–148	144–159	153–173

* *1-inch heels for men and 2-inch heels for women.*
Note: Prepared by the Metropolitan Life Insurance Company. Derived primarily from data of the Build and Blood Pressure Study.

Estimating obesity: For 18-year-old males the standard is 15%–18% of total weight as body fat, and for 18-year-old females, it is 20%–25% of total weight as body fat. Since accurate measurements of body fat require sophisticated equipment, obesity is generally estimated from weight standards that are adjusted for body size. Two methods are commonly used to estimate obesity: relative weight and body mass index. *Relative weight* is defined as the actual body weight divided by the desirable weight for a person of medium frame, as given by the Metropolitan Life Insurance Company. The term "desirable weight" is based on the weight that has been found to have the lowest mortality for a given height (see chart). *Body mass index* is defined as a person's body weight in kilograms divided by their height in meters, squared $(w/h)^2$. Both relative weight and body mass index correlate roughly with health risk and longevity. Relative weight is an easy index for people to derive from charts, while body mass index is a more cumbersome but more precise measurement, and is therefore used in studies. Another way of estimating obesity is measuring skin fold thickness with calipers. Generally, the measurement used is the skin thickness over the triceps, the muscle at the back of the upper arm.

Based on body weight and skin fold measurements, a significant percentage of Americans are obese: at least 20% of middle-aged men and 40% of middle-aged women. Since individuals generally tend to put on weight as they grow older, the percentage of people who are overweight rises with age, peaking at around age 50. This is thought to be due to the fact that people require less calories as they grow older because they tend to be less active, but they do not decrease their calorie consumption. On the average, with each decade, the daily caloric requirement for maintaining a given weight drops 43 calories per square meter of surface area in men, and 27 calories in women.

Researchers have identified two types of obe-

sity: lifelong obesity and adult-onset obesity. *Lifelong obesity* applies to people who are heavy as children, gain significant weight during puberty, and continue to gain weight as they enter middle age. In most cases, people with lifelong obesity are fat in their limbs and their trunk. These people actually have a greater than average number of fat cells, and their fat cells tend to be larger than average. People with lifelong obesity have a difficult time losing weight, and they tend to put weight back on easily. *Adult-onset obesity*, which is much more common, applies to people who maintain a normal weight until they are over 20, but then begin to gain weight. These people tend to put on weight mostly in their abdomen, so this type of obesity is often referred to as *middle-aged spread*. People with adult-onset obesity have a normal number of fat cells, but their fat cells are larger than normal. In general, they do not tend to be as obese as those people who have been overweight all their lives. Moreover, they tend to have an easier time losing weight when they alter their diet and exercise patterns, and they are more successful at keeping their weight down after dieting.

New studies have shown that the location of excess fat on a person's body is an important predictor of the health hazard of obesity. Fat cells around the waist or abdomen are more active metabolically, and are therefore more dangerous than those on the thighs, buttocks, and limbs. As a result, researchers have developed a *waist to hip circumference ratio* to use as an index of the hazards of excess fat.

The causes of obesity: Obesity has many causes, including genetic, social, environmental, and exercise factors. Only in infrequent cases is obesity due to endocrine or physiological problems. In terms of social and cultural factors, it has long been recognized that the society a person lives in has a profound effect on patterns of obesity.

For example, a 1965 study found that lower-class women had the greatest percentage of obesity. People's food habits are profoundly affected by the advertising and cultural norms to which they are exposed. Key elements in the general development of obesity in our society are the great value placed on high-calorie foods, the use of many labor-saving devices, and the increasingly sedentary life-style most people lead. To put it simply, we eat foods that are too fattening, and we exercise too little.

The most important factor affecting obesity is *nutrition*. Striking examples of the link between dietary habits and obesity have been demonstrated by an animal experiment that studied the effects of different diets on animals who had the same genetic weight tendencies. A study on rats showed that the diet that most increased the weight of rats from all genetic backgrounds was a diet that was high in sugar, high in fat, and varied, a combination which the researcher, Anthony Sclafani, termed *the supermarket diet*. The diet consisted of human foods such as salami, cheese, peanut butter, chocolate chip cookies, bananas, marshmallows, and chocolate milk. The rats had at least seven different foods available at all times, including normal rat chow, and the menu was changed frequently. Interestingly, the rats got only 3% of their calories from the rat chow. Rats on the supermarket diet gained 269% more weight in two months than did a control group that was fed only rat chow. Rats that were genetically resistant to obesity went from 10% to 14% body fat on the supermarket diet, while obesity-prone rats went from 13% to 40% body fat. Such obesity is referred to as *palatability obesity*; it is caused by the fact that animals (and humans) sometimes eat more food simply because it tastes so good. Culturally, modern humans are much like supermarket-fed rats, in that they have ready access to a wide variety of high-sugar, high-fat foods. As obesity researcher Albert Stunkard notes, such a diet can make any animal fat, and any fat animal

fatter still. Anthropologists speculate that early humans evolved to handle a diet very different from the one that most people currently eat (see p. 91).

New studies have shed striking light on the relationship between *genetics* and obesity. A study of adopted children in Denmark has shown a clear relationship between the body mass index of adopted children and their natural parents, and little relationship between the children and their adoptive parents. This careful study points up the great signficance of genetics in relation to all degrees of obesity. However, not all people with the genetic tendency for obesity are doomed to be overweight. Studies of genetically obese animals have shown that obesity is greatly increased when an animal is fed a high-fat diet, whereas animals with the same background did not become fat on a balanced diet. Researchers conclude that people with obese genetics need to be careful about their diet in order to avoid becoming overweight.

People with a genetic predisposition to gain weight probably have the ability to produce a greater than average number of fat cells, and have a less efficient metabolism for processing fat. There used to be a prevailing view that the number of fat cells was fixed fairly early in life, hence the concern over keeping babies from becoming fat in the first year or two of life. Now some researchers believe that the number of fat cells can increase throughout life. No definitive studies have yet proved one point of view or the other.

Another factor in obesity lies in why some people continue to eat, while others become satiated and stop. There are several theories about why some people are unable to stop eating. Many researchers believe the body has a regulator or "thermostat," referred to as the *body weight set point*. This theory is based on the fact that people's weight often increases or decreases, but then levels off. Researchers believe that dietary set points may interact with people's ability to refrain from eating when they do not physically need the food. Some scientists attribute overeating to chronic stress of any kind. They believe that stress actually affects the brain's hypothalamus by producing an excess of the neurotransmitter *dopamine*, which causes people to overeat. This theory has been supported by a study which found that animals who underwent frequent tail-pinching became obese. One psychological theory holds that obese people respond abnormally strongly to food stimuli, and weakly to internal satiation cues. Finally, some psychologists believe that the cycle of being overweight and dieting acts as a kind of chronic stressor that puts the body out of balance in relation to its weight-control thermostat, so that people feel hungry all the time.

Physical activity has a direct correlation with obesity because activity uses calories. All studies show that obese people are less active than thin people, but current data suggests that exercise by itself does not produce significant weight loss. A regular exercise program will only account for up to 5% weight loss, or .3 pounds per week. Moreover, in terms of weight, the beneficial effects of exercise stop as soon as the exercise stops. This fact can be discouraging to people who are trying to lose weight. It is important to realize that the beneficial effect of exercise is long-term: while exercise only helps people to lose small amounts of weight, it definitely helps to prevent people from gaining weight as they grow older. Finally, exercise is especially important for obese people because they are at much greater risk for heart disease.

It would appear that the cause of obesity is probably a combination of genetics, number of fat cells, exercise habits, diet, and psychological inability to restrain one's food urges. In summary, one might say that modern humans are like rats on the supermarket diet who are having their tails pinched all the time, while being forced to diet against the urges of their own thermostat.

Health effects of obesity: Striking evidence has emphasized the negative effects of obesity. The National Institutes of Health, at a 1985 conference, concluded that obesity is clearly associated with high blood pressure, high blood cholesterol levels, adult onset diabetes, and a high incidence of certain types of cancer. Probably the most important of these is the link between obesity and coronary artery disease—obesity being associated with all five major risk factors for heart disease (see p. 260). A person who is obese is 2.9 times as likely to have high blood pressure, and 2.1 times as likely to have high cholesterol. An obese person is also 2.9 times as likely to develop *diabetes*. In fact, obesity is considered to be the single largest cause of adult-onset diabetes, because people who are genetically prone to diabetes cannot sustain the chronic overproduction of insulin required by excess fat cells. Among men, obesity is associated with higher mortality rates from cancer of the colon, rectum, and prostate. Among women, it is associated with higher mortality rates from cancer of the breast, uterus, gallbladder, and ovaries.

Obesity also correlates with a number of less common medical conditions. Gout and osteoarthritis, especially of the spine, are more common and more severe among obese people. Gallstones, a fatty liver, and general gastrointestinal discomfort are all strikingly related to obesity, because in people who are overweight the bile

Increased Chance of Death Due to Obesity in Men 20% Overweight	
CAUSE OF DEATH	PERCENT INCREASED RISK OF DEATH
Heart disease	18–28%
Stroke	10–16%
Cancer	0–5%
Diabetes	100%
Digestive diseases	25–68%
All causes	20%

from the gallbladder becomes supersaturated with cholesterol. Also, gallstones tend to become worse when people chronically gain and lose weight, because cholesterol is released from fat cells as weight is lost.

Each of the diseases associated with obesity has an adverse effect on longevity, and these effects are additive. Convincing evidence to this effect has come from the highly regarded 30-year follow-up Framingham Study and a huge study by the American Cancer Society that dealt with over 1 million men and women, as well as from a number of major insurance studies. All the results point to the fact that the more overweight people are, the greater their chance of dying prematurely. The mortality rates rise with each percent a person is overweight and each year a person remains overweight. The Build Study, a large-scale insurance study, found that people whose weight was 125% of the desirable at 15–39 years of age had 10% greater than normal rate of mortality during the next five years. After 15–22 years, the mortality rates among people who had been at 125% of the desirable weight were 69% higher than normal. On the average, people at 145% of the desirable weight have an average mortality that is more than twice as high as people who are not overweight. The negative effects of obesity are not immediately apparent, but they accumulate inexorably. However, insurance studies do show that longevity quickly approaches normal when obese people diet and achieve the desirable weight for their height and build.

Due to the excess mortality associated with obesity, the National Institutes of Health consensus panel recommended weight reduction for any person with a weight 20% above the desirable, or for any man with a body mass index above 27.2 and any woman with a body mass index above 26.9. Analysis of the mortality-versus-weight chart included here shows that the optimum longevity rates are achieved at 85%–95% of desirable weight. This fact has led

How Mortality Increases with Increases in Weight	
PERCENT OVERWEIGHT	PERCENT INCREASED RISK OF DEATH
−20%	0–10%
−10%	−10– 0%
10%	7–13%
20%	10–25%
30%	30–42%
40%	36–67%
50%	50–100%

some researchers to state that the so-called desirable weights are not as desirable as they should be. It also shows that it is clearly beneficial for people to lose weight even if they are between 105%–125% of their desirable weight.

The NIH consensus panel defines four categories in terms of importance of losing weight. The first category, *lifesaving*, applies to anyone who is twice their desirable weight, or anyone 100 pounds or more overweight. The second category, *recommended*, applies to anyone that is 120% or more of the desirable weight. The third category, *highly desirable*, applies to people who are 105%–120% of the desirable weight and who also have hypertension, high blood triglyceride or cholesterol levels, or diabetes or a family history of diabetes (including women who developed gestational diabetes or even had a baby that was large for gestational age). The fourth and last category is *helpful*. It includes people who are 105%–120% of the desirable weight and have heart disease, gout, or osteoarthritis.

Self-Care

Dieting is perhaps the most common self-care treatment of any kind. Over the last hundred years, numerous diets that have been set forth in magazines and books have become popular for a time, only to be succeeded by new and more "effective" diets. In addition, various diet pills, health spas, and weight watching organizations have claimed to yield good results over the years.

From a medical standpoint, the most highly recommended self-help for the average, slightly obese person involves a diet that lowers the daily intake of calories until it is below the amount of energy the person expends each day. Because so many people have little or no success dieting, doctors have come to recognize that something more than a list of low-calorie foods is needed. Behavior modification techniques and exercise recommendations have therefore been added to many of the self-care regimens for dieting. In recent years, support groups have become a popular aspect of the fight against obesity.

From a medical standpoint, diets can be divided into two groups: diets that simply restrict calories and diets that structure meals and the circumstances under which they are eaten. The first group has been referred to as *the substitution* or *"the eat-less-of-everything"* type of diet. This kind of diet is balanced in terms of the normal amounts of protein, carbohydrates, fats, and vitamins that are recommended for a given height, but they use foods that are low in calories and they often decrease portion size, and/or the number of daily meals or snacks. By eating 500 calories less than required per day, a person will lose one pound per week. Likewise, eating 1,000 calories less will lead to a loss of two pounds per week. To use this basic type of diet, people find out what their ideal weight should be, and set the discrepancy between their actual and ideal weights as their goal for weight loss. After deciding how much weight they want to lose per week, they then select a balanced diet that will add up to the number of calories needed to create the necessary daily deficit. As an alternative to estimating the necessary calorie deficit needed, people can simply go on a daily diet of 800–1,500 calories, which will produce a moderate weight loss for the average person. To ac-

Guide for Losing Weight

- eat fewer total calories: in general, 100 extra calories a day over a long period gains 1 pound per month, 10 pounds per year
- eat smaller portions; don't eat seconds
- substitute low-calorie foods for high-calorie foods
- rid the house of junk foods
- have available low-calorie snacks such as carrots, celery, fruits, and unbuttered popcorn
- avoid sugary or fatty desserts such as cakes, pies, and ice cream
- use low-fat or non-fat dairy products instead of regular ones
- remove fat from meat, skin from poultry
- avoid fatty, marbled meats such as duck, goose, frankfurters, sausage, and regular hamburger
- avoid butter, oil, shortening, lard, mayonnaise, and fat
- avoid fried food, cream sauces, chocolate, alcohol, non-dairy creamers, and most packaged meals
- keep an honest food record for 1 week
- check the foods you eat against a calorie list
- exercise at least 3 times a week; avoid long sedentary periods

tually follow this type of diet, people have to reduce their food intake and/or alter the type of foods they eat (see p. 105).

From a medical point of view, a well-balanced, calorie-restricted diet is the optimum way to lose weight because it has the least negative medical side-effects. It also has the advantage of easily being modified into the lifelong maintenance habits that people need to establish in order to prevent regaining weight after they have achieved their ideal weight. Unfortunately, a calorie-restricted diet is very difficult for the average person to stick to because monitoring calories and portion size is tedious and difficult, and the variety allowed in this type of diet is tempting. In addition, these diets assume a degree of behavioral control that is often a problem for an obese person. As a result, people are often initially successful with a calorie-restricted diet, but unsuccessful in the long run.

Because the "reasonable eating approach" has failed so often, a number of *structured diets* have been designed to overcome the shortcomings of diets that are simply calorie-restricted. Structured diets prohibit certain food items or are so highly regimented that people are given little or no choice in what they eat. In some of these diets, there is no limit on portion size, but the foods allowed are repeated so often that people naturally cut down the amount they eat. Human and animal studies have shown that obese subjects lose weight much more rapidly on restricted diets than do non-obese people on the same diets. One can speculate from this that the people who were overweight were generally more tempted by variety and palatability than were their more slender counterparts.

The majority of structured diets are nutritionally unbalanced and are not suitable for long-term use. The ones that are most unbalanced are the so-called "crash diets" that are designed to be followed only for a certain number of days or weeks. One subgroup of this category, the *high-protein, low-carbohydrate diet*, causes a natural water loss which leads to a dramatic temporary weight loss that is reversed as soon as people go off the diet. Structured diets are often fairly effective, at least in the short run, due to their lack of variety, lack of palatability, and simplicity. It is important that people realize that there is nothing magic about such diets—like a well-balanced diet, they cause weight loss simply by restricting calories. Structured diets vary widely in how dangerous they are and how long they can safely be adhered to.

The most extreme of the structured diets are the *fixed-composition liquid formula diets* which are so unpalatable and boring that studies show that the majority of both people and experimental animals lose weight on them. Many of these nutritional formulas are completely unbalanced nutritionally and can be dangerous if they are not monitored by a doctor. Similarly, extended *fasting* can be dangerous. Although many people have fasted for varying periods without harm, there are uncommon life-threatening side effects that can occur with extended use of unbalanced formulas or fasting. After a relatively short time on a strict water fast, the body begins to break down the protein from muscle cells for energy. This throws people into negative nitrogen balance, which can cause their heart to go into fibrillation. In addition, fasting and unbalanced formulas can lead to vitamin and potassium deficiencies. Deaths have been reported when these techniques have been used without proper medical supervision.

Second to dieting, exercise is the most important component of most weight-loss plans. Although exercise by itself does not cause a significant weight loss, over a long period exercise does help to keep people from exceeding their calorie requirements, and studies suggest that exercise decreases appetite. The activities that cause the greatest calorie expenditure are jogging, walking, swimming, bike riding, and aerobic workouts. These are also the types of exercise which are of greatest benefit in terms of cardiovascular fitness (see p. 112).

Behavior therapy is playing an increasing role in weight-loss regimens and can increase the effectiveness of a good diet and exercise program. A typical behavior program involves a number of aspects: self-monitoring, stimuli control, developing of self-control, reward, changing beliefs, and reducing stress. *Self-monitoring* involves having people keep careful records of when and what they eat. Although boring, this technique vastly increases people's awareness of their food consumption, which is almost always something of a shock. To achieve *stimuli control*, diets may recommend limiting the amount of tempting, high-calorie foods that are kept in the house, and putting any remaining ones out of sight. Also, the diet may restrict people to eating only at the table, and in some cases only from one plate or bowl, in order to break compulsive-eating habits and reinforce good ones.

To help in *developing self-control*, many diets suggest techniques such as chewing each mouthful a certain number of times, or putting eating utensils down between bites. The goal is not only to slow down the rate at which people eat, but to make them savor what they do eat. Some diets stipulate that at designated intervals, such as when a specified weight loss has been achieved, people should give themselves a pre-arranged, nonfood *reward* in order to motivate and reinforce their weight loss. The point of *changing beliefs is* to help people identify their negative thoughts about weight loss, and then to consciously counter them with opposing arguments whenever such negative thoughts arise. Some diets have plans for *reducing stress* by doing relaxation exercises and restructuring key stress situations (see p. 60). The goal is to relieve the need to eat as a means of feeling good.

In recent years, a number of weight-loss *support groups*, such as Weight Watchers and TOPS (Take Off Pounds Sensibly), have been organized to help people stay on their diet until they achieve their desired weight loss, and to help maintain their goal weight thereafter. People pay a registration fee, set a weight loss goal, and then attend weekly meetings to chart their weight and have supportive discussions. These groups work very well for people who faithfully stick to the program, but like all other diet plans, they have a definite drop-out rate.

The Doctor

Surprisingly, obesity is the fifth most commonly diagnosed disease and is among the top 20 reasons that people consult a doctor. Currently, many doctors and clinics have well-designed weight-loss programs that involve diet, exercise, and various behavioral techniques. As discussed, medical supervision for dieting should be sought by anyone who has a serious medical condition or is very overweight. A supervised program often helps to keep a dieter on track, much like a support group, as well as provide an authoritative structure. Well-managed medical programs have the highest success rate in treating moderate obesity.

In addition to the conservative dieting methods discussed above, doctors can safely supervise very low-calorie diets and modified fasting diets. These diets can lead to significant, short-term weight loss, and are often prescribed by doctors when individuals are way above ideal weight. People are put on a high-protein, very low-calorie diet that uses natural foods or food supplements; then they are carefully monitored as to weight loss, blood pressure, and blood levels of potassium, sodium, etc. These plans result in an average loss of three pounds per week for women, and two pounds per week for men. Generally, such plans are not recommended for people who are not severely obese. Like any diet, these plans will ultimately fail if they are not succeeded by a well-balanced maintenance diet that involves a moderate calorie intake.

Currently, amphetamine-type *diet pills* are not recommended by most doctors. Their use is controversial; they do not produce permanent weight loss, they can be addictive, and they have other significant side effects including insomnia, agitation, excitement, tremor, and headache. Although some doctors do prescribe diet pills for selected patients for a short time, the trend is definitely away from their use.

In cases where obesity is life-threatening, as a last resort a doctor may prescribe a surgical procedure in which part of the small intestine is by-passed so that food absorption is minimized. This operation is recommended only for people who weigh more than twice their ideal weight and have not been able to successfully follow any other dieting regimen.

Ruling Out Other Diseases

Over 99% of all cases of obesity are *essential*; that is, they are caused by a combination of genetics, overeating, lack of exercise, and the temptation of a wide variety of foods. However, a very small number of cases—under 1%—are caused by, or associated with, endocrine diseases and metabolic conditions such as *thyroid disease*, (see p. 389) and *adrenal disease*. These diseases have other symptoms in addition to obesity and can generally be identified from abnormal values on a panel of blood tests.

Prevention

Obesity is best prevented by lifelong good nutritional habits, a well-balanced diet, and regular exercise. Such a goal is not always easily attained when people live in a rich society that spends billions of dollars to advertise high-fat, high-calorie foods (see p. 95). Doctors increasingly feel that good nutrition starts at the beginning of life—and even earlier, with the mother's diet during pregnancy. It is now believed that to a large extent the number of fat cells in a person's body is determined in the first several years of life. Healthy eating habits in the first few years of life and health education at school can do much to counter the high-sugar, high-fat diet that is constantly presented to the public in this country.

The Department of Health and Human Services now advises a national goal of weight management for life. In particular, it is recommended that people avoid the type of obesity referred to as middle-aged spread. Gaining 10 pounds a decade is not a normal part of growing older; it is the result of a mixture of diet and exercise habits that are ultimately unhealthy. Regular exercise can prevent a gain of .3 pounds per week without any change in food consumption, which amounts to 15 pounds per year. The best way to avoid middle-aged spread is a combination of a moderate diet and regular exercise. Not only will this prevent obesity, it will help to prevent a number of other serious medical conditions.

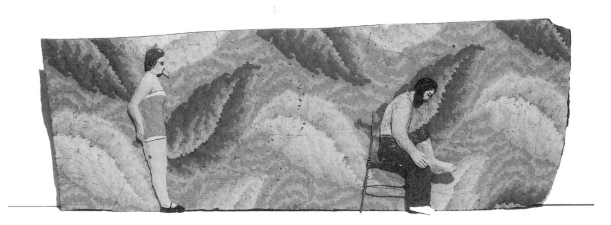

Symptoms

incomplete blockage
- difficulty breathing—ranging from near normal to very labored
- noisy breathing—gurgling, wheezing, etc.
- ability to cough and talk
- skin may start to turn blue

complete blockage
- inability to talk, cough, or breathe
- person may point to or hold throat
- person rapidly loses consciousness, can't be aroused
- no sign of breathing:
  chest or abdomen doesn't rise and fall
  air is not moving in or out of the mouth or nose
- skin turns blue

Description

Airway obstruction or blockage of the airway is a MEDICAL EMERGENCY that requires immediate treatment. To sustain life, the brain and heart need a constant supply of oxygen. To prevent death or permanent brain damage from occurring, a blocked airway must be cleared within *three to four minutes*. The sooner the blockage is eliminated, the less likely damage is to occur.

Choking takes place when a large object gets caught in the *pharynx*, the area where the back of the mouth joins the windpipe. People usually choke on food; in particular, large pieces of un-chewed meat. Although small amounts of liquid or crumbs can cause prolonged coughing and inability to catch one's breath, they will not ac-tually block the windpipe. Airway obstruction most often occurs in elderly people, especially those who wear dentures, and in people who are eating while inebriated. Once people start to choke, they usually become very frightened and agitated. If people are eating, food obstruction should be suspected first, although it is possible that the symptoms could be those of a heart at-tack (see p. 284) or, more rarely, a drug overdose.

If people can cough and speak, their airway is only partially blocked. Although very upsetting, this is not an immediately life-threatening situa-tion. With incomplete blockage of the airway, there may be either good or poor air exchange. People with good air exchange can produce a forceful cough even though they may make wheezing noises between coughs. However, a choking person can progress from good to poor air exchange or vice versa, and should be watched closely until the object is removed. Peo-ple with poor air exchange have difficulty breathing; they exhibit a weak, ineffective cough; and they make gasping, wheezing, or gurgling sounds. Often they make high-pitched crowing noises when they inhale, and they may start to turn blue around their lips, inside of their mouth, fingernails and skin.

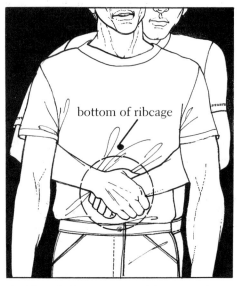

To do the Heimlich maneuver without causing internal injury, the rescuer's hands must be positioned across the middle of the belly, well below the victim's breastbone.

If the airway is completely blocked, people are unable to cough or talk at all. In this situation, people almost always grasp their throat, either in a reflexive gesture of distress or in a conscious effort to alert those nearby. Unlike people with a partial blockage, they will not exhibit any breathing sounds such as gurgling or wheezing. They will also not make any breathing motions in the chest or abdomen, and no air will move in or out of their nose or mouth. Lack of oxygen will cause their skin, lips, and fingernails to turn blue. If efforts to remove the blockage are not successful, a choking person will lose conscious-ness rapidly and die within minutes.

Self-Care

To assess whether the blockage is partial or complete, the choking person should be asked to speak or cough forcefully. If the person can do this, the obstruction is not complete and he or she should be encouraged to continue coughing. Often, coughing will dislodge the object. The person's efforts should not be interfered with and a Heimlich maneuver should *not* be attempted at this time (see below).

If chokers show signs of complete blockage or a partial blockage with poor air exchange as indicated by a weak cough, the American Heart Association recommends doing the *Heimlich maneuver*. This procedure, which doctors used to refer to as *abdominal thrusts*, is designed to force a large burst of air out of the lungs. Essentially, it produces an artificial cough when the choking person is unable to. The helper stands behind the choker and slides his or her arms around the choker's waist. Making a fist with one hand, the helper puts the thumb side of the fist against the middle of the choker's belly, slightly above the navel and well below the tip of the breastbone (see illustration). It is very important *not* to press on the ribs or bottom of the breastbone because it can cause serious internal damage. With the free hand, the helper pulls the fist sharply back and up, with "piston-like upward thrusts." Each thrust should be made with the intent of dislodging the obstruction immediately. The Heimlich maneuver should be repeated until the blockage is dislodged.

If the choker is an infant, a small child, a pregnant woman in the third trimester, or a markedly obese person, the helper should press his or her fist straight back against the middle of the breastbone. In either case, the fist should *not* be thrust against the bottom of the breastbone or the bottom of the ribcage because this can break ribs and/or damage the liver. If choking people happen to be alone, they can do a manual thrust on themselves by pressing their own fist into their abdomen with a quick upward thrust, or by leaning forward and pressing their abdomen sharply against a bedpost, chairback, or railing.

If efforts at the Heimlich maneuver fail and the choker loses consciousness, then the helper or another person should attempt to remove the blockage using a finger. Grasping the victim's tongue and chin with the thumb and forefinger of one hand, the rescuer opens the victim's mouth wide. This maneuver clears the tongue away from the blockage. Next the rescuer should insert the index finger of the other hand into the victim's mouth, sweeping down one cheek then deep into the throat at the base of the tongue, *taking care not to push the blockage further down*. With a hooking action, the rescuer should attempt to sweep the blockage up into the victim's mouth.

Next the rescuer should open the victim's airway and attempt rescue breathing. To do this, the unconscious person should be laid on the floor, and his or her head tilted back by pushing down on the forehead and lifting up on the chin, which will straighten out the airway (if the victim has been in an accident and appears to have a neck or spinal injury, the rescuer should simply grasp the back of the victim's jaw on either side and lift the jaw forward and up, while the head tilts backward). Then the rescuer should use the hand that was on the forehead to pinch the choker's nose closed, take a deep breath, hold it, and with mouth wide open, seal his or her mouth around the victim's mouth and blow air into the victim's mouth. In quick succession, the rescuer should blow air into the choking person's mouth 2 times for 1–1½ seconds each. If air can be gotten past the blockage, the victim can be kept alive (see p. 458).

If the rescuer has still not been able to dislodge the blockage, the emergency steps should be repeated in the same order: (1) *6–10 Heimlich maneuvers in a row*, (2) *a finger sweep*, and (3) *rescue breathing*. To do the Heimlich maneuver on an unconscious person, the rescuer kneels next to the person's thighs and positions the heel of one hand above the victim's navel, but below the ribcage, then puts the heel of the other hand on top of the first, and presses into the abdomen with a quick, upward thrust. The steps should be repeated as long as necessary, and a second person should *call 911* for help, if possible. Although severe choking is not that common, these steps save many lives every year.

If a rescuer initially finds the victim unconscious, and the cause is unknown, he or she must establish whether the person has simply fainted, is having a heart attack, or is choking. The first step is to try to arouse the person by yelling at or tapping on him. If the person is unresponsive, the rescuer should call for help, and then straighten out the person's airway using the head-tilt chin-lift procedure described above. If the victim does not make breathing motions and/or sounds, the rescuer should try rescue breathing. If air does not inflate the victim's chest, another effort should be made to straighten the person's airway, and rescue breathing should be repeated. If air still does not pass, 6–10 Heimlich maneuvers should again be done in rapid succession, followed by a finger sweep and rescue breathing, and then the whole series repeated until help arrives.

The techniques described here in *Self-Care* constitute the respiratory part of *Adult Basic Life Support*. Although they require no equipment or extensive training, these simple, effective techniques can save lives. Basic Life Support can be done from these instructions, which were derived from the American Heart Association Guidelines, but it is much better to learn the skills in a brief instructional course that involves hands-on practice with mannequins. Such courses are given frequently by local fire departments, the Red Cross, and other community organizations. It is estimated that almost 3,000 people a year die of choking. Although this figure does not approach the number that die of heart attacks annually (650,000), it is still a significant number.

The Doctor

In addition to doing Basic Life Support techniques, an *Emergency Medical Technician*

(EMT) working in conjunction with a doctor can perform *Advanced Life Support* techniques, which require medical equipment and training. Advanced techniques should not be attempted by untrained people because in some cases it might make the situation worse. For untrained people, the most important thing is for them to act quickly when a choking person has poor air exchange, and to persist in their efforts until help arrives.

An EMT will assess the victim's breathing and continue basic life support techniques. In addition, an EMT is trained to use an airway, portable suction units, and oxygen to assist the person's breathing once the object is removed. If the object cannot be removed, but the person can be kept alive, a doctor can perform a *cricothyrotomy*, a procedure in which an incision is made directly in the windpipe below the level of the blockage.

Ruling Out Other Diseases

A number of conditions other than choking can cause people to stop breathing—including *heart attack* (see p. 284), *stroke, electric shock, drowning,* and *drug overdose*. If witnesses are present, some of these conditions can be ruled out. If the victim is unconscious, attempts to open the airway and blow air into the lungs will immediately establish whether the airway is blocked. If the airway is not blocked, the rescuer should begin *cardiopulmonary resuscitation* if necessary (see below).

Prevention

Most choking incidents occur during eating. Often they involve gristly or stringy pieces of meat. As stated, choking is more likely when people wear dentures and/or are inebriated. Choking can be prevented by cutting food into small pieces and chewing them thoroughly. Excessive alcohol intake should be avoided before and during meals, and people should avoid laughing or talking while chewing.

Cardiopulmonary Resuscitation (CPR), or Basic Life Support (BLS)

When to Use CPR

- person is unconscious, doesn't respond to questions
- person is not breathing
- person's heart may not be beating
- person may have experienced a heart attack, stroke, drowning, drug overdose, or electric shock

Description

Cardiopulmonary resuscitation (CPR), or *basic life support* (BLS) is a system that has been devised to externally support breathing and blood circulation in an emergency until medical help arrives. It is a technique that can potentially save hundreds of thousands of lives, because almost 1 million people in the U.S. have a heart attack each year. Heart attacks are the number one medical emergency in this country: 350,000 die annually—outside the hospital— within two hours after experiencing heart attack symptoms. A grossly irregular heart rhythm, called *ventricular fibrillation,* is the cause of most of these deaths. In this situation, the heart muscle itself may only be minimally damaged and the person could recover if kept alive by means of medical intervention. Ventricular fibrillation can occur without heart attack symptoms, in which case it is referred to as *sudden death.* Although sudden death victims do not experience heart attack symptoms, they do have

coronary artery blockage. Studies have demonstrated that as many as 40–60% of people who experience ventricular fibrillation *outside* the hospital could be saved each year by prompt CPR.

If CPR were immediately available, 100,000 to 200,000 lives per year would be saved in the U.S. alone. This represents such a significant public health advance that the American Heart Association has encouraged CPR to be taught widely to lay people in every community, especially to those people who know someone with a heart condition. CPR is a physical skill that should be learned and practiced in a recognized course. It cannot be overemphasized how valuable this training is, even if it only has to be used once in a lifetime. In an emergency, basic life support measures can be performed from the instructions below, which are based on the American Heart Association's 1986 Guidelines (see chart and illustrations), but they do not serve as a substitute for proper training.

Self-Care

In an emergency, CPR should be started as soon as possible and the steps should be done in the proper order. The less time that elapses before CPR is started, the better the person's chances of surviving without permanent injury. Once breathing stops, brain damage or death occurs in four to six minutes.

The first step is to determine whether or not CPR is needed. If a victim has apparently sustained a head or neck injury, do not move him or her unless absolutely necessary. Tap the person and ask loudly if he or she is all right. A person will respond or move unless unconscious. If the victim doesn't respond, ask for additional help if someone is available. Position the person on his/her back on a flat hard surface and follow the *ABCs of cardiopulmonary resuscitation: airway, breathing, and circulation.*

Opening the airway: Opening the airway is the

Basic-Life Support Steps

1. Does the person respond to question, "Are you o.k.?"
2. If not, call for help immediately.
3. Unless the person has sustained serious trauma to the head and neck, position the person on his/her back on a firm, flat surface.
4. Kneel at the person's shoulders.
5. Open the person's airway by pushing the forehead back and lifting the chin (see illustration).
6. Place ear over the person's mouth and watch the chest to determine if there is breathing.
7. If not, perform rescue breathing; inhale, seal your lips around the person's mouth, pinch the person's nose closed and blow in. Repeat.
8. Now check for pulse in neck (see illustration).
9. If person is still unresponsive, get help if it has not already been summoned.
10. Chest compression: locate correct hand positions on person's chest (see illustration), lock elbows, and press the sternum down 1½ inches to 2 inches. Perform 15 chest compressions in a row, at a rate of 80–100 per minute (a little over 1 per second).
11. Open the airway and deliver two more rescue breaths.
12. Repeat cycles of 15 chest compressions, followed by 2 rescue breaths, 4 times.
13. Check for return of pulse. If absent, continue rescue cycle. If pulse is present, check to see if person is now breathing. If he or she is breathing, stop rescue efforts but continue to watch the victim. If the person is not breathing but has a pulse, continue rescue breathing alone.

Source: Adapted from the "Standards and Guidelines for Cardiopulmonary Resuscitation."

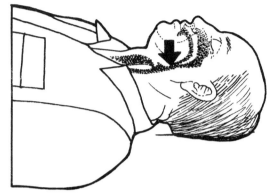

The most common reason an unconscious person is unable to breathe is that the airway is blocked by the tongue. Pushing down on the victim's forehead and lifting up on the chin opens the airway. Opening the airway should always precede mouth-to-mouth breathing.

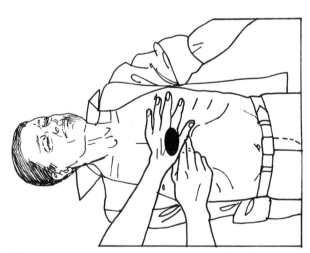

To prevent injury, it is very important that the rescuer's hands be correctly positioned on the victim's breastbone before starting chest compression. Chest compression is most effective when the rescuer is positioned directly over the victim's chest, with arms straight.

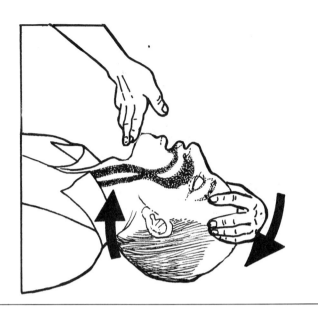

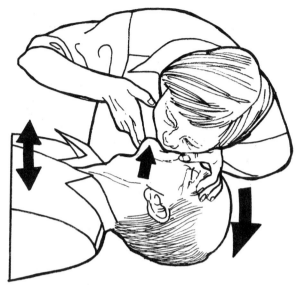

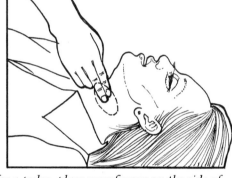

To check for a pulse, place your fingers on the side of the victim's neck, in the groove between the windpipe and the muscles of the neck. Press lightly to avoid compressing the artery and temporarily shutting off the pulse.

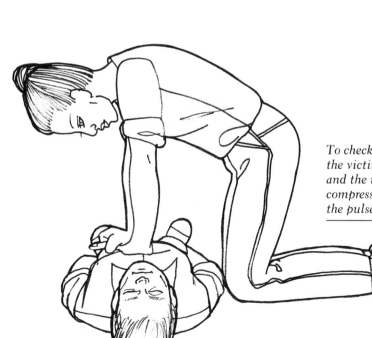

most important part of CPR. When a person loses consciousness, the jaw muscles relax and the tongue may fall into the back of the throat. The airway being blocked by the tongue is the most common reason that an unconscious person is unable to breathe. To open the airway, place one hand on the person's forehead, and apply firm backward pressure to tilt the head back. Place the other hand under the bony part of the chin, supporting it and lifting it slightly so the teeth are nearly together. This position straightens out the airway and ensures that the tongue is not blocking it. A head-tilt chin-lift maneuver should not be attempted if there is any question of a neck or spinal injury, as in an accident. In this case, the rescuer should kneel at the top of the victim's head, and leaning on his or her elbows, put a hand on either side of the victim's chin and push the jaw open to make mouth-to-mouth ventilation possible.

The next step is to determine whether or not the person is breathing. While maintaining the open airway position, the rescuer puts an ear next to the person's mouth to listen for breath sounds and feel if air is moving; at the same time the rescuer watches the victim's chest and abdomen to see if they are rising and falling.

Mouth-to-mouth breathing: If the victim is not breathing the rescuer must give *mouth-to-mouth ventilation* to keep the person alive. To do this, the rescuer should use the thumb and index finger of the hand on the forehead to gently pinch the victim's nose closed. Then the rescuer should take a deep breath, hold it, and with mouth open very wide, seal his or her lips around the other person's, and blow air into the victim's mouth. In quick succession, the rescuer should blow in two full breaths, each lasting 1–1½ seconds. After each breath, the rescuer should break contact with the person's mouth to take in another breath and to allow the victim to passively exhale. With each breath, the rescuer should watch to see if the person's chest is actually rising. If the first two breaths do not cause

the chest to rise, the rescuer should reposition the person's head and try again. Improper positioning of the chin is the most common cause of problems in rescue breathing. If the second attempt is not successful, the rescuer should check for an obstruction in the throat, and apply the Heimlich maneuver and a finger sweep if necessary (see p. 452).

When two breaths have successfully inflated the lungs, the rescuer should maintain one hand on the victim's forehead, but remove the other hand from the chin, and, using the index and third finger, feel for a pulse in one of the carotid arteries that lie to either side of the Adam's apple, between the windpipe and the muscles of the neck. This should be done with very little pressure since pushing too hard can actually compress the artery and temporarily stop the pulse. Since this step can be difficult, it is most effectively done if practiced in a course.

Calling for help: When the rescuer has established the presence or absence of breathing and pulse, 911 or the local emergency phone number should be called to request trained emergency help. The dispatcher at the emergency number will want to get a brief description of the

---

First Aid for Drowning

1. Get victim out of water; use a flotation device if available.
2. If possible, start mouth-to-mouth breathing even before getting to shore (see Basic Life Support chart).
3. Check neck for pulse. If pulse is absent, start chest compressions and continue rescue breathing.

Note: Experts do not advise trying to get water out of drowning victims. This can be dangerous for them, and they do not actually inhale much water.

Source: Adapted from the "Standards and Guidelines for Cardiopulmonary Resuscitation."

situation, including whether the victim has spontaneous breathing and a pulse, and a complete address with any special instructions about finding the exact location. If the rescuer is alone, he or she should make the phone call either after the pulse check or after doing CPR for one minute. If a phone is not close by or the interruption would take more than 30 seconds, the rescuer should simply maintain CPR efforts and yell for any nearby help that might be available.

Artificial circulation or external chest compression: Artificial circulation involves making the heart pump by rhythmically pressing on the lower part of the victim's *sternum,* or breastbone. Properly done, chest compression can circulate the blood, producing a carotid pulse and a blood pressure as high as 100/40. This pressure is not as high as the normal blood pressure of 120/80, but it maintains sufficient blood flow to the brain to prevent damage.

Chest compression is best done with the victim lying back down on a firm surface such as the floor or the ground. The victim's head should not be higher than the feet. If possible, someone should place a small pillow or object under the victim's heels. The rescuer should kneel to the side of the victim's chest. Using the index and middle fingers of the hand nearest the victim's feet, the rescuer should locate the bottom of the victim's ribcage, then slide up to the center notch in the ribcage where the ribs meet the breastbone (see illustration). Holding the middle finger in the notch and the index finger on the sternum, the rescuer positions the free hand across the victim's chest—with the heel of the hand on the middle of the victim's breastbone, and the thumb of this hand touching the index finger of the lower hand. The correct position enables the rescuer to press on the victim's chest without lacerating the liver with the bottom of the breastbone, and is least likely to crack the victim's ribs.

The rescuer's lower hand is now removed from the notch, and the heel is placed on top of the heel of the other hand. The fingertips of both hands should be pointing directly away from the rescuer. The fingers may lie on top of each other or be interlaced, but they should be lifted slightly off the victim's chest to prevent unnecessary injury.

To make the compressions most effective, the rescuer must not only position the hands correctly, but have his or her body in the right position to press directly down on the victim's chest. With arms straight and elbows locked, the rescuer leans slightly forward, with shoulders directly over the victim's breastbone. In this position the rescuer presses straight down with sufficient force to compress the victim's chest 1½"–2" or 4–5 cm (less for a child) for less than half a second. Then the rescuer releases the pressure completely for a similar interval so that the heart can refill with blood. Care should be taken not to change the position of the hands or bend the elbows. Chest compression should be repeated in a smooth regular rhythm at a rate of 80–100 compressions per minute (see below).

The rhythms for mouth-to-mouth ventilation and chest compression are completely different depending on whether there are one or two rescuers. Two-person CPR is much more effective because there is no break in chest compressions or the delivery of oxygen through mouth-to-mouth ventilation, but two-rescuer CPR is now recommended only for professional rescuers and EMT workers. One-rescuer CPR is the only type recommended for lay people. A single rescuer has to do both rescue breathing and artificial circulation alternately.

One-rescuer CPR: The rescuer does 15 chest compressions at the rate of 80–100 per minute ("1-and, 2-and, 3-and . . . 15-and"). At that point the rescuer repositions hands on the victim's forehead (nose) and chin and gives two quick breaths, 1½ seconds each, not allowing the victim's lungs to deflate completely in between. Without pausing, the rescuer immediately starts another set of 15 chest compressions.

After four rounds of ventilations and compressions, the rescuer stops to determine if a carotid pulse is present and to see if the victim is making spontaneous breathing motions. Ventilation and compression should never be discontinued for more than seven seconds. Most victims will not evidence spontaneous breathing or a pulse, and generally the rescuer will need to maintain CPR efforts until medical help arrives. In this case, a check for pulse and breathing need only be done every few minutes.

When CPR is done in real life, not in a classroom, it is a frightening, upsetting, and messy situation. Everyone feels a sense of panic, there is frenetic activity on every side. The victim looks terrible and often vomits. The reality of the situation may be so overwhelming as to hamper the efforts of an untrained helper, which is another reason why CPR instruction is of such importance.

The Doctor

Generally an emergency medical technician (EMT) will be the first medical person to see the victim. The EMT has the necessary training and equipment to perform advanced life support techniques. He or she will be in radio contact with a doctor who determines what medications and treatment should be given.

When heartbeat and breathing stop because of cardiac arrest, basic CPR will keep the victim alive, but specialized medical care is generally necessary to restore spontaneous heartbeat and breathing. First the EMT will rapidly assess the situation by asking the rescuer questions and checking the victim over. Emergency personnel will have oxygen, masks, and special airway tubes that will enable them to give the victim more oxygen.

Depending on the medical services available, the victim may be hooked up immediately to an electrocardiogram to monitor heart rhythm. An intravenous line will likely be started so that emergency medication can be given if necessary. There are a variety of drugs that can be used to correct arrhythmias, strengthen heartbeat, and correct pH imbalances. If necessary, at some point the EMT or a doctor may give the victim a brief electroshock to start the heart beating again. At the hospital, the person will be treated in the Emergency Room and taken to an Intensive Care Unit when stabilized. X-rays will be done to determine if any ribs were cracked during CPR efforts.

Ruling Out Other Diseases

By far the most common reason for people to go into cardiac arrest is some form of *heart disease* (see p. 255). Other causes include *drowning*, *electrocution*, *drug overdose*, and *accidents*. Drowning and electrocution are usually obvious. Bruises on the face or head may indicate a head, neck, or spinal injury. If the arrest is caused by airway obstruction (choking), artificial ventilation will not be effective until the obstruction is cleared (see p. 451). Heart disease or drug overdose will be definitely established by tests at the hospital.

Prevention

Most heart disease can be prevented early on through life-style changes that include a low-fat, low-cholesterol diet, not smoking, treating high blood pressure, getting regular exercise, and learning stress reduction techniques (see p. 60). Drowning and electrocution are often avoidable by taking appropriate safety precautions in situations involving electricity or water.

CPR training is the most important second line of defense in preventing death due to cardiac arrest. Ideally, every person should have a well-formulated plan for such emergencies, taking into account the local community resources.

People should know the early signs of a heart attack and who to call in case of emergency. This is especially crucial if a family member has heart disease or is at risk (see p. 260). Even when people are not sure if it's a true emergency, it is better to call an EMT, who is trained at evaluating medical situations and has the backup of a doctor.

Cuts, Abrasions, Puncture Wounds, Nosebleeds, Bleeding Under the Fingernail or Toenail, and Burns

Description

Soft tissue injuries are among the most common accidents that happen to adults. Although *scrapes* or *abrasions* are generally the most minor of this group, large abrasions can be uncomfortable and result in big scabs that take as long as a cut to heal. Whereas abrasions merely scratch the surface of the skin, *cuts* or *lacerations* go through the skin, and in more serious cases can even involve underlying tissues and structures. *Puncture wounds* can also be very deep, although they involve only a small opening on the skin. *Animal* or *human bites* constitute a special type of cut or puncture wound. In addition to the cut itself, they are of concern because of the possibility of infection, tetanus, or rabies. Infection is more likely if a wound is very dirty. Ironically, human bites are more likely to cause infection than animal bites, because people are more susceptible to human bacteria, and the mouth is a fertile breeding ground for germs. Rabies is very rare in the U.S. at this point, with

only one to two human cases per year. The chances of tetanus are more likely if a wound is contaminated with soil. Fortunately, most people in the U.S. receive tetanus immunization before they are two years old as part of the DPT series. This immunization requires a booster every 10 years, but is routinely given after only 5 years if a person has a serious wound or one that is contaminated with dirt.

How much a wound bleeds depends on several factors. Some areas of the body, such as the scalp, have more capillaries than others; these tissues can bleed profusely even though a wound is minor. The amount of bleeding also depends on the depth of the cut and its proximity to veins or arteries. Generally cuts are minor, but even when they are more serious, almost all bleeding can be stopped or controlled with direct pressure on the wound.

Nosebleeds are caused either by a blow to the nose or irritation of the thin, vascular lining of the nasal passages. Although nosebleeds can cause profuse bleeding, they can usually be stopped readily with pressure. Bleeding that results from injuring a *fingernail* or *toenail* is similar to a bruise in that the blood is trapped under the skin. The nail not only prevents blood from getting out, it doesn't stretch like skin in response to the pressure from swelling. This lack of elasticity, in conjunction with many nerve

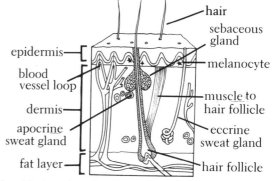

The skin has three layers. Burns are categorized by the number of layers they affect.

endings under the nail, can cause this type of injury to be very painful; fortunately however, it is easily treated (see below).

Burns, which are less common than cuts, can be caused by heat or by caustic chemicals. Burns are serious if they are deep or cover large areas of the body. Doctors classify burns according to their depth. A *first-degree burn* is superficial, involving only the top layer of skin (see illustration). The burn appears red or pink, swells, and is painful. A *second-degree burn* involves the top two layers of skin, but does not affect underlying tissues. It causes blistering, a red or mottled appearance, and more significant pain. A *third-degree burn* involves all three layers of skin and can affect underlying structures. Third-degree burns can be less painful than second-degree burns if they destroy nearby nerve endings. Third-degree burns look similar to second-degree burns, but have areas of charred black or white as well.

Self-Care

Soft tissue injuries must be evaluated to see if they need to be seen by a doctor. If not, they can be dealt with at home. Proper first-aid will help to prevent infection and speed healing.

Abrasions: Like any open injury, an abrasion should be flushed or soaked with copious amounts of cool water. If foreign matter remains in the scrape, it should be gently removed with a clean washcloth, and the wound should be rinsed again. Strong soaps and skin disinfectants like iodine should not be used because they can irritate or damage the tissue. However, many doctors recommend applying *1% hydrogen peroxide* because its foaming action helps to remove dirt and clotted blood. If a significant amount of foreign matter cannot be removed, the abrasion should be seen by a doctor. A clean abrasion can be left open to the air, or it can be covered with gauze if it is likely to get dirty. Some doctors advise applying an antiseptic ointment, such as

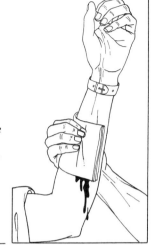

Almost all bleeding can be stopped with direct pressure. A sterile dressing or clean cloth should be pressed firmly and continuously against the wound until bleeding stops.

Bacitracin or *Neosporin*. These preparations are not only antiseptic, they may make the scab more comfortable by keeping it soft. An abrasion should be checked occasionally during the first 24 hours. If signs of infection such as pus, swelling, heat, or severe redness develop, the abraded area should be soaked in warm water or covered with warm washcloths for 15-minute intervals, three times a day. Because hot soaks increase circulation which brings in more white blood cells, they are amazingly effective at clearing up infections. However, if a person develops a fever, significant pus, or red streaks leading away from the wound, he or she should see the doctor.

Cuts: Cuts are generally more upsetting than abrasions because they bleed more and they may require stitches. With cuts, the first step is to stop the bleeding by covering the wound with sterile gauze pads and applying constant firm pressure for 5–30 minutes, as necessary. If the bleeding is significant, the pressure should not be relieved and the dressing should not be removed until the bleeding appears to stop. If such pressure is applied firmly for a long enough time, it will stop all but the most severe bleeding. If necessary, extra dressings can be applied on top of the initial ones and pressure can be maintained while the person is taken to the doctor. For lacerations that are serious or even for those that may possibly be, emergency help should be summoned by calling 911. In this case, continuous pressure should be maintained and the injured area should be elevated above the person's heart if possible. Tourniquets are no longer recommended because they can cause severe damage if not used correctly.

Once the bleeding has stopped or slowed, the laceration or cut can be evaluated. The treatment of a cut depends on how deep it is, where it is located, and how dirty it is. If the cut doesn't go through all the layers of skin, it can simply be cleaned and carefully bandaged in the same manner as an abrasion. If signs of infection develop after a day, the cut should be treated with warm compresses or soaks for 15-minute periods three times a day.

If a cut goes through all skin layers, it may gape enough to require stiches, and it can affect underlying structures. If the edges of the cut do not stay together easily, or if the cut is on the person's face or across a joint, it should be seen by a doctor to determine whether stitches are necessary or preferable. Stitches have advantages and disadvantages. They are not crucial for healing, but they hold the edges of the cut together, resulting in a narrower scar that can heal more quickly. The face has many vulnerable structures, and plastic surgery stitches can minimize scarring. Since lacerations near joints are subject to tension every time the joint is moved, stitches prevent the wound from reopening and thereby speed healing. Wounds should be sutured within six hours after the injury takes

place. Generally, after more than six hours have elapsed, the wound should be kept open and draining due to the possibility of bacterial infection. If a flap of skin or the end of a finger is actually cut off, the severed part should immediately be put in a clean plastic bag, put on ice, and rushed with the person to the doctor. Often the flap or part can be sewn back on.

If the edges of a cut can be kept together with an adhesive bandage, a butterfly bandage, or a steristrip, it's better to avoid stitches because they also act like a foreign body and can delay healing. A small cut that goes through the skin but does not involve underlying structures or lie near the face or a joint, can be washed carefully and taped shut with an adhesive bandage or an improvised butterfly bandage (see illustration).

Signs of a more serious laceration are profuse bleeding that doesn't respond to pressure (possible lacerated blood vessel), numbness or tingling past the wound (possible nerve damage), or difficulty moving fingers or toes (possible injured tendon). Any of these situations should be evaluated by a doctor. Likewise, any deep wound in the back, chest, or abdomen should be seen by a doctor because of the possibility of damage to internal organs.

Punctures: Most puncture wounds are minor and generally affect the hands or feet. Puncture wounds involve some special considerations. First, if a puncture wound is deep, or is located on the head, abdomen, or chest, underlying structures may have been damaged. This possibility is suggested by profuse bleeding or tingling, or by difficulty with movements in the affected area. Second, cleaning the wound is

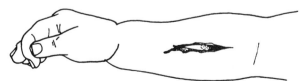

If a cut gapes, it should be evaluated by a doctor to see if stitches are advisable.

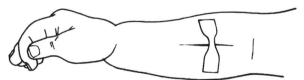

Sometimes the edges of a cut can be kept together with a butterfly bandage or a steristrip.

very important in order to prevent infection, which is somewhat more likely than with a simple cut because puncture wounds are often hard to clean and they tend to close up, which prevents them from draining. Minor puncture wounds on the feet should be rinsed thoroughly and allowed to bleed for several minutes in order to wash out any dirt or foreign matter. Puncture wounds on the hand should be seen by a doctor because infections of the hand can be difficult to treat.

To prevent infection, the wound should be soaked in warm water for 15 minutes, three times a day, for three to five days. Soaking helps to increase circulation, keep the wound open, and maintain drainage to remove germs naturally. It is common for puncture wounds to become slightly red and tender after 24 hours. A fever, swelling, severe redness, or pus are signs of a more serious infection, in which case the doctor should be seen.

Bites: Animal bites constitute a special type of puncture wound, or cut. Provided the animal has known rabies immunization, the bite will be treated like other cuts, although special emphasis should be put on cleaning the wound properly and soaking it three times a day thereafter. With an unprovoked attack by a wild animal or an unfamiliar animal that escapes, the doctor should be seen and the possibility of rabies immunization considered if the animal can't be located and certified as healthy.

Nail injuries: When a blow or severe pinch causes *bleeding under a finger- or toenail* to occur, treatment is often necessary to relieve the pain. If the finger or toe does not look broken and can be moved (see p. 469), the injury can often be treated at home. Immediate relief will be provided by making a small opening in the nail itself. This can be done by heating a straightened paper clip until it's very hot, and then holding the heated end against the nail bed above the discolored area (see illustration). Because it's hot, the paper clip should be held with

If a blow causes bleeding under a nail, the pressure can be relieved by making a tiny hole in the nail with a paperclip that has been heated.

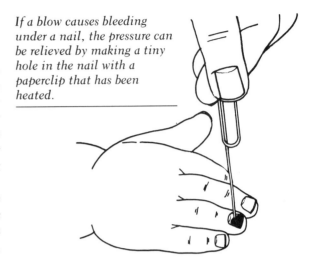

pliers. Only slight pressure should be applied against the nail; when the paperclip is through the nail, the blood will spurt out by itself. If necessary, the paper clip can be reheated and reapplied. The procedure shouldn't hurt (except for pressure) because the nail has no sensation, and the skin underneath is protected by the pool of blood.

Nosebleeds: Spontaneous nosebleeds can almost always be dealt with at home. If there is no question of head injury, all that's necessary is to stop the bleeding with sustained direct pressure on the cartilage at the bottom of the nose. Often nosebleeds are stubborn and require three to five minutes of firm pressure before clotting takes place. A doctor should be seen if a person has recurrent nosebleeds or high blood pressure.

Burns: Minor burns, that is, first-degree and small second-degree burns that are less than two inches by two inches, can usually be treated at home. Second-degree burns that are large or are located on the face or hands should be treated by a doctor because they can result in problematic scarring. Third-degree burns should always be treated by a doctor due to concern about infection as well as scarring.

The immediate treatment for any burn is to immerse the area in very cold water. The in-

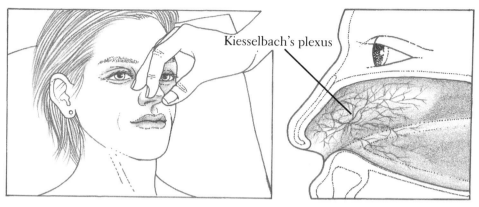

Kiesselbach's plexus

Most nosebleeds occur in Kiesselbach's plexus, an area of the cartilage at the bottom of the nose. Direct pressure, applied for up to 5 minutes, will stop almost any nosebleed.

crease in the temperature of the skin and underlying tissues caused by the burn can persist for up to 45 minutes after the flame or hot object has been removed, unless some cooling action is initiated. During this time, the damage being done by the heat will continue and will injure more cells. Any burn should be immersed in cold water for a minimum of 5–10 minutes, and for as much as 60 minutes. Ice cubes should not be used because they can actually cause frostbite if applied for long intervals, but the water should be changed when it begins to warm up. If the water feels very uncomfortable, the person can remove the burned area from the water for short periods. When the injured area can't be immersed, cold wet towels or a bag of ice water should be applied to it. Butter, petroleum jelly, or anesthetic sprays should not be applied because they can increase the chance of infection if the burn is open; however, once the burn no longer needs a dressing, nonprescription *aloe cream* or *Vitamin E oil* can be applied and may lessen scarring.

Often a person can't distinguish a first-degree from a second-degree burn for several minutes until blisters form. Blisters should not be removed because, in effect, they constitute a sterile dressing and help to prevent infection. Any large burn should be kept cool while the person is transported to the doctor. *Acetaminophen* (e.g., *Tylenol*) or *aspirin* can be taken for pain.

The Doctor

For soft tissue injuries, the doctor does additional first aid if necessary, assesses the severity of the injury, determines whether there is damage to underlying structures, and decides what treatment should be given. The doctor will also give a tetanus booster if the person has not had one for ten years; for a dirty injury or a deep puncture wound, a booster is given after five years.

Abrasions: The doctor is only necessary if the wound can't be cleaned, if there is a question of damage to underlying structures, or if the wound appears to be getting infected. For a large, dirty abrasion, the doctor may give a local anesthetic before cleaning the wound with a high pressure stream of water or a brush, and then will apply an antibacterial ointment and a dressing. If an infection develops, antibiotics will be prescribed and a culture may be done. X-rays will be taken if there is any question of a broken bone.

Lacerations: First the doctor will make sure the bleeding is under control. In addition to elevating the wound and putting direct pressure on it, for severe cuts the doctor can use a blood pressure cuff as a tourniquet, administer drugs that constrict the blood vessels, and tie off a torn vein or artery if necessary. The doctor will determine if any major blood vessel, tendon, or nerve has been affected, and flush any foreign bodies from the wound with saline solution (mild salt water). The area around the laceration is generally shaved to prevent infection and to make it easier to suture or tape the wound.

If sutures (stitches) are necessary, the doctor will inject a local anesthetic (e.g., *lidocaine*) into the edges of the wound with a very thin needle. The anesthetic rapidly takes effect and generally only the first injection is a little uncomfortable. For a large laceration, the doctor may do a *nerve block*, injecting the anesthetic around the major nerve that leads to the area. If the edges of the wound are rough or there is dead tissue around the edges, the doctor may trim them so the wound will heal with less scarring. Depending on how deep the laceration is, the doctor will either put in sutures or hold the sides together with a steristrip (clear reinforced tape that is held in place with an adhesive). Sutures are put in with a small curved needle, and are knotted off individually. The number of stitches does not affect the speed of healing, since the wound basically heals from side to side. For a laceration on the face or hands, very fine thread and many stitches may be used in order to minimize the degree of scarring.

For the first 48 hours, a large wound should be kept dry and clean until the initial healing has taken place. Depending on the location, a laceration may be left open to the air or be covered with a dressing that will not adhere to the wound. Exposed lacerations should be cleaned two to three times per day with *dilute hydrogen peroxide* to prevent infection. In some cases, an antiseptic cream such as *Bacitracin* is also applied. Any signs of infection should be reported immediately to the doctor (see chart).

Skin sutures are not dissolvable, and must be removed after four to eight days. The exact timing depends on where the laceration is. Although doctors often check on wound healing when the stitches are removed, they sometimes allow people to remove their own stitches if the

Signs of Infection in a Cut or Burn
• increased redness
• increased heat
• increased swelling
• increased pain
• red streaks
• pus
• swelling of nearby lymph nodes

laceration is small and uncomplicated. To do this, the sutures should be pulled up away from the skin with tweezers, and cut off close to the skin on one side. Once the cut is made, the sutures can be pulled out with a gentle tug. This procedure usually does not hurt, but may be made easier if any scab is removed with hydrogen peroxide first. The scar from a laceration generally flattens out after three months and loses its redness within three to six months.

Puncture wounds: Although shallow puncture wounds on the feet, legs, or arms generally don't need to be seen by a doctor, deep puncture wounds or any puncture wound on the hands, face, or torso should be seen. The doctor will examine the wound to rule out underlying damage, and with a hand puncture, will prescribe antibiotics to prevent infection. Animal bites, in particular, will be flushed out thoroughly. Antibiotics are given for either human or cat bites because both types have a high risk of infection. In general, bites are left open or are loosely sutured in order to allow drainage and lessen the risk of infection. If there is a risk of rabies, the person will be given a rabies immunization series.

Bleeding under the nail: Although pressure can be relieved at home, many people are not comfortable relieving the pressure by themselves. The doctor uses a dental hand drill or a needle to make a hole in the nail, and may give a local anesthetic to relieve the pain caused by pressing on the nail. If a break is suspected, the doctor will x-ray the finger, and splint it if necessary.

Nosebleeds: A nosebleed that can't be stopped with direct pressure, or a recurrent nosebleed, should be seen by a doctor. Often the doctor will reattempt direct pressure first. If this fails, the doctor will apply a medicated compress that will shrink the blood vessels in the area. The doctor may also coagulate the torn capillaries with a drop of *silver nitrate solution,* or cauterize them electrically. If this is not successful, the nostril will be packed with *petroleum-impregnated gauze* to apply pressure.

Burns: First the doctor establishes the extent and degree of the burn. For minor burns, the doctor will cool the area if this has not already been done, and apply antibacterial ointment. A small third-degree burn will be treated with one of several more powerful antibacterial agents (e.g., *1% silver sulfadiazine cream*), and then covered with nonadherent gauze. The dressing should be changed every four to five days. Oral antibiotics may be given to prevent infection. For larger burns, the doctor will recommend keeping the area elevated or in a sling. If a large area has second- or third-degree burns, the person will be hospitalized in order to give intravenous fluids and antibiotics. If necessary, skin grafting will be done.

Before changing a dressing on a second-degree burn, people should wash their hands to lessen the chances of infection. If the dressing sticks to the wound, the area can be soaked in warm water for a few minutes. Once the bandage is off, the area should be cleaned with warm, soapy water, and patted dry with a clean towel. The doctor should be called if there is pus, swelling, or increased redness. Provided there is no sign of infection, the burn should be covered with an antibacterial cream and a new dressing.

Ruling Out Other Diseases

With many soft tissue injuries, *broken bones* have to be ruled out as well (see p. 469). It is especially important to rule out head or spinal injuries before beginning first aid. This is best done by a trained person who can be reached by calling 911 or the local emergency number. Head or spinal injuries are most likely in the event of a motor vehicle accident, a fall from a great height, a blow to the head, or if there are lacerations about the face.

Prevention

A significant number of accidents are preventable. Many are due to inattention caused by stress or haste. This is only common sense—everyone can recall injuring themselves because of hurrying, being upset, or being too tired.

Other important causes of accidents are unsafe working conditions, dangerous habits, or faulty tools. Common examples are leaving boards on the ground with nails sticking out or leaving pot handles sticking out on the stove. Knives should always be used carefully; fingers should be *behind* the blade, no matter what the task. Like cuts, burns often take place in the kitchen. Proper care (as well as potholders) should always be used during cooking tasks at the stove or the barbecue.

The most severe cuts and abrasions occur in auto accidents. An enormous percentage of these injuries could be prevented simply by wearing seat belts. Also, people should not drive after drinking or when sleepy.

Keeping up to date on tetanus immunizations and pets' rabies shots can prevent the possibility of these infections following a laceration or puncture wound.

Bruises, Sprains, Dislocations, Fractures, and Head Injuries

Description

Adults get musculoskeletal injuries most often during sports activities or accidents. The variety of injuries and areas injured are numerous, but in general, the greater the force with which the injury takes place, the more likely a fracture or bad sprain will occur. When either muscles or bones are hurt, many nearby blood vessels are damaged and the resultant bleeding causes bruising and swelling. The swelling in turn puts pressure on nearby nerves and can cause considerable pain.

Musculoskeletal injuries: In the case of a *fracture*, a bone is either broken or cracked. With a *simple fracture*, the skin is unbroken; with a *compound fracture*, which is much less common, the skin is broken. This is much more serious because the chances of infection are much greater. With an *undisplaced fracture*, the normal anatomical configuration of the bone is maintained. With a *displaced fracture*, the bone fragments are separated enough to make the bone appear visibly misshapen. Several other terms apply to fractures: *angulated* refers to a displaced break which produces an obvious bend, while *comminuted* refers to a fracture in which the bone is broken into more than two pieces.

A *dislocation*, though painful, does not involve any broken bones; rather, the bones that meet at a joint are out of alignment. Under great force, bones can actually separate or pop out of the *joint capsule*. Often there is damage to the *ligaments*, the fibrous bands that attach one bone to another and hold the joint in place. An incomplete dislocation is often referred to by doctors as a *subluxation*.

The most common musculoskeletal injuries are sprains and strains. *Sprains*, like dislocations, involve damage to ligaments. In the case of a sprain, the joint is not dislocated, but a ligament is torn. There are three grades of sprains: mild, moderate, and severe. With a *Grade 1 sprain*, there is a minor, incomplete tear of a ligament, resulting in pain and tenderness in the joint, along with minimal swelling and discoloration, or bruising. In a Grade 1 sprain, there is no abnormal slackness when the joint is moved. With a *Grade 2 sprain*, there is a more significant, but incomplete tear of a ligament. Swelling, discoloration, and pain are more pronounced, and the joint has excessive mobility when moved. With a *Grade 3 sprain*, the ligament is torn completely, so the joint opens or moves past its normal range. A *strain*, by comparison, is a partial or complete tear of a muscle or *tendon*, a fibrous band that connects a muscle to a bone. Like sprains, strains are graded 1, 2, and 3, depending on the degree of tearing involved.

Head injuries: Blows to the head generally don't cause fractures, but they can cause serious internal damage. A *concussion* is defined as any shock to the brain that causes grogginess or loss of consciousness. A concussion can be as mild as a bump that makes a person momentarily woozy, or as serious as a blow that causes a person to lose consciousness for a period of time. Generally there is some loss of memory around the time of the accident.

A *simple concussion* causes no permanent damage to the brain—it just briefly lowers the functioning of the *reticular activating system*, the portion of the brain that maintains consciousness. With a simple concussion the symptoms are worst right after the accident, and improve progressively thereafter. In a more severe injury, called a *contusion*, the brain is actually bruised and internal bleeding puts pressure on the brain because the skull cannot expand. Such internal bleeding and swelling is not apparent on the outside, but can be determined on the basis of other symptoms. The symptoms of a contusion are more severe than those of a concussion; they do not improve right away and may even worsen (see p. 472). In some cases, bleeding does not occur immediately, but begins within a day after the accident. The most common type of slow bleeding takes place under the membrane that surrounds the brain; it is referred to as a *subdural hematoma*. In this case the symptoms may not be apparent immediately after the accident, but will become more pronounced in the hours following the accident (see section on *Self-Care*).

Self-Care

Minor sprains and strains can be treated at home, but if great force was involved and it's likely the injury is a severe strain or sprain, and there is obvious looseness in the joint, the doctor should be seen. Likewise, with a dislocation or an obvious fracture, the doctor should be seen. Often it is difficult to tell a sprain from a fracture or dislocation because a minor sprain can have as much swelling, discoloration, and pain as a minor fracture or dislocation. If there is any doubt, it is best to have the injury looked at.

Fractures: Fractures require medical treatment. Any suspected fracture should be seen by a doctor. Several signs indicate a possible fracture. A *cracking sound* may occur at the time of injury and/or grating noises, called *crepitus*, may occur when the broken bone is moved. There may be an obvious *deformity* in the bone—a difference in size, shape, or length which is readily seen in an arm or leg if it is compared with the opposite side. There may be significant *swelling, tenderness*, and *pain*. Usually the pain is severe with a break, and the bone is "point tender" right over the fracture. *Motion may be limited*, and moving the bone may cause pain.

Unless the spine, head, or rib cage is involved, most fractures are not a medical emergency in the sense that time is critical.

Immediate treatment is important if there is a serious laceration, an open fracture, numbness (nerve damage), or the possibility of damage to an artery (paleness and coldness of an affected limb). Injuries to the pelvis or thigh can involve significant internal bleeding and should also be seen by a doctor quickly. A severely angulated break should be straightened before it's splinted to prevent nerve or artery damage, but this is best done by a trained person who has proper splinting equipment. For any of these more serious conditions, local emergency help should always be summoned.

If a fracture is suspected, the most important thing is to take the time to immobilize the bone,

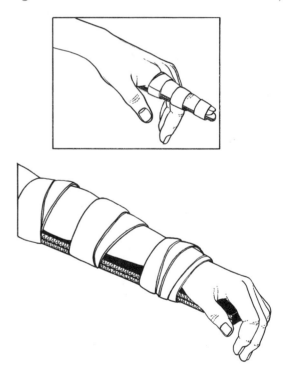

Rigid splints can be made from a tongue depressor (finger-size), several layers of cardboard, or rolled newspaper or magazines. A rigid splint prevents movement of a broken bone and makes a person much more comfortable while being transported to the doctor.

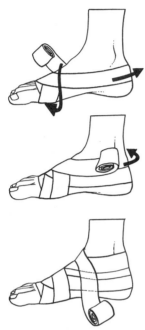

A sprained ankle should be iced, wrapped with an elastic bandage, and elevated.

both to prevent further injury and to make the injured person more comfortable while being transported to the doctor. Most of the pain following a fracture is associated with moving the injured bone. An untrained person can put a homemade splint on an uncomplicated fracture and take the injured person to the doctor, although some people may be more comfortable calling the local emergency number for help. EMTs are trained in evaluating and splinting suspected fractures, and have special splints for different parts of the body.

Splints can be made with rolled newspapers or magazines, boards, canes, umbrellas, kitchen utensils, etc. The splint must be long enough to immobilize the joints *above* and *below* the fracture. A rigid splint should be wrapped with gauze or a towel to soften it. To put the splint in place, the bone should be supported on both sides of the break. Either gauze or tape can be used to hold the splint in place. Injuries of the shoulder are usually put in a sling; breaks of the upper or lower arm are splinted and then put in a sling (see illustrations). Fingers are splinted

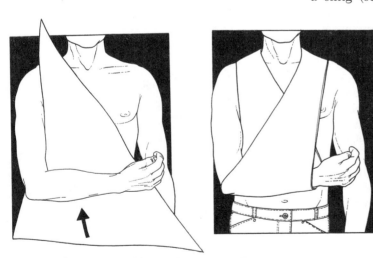
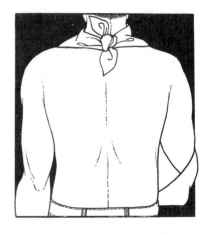

An injured arm or shoulder can be temporarily immobilized in a sling while a person is transported to the doctor. If a bone appears to be broken, a rigid splint should be applied first.

Self-Care for Sprained Ankles

For the first 48 hours:
- apply ice pack for two hours or more except for short respites; thereafter for two hours, three times a day, as necessary
- keep the ankle elevated as much of the time as possible
- immobilize the ankle with elastic bandages, and wear shoes with good support unless the doctor recommends crutches or bedrest
- take aspirin or ibuprofen (e.g., *Advil*) to reduce pain and swelling

During the healing period:
- soak ankle in warm water for 15–20 minutes three times a day
- after soaking, do ankle exercises unless painful: turn ankle in circles while lying down when the ankle can bear weight, stand on toes, then roll back on heels a number of times when you can walk, sit in a chair and "write" the alphabet with your big toe

---

with a pencil, or taped to the adjoining finger. Injuries of the lower leg or ankle are splinted. The ankle or wrist can also be soft-splinted with tape and a rolled up pillow.

Sprains and strains: Mild sprains and strains can be treated with self-help. However, if the joint is wobbly, can be moved past the normal range of motion, is obviously deformed in comparison to its counterpart, or if the pain is too severe to permit regular use, the doctor should be seen to make sure that the ligaments have not been badly torn. This is especially important with a knee or shoulder injury because ligaments are commonly torn in the knee, and the shoulder is more likely to be dislocated than are other joints.

Serious sprains and strains can be the source of more persistent discomfort than a fracture because they often are not treated seriously enough. The initial treatment for sprains and strains is covered by the acronymn *R-I-C-E: rest,* *ice, compression,*and *elevation.* Initially, the injured joint should be chilled with an ice pack and elevated above the level of the heart for at least 30 minutes to minimize swelling. If the joint is still painful, ice should be applied for 15 minutes every hour for the next several hours. If necessary, the joint should continue to be iced, elevated, and rested for two to three days. The doctor should be seen if the joint is not much better after one day.

As pain subsides, normal use can gradually be resumed. At first, an elastic bandage should be worn to give the joint support and aid healing. Care should be taken to see that the bandage is not too tight, causing pain, tingling, numbness, or coldness. Once the initial swelling is down, the joint may be soaked in warm water to promote healing. If pain returns, use should be decreased temporarily.

With all but the most minor sprain or strain, it will take one to two weeks for the joint to feel comfortable, and six to eight weeks to heal fully. Complete healing of a moderate sprain or strain is helped by appropriate exercise once movement becomes possible. Each joint has a specific set of recommended exercises. At no time should these exercises be painful. Physical therapy programs are credited as the reason why professional athletes recover from injuries as quickly as they do.

Head injuries: Most head injuries are mild and do not do any serious damage. For a mild injury in which a person does not lose consciousness and acts normally afterward, home treatment is generally adequate. An ice bag can be applied at the point of impact, and *aspirin* or *acetaminophen* (e.g., *Tylenol*) can be taken for a headache. If the blow is significant, the person should be observed for a day or so. Emergency help or the doctor should be called whenever a person loses consciousness during an accident; experiences bleeding from the eyes, ears, or mouth; or has a seizure at any time. Internal bleeding may be signalled by a number of symptoms: loss of alertness or increasing sleepiness; changes in behavior such as confusion, irritability, irrational behavior or personality changes; vomiting three or more times; a severe or increasing headache; a decrease in vision; and/or a difference in the size of the two pupils that was not present before the accident. These symptoms indicate a serious medical situation, for which the doctor should be called immediately.

The Doctor

Musculoskeletal injuries should be seen by a family practitioner or an orthopedic surgeon. The doctor will take a history, eliciting details of the injury in order to determine the intensity and direction of the forces. Then the doctor will do a physical exam, checking for misshapenness, swelling, tenderness, and excessive range of motion. The doctor will not move an obvious fracture, but will generally check for a pulse and sensation past the injured joint to be sure there is no nerve or blood vessel damage. If a sprain is suspected (especially in the knee), the doctor will move the joint through its range of motion in order to make sure there is no wobbliness in the joint.

Fractures: If a fracture is suspected, x-rays will be taken. Several views are needed because a fracture is not always visible from every angle. To make the person more comfortable, the area may be splinted before going to x-ray. If a fracture is found, it will be *reduced*, or aligned in proper position, and then casted. Appropriate pain medication is given before this is done. Most fractures can be aligned rapidly with manual traction. Currently, plaster and fiberglass casts and splints are used for fractures. The particular cast or splint chosen depends on where the break is and how serious it is.

A dislocated shoulder is put back in place with manual traction, and then the arm is put in a sling. Often severe sprains and strains are splinted as well as fractures. A cast doesn't cause healing or speed it; a cast simply holds the broken bone or torn ligament or tendon in place while it is healing. Sometimes serious tears of tendons or ligaments have to be repaired surgically.

After the fracture has been set, it is important that the person keep the area elevated in order to minimize swelling. Not only does swelling increase pain, it can slow or shut off blood flow. If there is a great deal of swelling, the cast may have to be loosened or even changed. Signs of severe swelling are blueness, numbness, coldness, and tingling of the extremities past the break, as well as constant severe pain, especially in one area, that is not relieved by the prescribed pain medication. A person with a fracture often runs a fever and is in a fair amount of pain—enough to require medication—for the first several days. Generally the doctor will prescribe *meperidine* (e.g., *Demerol*), *codeine*, or *propoxyphene* (e.g., *Darvon*) for pain, but by the third day the pain has usually subsided and the person feels much better.

Although sweating under the cast often causes itching, people are warned not to scratch the area by putting anything under the cast because this can irritate the skin or cause infection. Air can be blown under the cast with a hair dryer set on cool. Because plaster casts will weaken and dissolve if they get wet, they must be wrapped in plastic when a person showers. Fiberglass casts can be submerged in water, but they must be dried completely in order to avoid skin irritation and infection. Drying takes 30–60 minutes with a hair dryer, which should be set on "warm," because a high setting can burn the skin. The cast is dry when it no longer feels cool.

Casts are kept on for varying lengths of time depending on the break. Often the break will be re-x-rayed after several weeks and a new cast put on. Whenever the cast is finally removed, the bone is vulnerable to rebreaking for several weeks because a natural mineral loss takes place when a bone is immobilized for such a long time. Mineral is redeposited in response to the stress of normal use. If a joint has been immobilized by the cast, it will naturally be somewhat stiff, and the muscles will be weaker than normal due to lack of use, but flexibility and strength gradually returns to normal. Specific exercises may speed this process.

Head injuries: In the case of a head injury that needs medical evaluation (see section on *Self-Care*), the doctor will do a history, with particular emphasis on the length of time the person was unconscious and whether he or she experienced a seizure. The doctor will do a careful physical exam of the head, paying special attention to bruises and bumps, as well as any bleeding or fluid discharge from the nose, ears, or eyes. The doctor will also do a full neurological exam, emphasizing the person's alertness, ability to move, and pupil reactivity to light.

If the person has sustained a significant blow to the head but does not need to be hospitalized, the doctor will want the person to be observed for alertness and pupil size every 2 hours during the first 24 hours, and every 4 hours during the second 24 hours. The doctor will want to know if the person is groggy or disoriented, or if the person's pupils do not react equally to light. De-

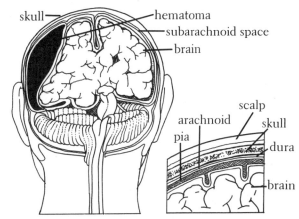

When a severe head injury takes place, there may be bleeding under the skull which puts pressure on the brain. Since the skull cannot swell, the pressure has to be relieved surgically.

pending on the severity of the blow, the doctor may or may not advise that the person be aroused from sleep to make these checks.

If the exam reveals cause for concern, the doctor will order x-rays of the head and neck for fractures. If the person had a definite period of unconsciousness, a seizure, a skull fracture, or abnormal neurological findings, he or she will be hospitalized for one to two days for close observation. The nurses will check the person's pulses, blood pressure, pupils, and alertness on an hourly basis. In most cases a CT-scan will be done to rule out bleeding under the skull. In the great majority of cases, people hospitalized for observation after a head injury get better without any problem. Occasionally, people's symptoms get worse, in which case a neurosurgeon will be called in to evaluate the situation. If a person has a subdural hematoma, surgery will be done to relieve pressure inside the skull.

Ruling Out Other Diseases

As discussed above, the doctor differentiates between a sprain, a fracture, and a dislocation on the basis of the physical exam and an x-ray. Occasionally joint pain can be caused by an *arthritis* (see p. 333), *bursitis*, or *tendinitis* (see p. 310). Usually these conditions are not associated with a specific injury, and they exhibit signs of inflammation such as redness, heat, and swelling.

Prevention

Most fractures and head injuries in the U.S. are the result of car accidents. Auto accidents account for about 50% of the annual 100,000 trauma deaths that occur each year, and are the fifth leading cause of death for 40-year-old men. Approximately two-thirds of all accidents are caused by human error, but alcohol is involved in more than half of all the fatal accidents. Seat belts are effective in preventing serious injury 42% of the time, yet ironically 98% of people killed in car crashes are not wearing their seat belts.

Athletics is another cause of musculoskeletal injuries. The people who are most likely to sustain sports injuries are those who are out of condition or are attempting sports that require great balance. Preventive measures include getting into shape with a graduated training program and using protective equipment. Accidental falls also account for a good number of fractures and sprains among adults; they are best prevented by removing environmental dangers and practicing good safety habits.

Anaphylactic Shock, Insect Stings, and Allergic Reactions

Symptoms

skin
• rash or hives
• itching
• flushing
• swelling of the eyes, lips, or tongue

respiratory
• difficulty breathing
• constriction of the throat and chest
• wheezing
• hoarseness and choking

other
• restlessness
• dizziness
• nausea, bowel cramps, and diarrhea
• unconsciousness

Description

An *anaphylactic reaction* is an extreme allergic response that causes shock-like symptoms within minutes of exposure to a substance that a person is allergic to. Such a reaction is potentially dangerous and constitutes a true MEDICAL EMERGENCY. Fortunately, most allergic reactions are not severe, and do not cause anaphylactic shock. Life-threatening anaphylactic reactions are relatively uncommon, causing less than 100 deaths per year in the U.S.—mostly in elderly people with heart conditions.

Anaphylactic shock most commonly occurs as a reaction to insect venom, food, and medications. The largest insect group that causes anaphylactic shock is *Hymenoptera*, which includes honeybees, bumblebees, yellow jackets, hornets, wasps, and fireants. Less commonly, reactions occur in response to pollens (ragweed or

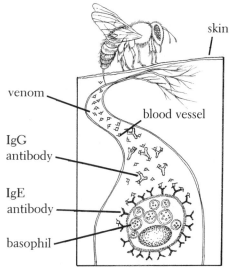

When people are stung by an insect, the white blood cells called basophils *produce an allergic reaction in response to chemicals in the venom.*

grasses) or various foods (eggs, seafood, nuts, grains). Anaphylactic shock also occurs in reaction to penicillin and other drugs, and infrequently, to the allergens in allergy shots (see p. 253).

All of these substances contain an *antigen*, a protein that causes some people's bodies to produce antibodies in response to an initial exposure. On subsequent exposure when the body picks up the antigen, it binds the antigen to antibodies on the surface of special blood cells called *basophils*. In response, the basophils release massive amounts of chemicals which cause the allergic reaction (see p. 248). One of these chemicals, *histamine*, causes smooth muscle in the throat, bronchi, and gastrointestinal tract to contract, and blood vessels to dilate throughout the body, which explains the general nature of anaphylactic symptoms.

Anaphylactic shock generally occurs within two or three minutes after exposure to a particular antigen. Symptoms can range from very mild to very severe. Mild symptoms involve the skin and are often localized; they include flush-

Drugs That Most Commonly Cause Immediate Allergic Reactions

ampicillin
corticotropin
erythromycin
penicillin
sulfamethoxazole

Foods That Most Commonly Cause Immediate Allergic Reactions

chicken
eggs
fish
milk
nuts
peanuts
shellfish
soybeans
wheat

ing and redness of the skin, itching, hives, and swelling around the eyes, lips, and tongue. Mild symptoms do not constitute a medical emergency, but in some cases they progress to more severe symptoms which involve the whole body. Severe symptoms, which are a MEDICAL EMERGENCY, include narrowing of the airway, diversion of blood from the organs, and pooling of blood in the capillaries. Respiratory symptoms cause difficulty breathing, tightness of the throat and chest, hoarseness, wheezing, and choking. Blood pooling causes dizziness, nausea, abdominal cramps, diarrhea, and sometimes unconsciousness.

It is difficult to predict the course of a reaction when it first starts, but difficulty breathing is definitely a sign of an emergency. For a person who has a history of anaphylactic reactions, even skin symptoms can be cause for concern. A study has shown that approximately 60% of people who have had a previous systemic reaction to insect stings had another systemic reaction when stung again. Contrary to popular myth, systemic reac-

tions do not necessarily get worse with each sting. Unless people have multiple stings, they tend to react as they did previously. Approximately 4% of the population has some immediate, systemic allergic reaction to insect stings, but most reactions are mild. Insect sting reactions are unrelated to other allergies, so people with allergies are not necessarily more reactive to insect bites than are nonallergic people. But like other allergies, insect sting reactions tend to be inherited and occur more often among members of the same family.

Local reactions to insect bites vary widely in degree—a small amount of swelling constitutes a "normal" reaction, whereas an allergic reaction can result in sufficient swelling to make movement difficult near the bite. As disconcerting as such a marked local reaction may be, it does not usually progress to a systemic reaction. Less than 10% of people with significant local reactions ever develop symptoms of anaphylactic shock.

Self-Care

Anaphylactic shock is a MEDICAL EMERGENCY that requires immediate treatment. Emergency help should be sought by calling 911, or the local emergency number. The person should be taken to a doctor for treatment unless they have had previous attacks and have their own emergency injectable medication (see below). Although an anaphylactic reaction needs treatment, it is rarely life-threatening if treated.

Mild reactions to insect stings can be treated at home. Local reactions should be iced as soon as possible to minimize swelling. If the bite is from a bee and the stinger is left behind, tweezers or a knife blade should be used to pull or scrape the stinger out, which will lessen the reaction. Ice should be applied over the affected area for 15–30 minutes or longer if the person is very uncomfortable or has significant swelling or pain. Calamine lotion can be applied to reduce itching (see p. 175). *Aspirin* or *acetaminophen* (e.g., *Tylenol*) can be taken to control pain, and an *antihistamine* (e.g., *Chlor-Trimeton, Benadryl*) can be taken to reduce itching and diminish the local reaction. Antihistamines should not be taken before driving because they can cause drowsiness.

The Doctor

The doctor diagnoses an anaphylactic reaction from a skin rash, swelling, and difficulty breathing following exposure to an insect bite, allergic food, pollen, or drug. The treatment for an anaphylactic reaction is an injection of *epinephrine*, which is a natural stress hormone that widens the airway and constricts peripheral blood vessels, sending blood back to the brain and heart. Epinephrine is rapidly used up by the body, and the injection can be repeated twice at 10–15 minute intervals if necessary. The doctor will also give the person an *antihistamine* shot or tablet to help reduce the local skin reaction.

In some cases the doctor may put a constriction band above the bite to prevent the antigen from spreading to the rest of the body. The band must be released for 30 seconds every three minutes to prevent permanent damage to the limb. In the rare case that a person has extreme difficulty breathing or goes into true shock and experiences a drop in blood pressure, the doctor will make sure the airway is open, give oxygen, start intravenous fluids, and sometimes administer drugs to further constrict the blood vessels and raise blood pressure. Most often, people respond well to the epinephrine and do not require further treatment.

Once people have experienced an anaphylactic reaction, they will be given an emergency kit containing premeasured doses of epinephrine. The kits often contain *ephedrine sulfate*, an *antihistamine*, and a tourniquet as well. The people will be instructed in their use and told to administer them at the first sign of anaphylactic shock. Early self-treatment will prevent a severe reaction. These kits must be replaced annually because the epinephrine loses its effectiveness.

If people have a history of life-threatening reactions or are likely to be stung in their daily activities, the doctor may recommend *venom immunotherapy*. After skin-testing to establish whether the person is truly allergic, the doctor will give weekly venom shots for six to eight weeks and maintenance shots every six to eight weeks thereafter for an indefinite period. By gradually desensitizing the individual to the venom, this program lowers people's chances of a subsequent anaphylactic reaction from 60% to 3%. Children are not usually given the series because they generally only get skin reactions.

Ruling Out Other Diseases

Anaphylactic shock is usually easy to diagnose from a history of systemic reaction immediately following exposure to an allergen. Occasionally the condition has to be differentiated from an *asthma* attack (see p. 294) or a *heart attack* (see p. 284), both of which can produce difficulty breathing. An asthma attack is differentiated by wheezing, a heart attack by chest pain. Neither of those conditions will produce a local skin reaction.

Prevention

The most successful prevention is avoidance of the allergic substance. The success of this approach varies with the allergen. Food allergens can generally be readily avoided, although certain allergic substances, like sesame seeds, are sometimes "hidden" in baked or processed foods. People who are allergic to particular drugs should always mention this fact when they see a doctor for any reason. This is particularly important if people are allergic to penicillin, because penicillin is so widely used, and can produce an anaphylactic reaction in a susceptible person.

People who are allergic to insects should avoid areas where those insects are likely to be. If nests are identified near the house, they should be destroyed. Highly allergic people might even consider removing plants and shrubs that are especially attractive to the insects. Finally, people can lessen the chance of being stung if they avoid wearing bright colors and perfumes or aftershave lotions, all of which are attractive to insects. Protective clothing such as long pants and gloves can also help to minimize the risk of being stung.

People who have had an anaphylactic reaction should always carry their emergency medical kit with them when they travel, or in any situation where they could be stung. It is also advisable for these people to carry an identification card or wear a medical I.D. bracelet, e.g. *Medic-Alert*, especially if they happen to be allergic to a drug.

Eye Injuries and Foreign Objects in the Eye

Symptoms

- pain in eye
- feeling of something in the eye
- eye appears bloodshot
- eye tears by itself
- affected eye is sensitive to light
- blood in the eye

Description

A foreign body in the eye or injury to the eye should be taken seriously because of the chance of infection or permanent damage to the eye, but generally a foreign body in the eye is a minor incident that can be dealt with at home. Most often the offending substance is dirt, dust, sand, or sawdust. Particles often lodge under the

When to See an Ophthalmologist

- there is severe and persistent pain in one or both eyes
- a foreign body cannot be removed with water or a cotton swab
- a foreign body is stuck on the cornea
- the eye has possibly been penetrated by any sharp object, even a tiny one
- the eye itself has been hit with significant force; the lid may even be swollen shut
- blood can be seen in the anterior chamber of the eye
- there is blurriness or loss of vision after the object has been removed and the tears have cleared
- the pupil doesn't close down in response to light or has an irregular shape

upper eyelid or move about. When the eye is rolled back and forth, there will be pain at some points and not at others. The pain is most intense when the cornea, the clear area over the pupil, comes in contact with the foreign body. If the object is actually stuck over the cornea, it will cause continuous pain in one place that is unaffected by eye movement. Sometimes the tears will naturally wash particles into the back of the nose (see illustration).

Eye injury can occur if the *cornea*, the clear area in front of the lens, is scratched by a foreign body in the eye (including dirt caught under a contact lens) or by a sharp object outside the eye, such as a branch, a fingernail, or a piece of paper. Even if the foreign body is washed out, the cornea may be scratched. In that case, the person will continue to feel as if something is in the eye even after the object is gone. Often a corneal abrasion is very painful and produces sensitivity to light, causing people to dim the lights or close their eye. Corneal abrasions usually heal within a week.

Occasionally metal chips from hammering or drilling penetrate the eye. If there is any possibility of a corneal abrasion or penetration, the

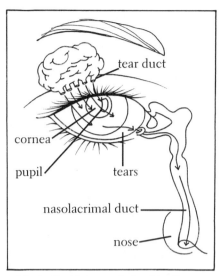

Foreign objects that become lodged in the eye are often washed by the tears down into the back of the nose.

injury should be seen by an eye doctor, or *ophthalmologist*. If there is a penetrating object, it should not be touched. The eye should be covered and the person should immediately be taken to the eye doctor.

Another type of eye injury involves a large blunt object, such as a ball, hitting the eye with real force. This often results in a black eye due to bruising, or bleeding under the skin. If the eye itself is hit, there can be bleeding in the *anterior chamber*, the area between the front of the eye and the iris (see illustration), or the eye can be injured behind the pupil. Any serious blow to the eye should be evaluated by an eye doctor.

Self-Care

Small, non-sharp foreign bodies can often be successfully removed at home. First, someone should inspect the eye, shining a bright light at the eye directly and from the side. Side illumination shows variation in the surface and is especially useful in distinguishing something that is over the cornea.

Even if the object cannot be seen, the eye should be gently flushed with water, either by holding the eye open under the tap or by using an eye cup. If the object seems to be under the upper eyelid, the person should try to pull the eyelid back while flushing out the eye. The upper eyelid should not be rubbed if the foreign body is over the cornea, since the cornea is easily scratched, but the lid may be pulled out and down, which will sometimes dislodge a foreign body.

If the object is not removed by flushing, but is visible, it can often be removed by lightly touching it with a wet cotton swab. This is easily done if the object is on the lining of the lid or on the *sclera*, the white part of the eye. It is not recommended if the object is over the cornea because the pressure may scratch the cornea. Sometimes flushing will move the object off the cornea to an area where it can safely be removed with a cotton swab.

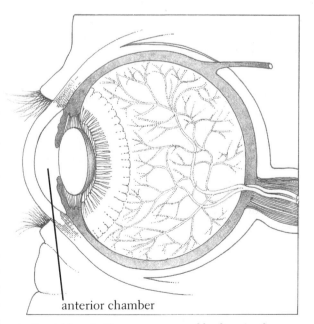

A direct blow to the eye can cause bleeding in the anterior chamber.

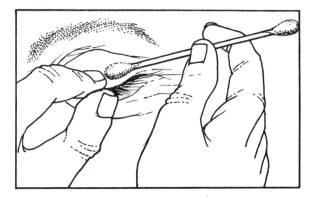

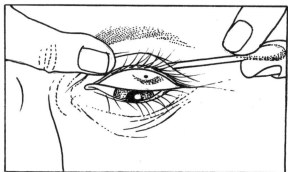

If a foreign object in the eye cannot be readily seen, the eyelid can be flipped back over a cotton-tipped applicator.

If the object can't be visualized and seems to be caught under the eyelid, the lid can be carefully flipped back. While the person looks down, the helper gently but firmly grasps the edge of the lid with thumb and forefinger, drawing it downward and outward (see illustration). With the other hand, the helper lays a cotton swab along the center of the lid, and lifts the eyelid back over the swab with the thumb and forefinger. Once the lid is flipped, the swab can be gently slid out and used to remove the foreign body. To return the lid to normal position, the person simply has to look up.

If the helper can see a small scratch on the cornea, the person has a corneal abrasion. Provided the scratch is very small and the object has been removed, the eye can simply be patched

closed with gauze and adhesive tape for a day. Resting the eye will diminish the person's discomfort and allow the eye to heal a minor abrasion. For a simple black eye, in which the eye itself was not injured, ice packs should be applied to the eye to keep down swelling and minimize bruising. Whenever people experience *any* kind of eye injury, it is very important to make sure that their vision is unimpaired. This can be done by closing or covering the uninjured eye and asking them to read with the injured eye.

The Doctor

The doctor, an ophthalmologist, takes a history to help determine whether the injury was a penetrating or impact injury, and then does a brief vision check. Next, using a bright light and a magnifier, or a special magnifying lamp called a *slit lamp*, the doctor will examine the eyelids, the *conjunctiva* (the lining of the eyelids), the cornea, and the anterior chamber.

If there is a suspected foreign body on the cornea, the doctor will give the person anesthetic eyedrops and then put in a drop of fluorescent dye which will make a foreign body or corneal abrasion easier to see. If a foreign body is found, the doctor will lift it off with a cotton swab or a needle. An antiseptic ointment will be put in the eye and the eye will be patched for several days if necessary. The treatment will be the same for a minor corneal abrasion.

If people have a penetrating injury or blood in the anterior chamber, they will possibly be hospitalized. Bed rest for several days will help to prevent further bleeding and damage to the eye. In some cases penetrating injuries require surgery.

Ruling Out Other Diseases

A history of injury or a foreign body in the eye eliminates other eye conditions such as *con-*

junctivitis (see p. 229), *corneal infection* (see p. 230), or *acute glaucoma* (see p. 233)—any of which can cause blurred vision, light sensitivity, and eye pain.

Prevention

Two factors are key to preventing eye injuries: 1) awareness, and 2) protective eye equipment. Special types of eyewear are designed to protect the eyes in industrial, hobby, or sports situations that carry a risk of eye injury. Situations in which small particles are being blown by the wind or by a machine are also potentially hazardous for the eyes. Safety glasses should be used for carpentry or metalwork involving sawing, drilling, and sanding.

In the area of sports, baseball and basketball are the leading causes of eye injuries. Sports doctors recommend that a baseball face protector always be worn during batting. Basketball injuries are usually caused by fingers or elbows, and are difficult to prevent. Racquet sports such as squash, racquetball, tennis, and badminton cause 30%–40% of all sports-related eye injuries. Sports physicians advise that all the people involved in racquet sports wear protective eye gear. Bike riders can avoid foreign objects in the eye by wearing sunglasses; skiers can avoid getting twigs in their eyes by wearing goggles.

NOTES

CHAPTER 2: PREVENTIVE MEDICINE

1. U.S. Dept. of Health, Education, and Welfare. 1979. *Healthy People.* DHEW Publication No. 79-55071, p. VIII–IX.
2. *Ibid.*, p. 10.
3. Knowles, J. 1977. "The Responsibility of the Individual." *Daedalus* Winter: 106.
4. Eisenberg, L. 1977. "The Perils of Prevention: A Cautionary Note." *New England Journal of Medicine* 297:1231.
5. Kervasdoue, J. 1984. *The End of an Illusion.* University of California Press, p. 69.
6. *Ibid.*, p. 76.
7. McKinlay, J. 1979. "A Case for Refocusing Upstream: The Political Economy of Illness." *Patients, Physicians, and Illness*, E. Jaco, ed. Free Press, p. 9.
8. *Ibid.*

CHAPTER 3: STRESS AND HEALTH

1. Cohen, S. 1986. *Behavior, Health, and Environmental Stress.* Plenum Press, p. 3.
2. Kaplan, M. 1986. "Social Support and Health." *Medical Care* 15:47.
3. Ornstein, R. 1987. *The Healing Brain.* Simon & Schuster, p. 206.
4. Kobasa, S. 1983. "Effectiveness of Hardiness, Exercise, and Social Support As Resources Against Illness." *Journal of Psychosomatic Research* 29:525.
5. Luthe, W. 1969. *Autogenic Therapy, Vol. I.* Grune & Stratton, p. 7.

CHAPTER 4: FULFILLMENT AND HEALTH

1. Jung, C. 1971. "The Stages of Life." *The Portable Jung*, J. Campbell, ed. Penguin Books, p. 17.

2. *Ibid.*, p. 20.
3. Erikson, E. 1963. *Childhood and Society.* W. W. Norton, p. 267.
4. Jaques, E. "Death and the Mid-Life Crisis." *International Journal of Psychoanalysis* 46: 505.
5. *Ibid.*, p. 513.
6. Levinson, Daniel. *The Seasons of a Man's Life.* Knopf, 1978.

CHAPTER 5: NUTRITION AND HEALTH

1. Eaton, B., and Konner, M. 1985. "Diet: Paleolithic Genes and 20th Century Health." *Anthroquest* 33:1.
2. McKinlay, J. *op. cit.*, p. 15.
3. *Ibid.*, p. 16.
4. *Ibid.*, p. 12.

CHAPTER 7: CHEMICALS AND HEALTH

1. Ashford, N. 1987. "New Scientific Evidence and Public Health Imperatives." *New England Journal of Medicine* 316:1084.
2. Burns. D. 1985. "Tobacco and Health." *Cecil Textbook of Medicine*, Wyngaarden, J., ed., p. 46.
3. Task Force on Smoking. 1982. *Smoking and Health in Ontario.* Ontario Council of Health, p. 1.
4. *Ibid.*, p. 4.
5. U.S. Department of Health, Education, and Welfare. *op cit.*, p. 67.
6. Millman, R. "Drug Abuse and Dependence." *Cecil Textbook of Medicine*, Wyngaarden, J., ed. p. 2015.

BIBLIOGRAPHY

PART I

Chapter 1: Taking Control of Your Health

Antonovsky, A. 1984. "A Sense of Coherence as a Determinant of Health." *Behavioral Health*, J. Matarazzo, ed. John Wiley & Sons, pp. 114–129.

Bandura, A. 1977. "Self-Efficacy." *Psychological Review* 84:191-215.

Bandura, A. 1985. "Catecholamine Secretion as a Function of Perceived Coping Self-Efficacy." *Journal of Consulting and Clinical Psychology* 53:3, pp. 406–414.

Cypress, B. 1980. *National Health Survey Pattern of Ambulatory Care*. DHHS Publication.

Feinstein, D. 1987. "The Shaman Within: Cultivating a Sacred Personal Mythology." *Shamanism*, S. Nicholson, ed. Theosophical Publishing House, pp. 207–279.

Kobasa, S. 1981. "Personality and Constitution as Mediators in the Stress-Illness Relationship." *Journal of Health and Social Behavior* 22:368-378.

Langer, E. J. 1976. "The Effects of Choice and Enhanced Personal Responsibility for the Aged." *Journal of Personal and Social Psychology* 34:191-198.

Langer, E. J. 1977. "Long-Term Effects of a Control-Relevant Intervention with Institutionalized Aged." *Journal of Personal and Social Psychology* 35:897-902.

O'Leary, A. 1985. "Self-Efficacy and Health." *Res Ther* 23:437-451.

Thoresen, C. 1984. "Overview." *Behavioral Health*, J. Matarazzo, ed. John Wiley & Sons, p. 297.

U.S. Department of Health, Education, and Welfare. 1979. *Healthy People*. DHEW Publication.

Vickery, D. M. 1983. "Effect of a Self-Care Education Program on Medical Visits." *Journal of the American Medical Association* 250:21:2952.

Zautra, A. 1984. "Subjective Well Being and Physical Health." *International Journal of Aging and Human Development* 19:95-110.

Chapter 2: Preventive Medicine

Belloc, N. B. 1972. "Relationship of Physical Health Status and Health Practices." *Preventive Medicine* 1:409-421.

Breslow, L. 1980. "Persistence of Health Habits and Their Relationship to Mortality." *Preventive Medicine* 9:469-483.

Dawber, T.R. 1957. "Coronary Heart Disease in the Framingham Study." *American Journal of Public Health* 47:4-24.

Eisenberg, L. 1977. "The Perils of Prevention: A Cautionary Note." *New England Journal of Medicine* 297:1231.

Farquhar, J. W. 1984. "Community Application of Behavioral Medicine." *Handbook of Behavioral Medicine*, Guilford Press.

Geller, H. 1974. *The 1974 Probability Tables of Dying in the Next 10 Years from Specific Causes*. Methodist Hospital of Indiana.

Hall, J. 1979. *Prospective Medicine*. Methodist Hospital of Indiana.

Hammond, E. C. 1954. "The Relationship Between Human Smoking Habits and Death Rates: A Follow-Up Study of 187,766 Men." *Journal of American Medical Association* 155:1316-1328.

Kervasdoue, J. 1984. *The End of An Illusion*. University of California Press.

Kitagawa, E. 1973. *Differential Mortality in the U.S.* Harvard University Press.

McKinlay, J. 1979. "A Case For Refocusing Upstream: The Political Economy of Illness." *Patients, Physicians, and Illness*, E. Jaco, ed. Free Press, p. 9.

McKinlay, J. 1979. "The Questionable Contribution of Medical Measures to the Decline of Mortality in the U.S. in the 20th Century." *Millbank Memorial Fund Quarterly* 55:405-428.

Multiple Risk Factor Intervention Trial Research Group. 1982. "Multiple Risk Factor Intervention

Trial." *Journal of the American Medical Association* 248:12, 1465.

Puska, P. 1981. *The North Karelia Project*. WHO Monograph.

Robbins, L. 1970. *How to Practice Prospective Medicine*. Methodist Hospital of Indiana.

Slater, C. 1985. "Behavior, Lifestyle, and Socioeconomic Variables as Determinants of Health Status." *American Journal of Preventive Medicine* 15:25.

U.S. Department of Health, Education, and Welfare. 1979. *Healthy People*. DHEW Publication.

Chapter 3: Stress and Health

Achterberg, J. 1985. *Imagery and Healing: Shamanism and Modern Medicine*. Shambala.

Ader, R. 1981. *Psychoneuroimmunology*. Academic Press.

Antonovsky, A. 1984. "A Sense of Coherence as a Determinant of Health." *Behavioral Health*, J. Matarazzo, ed. John Wiley & Sons, pp. 114–129.

Bandura, A. 1977. "Self-Efficacy." *Psychological Review* 84:191–215.

Bandura, A. 1985. "Catecholamine Secretion as a Function of Perceived Coping Self-Efficacy." *Journal of Consulting and Clinical Psychology* 53:3, pp. 406–414.

Benson, H. 1976. *The Relaxation Response*. Avon Books.

Berkman, L. 1979. "Social Networks, Host Resistance, and Mortality: A 9-Year Follow-Up Study of the Alameda County Residents." *American Journal of Epidemiology* 109:186–204.

Cohen, S. 1986. *Behavior, Health, and Environmental Stress*. Plenum Press, p. 3.

Cohen, S. 1985. *Social Support and Health*. Academic Press.

Elliot, R. S. 1984. *Is It Worth Dying For?* Bantam.

Friedman, M. 1974. *Type A Behavior and Your Heart*. Knopf.

Goldstein, J. 1983. *The Experience of Insight: A Simple and Direct Guide to Buddhist Meditation*. Shambala Publications.

Henry, J. P. 1977. *Stress, Health, and the Social Environment*. Springer-Verlag.

Holmes, T. H. 1967. "The Social Readjustment Rating Scale." *Journal of Psychosomatic Research* 1:213–218.

Kaplan, M. 1986. "Social Support and Health." *Medical Care* 15:47.

Jacobson, E. 1962. *You Must Relax*. McGraw-Hill.

Kobasa, S. 1983. "Effectiveness of Hardiness, Exercise, and Social Support As Resources Against Illness." *Journal of Psychosomatic Research* 29:525–533.

Locke, S. 1987. *The Healer Within*. E. P. Dutton.

Lynch, J. 1977. *The Broken Heart*. Basic Books.

Lynch, J. 1985. *The Language of the Heart*. Basic Books.

Muktananda, S. 1980. *Meditate*. State University of New York.

Nuckolls, K. 1972. "Psychological Assets, Life Crises, and the Prognosis of Pregnancy." *American Journal of Epidemiology* 95:431–441.

Ornstein, R. 1987. *The Healing Brain*. Simon & Schuster.

Pelletier, K. 1977. *Mind as Healer, Mind as Slayer*. Dell.

Rosenman, R. 1975. "Coronary Heart Disease in the Western Collaborative Study." *Journal of the American Medical Association* 223:872–877.

Rossman, M. 1987. *Healing Yourself: A Step-By-Step Program for Better Health Through Imagery*. Walker.

Samuels, M. and N. 1975. *Seeing with the Mind's Eye*. Random House.

Seligman, M. 1975. *Learned Helplessness*. W. H. Freeman.

Selye, H. 1956. *The Stress of Life*. McGraw-Hill.

Siegel, B. 1986. *Love, Medicine, and Miracles*. Harper & Row.

Simonton, C. 1978. *Getting Well Again*. Bantam Books.

Weiss, S. 1986. *Perspectives In Behavioral Medicine*. Academic Press.

Wood, C. 1987. "Are Happy People Healthier?" *Journal of the Royal Society of Medicine* 80:354–356.

Chapter 4: Fulfillment and Health

Borysenko, J. 1987. *Minding the Body, Mending the Mind*. Addison Wesley.

Erikson, E. 1963. *Childhood and Society*. W. W. Norton.

Gould, R. L. 1978. *Transformations*. Simon & Schuster.

Jampolsky, G. 1979. *Love Is Letting Go of Fear*. Celestial Arts.

Jaques, E. 1965. "Death and the Mid-Life Crisis." *International Journal of Psychoanalaysis* 46:502–514.

Jung, C. 1971. "The Stages of Life." *The Portable Jung*, J. Campbell, ed. Penguin Books, p. 3–22.

Jung, C. 1968. *Man and His Symbols*. Dell.

Levinson, D. 1978. *The Seasons of a Man's Life*. Ballantine.

Lynch, J. 1977. *The Broken Heart*. Basic Books.

Milsum, J. H. 1985. *Health, Stress, and Illness*. Praeger.

Selye, H. 1974. *Stress Without Distress*. Signet Books.

Sheehy, G. 1976. *Passages: Predictable Crises of Adult Life*. E. P. Dutton.

Siegel, B. 1987. *Love, Medicine, and Miracles*. Harper & Row.

Steinberg, L. 1987. *The Life Cycle*. Columbia University Press.

Vaillant, G. 1977. *Adaptations to Life*. Little, Brown & Co.

Ziegler, A. J. 1983. *Archetypal Medicine*. Spring Publication.

Chapter 5: Nutrition and Health

American Heart Association Committee. 1982. "Rationale for the Diet-Heart Statement of the American Heart Association." *Circulation* 65:839A–851A.

Dawber, T. R. 1980. *The Framingham Study*. Harvard University Press.

DeBakey, M. 1984. *The Living Heart Diet*. Raven Press.

Doll, R. 1981. "The Causes of Cancer." *Journal of the National Cancer Institute* 66:1191–1308.

Eaton, B. 1985. "Paleolithic Genes and 20th Century Health." *Anthroquest* 33:1.

Iacono, J. M. 1987. "Recommendations of the Fat and Fiber Groups From the Workshop on New Developments on Fat and Fiber in Carcinogenesis." *Preventive Medicine* 16:592–595.

Levy, R. I. 1979. *Nutrition, Lipids, and Coronary Heart Disease*. Raven Press.

Levy, R. I. 1986. "Cholesterol and Coronary Artery Disease." *Journal of the American Medical Association* 80, suppl. 2A, p. 18.

Lipid Research Clinics Program. 1984. "The Lipid Research Clinics Coronary Primary Prevention Trial Results." *Journal of the American Medical Association* 251:351–374.

McKinlay, J. 1979. "A Case For Refocusing Upstream: The Political Economy of Illness." *Patients, Physicians, and Illness*, E. Jaco, ed. Free Press, p. 9.

National Academy of Science/National Research Council Food and Nutrition Board. 1980. *Recommended Dietary Allowances, 9th Edition*. NAS/NRC.

National Research Council. 1982. *Diet, Nutrition, and Cancer*. National Academy Press.

Senate Select Committee on Nutrition and Human Needs. 1977. *Dietary Goals for the U.S.* U.S. Government Printing Office.

U.S. Department of Health, Education, and Welfare. 1979. *Healthy People*. DHEW Publication.

U.S. Department of Health, Education, and Welfare. 1986. *1990 Health Goals For the Nation*. DHEW.

Chapter 6: Exercise and Health

Boger, J. L. 1970. "Exercise, Therapy, and Hypertensive Men." *Journal of the American Medical Association* 211:1668.

Cassel, J. 1971. "Occupation, Physical Activity, and Coronary Heart Disease." *Archives of Internal Medicine* 128:920.

Chalmers, J. 1970. "Geographic Variations in Senile Osteoporosis: The Association of Physical Activity." *Bone and Joint Surgery* 52:667.

Cooper, K. H. 1976. "Physical Fitness Levels Versus Selected Coronary Risk Factors." *Journal of the American Medical Association* 236:166.

Eaton, B. 1985. "Paleolithic Genes and 20th Century Health." *Anthroquest* 33:1.

Hicky, N. 1975. "Studies of Coronary Risk Factors Related to Physical Activity in 15,171 Men." *British Medical Journal* 5982:507–509.

King, H. 1984. "Non-Insulin-Dependent Diabetes in a Newly Independent Nation." *Diabetic Care* 7:409–415.

Morris, J. N. 1980. "Vigorous Exercise in Leisure-

Time: Protection Against Coronary Heart Disease." *Lancet* 8206:1207–1210.

Paffenberger, R. S. 1975. "Work Activity and Coronary Heart Disease Mortality." *New England Journal of Medicine* 292:545–550.

Paffenberger, R. S. 1978. "Physical Activity as an Index of Heart Attack In College Alumni." *American Journal of Epidemiology* 108:161–175.

Paffenberger, R. S. 1983. "Physical Activity and the Incidence of Hypertension in College Alumni." *American Journal of Epidemiology* 117:245–256.

Powell, K. E. 1985. "Workshop on Epidemiological and Public Health Aspects of Physical Activity and Exercise: A Summary." *Public Health Reports* 100:118.

Richter, E. A. 1981. "Diabetics and Exercise." *American Journal of Medicine* 70:201–209.

Sallis, J. R. 1986. "Moderate Intensity Physical Activity and Cardiovascular Risk Factors: the Stanford Five-City Project." *Preventive Medicine* 15:561–568.

Siscoveck, D. S. 1985. "The Disease-Specific Benefits and Risks of Physical Activity and Exercise." *Public Health Reports* 100:180.

Taylor, T. B. 1985. "The Relationship of Physical Activity and Exercise to Mental Health." *Public Health Reports* 100:195.

Chapter 7: Chemicals and Health

American Heart Association. 1978. "Report on the Ad Hoc Committee of the Institute of Medicine; Division of Health Science Policy. 1982. *Marijuana and Health*. National Academy Press.

Committee on Cigarette Smoking and Cardiovascular Disease." *Circulation* 57:404A.

Epstein, S. S. 1979. *The Politics of Cancer*. Anchor Doubleday.

Frameni, J. 1975. *Person at High Risk for Cancer*. Academic Press.

Highland, J. 1980. *Malignant Neglect*. Random House.

Isner, N. 1986. "Acute Cardiac Events Temporally Related to Cocaine Abuse." *New England Journal of Medicine* 315:23:1438.

Kissin, B. 1985. "Alcohol Abuse and Alcohol-Related Illnesses." *Cecil Textbook of Medicine*, W. B. Wyngaarden, ed. W. B. Saunders.

Lave, L. 1977. *Air Pollution and Human Health*. Johns Hopkins University Press.

Mason, T. J. 1975. *Atlas of Cancer Mortality for U.S. Counties*. U.S. Government Printing Office.

Millman, R. 1985. "Drug Abuse and Dependence." *Cecil Textbook of Medicine*, W. B. Wyngaarden, ed. Saunders.

Mittleman, R. E. 1985. "Death Caused by Recreational Cocaine Use." *Journal of the American Medical Association* 252:1889.

Royal College of Physicians. 1977. *Smoking or Health?* Putnam Medical.

Samuels, M. 1983. *Well Body, Well Earth*. Sierra Club Books.

Siegel, B. 1987. *Love, Medicine, and Miracles*. Harper & Row.

Task Force on Smoking. 1982. *Smoking and Health in Ontario*. Ontario Council of Health.

U.S. Department of Health, Education, and Welfare. 1979. *Healthy People*. DHEW.

U.S. Department of Health, Education, and Welfare. 1982. *The Health Consequences of Smoking: Cancer*. DHEW.

U.S. Department of Health, Education, and Welfare. 1984. *Smoking and Health*. DHEW.

U.S. Department of Health, Education, and Welfare. 1986. *1990 Health Objectives for the Nation*. DHEW.

PART II

General References (see current editions)

Braunwald, E. 1987. *Harrison's Principles of Internal Medicine*. McGraw-Hill.

Dunphy, J. E. 1988. *Current Surgical Diagnosis and Treatment*. Appleton and Lang.

Krup, M. 1988. *Current Medical Diagnosis and Treatment*. Appleton and Lang.

Wyngaarden, J. B. 1985. *Cecil Textbook of Medicine, 17th Edition*. W. B. Saunders.

Specialty Textbooks (see current editions)

Berk, J. E. 1985. *Bochus Gastroenterology*. W. B. Saunders.

Braunwald, E. 1984. *Heart Disease: A Textbook of Cardiovascular Medicine.* W. B. Saunders.

Danforth, D. M. 1986. *Obstetrics and Gynecology.* Lippincott.

Diamond, S. 1982. *The Practicing Physician's Approach to Headache.* Williams & Wilkins.

Domonkos, A. N. 1982. *Andrew's Diseases of the Skin.* W. B. Saunders.

Genest, J. 1983. *Hypertension.* McGraw-Hill.

Jones, A. W. 1985. *Novak's Textbook of Gynecology.* Williams & Wilkins.

Kelly, W. 1985. *Textbook of Rheumatology.* W. B. Saunders.

Marble, A. 1985. *Joslin's Diabetes Mellitus.* Lea & Febriger.

McCarty, D. J. 1985. *Arthritis and Allied Disorders.* Lea & Febriger.

Newell, F. W. 1986. *Opthalmology: Primary Concepts.* C. V. Mosby.

Sleisenger, M. H. 1983. *Gastrointestinal Diseases.* W. B. Saunders.

Turek, S. C. 1984. *Orthopaedics.* Lippincott.

Vaughan, D. 1986. *General Opthamology.* Appleton & Lang.

Weiss, E. B. 1985. *Bronchial Asthma.* Little Brown.

Wilson, J. D. 1985. *William's Textbook of Endocrinology.* W. B. Saunders.

Selected Periodical References

Skin:

Adams, R. M. 1986. "Contact Allergen Alternatives." *Journal of the American Academy of Dermatology* 14:951.

Becker, T. M. 1985. "Genital Herpes Infections in Private Practice in the United States, 1966–1981." *Journal of the American Medical Association* 253:1601.

Hanifin, J. M. 1982. "Atopic Dermatitis." *Journal of the American Academy of Dermatology* 6:1.

Head:

Crouch, R. 1984. "The Common Cold." *Journal of Infectious Diseases* 150:2:167.

"Glaucoma." 1981. *Ophthalmology* 88:175.

Gwaltney, J. 1982. "Transmission of Experimental Rhino Virus Infection By Contaminated Surfaces." *American Journal of Epidemiology* 116:3:828.

Jackson, G. 1960. "Susceptibility and Immunity to Common Upper Respiratory Infections–The Common Cold." *Annals of Internal Medicine* 53:2.

Norman, P. S. 1985. "Allergic Rhinitis." *Journal of Allergy and Clinical Immunology* 75:531.

Totman, R. 1980. "Predicting Experimental Colds in Volunteers from Different Measures of Recent Life Stress." *Journal of Psychosomatic Research* 24:155.

Wannamaker, L. W. 1979. "Changes and Changing Concepts in the Biology of Group A Streptococci and in the Epidemiology of Streptococcal Infections." *Review of Infectious Diseases* 1:967.

Chest:

Burish, T. G. 1981. "Effectiveness of Relaxation Training in Reducing Adverse Reactions to Cancer Chemotherapy." *Journal of Behavioral Medicine* 4:1:65.

Crique, M. 1986. "Epidemiology of Atherosclerosis: An Updated Review." *American Journal of Cardiology* 57:18C.

Detre, K. 1988. "Percutaneous Transluminal Coronary Angioplasty in 1985–1986 & 1977–1981: The National Heart, Lung, and Blood Institute Registry." *New England Journal of Medicine* 318:5:265.

Goldstein, R. A. 1985. "Advances in the Diagnosis and Treatment of Asthma." *Chest* 87:1 (supplement).

Gruentzig, A. 1987. "Long-Term Follow-Up After Percutaneous Transluminal Coronary Angioplasty." *New England Journal of Medicine* 316:18:1127.

Grumm, R. 1986. "Lipids and Hypertension." *American Journal of Medicine* 80 (Supplement 2A).

Hypertension Detection and Follow-Up Program. 1979. "Five-Year Findings of the Hypertension Detection and Follow-Up Program." *Journal of the American Medical Association* 242:2562.

Kaplan, N. M. 1987. "Non-Pharmocologic Therapy of Hypertension." *Medical Clinics of North America* 71:5:921.

Leaf, A. 1988. "Cardiovascular Effects of No-3 Fatty Acids." *New England Journal of Medicine* 318:9:549.

Levy, R. 1986. "Cholesterol and Coronary Artery Disease: What Do Clinicians Do Now?" *American Journal of Medicine* 80 (Supplement 2A), p. 18.

McCanon, D. 1984. "Diuretic Therapy for Mild Hypertension: The Real Cost of Treatment." *American Journal of Cardiology* 53:9A.

Medalie, J. H. 1976. "Angina Pectoris Among 10,000 Men." *American Journal of Medicine* 60.

National Heart, Lung, and Blood Institute. 1985. "Lowering Blood Cholesterol to Prevent Heart Disease." *Journal of the American Medical Association* 253:14:2080.

Ragland, D. 1988. "Type A Behavior and Mortality for Coronary Artery Disease." *New England Journal of Medicine* 318:2:65.

Ross, R. 1976. "The Pathology of Atherosclerosis." *New England Journal of Medicine* 299:369.

Rozanski, A. 1988. "Mental Stress and the Induction of Silent Myocardial Ischemia in Patients with Coronary Artery Disease." *New England Journal of Medicine* 318:16:1005.

Shepherd, J. T. 1987. "Conference on Behavioral Medicine and Cardiovascular Disease." *Circulation Monograph* #6, 76 (Supp. I).

Musculoskeletal:

Bellamy, N. 1986. "The Clinical Evaluation of Osteoarthritis in the Elderly." *Clin. Rheumatic Diseases* 12:131.

Deyo, R. 1986. "How Many Days of Bed Rest for Acute Low Back Pain?" *New England Journal of Medicine* 315:17:1064.

Million, R. 1984. "Long-term Study of Management of Rheumatoid Arthritis." *Lancet* 1:812.

Post, M. 1983. "The Painful Shoulder." *Clinical Orthopedics* 173:1.

Reuler, J. B. 1985. "Low Back Pain." *Western Journal of Medicine* 143:259.

Sobel, D. 1986. "Oh, Your Aching Back." *New York* Magazine, March 10, 1986, p. 42.

Gastrointestinal:

Hackford, A. W. 1985. "Diverticular Disease of the Colon." *Surgical Clinics of North America* 65:347.

Legerton, C. W. 1984. "Symposium on Management of the Ulcer Patient." *American Journal of Medicine* 17 (Supplement I).

Richter, J. E. 1982. "Gastroesophageal Reflux." *Annals of Internal Medicine* 97:93.

Sackmann, M. 1988. "Shock-Wave Lithotripsy of Gallbladder Stones: The First 175 Patients." *New England Journal of Medicine* 318:7:393.

"Third International Symposium on Colorectal Cancer." 1984. *CA* 34:130.

Endocrine:

Feingold, K. R. 1986. "Diabetic Vascular Disease." *Advances in Internal Medicine* 31:309.

Kaplan, M. M. 1985. "Thyroid Disease." *Medical Clinics of North America* 69:5.

Lean, M. E. 1986. "The Prescription of Diabetic Diets in the 1980s." *Lancet* 1:723.

Genitourinaray:

Colditz, G. 1987. "Menopause and the Risk of Coronary Heart Disease in Women." *New England Journal of Medicine* 316:18:1105.

Fisher, B. 1985. "Five-Year Results of a Randomized Clinical Trial Comparing Total Mastectomy And Segmental Mastectomy With or Without Radiation in the Treatment of Breast Cancer." *New England Journal of Medicine* 312:665.

Friedland, G. 1987. "Transmission of the Human Immunodeficiency Virus." *New England Journal of Medicine* 317:18:1125.

Hoff, R. 1988. "Seroprevalence of Human Immunodeficiency Virus Among Childbearing Women." *New England Journal of Medicine* 318:9:525.

Mass, L. 1987. *Medical Answers About AIDS.* Gay Men's Health Crisis, Inc., New York.

Meares, E. M. 1983. "Prostatitis. *Seminars in Urology* 1:146.

Mishell, D. 1984. "Menorrhagia." *The Journal of Reproductive Medicine* 29:10 (supplement):763.

O'Malley, M. S. 1987. "Screening for Breast Cancer with Breast Self-Examination." *Journal of the American Medical Association* 257:2197.

Schatzkin, A. 1987. "Alcohol Consumption and Breast Cancer in the Epidemiologic Follow-Up Study of the First National Health and Nutrition

Examination Survey." *New England Journal of Medicine* 316:19:1169.

Obesity:

Hirsch, J. 1988. "New Light on Obesity." *New England Journal of Medicine* 318:8:509.

National Institutes of Health. 1985. "Health Implications of Obesity." *Annals of Internal Medicine* 103:147.

Simopolulos, A. P. 1984. "Body Weight, Health, and Longevity." *Annals of Internal Medicine* 100:285.

Stunkard, A. J. 1986. "An Adoption Study of Human Obesity." *New England Journal of Medicine* 314:4:193.

Emergency Medicine:

Beall, G. N. 1986. "Anaphylaxis—Everyone's Problem." *Western Journal of Medicine* 144:329.

Behrendt, T. 1982. "Eye Emergencies." *Family Practice Recertification* 4:23.

Montgomery, H. 1986. "1985 National Conference on Standards and Guidelines for Cardiopulmonary Resusitation and Emergency Cardiac Care." *Journal of the American Medical Association* 255:21:2845.

I N D E X

— **495**
Index

ABOUT THE AUTHORS

Mike Samuels is a physician and author. He attended Brown University and New York University College of Medicine, during which time he did research in immunogenetics. He has always been interested in preventive medicine and healing. After internship he worked on the Hopi Indian Reservation for the U.S. Public Health Service and then worked for the Marin County Health Department. During this time he helped set up one of the first holistic medicine clinics in northern California, and wrote the pioneering self-help medical book, *The Well Body Book*, with Hal Z. Bennett. Throughout his career, Mike has been especially interested in how the mind affects health, and how imagery can be used to stay well and heal illness.

Nancy Harrison Samuels is an author and former nursery school teacher. She attended Brown University and Bank Street College of Education. After several years of teaching she did editing on *The Well Body Book*, and began to write with Mike. Together they have written *Seeing with the Mind's Eye*, a book on relaxation and mental imagery, and four books in a self-help series, *The Well Baby Book*, *The Well Child Book*, *The Well Child Coloring Book*, and *The Well Pregnancy Book*. *The Well Adult*, which is the most recent in this series of self-help books, deals with the health concerns of midadulthood. The Samuelses believe that self-help medical books are preventive medicine *tools* for learning that provide valuable information which can relieve concerns and help to bring about changes in habits and attitudes that promote health and healing. Although they are unable to answer all letters individually, they appreciate hearing about readers' experiences and suggestions.

Mike and Nancy Samuels live in a small seacoast town in northern California in a house they built themselves and continue to work on, much like their series of self-help books. They have a close family life and spend much of their free time doing projects with their growing sons, Rudy and Lewis. Together the family enjoys building, gardening, traveling, and camping.

About the Illustrator

Wendy Frost left Australia in 1965 to live in London where she worked for *The Observer* and various magazines and publishers. Since 1969 she has lived mainly in New York, with sojourns in Italy and Australia. She has also had numerous exhibitions of her paintings in Europe, the U.S.A., and Australia. Mike and Nancy Samuels have worked with her on four previous books. She now lives in New York with her son, Darcy Darwin.